bioethics

A Nursing Perspective

7e

Dedication

To Olga

bioethics

A Nursing Perspective

7e

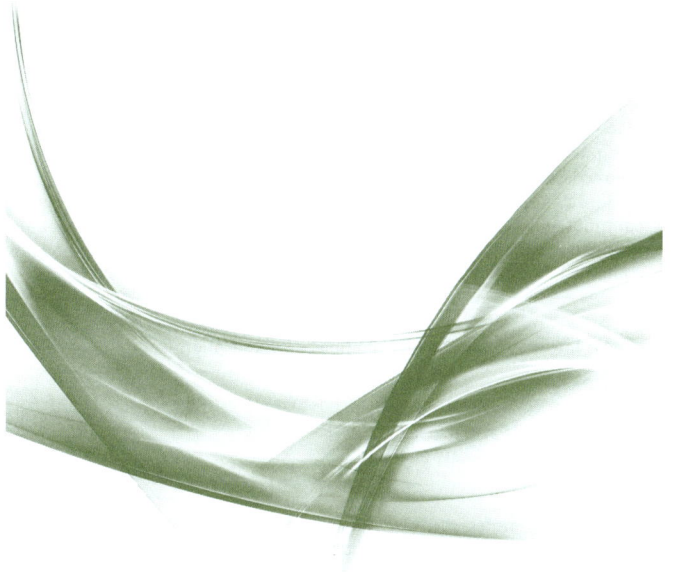

Megan-Jane Johnstone PhD, BA, RN
Independent Scholar
Formerly Professor of Nursing, School of Nursing and Midwifery, Faculty of Health, Deakin University, Victoria, Australia
Currently Adjunct Member, Alfred Deakin Institute for Citizenship and Globalisation, Deakin University, Melbourne

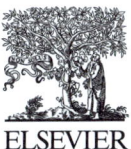

ELSEVIER

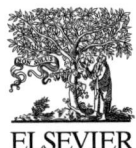

Elsevier Australia. ACN 001 002 357
(a division of Reed International Books Australia Pty Ltd)
Tower 1, 475 Victoria Avenue, Chatswood, NSW 2067

Copyright 2019 Elsevier Australia. 6th edition © 2016; 5th edition © 2009; 4th edition © 2004; 3rd edition © 1999; 2nd edition © 1994; 1st edition © 1989 Elsevier Australia. Reprinted 2020

All rights reserved. No part of this publication may be reproduced or transmitted in any form or by any means, electronic or mechanical, including photocopying, recording, or any information storage and retrieval system, without permission in writing from the publisher. Details on how to seek permission, further information about the Publisher's permissions policies and our arrangements with organizations such as the Copyright Clearance Center and the Copyright Licensing Agency, can be found at our website: www.elsevier.com/permissions.

This book and the individual contributions contained in it are protected under copyright by the Publisher (other than as may be noted herein).

ISBN: 978-0-7295-4322-4

Notice

Practitioners and researchers must always rely on their own experience and knowledge in evaluating and using any information, methods, compounds or experiments described herein. Because of rapid advances in the medical sciences, in particular, independent verification of diagnoses and drug dosages should be made. To the fullest extent of the law, no responsibility is assumed by Elsevier, authors, editors or contributors for any injury and/or damage to persons or property as a matter of products liability, negligence or otherwise, or from any use or operation of any methods, products, instructions, or ideas contained in the material herein.

National Library of Australia Cataloguing-in-Publication Data

 A catalogue record for this book is available from the National Library of Australia

Senior Content Strategist: Libby Houston
Content Project Manager: Fariha Nadeem
Edited by Christine Wyard
Proofread by Tim Learner
Cover by Natalie Bowra
Internal design: Non-Standard
Index by Innodata Indexing
Typeset by Toppan Best-set Premedia Limited
Printed in China by RR Donnelley

Last digit is the print number: 9 8 7 6 5 4 3 2

Contents

Preface	xiii
Acknowledgments	xiv
List of abbreviations	xv

Chapter 1 Professional standards and the requirement to be ethical — 1
Introduction — 1
The requirement to uphold exemplary standards of conduct — 4
Unprofessional conduct and professional misconduct — 4
   Ethical professional conduct — 5
   Unprofessional conduct — 5
   Professional misconduct — 5
   Unsatisfactory professional performance — 5
   Unethical professional conduct — 6
Questioning the requirement to be morally exemplary — 6
Nursing as a moral project — 7
Conclusion — 7

Chapter 2 Ethics, bioethics and nursing ethics: some working definitions — 11
Introduction — 11
The importance of understanding ethics terms and concepts — 12
The need for a critical inquiry into ethical professional practice — 13
Understanding moral language — 13
What is ethics? — 14
What is bioethics? — 15
What is nursing ethics? — 17
What ethics is not — 18
   Law — 18
   Codes of ethics — 22
   Codes of conduct — 24
   Hospital or professional etiquette — 25
   Hospital or institutional policy — 26
   Public opinion, populism or the view of the majority — 27
   Ideology — 30
   Following the orders of a supervisor or manager — 31
The task of ethics, bioethics and nursing ethics — 31
Conclusion — 34

Chapter 3 Moral theory and the ethical practice of nursing — 37
Introduction — 37
Moral justification — 38
Theoretical perspectives informing ethical practice — 40
    Ethical principlism — 41
        What are ethical principles? — 41
        Autonomy — 41
        Non-maleficence — 42
        Beneficence — 43
        Justice — 45
        Moral rules — 48
        Problems with ethical principles — 49
    Moral rights theory — 49
        Moral rights — 50
        Moral rights based on natural law and divine command — 50
        Moral rights based on common humanity — 50
        Moral rights based on rationality — 51
        Moral rights based on interests — 51
        Moral rights based on human experiences of grievous wrongs — 52
        Different types of rights — 53
        Making rights claims — 54
        Rights and responsibilities — 54
        Problems with rights claims — 55
    Virtue ethics — 56
        The notion of virtue — 58
        The virtuous person — 58
        Virtue theory, an ethic of care and nursing ethics — 59
        Virtue ethics and an ethic of care in nursing – some further thoughts — 61
        Problems with virtue ethics — 62
    Deontology and teleology — 63
        Deontology — 63
        Teleology — 63
    Moral duties and obligations — 64
        Moral duties — 64
        Moral obligations — 65
        Clarifying the difference between rights and duties — 66
    Limitations and weaknesses of ethical theory — 66
    Moral justification and moral theory – some further thoughts — 67
Conclusion — 68

Chapter 4 Cross-cultural ethics and the ethical practice of nursing — 71
Introduction — 71
Cross-cultural ethics and nursing — 73
Culture and its relationship to ethics — 74
The nature and implications of a cross-cultural approach to ethics — 75
Moral diversity and the challenge of moral pluralism — 82

Dealing with problems associated with a cross-cultural approach to ethics in health care	83
Ethics, cultural competency, cultural safety and cultural humility	86
Cultural competency	87
Cultural safety	88
Cultural humility	90
Conclusion	90

Chapter 5 Moral problems and moral decision-making in nursing and health care contexts — 93

Introduction	94
Distinguishing moral problems from other sorts of problems	94
Identifying different kinds of moral problems	95
Moral unpreparedness / moral incompetence	96
Moral blindness	98
Moral indifference and insensitivity	101
Moral disengagement	102
Moral fading / ethical fading	103
Amoralism	104
Immoralism	105
Moral complacency	105
Moral dumbfounding / stupefaction	106
Moral fanaticism	106
Moral disagreements	107
Internal moral disagreement	107
Radical moral disagreement	108
Moral conflict	109
Moral dilemmas	110
'Moral distress'	114
Making moral decisions	115
Moral decision-making – a working definition	116
Processes for making moral decisions	116
Reason and moral decision-making	118
Emotion and moral decision-making	118
Intuition and moral decision-making	121
Life experience and moral decision-making	123
Reason, emotion, intuition and life experience – some further thoughts	124
Dealing with moral disagreements and disputes	124
Being accepting of different points of view	124
Everyday moral problems in nursing	126
Conclusion	127

Chapter 6 Ethics, dehumanisation and vulnerable populations — 131

Introduction	131
Vulnerability	132
Identifying vulnerable populations	132
Vulnerability as a guide to action	133
Vulnerability and nursing ethics	133

Humanness, dehumanisation and vulnerability	134
Humanness	134
Dehumanisation	135
Forms of dehumanisation	135
Explicit and subtle expressions of dehumanisation	136
Why dehumanisation occurs	137
Consequences of dehumanisation	138
Deterring dehumanisation	139
Stigma	142
Prejudice and discrimination	143
Disadvantage	144
Identifying vulnerable individuals and groups	144
Older people	145
People with mental health problems and illness	148
Immigrants and ethnic minorities	150
Refugees, asylum seekers, displaced people, stateless people and returnees	152
People with disabilities	154
Indigenous peoples	156
Health status of Australia's indigenous peoples	157
Health status of New Zealand Māori	157
Global call to redress indigenous health disparities	158
Prisoners and detainees	159
Homeless people	162
What is homelessness?	163
Causes of homelessness	164
Homelessness and the right to health	165
Sexual minorities (LGBTIQ people)	165
Conclusion	169
Chapter 7 Patients' rights to and in health care	**173**
Introduction	174
What are patients' rights?	175
The right to health and health care	176
The right to equal access to health care	178
The right to have access to appropriate care	179
The right to quality care	179
The right to safe care	180
Challenges posed by the right to health and health care	180
The right to make informed decisions	181
What is informed consent?	182
The analytic components and elements of an informed consent	183
Informed consent and ethical principlism	184
The right not to know	184
Informed consent and the sovereignty of the individual	186
Paternalism and informed consent	186
Is paternalism justified?	188

Applying the 'paternalistic principle' in health care	189
Informed consent and nursing care	190
The right to confidentiality	190
Confidentiality as an absolute principle	191
Confidentiality as a prima-facie principle	193
The right to be treated with dignity	195
What is dignity?	195
Dignity and the right to dignity	197
Dignity violations	197
The right to be treated with respect	198
The right to cultural liberty	200
Conclusion	200

Chapter 8 Ethical issues in mental health care — 203

Introduction	204
Vulnerability, human rights and the mentally ill	205
Competency to decide	207
Psychiatric advance directives	215
Striking a balance between promoting autonomy, supporting decision-making and preventing harm	215
Origin, rationale and purpose of psychiatric advance directives	216
Forms and function of psychiatric advance directives	217
Anticipated benefits of psychiatric advance directives	218
Anticipated risks of psychiatric advance directives	219
Current trends in the legal regulation of psychiatric advance directives	220
Ethical issues in suicide and parasuicide	221
Scope of the problem	221
Cybersuicide	221
The moral challenge of suicide	222
Defining suicide	224
Distinguishing suicide from euthanasia	228
Ethical dimensions of suicide	228
Autonomy and the right to suicide	229
The ethics of suicide prevention: some further considerations	232
Conclusion	234

Chapter 9 Ethical issues in end-of-life care — 237

Introduction	237
Not For Treatment (NFT) directives	239
The problem of treatment in 'medically hopeless' cases	239
Who decides?	240
Not For Resuscitation (NFR)/Do Not Resuscitate (DNR) directives	241
Issues raised	243
Problems concerning NFR/DNR decision-making criteria, guidelines and procedures	244
Criteria and guidelines used	244
The exclusion of patients from decision-making	245
Misinterpretation of directives	245

Problems concerning the documentation and communication of
  NFR/DNR directives 246
Problems concerning the implementation of NFR/DNR directives 246
Improving NFR/DNR practices 247
Medical futility 248
Quality of life 251
  Origin of the phrase 251
  Defining quality of life 251
    Why defining quality of life is difficult 252
  Different conceptions of quality of life 252
  Using quality-of-life considerations to inform treatment choices 254
  Three senses of quality of life 254
    Descriptive sense of quality of life 254
    Evaluative sense of quality of life 254
    Prescriptive sense of quality of life 255
Advance directives 256
  What is an advance directive? 256
  How do advance directives work? 257
  Risks and benefits of advance directives 258
Advance care planning 260
  Respecting patient choices 261
Rethinking 'end-of-life care' 262
Conclusion 263

Chapter 10 The moral politics of abortion and euthanasia 267
Introduction 268
Morality policy 268
Moral politics 269
Abortion 270
  What is abortion? 273
  Arguments for and against the moral permissibility of abortion 273
    The conservative position 273
    The moderate position 274
    The liberal position 276
  Abortion and the moral rights of women, fetuses and fathers 277
  Abortion, politics and the broader community 281
Euthanasia 282
  Euthanasia and its significance for nurses 283
  Definitions of euthanasia, assisted suicide and 'mercy killing' 284
    Euthanasia 284
    Assisted suicide 286
    'Mercy killing' 286
  Views for and against euthanasia/assisted suicide 286
    Views in support of euthanasia 286
    Counter-arguments to views supporting euthanasia 288
    Specific arguments against euthanasia 291
  The doctrine of double effect 297

Palliative sedation	298
Definition, purpose and intention of palliative sedation	299
Palliative sedation in existential suffering	300
Nurses' attitudes and experiences	300
Withholding or withdrawing clinically assisted nutrition and hydration	301
Position statements and the nursing profession	303
Taking a partisan stance	304
Taking a non-partisan (neutral) stance	304
The need for a systematic response	306
'The quandary of uncertainty' – one nurse's story	307
Conclusion	307

Chapter 11 Professional judgment, moral quandaries and taking 'appropriate action' — 311

Introduction	311
Moral conflict and professional judgment	312
Making 'correct' moral judgments	313
Common situations involving moral conflict	314
Professional judgment	314
The nature and moral importance of professional judgment	315
Conscientious objection	316
The nature of conscience explained	319
Conscience as moral reasoning	319
Conscience as moral feelings	320
Conscience as moral reason and moral feelings	320
How conscience works	320
Bogus and genuine claims of conscientious objection	321
Conscientious objection to the lawful but morally controversial directives of an employer/manager	322
Conscientious objection and the problem of conflict in personal values	323
Conscientious objection and policy considerations	324
Whistleblowing in health care	327
The Moylan case (Australia)	329
The Pugmire case (New Zealand)	329
The Bardenilla case (US)	330
The MacArthur Health Service case (Australia)	330
The Bundaberg Base Hospital case (Australia)	332
The notion of whistleblowing/whistleblowers	332
The act of whistleblowing	333
Deciding to 'go public'	333
Risks of whistleblowing	334
Whistleblowing and clinical risk management	335
Whistleblowing as a last resort	336
Preventing ethics conflicts	336
The ethics–quality linkage	337
Appropriate disagreement	337
Conclusion	338

Chapter 12 Professional obligations to report harmful behaviours: risks to patient safety, child abuse and elder abuse — 341

Introduction — 342
Reporting notifiable and health-impaired conduct of practitioners and students — 342
    Legal requirements to report wrongdoing — 342
    Professional requirements to report wrongdoing — 345
    'No blame' culture and patient safety — 347
    Attitudes and experiences of reporting patient safety concerns — 348
Reporting child abuse and elder abuse — 351
Child abuse and neglect — 352
    Defining child abuse — 353
    Incidence of child abuse — 353
    Redressing child abuse — 354
Elder abuse and neglect — 355
    Defining elder abuse — 356
    Incidence of elder abuse — 357
    Redressing elder abuse — 357
Ethical issues associated with protecting children and elderly people from abuse — 359
    Why the maltreatment of children and elderly people constitutes a moral issue — 360
    The ethical implications of maltreating children and elderly people — 360
The moral demand to report child and elder maltreatment — 361
The notion of harm and its link with the moral duty to prevent child and elder abuse — 361
Considerations against reporting the maltreatment of children and elderly people — 362
    The professional–client relationship — 363
    Families — 363
    Maltreated children and elderly people — 364
Response to the criticisms — 365
    The problem of maintaining confidentiality — 365
    The problem of being 'the arm of the state' — 367
    Preserving the integrity of the professional–client relationship — 367
    Upholding the interests of families — 367
The importance of a supportive socio-cultural environment in abuse prevention — 368
Conclusion — 368

Chapter 13 Nursing ethics futures – challenges in the 21st century — 371

Introduction — 371
Public health emergencies — 372
Climate change — 373
Pandemic influenza — 375
Antimicrobial resistance — 377
Inequalities in health and health care — 378
Emergency preparedness — 382
Conclusion — 384

Bibliography — 387
Index — 451

Preface

In the 30 years since this book was first published the world has changed in unimaginable ways such that the study, understanding and application of ethics in our everyday and professional lives have never been more important or more pressing.

At the time of its 1989 publication, *Bioethics: a nursing perspective* stood as the first text of its kind to be written from an Australasian perspective. Both the first and second editions of this book were largely apologist in nature in that they sought to advance a robust defence of nursing ethics and why it should be taken seriously. As the years passed this 'defence' became no longer necessary as, due to the ongoing work of nursing ethics scholars around the world, the field of nursing ethics developed as a distinct and authoritative discipline in its own right. Accordingly, the focus of the subsequent editions of this book shifted to examining critically emerging ethical issues of the day and explored how nurses and the nursing profession might best respond to these.

The respective editions of this book have contributed significantly to the development of nursing ethics by consistently providing a critical examination of the ethical concepts, values and theories that are pertinent to the profession and practice of nursing, and by exploring in meaningful ways the relationship between nursing ethics and the various fundamental traditions in philosophical ethics. They have also advanced understanding of the relevance and *practical application* of ethical concepts, values and theories to the profession and practice of nursing.

The unwavering key aims of all editions of this book (including this revised edition) have been twofold: first, to remind nurses that the ultimate goal of nursing ethics is – and has always been – to promote the wellbeing of patients through the delivery of *good nursing care*; second, to provide nurses with a guiding framework to enable them to successfully navigate the moral terrains of their everyday practice, and to develop the capacities necessary to articulate clearly the ethical issues they encounter in health and social care contexts *as well as* to provide sound reasons and sound justifications for their decisions and action. It is hoped that by studying the ideas, discussions and case scenarios advanced in this book these aims will be achieved.

This seventh revised edition of *Bioethics: a nursing perspective* builds on the discussions and thought advanced in the sixth edition and reflects the increasing maturity and sophistication of nursing ethics discourse, locally and globally. It also provides a reminder to those both inside and outside of the profession that nursing ethics is an ongoing endeavour and, as such, will be a lifelong project – in short, it will never be 'done'.

The substantial review and revision of the book's chapters has highlighted a number of important concerns and challenges which lie ahead. Of particular concern is that – despite developments in the field – like the general public, nurses are vulnerable to being swayed by public opinion, dogmatic moralising and high-sounding rhetoric rather than reasoned argument when it comes to taking a stand on controversial ethical issues. The reasons for this are complex. As I have noted elsewhere,[1] nurses are living in a time when old certainties are shifting and where identifying the 'right' position to take on given moral issues has become increasingly difficult. Deciding a right course of action can be especially difficult in contexts where a clear-eyed view of the world is muddied by populist opinion and personal dogma masquerading as 'fact'. In this new era of shameless authoritarian populism, 'fake news' and post-truth politics, it is perhaps understandable that nurses face new quandaries when it comes to deciding what to do and even whether to do anything at all. Being morally passive bystanders to questionable activities and events, however, is not an option.

The ultimate message of this revised work, as it was with the previous edition, is that what we, as nurses, do about health care reflects what kind of profession we are, and what we think ought to be done about health care will ultimately reflect what kind of profession we think we ought to be. In making the revisions to this seventh edition, it is hoped that readers (nurses as well as those with whom they work) will cultivate new insights and a new moral wisdom about the ethical issues they face and will become inspired to be much more than mere 'morally passive bystanders' in the world of human affairs and to take a stand on the things that really matter.

Megan-Jane Johnstone

---

[1] Johnstone M-J (2017) Is nursing ethics good enough? *Australian Nursing and Midwifery Journal*, 25(3): 19

Acknowledgments

In writing and revising this book I have become indebted to a number of people. Foremost among them are Alfred Deakin Professor Fethi Mansouri and the Alfred Deakin Institute for Citizenship and Globalisation, of which he is the director. His assistant Cayla Edwards is also due acknowledgment. Without this support, which enabled generous access to the Deakin University library resources, the revision of this book would not have been possible. Thanks are also due to the many nurses, students, patients, colleagues and others whose generosity in sharing their experiences and views over the 30 years this book has been in print has, in many ways, made this book possible. My deep gratitude is also due to my good friend and colleague Dr Olga Kanitsaki, AM (now retired) who, as in the case of all the previous editions, has been a stalwart mentor and supporter of my work.

Finally, these acknowledgments would not be complete without thanks being given to Libby Houston, Senior Content Strategist from Elsevier, and members of the editorial team, Vanessa Ridehalgh (Content Development Specialist), Fariha Nadeem (Content Project Manager) and also Chris Wyard (Freelance Editor) for their contribution to the successful production of this book. The final work is, however, my own, as are any weaknesses and omissions.

Permissions acknowledgments

The author and publisher would like to thank the following for granting permission to reproduce material:

BMJ Publishing Group, London: Craig G (1994) On withholding nutrition and hydration in the terminally ill: has palliative medicine gone too far? *Journal of Medical Ethics*, 20(3): 140-2; and Wyatt J (2001) Medical paternalism and the fetus. *Journal of Medical Ethics*, 27 (supp ii): ii15-ii20

Cambridge University Press, Melbourne: Buchanan A & Brock D (1989) *Deciding for others: the ethics of surrogate decision making*

eContent Management Pty Ltd, Queensland: Johnstone M-J (2002) The changing focus of health care ethics: implications and challenges for the health care professions. *Contemporary Nurse* (www.contemporarynurse.com), 12(3): 213-24

Martin Benjamin: Benjamin M (2001) Between subway and spaceship: practical ethics at the outset of the twenty-first century. *Hastings Center Report,* 31(4): 22-31

Oxford University Press, New York: Beauchamp T & Childress J (2013) *Principles of biomedical ethics*, 7th edn

The Hastings Center Report, New York: Benjamin M (2001) Between subway and spaceship: practical ethics at the outset of the twenty-first century. *Hastings Center Report,* 31(4): 22-31

University of Chicago Press, Chicago: Wong D (1992) Coping with moral conflict and ambiguity. *Ethics*, 102(4): 763-84

List of abbreviations

ABC	Australian Broadcasting Corporation
ABS	Australian Bureau of Statistics
ACN	Australian College of Nursing
ACP	advance care plan / planning
ACSQHC	Australian Commission on Safety and Quality in Health Care
AHMAC	Australian Health Ministers Advisory Council
AHPRA	Australian Health Practitioner Regulation Agency
AIDS	acquired immunodeficiency syndrome
AIFS	Australian Institute of Family Studies
AIHW	Australian Institute of Health and Welfare
ALRC	Australian Law Reform Commission
AMA	Australian Medical Association
AMR	antimicrobial resistance
ANA	American Nurses Association
ANF	Australian Nursing Federation
ANH	artificial nutrition and hydration
ANPEA	Australian Network for the Prevention of Elder Abuse
CALD	culturally and linguistically diverse
CALDB	culturally and linguistically diverse background
CAHN	clinically assisted hydration and nutrition
CCP	Compassion Cultivation Program
CDC	Centers for Disease Control and Prevention
CLAS	cultural and linguistically appropriate services
CNA	Canadian Nurses Association
COAG	Council of Australian Governments
CPR	cardiopulmonary resuscitation
CRPD	Convention on the Rights of Persons with Disabilities
CSDH	Commission on Social Determinants of Health
DCS	deep continuous sedation
DNR	Do Not Resuscitate
DoH	Department of Health
DST	deep sleep therapy
EC	European Community
ECG	electrocardiograph
ECT	electroconvulsive therapy
ED	emergency department
ELP	English language proficiency
EN	enrolled nurse

GFC	Global Financial Crisis
GP	general practitioner
HAI	HelpAge International
HIV	human immunodeficiency virus
HPP	Homeless Persons Program
ICN	International Council of Nurses
IMR	infant mortality rate
IOM	Institute of Medicine (USA)
ISPCAN	International Society for the Prevention of Child Abuse and Neglect
IVF	in vitro fertilisation
IWGIA	International Work Group for Indigenous Affairs
LEF	low English fluency
LEP	limited English proficiency
LGBTIQ	lesbian, gay, bisexual, transgender, intersex, queer / questioning
LOTE	language other than English
MAD	medically assisted death
MAiD	medical assistance in dying
MAS	medically assisted suicide
NBV	Nurses Board of Victoria
NCHK	Nursing Council of Hong Kong
NCNZ	Nursing Council of New Zealand
NES	non-English speaking/native English speaker
NESB	Non-English speaking background
NFR	Not For Resuscitation
NFT	Not For Treatment
NGO	non-government organisation
NHS	National Health Service
NLCHP	National Law Center on Homelessness and Poverty
NMBA	Nursing and Midwifery Board of Australia
NMC	Nursing and Midwifery Council (UK)
NNA	National Nursing Association
NNES	non-native English speaker
NT	Northern Territory (Australia)
NWRO	National Welfare Rights Organisation
NZNO	New Zealand Nurses Organisation
OPA	Office of the Public Advocate
PAD	psychiatric advance directive
PAS	physician-assisted suicide
PBS	pharmaceutical benefits scheme
PDCC	Police Department's Communication Centre
PEG	percutaneous endoscopic gastrostomy
PHM	People's Health Movement
PPS	proportionate palliative sedation
PTSD	post-traumatic stress disorder
QLS	Queensland Law Society
RCNA	Royal College of Nursing, Australia
RDNS	Royal District Nursing Service

RN	registered nurse
RPC	respecting patient choices
SARS	severe acute respiratory syndrome
SBD	self-binding directive
SCRGSP	Steering Committee for the Review of Government Service Provision (Australia)
SNB	Singapore Nursing Board
SOGI	sexual orientation and gender identity
TMT	Terror Management Theory
TNMC	Thailand Nursing and Midwifery Council
TRC	Truth and Reconciliation Commission (South Africa)
UK	United Kingdom
UN	United Nations
UNDP	United Nations Development Programme
UNHCR	United Nations High Commissioner for Refugees
US	United States
WASP	White Anglo-Saxon person
WEIRD	Western, educated, industrialised, rich and democratic
WHA	World Health Assembly
WHO	World Health Organization
WMA	World Medical Association
WWII	World War Two

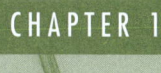

CHAPTER 1

Professional standards and the requirement to be ethical

KEYWORDS

ethical practice
ethical professional conduct
moral impairment
moral incompetence
professional boundaries
professional conduct
professional misconduct
professional practice
professional standards
unethical professional conduct
unprofessional conduct
unsatisfactory professional performance

LEARNING OBJECTIVES

Upon the completion of this chapter and with further self-directed learning you are expected to be able to:

- Locate the code of conduct, code of ethics and related standards of practice developed by the relevant nursing authority in the jurisdiction / state / country of your practice, and which you are expected to uphold as a professional nurse.
- Identify the ethical standards and moral competencies expected of professional nurses in the jurisdiction / state / country of your practice.
- Define ethical and unethical conduct.
- Discuss examples in which breaches of the expected ethical standards of the nursing profession might be deemed instances of unprofessional conduct, professional misconduct or unsatisfactory professional performance.
- Discuss why, if at all, nurses should uphold the standards of ethical conduct prescribed by national and international nursing authorities.
- Reflect critically on why, if at all, the practice of nursing is a moral undertaking.

Introduction

From the moment a nurse enters into professional practice she or he is bound by strict standards of professional conduct. The standards of conduct expected of professional nurses are stated publicly in a range of documents including formally endorsed professional codes of conduct, codes of ethics, competency standards and guidelines and position statements formulated on a range of issues relevant to the profession and ethical practice of nursing. For example, nurses in Australia are bound by the standards of conduct expressed in the following documents published by the Nursing and Midwifery Board of Australia (NMBA):

- *Code of conduct for nurses* (2018a)
- *Nurse practitioner standards for practice* (2014)
- *Registered nurse standards for practice* (2016).

(Note: These and other documents, such as policies, guidelines, case studies and position statements, can be viewed by visiting http://www.nursingmidwiferyboard.gov.au/ and following the links under 'Professional Codes & Guidelines' (https://www.nursingmidwiferyboard.gov.au/Codes-Guidelines-Statements/Professional-standards.aspx).)

Nurses in New Zealand, meanwhile, are bound by the standards of conduct expressed in various documents published respectively by the Nursing Council of New Zealand (NCNZ) and the New Zealand Nurses Organisation (NZNO), such as:

- *Code of conduct for nurses* (NCNZ 2012a)
- *Code of ethics* (NZNO 2013)
- *Competencies for nurse practitioners* (NCNZ 2012b)
- *Competencies for registered nurses* (NCNZ 2016)
- *Guidelines for cultural safety, the Treaty of Waitangi and Māori health in nursing education and practice* (NCNZ 2011)
- *Guidelines: professional boundaries* (NCNZ 2012c)
- *Guidelines: social media and electronic communication* (NCNZ 2012d).

(Note: This and other documents can be viewed by visiting: http://www.nursingcouncil.org.nz/Publications/Standards-and-guidelines-for-nurses and http://www.nzno.org.nz/resources/nzno_publications.)

Nurses working in other countries (e.g. Canada, Hong Kong(China), India, Korea, Singapore, Thailand, United Kingdom (UK) and the United States of America (USA)) are likewise bound by the standards of conduct and related policies and guidelines developed, endorsed and published by their respective national nurse organisations and regulating authorities, such as nursing associations, boards and councils (see Box 1.1).

In addition, in countries where national nursing organisations are also in membership with the International Council of Nurses (ICN) (currently the ICN represents over 20 million nurses worldwide in more than 130 countries), nurses are also bound by the codes, policy and position statements published and endorsed by the ICN. Of particular note are the ICN's:

- *The ICN code of ethics for nurses* (2012a)
- Position and policy statements on a range of issues relating to:
    - nursing roles in health care service
    - nursing profession
    - socioeconomic welfare of nurses
    - health care systems
    - social issues.

(Note: these can be viewed at: http://www.icn.ch.)

A range of resources including fact sheets, position statements, and guidelines have been devised in relation to each of the above issues, which can all be viewed via the ICN web pages. (For a comprehensive examination of *The ICN code of ethics for nurses* and related position statements, and their application as a guide to ethical decision-making in nursing, see Fry & Johnstone 2008.)

In Australia, the obligation to uphold the ICN Code and related guidelines is more specific owing to the NMBA, the Australian Nursing and Midwifery Federation (ANMF) and the Australian College of Nurses (ACN) conjointly agreeing to abandon the Australian *Code of ethics for nurses in Australia* (NMBA 2008a, first published in 1993) in favour of adopting *The ICN code of ethics for nurses* (2012a) as the guiding

BOX 1.1 Nursing codes of ethics and position statements pertaining to jurisdictions outside Australia

American Nurses Association (ANA)
- *Code of ethics for nurses* with interpretive statements (2015)
- Other resources on ethical issues (e.g. end-of-life issues, ethics and human rights, moral courage and moral distress, genetics and genomics)

   Available at: https://www.nursingworld.org/practice-policy/nursing-excellence/ethics/code-of-ethics-for-nurses/

Canadian Nurses Association (CNA)
- *Code of ethics for registered nurses* (2017)
- Other resources on ethical issues (e.g. end-of-life issues, ethics and human rights, moral courage and moral distress, genetics and genomics)

   Available at: https://www.cna-aiic.ca/html/en/Code-of-Ethics-2017-Edition/index.html#4

Korean Nurses Association (KNA)
- *Korean nurses' declaration of ethics* (nd)

   Available at: http://en.koreanurse.or.kr/about_KNA/ethical.php

Nursing Council of Hong Kong (NCHK)
- *Code of ethics and professional conduct for nurses in Hong Kong* (2015)

   Available at: https://www.nchk.org.hk/filemanager/en/pdf/conduct.pdf

New Zealand Nurses Organisation (NZNO)
- *Code of ethics* (2013)

   Available at: http://www.nzno.org.nz/resources/nzno_publications

Nursing Council of New Zealand (NCNZ)
- *Code of conduct for nurses* (NCNZ 2012a)
- *Competencies for registered nurses* (NCNZ 2016)
- *Competencies for nurse practitioners* (NCNZ 2012b)
- *Guidelines for cultural safety, the Treaty of Waitangi and Māori health in nursing education and practice* (NCNZ 2011)
- *Guidelines: professional boundaries* (NCNZ 2012c)
- *Guidelines: social media and electronic communication* (NCNZ 2012d)

   Available at: http://www.nursingcouncil.org.nz/Publications/Standards-and-guidelines-for-nurses

Nursing and Midwifery Council (NMC) (UK)
- *The code: professional standards of practice and behaviour for nurses and midwives* (2015)

   Available at: https://www.nmc.org.uk/globalassets/sitedocuments/nmc-publications/nmc-code.pdf

Singapore Nurses Board (SNB)
- *Code for nurses and midwives* (2018a)
- *Core competencies and generic skills for registered nurses* (2018b)
- *Core competencies of advanced practice nurses* (2018c)

   Available at: http://www.healthprofessionals.gov.sg/snb/nursing-guidelines-and-standards

Thailand Nursing and Midwifery Council (TNC)
- *Competencies of registered nurses* (includes competencies in ethics, code of conduct and the law) (nd)

   Available at: http://www.tnc.or.th/en

document for ethical decision-making for nurses in Australia. Due to the formal adoption of the ICN Code by the Australian nursing organisations, upon its coming into effect 1 March 2018 the extant *Code of ethics for nurses in Australia* (NMBA 2008a) and *Code of professional conduct for nurses in Australia* (NMBA 2008b), both of which had been developed specifically for application in the cultural context of Australia,[1] were superseded and are now redundant. (The NMBA's abandonment of its code of ethics and shift to a more managerial and regulatory approach to professional conduct will be considered further in Chapter 2 of this book.)

The requirement to uphold exemplary standards of conduct

The requirement for nurses to be ethical and to uphold the highest standards of conduct when practising in a professional capacity is not unique to nursing. It is generally expected that, when performing their duties and conducting their affairs, professionals (of all fields) will uphold exemplary standards of conduct – which is commonly taken to mean standards that are higher than, and not generally expected of, lay people or the 'ordinary person on the street'. A key reason underpinning this expectation relates to the potential vulnerability of clients and an associated expected 'special obligation' on the part of professionals to reduce this vulnerability by conforming to 'particularly high ethical standards both in their professional and non-professional lives' (Freckelton 1996: 142). This expectation also relates to what Mortensen (2002, p 166) describes in the context of the legal profession as the 'overarching principle' of qualifications to practise – notably, protecting the public and providing assurance to the public that those registered to practise can be trusted to do so safely. To this end a 'thicker' standard other than that set by law is required – notably, moral standards of character, competency and commitment involving a deep appreciation in moral terms of how the public interest is best served (Mortensen 2002, p 175). Such are these and related expectations that exemplary standards of ethical conduct have historically been cited as one of the key hallmarks of professionalism and indeed as a necessary feature of professions generally (Bayles 1981).

Nurses are also expected to uphold exemplary standards of ethical conduct in their personal or 'non-professional' lives. The main reason for this is that engaging in unethical conduct in their personal lives risks bringing both themselves and the nursing profession into disrepute, thereby losing the trust of the public.

A notable feature of the respective standards, policies and guidelines that have been operationalised by Australian, New Zealand and other national nursing organisations around the world is that they function as 'companion codes'. When taken together, these companion codes provide a framework for legally and professionally accountable and responsible nursing practice in all its domains including clinical, management, leadership, governance and administration, education, research, advice/consultation and policy development. The standards contained in the codes work by setting the 'ethical baseline' against which a nurse's conduct can be measured and evaluated. Thus, if a nurse engages in conduct that breaches the agreed standards of the profession (i.e. fails literally to 'measure up' to the standards in question), this may be deemed as unethical professional conduct or professional misconduct and may result in a notification being made to a nurse regulating authority. (The requirement to make notifications of unprofessional conduct or professional misconduct to a nurse regulating authority is discussed in more depth in Chapter 12 of this book.)

Unprofessional conduct and professional misconduct

In Australia, a nurse's activities deemed to be breaches of acceptable professional conduct may fall under three possible categories: *unprofessional conduct*, *professional misconduct* and *unsatisfactory professional performance*.

Each of these behaviours in turn may constitute *notifiable conduct*. All three categories are defined in the *Health Practitioner Regulation National Law Act* (2018) (to be referred to from here on as the 'National Law') as well as in the NMBA (2018a) *Code of conduct for nurses*. The category 'notifiable conduct' is also defined in the National Law and is comprehensively addressed in the Australian Health Practitioner Regulation Agency (AHPRA) (2014) National Board guidelines for registered health practitioners: *Guidelines for mandatory notifications* (to be considered in more detail in Chapter 12 of this book). Significantly, none of the above documents defines 'unethical conduct' or includes unethical conduct in its definitions of either professional misconduct, unprofessional conduct, unsatisfactory professional performance or notifiable conduct. Instead, the respective documents have framed their definitions as encompassing more breaches of law, rather than ethics. Although the National Law states as one of its objectives 'to provide for the protection of the public by ensuring that only health practitioners who are suitably trained and qualified to practise in a competent and *ethical* manner are registered' [emphasis added] (Section 3.2(a)), what constitutes an 'ethical manner' as such is not defined.

It is noted that reference is made in the NMBA Code to the ethical responsibility of nurses to: 'practise honestly and ethically', 'abide by relevant reporting requirements' and 'protect the privacy of people'. The Code stops short, however, of identifying the *ethical* responsibilities of nurses and of defining 'unethical conduct' despite this being an important component of both professional misconduct and unprofessional conduct. The AHPRA Guidelines also stop short of considering and defining 'unethical conduct', other than to clarify that it is not a breach of professional etiquette or ethics, or a departure from accepted standards of professional conduct, for a person to make notifications concerning the substandard conduct of a practitioner.

To help improve nurses' understanding of their responsibilities under a nurse regulating authority's provisions concerning breaches of acceptable professional conduct, working definitions of the notions ethical professional conduct, unprofessional conduct, professional misconduct, unsatisfactory professional performance and unethical professional conduct are required. These are considered briefly below.

Ethical professional conduct

Ethical professional conduct may be defined as conduct that accords with and upholds the accepted ethical principles and standards of a given profession and is thereby deemed to be 'right' and 'correct'.

Unprofessional conduct

Unprofessional conduct (from *un* – meaning *not; opposite of; contrary to*) may literally be defined as conduct that is contrary to the expected standards of a profession, or conduct that is not belonging to or of a lesser standard otherwise expected of a profession and thereby may be deemed 'wrong' and 'incorrect'.

Professional misconduct

Professional misconduct (from *mis* – meaning *wrong, bad or erroneous; a lack of*) may be defined literally as conduct or behaviour that is morally wrong, bad or erroneous. This form of conduct may pertain to behaviour that is improper and unbefitting a professional person or someone to be registered as a professional person albeit in a non-professional context (e.g. being drunk and disorderly in a public place, engaging in fare evasion while using public transport or engaging in criminal behaviour outside of a work-related context).

Unsatisfactory professional performance

In the National Law, *unsatisfactory professional performance* of a registered health practitioner is taken to mean 'the knowledge, skill or judgment possessed, or care exercised by, the practitioner in the practice of the health profession in which the practitioner is registered is below the standard reasonably expected of a health practitioner of an equivalent level of training or experience' (Section 5).

Unethical professional conduct

Unethical professional conduct is more complex than conduct that is merely contrary to the accepted ethical standards of a profession. Unethical professional conduct may be more comprehensively defined as an umbrella term that incorporates the following three related although distinct notions: (i) unethical conduct, (ii) moral incompetence and (iii) moral impairment (Johnstone 2012a). Here, *unethical conduct* may be defined as 'any act involving the deliberate violation of accepted or agreed ethical standards' and can encompass both 'moral turpitude' and 'moral delinquency' (Johnstone 2012a: 34). *Moral turpitude*, a legal concept that originates from the United States, refers to 'conduct that is considered contrary to community standards of justice, honesty or good morals' (*Legal dictionary*, 2016; see also Wikipedia 2018a). *Moral delinquency*, in turn, refers to any act involving moral negligence or a dereliction of moral duty. In professional contexts, moral delinquency entails a deliberate or careless violation of agreed standards of ethical professional conduct.

Moral incompetence (analogous to clinical incompetence) pertains to a person's lack of requisite moral knowledge, skills, 'right attitude' and soundness of moral judgment. The specific moral competencies expected of nurses in Australia are not defined. Although the NMBA (2016) *Registered nurse standards for practice* require nurses to use ethical frameworks when making decisions (Standard 1.5), such a framework or the knowledge and skills required to use it are not described. The NZCN *Competencies for registered nurses* (2016: 4), in contrast, is more explicit. A range of competencies nurses are expected to have are detailed, which require nurses being able to 'demonstrate knowledge and judgment and being accountable for own actions and decisions' (the issue of moral competence/incompetence will be discussed in more detail in Chapter 5 of this text).

Moral impairment meanwhile is generally distinguished from moral incompetence. Unlike moral incompetence (attributable to a lack of moral knowledge, skills, etc.), moral impairment entails a disorder (e.g. psychopathy) that interferes with a person's social and moral reasoning and hence capacity to behave ethically. More specifically, because of their impaired moral reasoning, such persons are unable to engage in the competent discharge of their moral duties and responsibilities towards others. Accepting the notion of moral impairment (a notion which has received little attention in the nursing literature), nurses could be judged morally impaired when, because of their disorder, they are unable to practise nursing in an ethically just and morally accountable manner.

Questioning the requirement to be morally exemplary

The demand placed on nurses to be ethical and to uphold exemplary ethical standards of conduct is not without controversy. One reason for this is that the expectation to be ethical seems to assume (without supporting evidence) that nurses, like other professionals, should as a matter of fact be ethical. This assumption raises a number of important questions, such as:

- What is ethics and ethical professional conduct?
- Is it the case that nurses 'should' be ethical?
- What does it mean to be an 'ethical practitioner'?
- Is it possible to be an ethical professional in health care environments, situations and circumstances that are not supportive of and may even be hostile to ethical conduct?
- How should ethics be practised in professional (e.g. nursing and health care) contexts?
- What moral 'competencies' and 'capabilities' does a professional person need in order to be able to practise ethics safely and effectively as an accountable and responsible professional?

Whatever the possible answers to these and related questions (and there are many), one thing is clear: nurses may be able to accept or reject the different viewpoints expressed, but they cannot ignore them. This is because, so long as nurses continue to work with and care for people – and strive to promote the health and wellbeing of people (a core purpose of nursing practice) – they will not be able to avoid the many and complex moral problems that will inevitably arise during the course of their work. Neither will nurses be able to avoid making decisions and taking action (including the 'action' of deliberately not taking action) in response to the problems they encounter. As Hinman (1994: 1–2) has classically explained in another context:

> We cannot avoid confronting moral problems, because acting in ways that affect the wellbeing of ourselves and others is as unavoidable as acting in ways that affect the physical health of our own bodies. We inevitably face choices that hurt or help people, choices that may infringe on their rights or violate their dignity or use them as mere tools to our own ends. We may choose not to pay attention to the concerns of morality such as compassion or justice or respect, just as we may choose to ignore the concerns of nutrition. However, that does not mean we can avoid making decisions about morality any more than we can evade deciding what foods to eat. We can ignore morality, but we cannot sidestep the choices to which morality is relevant, just as we cannot avoid decisions to which nutrition is pertinent even when we ignore the information that nutritionists provide for us. Morality is about living, and as long as we continue living, we will inevitably be confronted with moral questions – and if we choose to stop living that too is a moral issue.

Nursing as a moral project

Nursing is, without question, a moral undertaking. Its practice never occurs in a moral vacuum and is never free of moral risk. Even nursing care practices and procedures that might seem 'simple', 'basic' or 'trivial' (e.g. placing a person on a bedpan, or administering an aspirin tablet) could, potentially, have morally significant, harmful consequences. It is because of the potential to cause morally significant harm to others – not to mention the breach of trust that could occur as a consequence of such harm being caused – that nursing practice and the conduct of nurses warrant attention from an ethical point of view. It is the purpose of this book to provide such attention and to advance a critical examination of the moral role, responsibilities and rights of nurses as accountable and responsible health care professionals. To this end, in the chapters to follow, particular attention will be given to explaining what ethics is and why nurses 'should' be ethical – even in contexts which are not supportive of ethical conduct and where being ethical may be difficult. Issues and examples will be discussed critically to show that it is not enough just to be 'sensitive' to and have knowledge of certain ethical issues, but nurses also need to have the skills and wisdom (the moral 'know-how') to deal with them safely, competently and effectively and, equally important, to have the capacity to act in order to achieve morally desirable outcomes. It will also be suggested that it is not enough for nurses to simply comply with the law (Acts and regulations) governing their practice – and being what Snelling (2016) terms 'just-good-enough' nurses. In the interests of both sustaining and justifying the public's trust in the nursing profession, nurses need also to subscribe to 'thicker' standards of conduct, notably ethical standards of conduct, competency and commitment to practising nursing as a moral undertaking.

Conclusion

Nurses in all levels and areas of practice are bound by strict standards of professional conduct and are expected publicly to uphold the highest ideals of ethical professional practice. However, just why nurses should uphold the standards expected of them and how best to do so remains an open question. It is important, therefore, for nurses (whatever their level and area of practice, and whether working in clinical, managerial, administration, education, research and/or other related domains) to critically examine and reflect on such questions as:

- What is ethics?
- What is ethical professional conduct?
- Why should I be ethical?
- What should I do in situations where I know what the 'right' thing to do is, but I have no support to act on my judgment?
- Do I know enough about ethics in order to practise ethics safely and effectively as an accountable and responsible professional?
- What moral 'competencies' and 'capabilities' do I need to develop in order to fulfil my responsibilities as an ethical nurse?

It is hoped that, by studying this book and examining critically the ideas considered within its pages, nurses will be better enabled to address these questions in an informed and responsible way.

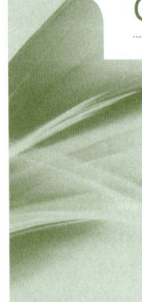

Case scenario 1

Over an 8-week period, while being treated as in-patients at a public hospital, two elderly patients were robbed of $23 000 and of $15 000 respectively by a nurse working at the hospital. The robbery took place after the nurse in question allegedly stole the patients' bank debit cards and personal identification numbers (PINs) from their wallets at the time of their admission to hospital. The patients realised that their money was missing from their accounts only when they each received a letter from their respective banks advising them that their accounts were overdrawn. The nurse subsequently resigned from the hospital and moved interstate. When later questioned about the matter she lied to investigating authorities and gave them false information. Ultimately, she was summonsed on a total of 46 counts of obtaining a benefit by deception and arrested to face charges in the local court of the city where the offences allegedly took place.

Case scenario 2

While on duty at a metropolitan hospital, a registered nurse of 3 years experience stole medication from the drug cupboard. The nurse had also engaged in a range of other unacceptable behaviours while on duty that included taunting an aphasic patient by making inappropriate comments that related to the patient, writing offensive descriptions of patients on their care plans (which were in full view of other staff working on the ward), giving patients offensive and derogatory names, and often acting in an aggressive way towards patients and co-workers. In addition, the nurse had administered an unauthorised and excessive amount of medication to a patient 'to keep the patient quiet'.

Following a formal investigation into the nurse's conduct by the regulating authority in the jurisdiction where the nurse was working, the nurse was found to have engaged in unprofessional conduct of a serious nature and had her registration cancelled.

> **CRITICAL QUESTIONS**
>
> 1 What standards of ethical professional conduct did the nurses breach in these scenarios?
> 2 If you were a nurse working in a hospital or a residential home care setting and you suspected or knew that a nurse was abusing, defrauding or derogating a patient or resident, what, if any, action would you take?
> 3 Upon what basis would you justify your actions (or non-actions, as the case may be)?
> 4 What might be the consequences both to the patients/residents and to yourself, in either case, of your taking action or not taking action?

Endnote

1 For an historical overview of the operationalisation of professional nursing ethics in Australia and its jurisdictions, including the relatively late development of the *Code of ethics for nurses in Australia*, see Johnstone (2016a).

CHAPTER 2

Ethics, bioethics and nursing ethics: some working definitions

KEYWORDS

bioethics
codes of conduct
codes of ethics
ethics
etiquette
ideology
law
moral issue
morality
nursing ethics
public opinion

LEARNING OBJECTIVES

Upon the completion of this chapter and with further self-directed learning you are expected to be able to:
- Define the following concepts:
  – ethics
  – morality
  – bioethics
  – nursing ethics.
- Discuss why it is important to have a correct understanding of the terms commonly used in discussions and debates about ethics and ethical issues in nursing and health care.
- Discuss why each of the following processes cannot be relied upon to guide sound and just ethical conduct in nursing and health care contexts:
  – law
  – codes of ethics
  – codes of conduct
  – hospital or professional etiquette
  – hospital or institutional policy
  – public opinion, populism or the view of the majority
  – ideology
  – following the orders of a supervisor or manager.

Introduction

Understanding the basis of ethical professional conduct in nursing requires nurses to have at least a working knowledge and understanding of the language, concepts and theories of ethics. One reason for this, as explained by the English philosopher, Richard Hare (1964: 1–2), is that:

> *in a world in which the problems of conduct become every day more complex and tormenting, there is a great need for an understanding of the language in*

which these problems are posed and answered. For confusion about our moral language leads, not merely to theoretical muddles, but to needless practical perplexities.

At first glance it might seem cumbersome spending time on clarifying and developing an understanding of the language, concepts and underpinning theories used in discussions and debates on ethics. Upon closer examination, however, it soon becomes clear that such an undertaking is crucial if nurses and their associates are to engage in a meaningful inquiry into what ethics is, what constitutes 'nursing ethics' and how, if at all, nursing ethics differs from other fields of ethics, what it means to be an 'ethical practitioner', why nurses have an obligation to practise their profession in an ethical manner and how to be an ethical professional. Furthermore, and not least, is the question of how best to proceed with the difficult task of identifying and resolving the many moral problems that nurses (like others in the health care team) will inevitably encounter during the course of their everyday practice.

The importance of understanding ethics terms and concepts

The terms 'ethics', 'morality', 'rights', 'duties', 'obligations', 'moral principles', 'moral rules', 'morally right', 'morally wrong' and 'moral theory', to name some, are all commonly used in discussions about ethics. Nurses, like others, may use some of these terms when discussing life events and practice situations that are perceived as having a moral/ethical dimension. These terms are not always used correctly, however, with the unfortunate consequence of communication and discussions about ethical issues sometimes becoming distorted and, as a consequence, giving rise to problems and perplexities that did not exist previously or which could otherwise have been avoided had they been dealt with more competently.

One notable example of the incorrect use of ethical terms can be found in the tendency by some nurses (scholars included) to treat the terms 'rights' and 'responsibilities' or 'duties' as being synonymous, and thus able to be used interchangeably. Examples of this are found in the view that nurses have the 'right' to practise within their codes of ethics and laws governing their practice, and the 'right' to act as patient advocates. When the nature of rights and duties is examined later, it will become clear that the term 'right' in these examples should, in fact, read 'duty'. The implications of confusing the meanings of the terms 'rights' and 'duties' and treating these two terms as being synonymous will be explored more fully in the chapters to follow.

Another common mistake is the tendency by some nurses to draw a distinction between the terms *'ethics'* and *'morality'*. They draw a distinction on the grounds that, in their view, morality involves more a personal or private set of values (i.e. 'personal morality') whereas ethics is more concerned with a formalised, public and universal set of values (i.e. 'professional ethics'). Thompson and colleagues (2006: 42), for example, acknowledge that the terms 'ethics' and 'morals/morality' mean the same thing and 'can be used more or less interchangeably'. Yet they perpetuate confusion about whether this is in fact correct by going on to argue:

> *A distinction has grown up between the two terms in more formal usage. Morals (and also morality) now tend to refer to the standards of behaviour actually held or followed by individuals or groups, while ethics refers to the science or study of morals – an activity, in the academic context, also often called moral philosophy.*
> (Thompson et al 2006: 42)

As will be shown shortly, there is, in fact, no philosophically significant difference between the terms 'ethics' and 'morality' and to distinguish between them, as Thompson and others have done, is both unnecessary and confusing.

The need for a critical inquiry into ethical professional practice

It is acknowledged that most people brought up in a common cultural context share what Beauchamp and Childress (2013: 3) call a 'common morality' – that is, a set of core norms and dimensions of morality that most people accept as being relevant and important (e.g. respect the rights of others, do not harm or kill innocent people, it is wrong to steal, it is wrong to break promises, and so forth) and about which philosophical debate would be 'a waste of time'. It would be a mistake, however, to assume or to accept that 'common morality' or 'commonsense morality' is in and by itself sufficient to enable nurses to deal with the many complex and complicated ethical issues that they will encounter in their practice. As examples to be presented in the following chapters will show, while our 'ordinary moral apparatus' may motivate and guide us to behave ethically as people, it is often quite inadequate to the task of guiding us to deal safely and effectively with the many complex ethical issues that arise in nursing and health care contexts. A much more sophisticated moral competency and capability is required than that otherwise provided by a 'commonsense' morality.

If nurses are serious about ethics and about conducting themselves ethically in the various positions, levels and contexts in which they work, then they must engage in a critical inquiry about what ethics is and how it can best be applied in the 'real world' of professional nursing practice. It cannot be assumed that just because we know of and use certain ethical terms in our conversations that we know what they mean or that we are using them correctly. As Warnock warns in his classic work *Contemporary moral philosophy* (1967: 75):

> When we talk about 'morals' we do not all know what we mean; what moral problems, moral principles, moral judgments are is not a matter so clear that it can be passed over as simple datum. We must discover when we would say, and when we would not, that an issue is a moral issue, and why; and if, as is more than likely, disagreements should come to light even at this stage, we could at least discriminate and investigate what reasonably tenable alternative positions there may be.

Understanding moral language

When discussing and advancing debates on ethical issues in nursing and health care it is vital that all parties involved have a shared working knowledge and understanding of the meanings of terms and concepts that are fundamental to the issues being considered. This imperative is captured by the philosophical adage 'there must first be agreement before there can be disagreement'. The reasoning behind this imperative is that unless there is a shared understanding of core terms and concepts it will be extremely difficult, if not impossible, to develop insight and understanding of the issues at stake and address, if not resolve, the disagreements and conflicts that may have arisen in relation to them. For example, if two dissenting parties do not share a common understanding about the nature and content of human rights (what these entail, the moral authority they have, what entities can validly claim human rights and so forth) they cannot even begin to debate the conditions under which human rights ought to be respected and when they might justifiably be overridden, and to take action accordingly. Similarly, if two dissenting parties do not share a common conception of what *nursing ethics* is, then they cannot meaningfully debate whether or not nursing ethics ought to be recognised as a distinctive field of inquiry and practice in its own right, or whether nurses are obliged to uphold the standards of ethical conduct developed as a result of focused nursing ethics inquiry.

In developing a shared understanding of core terms and concepts used in discussions and debates on ethical issues, it is important for nurses to be aware that, contrary to expectations, many of the terms commonly used in ethical debates are themselves 'ethically loaded' and thus, paradoxically, at risk of distorting if not corrupting the debates. The notion of 'quality of life' is a good example. Many writers on bioethics assume that when a life ceases to be 'independent' it has diminished worth. In instances where quality of life has been a criterion for decision-making at the end stage of life, euthanasia might be considered a right and proper course of action to take. Here the ethically loaded notion of 'dependence' imparts a sense of the permissibility of the euthanasia option and limits thought of, say, pursuing a rehabilitation option. It also overrides thought of the possibility that for some people dependence may be irrelevant to the notion of a worthwhile life. For example, consciousness, memory, love and friendship may be more important to a person's sense of 'quality of life' than being able to live it independently (Seachris 2013; Wolf 2010). Moreover, as has been well documented, in some traditional cultural groups, familial and friendly relationships are characteristically collective and interdependent, and thus any thought of individual independence is irrelevant to the assessment of 'a life worth living' (Johnstone & Kanitsaki 2009a).

Poorly or inappropriately defined ethical terms and concepts can seriously impinge upon and limit people's moral imagination, and the moral options and choices that might otherwise be identified, considered and chosen in the face of moral disagreement, conflict and adversity.

What is ethics?

It is appropriate to begin the task of defining commonly used ethical terms and concepts by first examining the terms 'ethics' and 'morality', and clarifying from the outset that there is no philosophically significant difference between the terms 'ethics' and 'morality'. As an examination of the etymology (the study of the origin of the words) of both these terms shows, 'ethics' comes from the ancient Greek *ethikos* (originally meaning 'pertaining to custom or habit') and 'morality' comes from the Latin *moralitas* (also originally meaning 'custom' or 'habit'). This means that the terms may be used interchangeably, as they are in the philosophical literature and in this book. With respect to deciding which terms should be used in ethics discourse (i.e. whether to use the term 'ethics' or the term 'morality'), this is very much a matter of personal preference rather than of philosophical debate – noting, however, that the terms ethics and morality have come to refer to something far more sophisticated than 'custom' or 'habit', as will soon be shown.

Having clarified that there is no philosophically significant difference between the terms 'ethics' and 'morality', it now remains the task here to define what 'ethics' is.

For the purposes of this discussion, ethics is defined as a generic term that is used for referring to various ways of thinking about, understanding and examining how best to live a 'moral life' (Beauchamp & Childress 2013). More specifically, ethics involves a critically reflective activity that is concerned with a systematic examination of living and behaving morally and 'is designed to illuminate what we ought to do by asking us to consider and reconsider our ordinary actions, judgments and justifications' (Beauchamp & Childress 1983: xii). For example, a nurse may make an 'ordinary' moral judgment that abortion is wrong and conscientiously object to assisting with an abortion procedure. Whether her conscientious objection ought to be respected, however, requires a critical examination of the bases upon which the nurse has made that judgment and a consideration of the justifications (moral reasons) she has put forward to support the position she has taken.

Ethics, as it is referred to and used today, can be traced back to the influential works of the Ancient Greek philosophers Socrates (born 469 BC), Plato (born c. 428 BC) and Aristotle (born 384 BC). The works of these ancient Greek philosophers were especially influential in seeing ethics established as a branch of philosophical inquiry which sought dispassionate and 'rational' clarification and justification of the basic assumptions and beliefs that people hold about what is to be considered morally acceptable and morally unacceptable behaviour. Ethics thus evolved as a mode of philosophical inquiry (known as moral philosophy) that asked people to question why they considered a particular act right or wrong, what the reasons (justifications) were for their judgments and whether their judgments were correct. This view of ethics remains an influential one and, although the subject of increasing controversy over the past several decades, retains considerable currency in the mainstream ethics literature.

It is important to clarify that ethics has three distinct 'sub-fields', namely: descriptive ethics, metaethics and normative ethics. Descriptive ethics is concerned with the empirical investigation and description of people's moral values and beliefs (i.e. values and beliefs concerning what constitutes 'right' and 'wrong' or 'good' and 'bad' conduct). Metaethics, in contrast, is concerned with analysing the nature, logical form, language and methods of reasoning in ethics (e.g. it gives consideration to meanings of ethical terms such as 'rights', 'duties' and so on). Normative ethics, in turn, is concerned with establishing standards of correctness by identifying and prescribing certain rules and principles of conduct and developing theories to justify the norms established. Unlike descriptive ethics and metaethics, normative ethics is evaluative and prescriptive (hortatory) in nature. In the case of the latter, ethics inquiry is not so much concerned with how the world is, but with how it *ought* to be. In other words, it is not concerned with merely describing the world (although, of course, a description of the world is necessary as a starting point for an evaluative inquiry), but rather with prescribing how it should be and providing sound justification for this prescription. Just what is to count as a 'sound justification', however, is an open question and one that will be considered in the following chapter. In this book, all three sub-fields are drawn upon in varying degrees to advance knowledge and understanding of ethical issues in nursing and health care.

What is bioethics?

Bioethics may be defined as 'the systematic study of the moral dimensions – including moral vision, decisions, conduct and policies – of the life sciences and health care, employing a variety of ethical methodologies in an interdisciplinary setting' (Reich 1995a: xxi). The term 'bioethics' (from the Greek *bios* meaning 'life', and *ethikos*, *ithiki* meaning 'ethics') is a neologism that first found its way into public usage in 1970–71 in the United States of America (Reich 1994; see also Jecker et al 2007). Although originally the subject of only cautious acceptance by a few influential North American academics, the new term quickly 'symbolised and influenced the rise and shaping of the field itself' (Reich 1994: 320). Significantly, within 3 years of its emergence, the new term was accepted and used widely at a public level (Reich 1994: 328). Interestingly, it is believed that the term 'bioethics' caught on because it was 'simple' and because it was amenable to exploitation by the media, which had placed a great premium 'on having a simple term that could readily be used for public consumption' (Reich 1994: 331).

It is worth noting that initially the term 'bioethics' was used in two different ways, reflecting both the concerns and ambitions of two respective academics each of whom, it is suggested, quite possibly created the word independently of the other. The first (and later marginalised) sense in which the word was used had an 'environmental and evolutionary significance' (Reich 1994: 320). Specifically, it was intended to advocate attention to 'the problem of survival: the questionable survival of the human species and the even more questionable survival of nations and cultures' (Potter 1971 – cited by Reich 1994: 321). In short, it advocated long-range environmental concerns (Reich 1995b: 20). Reich (1994: 321–2) explains that the key objective in creating this term was:

> to identify and promote an optimum changing environment, and an optimum human adaptation within that environment, so as to sustain and improve the civilised world.

The other competing sense in which the word 'bioethics' was used referred more narrowly to the ethics of medicine and biomedical research. The primary focus of this approach was (Reich 1995b: 20):

1 the rights and duties of patients and health care professionals
2 the rights and duties of research subjects and researchers
3 the formulation of public policy guidelines for clinical care and biomedical research.

Significantly, it was this last sense which 'came to dominate the emerging field of bioethics in academic circles and in the mind of the public' – and which remains dominant today (Reich 1994: 320). There are a number of complex reasons for this, not least the political climate at the time, which saw the rise of the civil rights movement (including women's rights and the legal right to abortion, which helped to keep bioethical issues 'before the public'). Given the significant shift in social and moral values that was occurring at the time, however, it is perhaps not surprising that this essentially medical/biomedical sense of bioethics prevailed (Jonsen 1993; Singer 1994). For instance, it is now almost certain that the ideas behind the development of the field of bioethics in its medical/biomedical sense had been simmering for almost a decade before the field was eventually named (Jonsen 1993: S3; see also Jecker et al 2007). Notable among the events inspiring the development of the field were: the renal dialysis events of the early 1960s, the publication in 1966 of Henry Beecher's legendary and confronting article on the unethical design and conduct of 22 medical research projects, the heart transplant movement and later the much-cited 1975 Karen Ann Quinlan case involving the removal of artificial life support from a patient who was deemed to be in a 'persistent vegetative state' and credited with spearheading the 'right to die' movement (Beecher 1966; Jonsen 1993; Singer 1994).

Today, the dominant concerns of mainstream Western bioethics are still essentially medically orientated, with the most sustained attention (and, it should be added, the most institutional support) being given to examining the ethical and legal dimensions of the 'big' issues of bioethics, such as abortion, euthanasia, organ transplantation (and the associated issue of brain-death criteria), reproductive technology (e.g. in vitro fertilisation (IVF), genetic engineering, human cloning, stem cell research and utilisation, and so forth), ethics committees, informed consent, confidentiality, the economic rationalisation of health care, and research ethics (particularly in regard to randomised clinical trials and experimental surgery). Not only has mainstream bioethics come to refer to and represent these issues but, rightly or wrongly, it has given legitimacy to them as the most pressing bioethical concerns of contemporary health care across the globe.

It is alleged that Potter (one of the authors of the term 'bioethics') was himself very frustrated with this narrow conception of bioethics and is reported as responding that 'my own view of bioethics calls for a much broader vision' (Reich 1995b: 20). Indeed, Potter feared (prophetically as it turned out) that 'the Georgetown approach would simply reaffirm medical professional inclination to think of issues in terms of therapy versus prevention' (Reich 1995b: 20–1). Whereas Potter viewed bioethics as a 'new discipline' (of science and philosophy) emphasising a search for wisdom, the Georgetown group saw bioethics as an old discipline (applied ethics) to resolve concrete moral problems – that is, 'ordinary ethics applied in the bio-realm' (p 21).

It has been claimed that 'bioethics is a native-grown American product' reflecting distinctively American concerns and offering distinctively American solutions and resolutions to the bioethical problems identified (Jonsen 1993, S3–4). Whatever the merits of this claim, there is little doubt that bioethics in its medical/biomedical sense has become an international movement. This movement (propelled along by a variety of processes) has witnessed a number of spectacular achievements, including:

- the development of an awesome international body of literature on the subject of bioethics (including the publication in 1978 of the first *Encyclopedia of bioethics* (Reich 1978a, revised in 1995, 2004 and 2014) and, in the 1990s and beyond, the development and dissemination of vast online bioethics resources)
- the global establishment of research centres devoted specifically to investigating ethical issues in health care and related matters
- the emergence in the 1990s of a new profession of hospital ethicists/consultant ethicists
- the establishment of prestigious university chairs in applied ethics

- the rise of a commercially viable and even lucrative bioethics education industry, and not least
- the stimulation of public and political debate on 'life and death' matters in health care which, in many instances, has had a positive effect on influencing long-overdue social policy and law reform in regard to these matters.

The medical/biomedical senses of the term 'bioethics' have indeed dominated intellectual and political thought over the past few decades. Nevertheless, this dominance has been called into question and is now seeing increasing attention being given to other important bioethical issues such as environmentalism, sustainability, climate change, public health emergency preparedness and responses, genetically modified foods, and chemical warfare and torture, to name some (see, for example, the introductions to the second edition (edited by Reich 1995a), the third edition (edited by Post 2004) and the fourth edition (edited by Jennings 2014) of the *Encyclopedia of bioethics*; the landmark work of Jonathan Mann and associates on the fundamental relationship between health and human rights (Anand et al 2004; Gruskin et al 2005; Mann 1996, 1997; Mann et al 1999); the rise of the 'new' public health ethics (see, for example, Bayer et al 2006; Beauchamp & Steinbock 1999; Beyrer & Pizer 2007; Daniels 2006; Powers & Faden 2006); and a new focus on 'global health ethics' (Pinto & Upshur 2013)). In light of these developments, there is considerable room to speculate that in the not too distant future the term 'bioethics' might once again hold an environmental, evolutionary and humanitarian significance, and have a much broader focus than it has had up until now.

What is nursing ethics?

Nursing ethics can be defined broadly as the examination of all kinds of ethical and bioethical issues from the perspective of nursing theory and practice which, in turn, rest on the agreed core concepts of nursing, namely: person, culture, care, health, healing, environment and nursing itself (or, more to the point, its ultimate purpose) – all of which have been comprehensively articulated in the nursing literature (too vast to list here). In this regard, then, contrary to popular belief, nursing ethics is not synonymous with (and indeed is much greater than) an ethic of care, although an ethic of care has an important place in the overall moral scheme of nursing and nursing ethics. Unlike other approaches to ethics, nursing ethics recognises the 'distinctive voices' that are nurses and emphasises the importance of collecting and recording nursing narratives and 'stories from the field' (Benner 1991, 1994; Bishop & Scudder 1990; Parker 1990). Collecting and collating stories from the field are regarded as important since issues invariably emerge from these stories that extend far beyond the 'paramount' issues otherwise espoused by mainstream bioethics. Analyses of these stories tend to reveal not only a range of issues that are nurses' 'own', as it were, but also a whole different configuration of language, concepts and metaphors for expressing them. As well, these stories often reveal issues otherwise overlooked in mainstream bioethics discourses. Given this, nursing ethics can also be described as, *methodologically and substantively, inquiry from the point of view of nurses' experiences*, with nurses' experiences being taken as a more reliable starting point than other locations from which to advance a rich, meaningful and reliable system and practice of nursing ethics.

Like other approaches to ethics, however, nursing ethics recognises the importance of providing practical guidance on how to decide and act morally. Drawing on a variety of ethical theoretical considerations, nursing ethics at its most basic could thus also be described as a practice discipline which aims to provide guidance to nurses on how to decide and act morally in the contexts in which they work (Johnstone 2015a, 2015b, 2015c).

The project of nursing ethics has many aspects to its nature and approach. Among other things, it involves nurses engaging in 'a positive project of constructing and developing alternative models, methods, procedures [and] discourses' of nursing and health care ethics that are more responsive to the lived realities and experiences of nurses and the people for whose care they share responsibility (adapted from Gross 1986: 195). In completing this project, nursing ethics has had – and continues to have – the positive consequence of allowing other 'weaker' viewpoints (including those of patients and nurses themselves) to emerge and be heard. In this respect, nursing ethics is also intensely political – although, it should be added, no more political than other role-differentiated ethics.

As in the case of moral philosophy, nursing ethics inquiry can be pursued by focusing on one or all of the following:

- *descriptive nursing ethics* (describing the moral values and beliefs that nurses hold and the various moral practices in which nurses engage across and within different contexts)
- *meta (nursing) ethics* (undertaking a critical examination of the nature, logical form, language and methods of reasoning in nursing ethics)
- *normative nursing ethics* (establishing standards of correctness and prescribing the rules of conduct with which nurses are expected to comply).

It is important to remember (as discussed in the 3rd edition of this work (Johnstone 1999a)) that nursing ethics has not always enjoyed the status that it has today. Its development, legitimation and recognition as a distinctive field of inquiry is testimony to the reality that nursing ethics is both necessary and inevitable. It is necessary because 'a profession without its own distinctive moral convictions has nothing to profess' and will be left vulnerable to the corrupting influences of whatever forces are most powerful (be they religious, legal, social, political or other in nature) (Churchill 1989: 30). Furthermore, as Churchill (1989: 31) writes, 'Professionals without an ethic are merely technicians, who know how to perform work, but who have no capacity to say why their work has any larger meaning.' Without meaning, there is little or no motivation to perform 'well'.

In regard to the inevitability of nursing ethics, as Churchill (1989: 31) points out, the 'practice of a profession makes those who exercise it privy to a set of experiences that those who do not practice lack'. By this view, those who practise nursing are privy to a set of experiences (moral experiences included) that others who do not practise nursing lack. So long as nurses interact with and enter into professional caring relationships with other people, they will not be able to avoid or sidestep the 'distinctively nursing' experience of deciding and acting morally while in these relationships. It is in this respect, then, that nursing ethics can be said to be inevitable.

What ethics is not

To further our understanding of what ethics (and its counterparts bioethics and nursing ethics) is, it would be useful also to give some attention to what ethics is not. For instance, ethics is not the same as law or a code of ethics. Neither is ethics something that can be determined by public opinion, ideology or following the orders of a supervisor or manager. Failure to distinguish ethics from these kinds of things could result in otherwise avoidable harmful consequences to people in health care domains.

Law

Ethics and law overlap in significant ways, but they are nevertheless distinct from one another. This distinction becomes particularly clear in instances where what the law may require in a given situation ethics might equally reject, and vice versa. Consider, for example, the issue of active voluntary euthanasia (commonly referred to by the colloquial term 'medically assisted death') and the plight of patients suffering intractable, intolerable and irremediable pain who request euthanasia as a 'treatment' option despite it being illegal in the jurisdiction where they live. With the notable exception of the Australian State of Victoria,[1] under Australian law it is a criminal offence 'to assist, encourage or aid a person to commit suicide or attempt to commit suicide' (Forrester & Griffith 2015: 247). Under these provisions, any nurse or doctor who administers a lethal substance to a patient with the sole intention of assisting that patient to die (suicide) would be committing a criminal offence and likely to be prosecuted accordingly. The fact that such an act was demonstrably in accordance with the patient's autonomous wishes would not be a legitimate defence. Regardless of the benevolence and voluntariness of an act of assisted death / euthanasia, it would still be deemed by law as illegal, and thereby *legally wrong*. This legal wrongness, however, is not necessarily synonymous with moral wrongness. Consider the following.

Ethics essentially requires that people be respected as self-determining choosers, and further that the considered preferences of autonomous persons be maximised. This requirement holds even in instances where a person's individual preferences might be considered mistaken or foolish by others. Ethics also requires that otherwise avoidable harm (such as the needless suffering of intractable and intolerable pain) should be prevented where this can be done without sacrificing other important moral interests. Returning to the euthanasia example, it soon becomes clear that an application of ethics (or, more particularly, the principles of bioethics) might, in this instance, permit the administration of a lethal injection to a suffering patient who has autonomously requested it. Not only might ethics permit such an act; it might actually require that it be done. Where sound moral justifications for the act can be shown, then the act of euthanasia in question could be deemed as having accorded with the principle of ethics and thereby as being *morally right* and justified.

Other compelling examples illuminating the difference between law and morality can be found by considering the laws enforced during wartime (such as those upheld by the Nazi and other despotic regimes), and the laws used to enforce apartheid (such as those upheld in early North America, and in South Africa circa 1948–91). The legal laws of the Nazis and of the apartheid-supporting regimes, although evil, still stand as constituting valid legal law (Hart 1958). We would presumably want to resist condoning the morality of these laws, however.

Law and ethics are quite separate action-guiding systems, and care must be taken to distinguish between them. Making this distinction may not only help to prevent moral errors, but also enforce moral and intellectual honesty about the undesirability of morally bad (evil) law (Hart 1958). Further, if we do not make this distinction we will not have an independent value system from which to judge the moral acceptability or unacceptability of valid legal law. For instance, if ethics were not distinct from legal law, we could not judge certain laws (e.g. Nazi laws) to be morally bad and wrong.

The question remains, however, of how the distinction between law and ethics can be made and, equally important, what the essential differences are between a legal decision and a moral / ethical decision, and, indeed, a clinical decision.

A very traditional view of law is that it is the command or order of a sovereign (e.g. a government) backed by a threat or sanction (e.g. punishment) (Hart 1961). For instance, governments around the world have formulated laws that command their citizens to pay taxes; if the citizens in question fail to pay their taxes they can expect to be punished in some way, such as by being fined or even sent to prison. The mere fact that they have not complied with the command – in essence, have broken the law – would probably be deemed sufficient justification for a sanction or punishment to be directed against them. Although this view of law does not capture its more political nature (see, for example, Johnstone 1994a; Kairys 1997), it is nevertheless sufficient for the purposes of this discussion in regard to distinguishing between law and ethics.

Accepting the above view of law, there is a fundamental sense in which the concept 'legal decision' as it is used by nurses probably refers to a type of decision that is made on the basis of what is required or prohibited by law – together with a desire to avoid a legal sanction or punishment for non-compliance. In this respect, the notion 'legal decision' is probably more aptly described as a 'legally defensive' decision. Consider the following example. A nurse who regards voluntary euthanasia as morally justified in cases of intolerable, intractable and irremediable suffering may nevertheless decline a patient's considered request for assistance to die in order to avoid any legal risk of receiving the penalty that would almost certainly be applied for assisting another's suicide should her actions be discovered. In this instance, the nurse's decision not to comply with the patient's request could be described as a 'legal decision' rather than a moral or clinical decision, and also as being 'legally defensive'. This is because her decision was influenced predominantly by considering the legal consequences of complying with the patient's request, rather than the moral or clinical consequences of doing so.

The question remains, however, of how a legal decision differs from an ethical decision. As is discussed more fully in the following chapter, ethics can be defined as a system of overriding rules and principles of conduct which function by specifying that certain behaviours are either required, prohibited or permitted. These principles are chosen autonomously on the basis of critical reflection, and are backed by autonomous moral reason (generally recognised in moral philosophy as the central organising principle of morality) and/or by feelings of guilt, shame, disgust, moral remorse and the like, which operate as kinds of moral sanctions. For example, we may choose autonomously to follow a moral principle which demands truth telling; if we fail to tell the truth in a given situation, we may then reason the act to be wrong and/or experience feelings of guilt, shame or moral remorse accordingly. Unlike what happens in instances involving a breach of legal law, however, we are not generally 'punished' for lying – for example, by being fined or sent to prison – unless, of course, our lying entails an act of perjury in a court of law.

Accepting this view of ethics, it is probably correct to say that the concept 'ethical decision', as it is used in health care contexts, refers to a type of decision that is guided by certain moral principles of conduct or other moral considerations (rather than by punitive legal laws) and a desire to achieve a given moral end. Thus, a doctor or a nurse tempted to tell a lie to either a colleague or a patient may choose instead to tell the truth in order to achieve some predicted overriding moral benefit and thereby also preserve her or his integrity as a morally autonomous professional (as distinct from, say, a law-abiding citizen).

In light of these basic views on law and ethics, and legal and ethical decision-making, what then is the nature of clinical (nursing and medical) decision-making? Primarily, nursing and medicine involve the skilful practice and application of tested principles of applied science and care to prevent, diagnose, alleviate or cure disease, illness and sickness and restore a person's health and sense of wellbeing. The practices of nursing and medicine are backed by legal and professional sanctions. For example, doctors and nurses can be found financially liable for negligence, and can be deregistered for professional misconduct as well as for civil misconduct unbefitting a professional person (see discussion on unprofessional conduct and professional misconduct in Chapter 1 of this book).

Accepting this, to say of a decision that it is a 'nursing decision' or a 'medical decision' in this context is probably to say little more than that it has been made by a nurse or a doctor respectively, and is based on an established body of evidence-based knowledge and 'reasonable' professional opinion on how this knowledge should or should not be applied in a clinical situation. For example, a doctor may venture the 'reasonable' medical opinion that if a certain life-saving treatment is stopped the patient will surely die. Or a nurse may venture the 'reasonable' nursing opinion that if a certain nursing care is not given the patient will suffer a particular type of harm. It must be understood here, however, that neither of the clinical opinions expressed in these instances is tantamount to expressing a valid moral judgment. For example, to say that a patient 'will die' if a certain drug or other treatment (e.g. surgery) is given or withheld says nothing about the moral permissibility or imperatives of giving or withholding the drug or other treatment in question. The ethics of a given clinical act is not implicit in the act itself; this is something that can be determined only by independent moral analysis.

Given these rough comparisons, it can be seen that legal, ethical and clinical decisions can be readily distinguished from one another (Fig. 2.1). What is also obvious is the enormous potential for the

FIGURE 2.1
Types of decisions in clinical settings

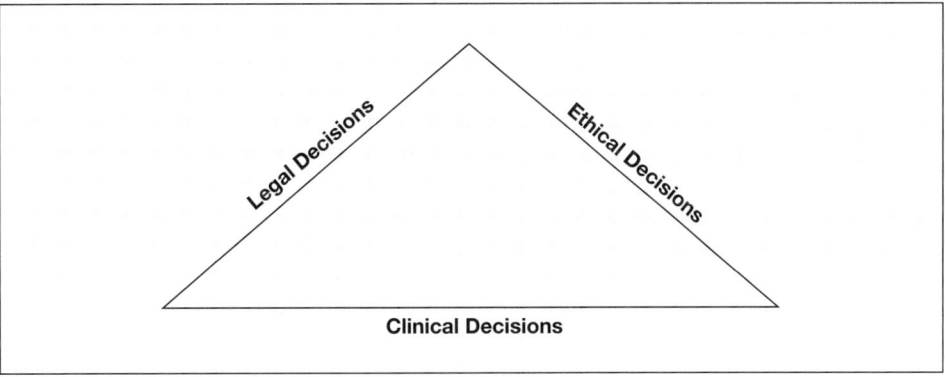

respective demands of each of these three types of decisions to come into conflict. For example, a medical decision not to resuscitate a patient in the event of a cardiac arrest (on the grounds that the patient's condition is 'medically hopeless') may be supported by an established body of medical opinion, but nevertheless be deemed morally unsound or even illegal, or both. For instance, the patient's autonomous wishes may not have been established before the medical decision was made, or the patient's legally valid consent may not have been obtained to withhold cardiopulmonary resuscitation (CPR) in the event of a cardiac arrest. Or, to take another example, a medical decision to continue treating a patient may accord with a 'reasonable body of medical opinion', be legal (as in cases where patients have been deemed rationally incompetent under a mental health act), yet be unethical if the patient has expressly stated a prior wish not to be treated, and if this expressed wish, contrary to popular medical opinion, is not 'irrational'.

We can also imagine cases where a medical decision to cease treatment accords with moral principles but may nevertheless invite legal censure – as in the case of withholding or withdrawing unduly burdensome life-prolonging treatment from severely brain-injured adults, poignant examples of which can be found in the much-publicised Terri Schiavo case in the United States (US) (discussed in Gostin 2005; Perry et al 2005; Quill 2005).

Although there is potential for conflict between ethical, legal and clinical decisions, it is not the case that these are always on a direct collision course; indeed, they may even complement or reinforce each other, as examples given in the following chapters show.

In drawing comparisons between legal, ethical and clinical decisions, there remains another crucial point to be observed: that it is conceptually incorrect to regard nursing or medical decisions per se as synonymous with either legal or moral decisions. This is not to say that we cannot meaningfully speak of nursing or medical decisions as being legally or morally correct or incorrect. On the contrary, it makes the point that, in asserting the legal or moral status of a given clinical (nursing or medical) decision, a judgment independent of the generally accepted scientific or indeed conventional standards of nursing or medicine must be made. In the case of ethics, the moral status of a clinical decision requires independent philosophical/moral analysis and judgment based on relevant moral considerations (e.g. moral rules and principles); in the case of law, the legal status of a clinical decision requires an independent legal analysis and judgment based on relevant legal considerations (e.g. legal rules and principles).

Codes of ethics

A code may be defined as a conventionalised set of rules or expectations devised for a select purpose. A code of professional ethics by this view could be described as a document that sets out a conventionalised set of moral rules and/or expectations devised for the purposes of guiding ethical professional conduct. It is important to understand, however, that codes of ethics are not ethics per se since they are not a fully developed system of ethics. Nevertheless, codes of ethics tend to reflect a rich set of moral values that have been expressed through a process of extensive consultation, debate, refinement, evaluation and review by practitioners over a period of time, and thus are well situated to function as meaningful action guides.

It is important to state at the outset that codes of ethics can be either prescriptive or aspirational in nature. In the case of prescriptive codes, provisions are 'duty-directed, stating specific duties of members' (Skene 1996: 111). In contrast, aspirational codes are 'virtue-directed, stating desirable aims while acknowledging that in some circumstances conduct short of the ideal may be justified' (Skene 1996: 111). Either way, codes of ethics have as their principal concern directing:

> *what professionals ought or ought not to do, how they ought to comport themselves, what they, or the profession as a whole, ought to aim at …* (Lichtenberg 1996: 14)

Codes of ethics are not, however, without difficulties – a point noted over 100 years ago by the distinguished North American nurse leader and scholar, Lavinia Dock. In a little-known but important essay entitled 'Ethics – or a code of ethics?', Dock (1900: 37) challenged:

> *What, exactly, could a Code of Ethics be? … What are ethics and can they be codified? Do we aim at ethical exclusiveness and shall our ethical development be bounded or limited by a code? 'Code' suggests statutes, infringements, penalties, antagonisms. If we have the ethics, we will not need a code. The code is to regulate those who have no ethics, and in proportion as ethical principles are made a part of our natures and lives, our codes and restrictions will shrivel away and die the death of inanition.*

Dock (1900: 38) goes on to explain that she is not advocating the total rejection of rules and regulations of professional conduct – on the contrary, particularly since such rules and regulations, as given in a code, could serve as helpful mechanisms 'to prop up the steps of those who are young in self-government or feeble in self-control'. Rather, the issue was not to call codes of rules and regulations *ethics* since, as she argued persuasively, there was a real risk that:

> *If we call them ethics we may perhaps come to believe that they are all there is of ethics, and presently be worshipping the code rather than the thing, so unreasoning a reverence is there in our souls for statutes, fines, and punishments; so exaggerated a notion of the potency of drafted laws; so strong a tendency to make rules the end and aim of life rather than simply conveniences, changeable contrivances.* (Dock 1900: 38)

Although written over a century ago, Dock's visionary words are applicable today. Nurses globally would be well advised to be cautious in their use of formally stated and adopted codes of ethics, and to be especially vigilant not to fall prey to 'worshipping the code' at the expense of being ethical – and not to fall into the trap of treating the requirements of a code as absolute, and as ends in themselves, rather than as prima-facie guides to ethical professional conduct.

It has long been recognised that a professional code of ethics is an important hallmark of a profession (Bayles 1981; Goldman 1980). Whether professional codes as such have succeeded in fulfilling their intended purpose of 'formulating the norms of professional ethics' (Bayles 1981: 25) and guiding ethical professional conduct is, however, another matter. Some have argued that codes of ethics have failed to ensure this; instead, codes of ethics have served to protect the interests of the professional group espousing them rather than the interests of the client groups whom the professionals are supposed to be serving (Beauchamp & Childress 2013: 6–10; Kultgen 1982: 53–69). Others have contended that codes may be little more than 'toothless tigers' and hence unable to serve their intended purpose – especially if barriers exist to their being used effectively in practice. Barriers can include constituents not having a working knowledge of the content of a given code or how to apply it in practice (Heikkinen et al 2006; Pattison 2001; Tadd et al 2006). Codes of ethics can also be problematic for disciplinary panels on account of their content being ambiguous and hence vulnerable to subjective interpretation (Snelling 2016). This, in turn, can make it difficult for disciplinary panels to take action and impose penalties for breaches of the code – particularly if involving the 'moral emotions' (e.g. failures to be compassionate) (Snelling 2016).

Despite the demonstrable shortcomings of professional codes of ethics, it is evident that many professional codes of ethics have been written with the principled intention of guiding ethically just professional practice and for providing a framework for dealing with code violations (see, for example, Sasso et al 2008). What needs to be understood, however, is that even the most scrupulously formulated and well-intended professional code of ethics is not without its limitations and, in the final analysis, may do little to either guide moral deliberation or ensure the realisation of morally just outcomes in morally problematic situations (see, for example, Page 2012). In the case of the nursing profession, owing to the complexity of nursing work and the complexity of the contexts in which nurses work, codes of ethics may be inadequate to the task of guiding ethical decision-making and conduct (see, for example, Numminen et al 2009). This is particularly so in environments where economic and legal considerations reign supreme and have dominance over other considerations (Meulenbergs et al 2004). Moreover, following a code of ethics will not necessarily protect nurses when they are called upon to defend their actions in, say, a court or disciplinary hearing (see Johnstone 1994b: 251–67).

For example, in an instructive 1990 Australian case involving the alleged unfair dismissal of a registered nurse involved in a case of suspected child sexual abuse, the deputy president of the Industrial Relations Commission of Victoria (where the case was heard) rejected the authority of the ICN (1973) *Code for nurses*, which was referred to in defence of the nurse's actions (*In re alleged unfair dismissal of Ms K Howden by the City of Whittlesea* 1990). In this case the deputy president of the commission pointedly criticised the ICN code as being 'imprecise' and lacking the ability to provide 'clear guidance' in matters requiring fine discretionary professional judgment. He also pointed out that the 'code in its terms cannot stand alone' and must be considered in relation to the guidance that is also offered by the law (*In re alleged unfair dismissal of Ms K Howden by the City of Whittlesea* 1990). The fact that the ICN code is widely accepted by professional nursing organisations around the world had little bearing on the deputy president's views in this case.

The legal authority of other codes of nursing ethics / conduct has also been called into question in other cases heard in jurisdictions outside Australia (Johnstone 1994b; see also *Irwin v Ciena Health Care Management Inc.* 2013).

One question which arises here is that, if codes of ethics are problematic, and have only limited legal (and, it should be added, moral) authority, should nurses adopt them? The short answer to this question is yes. One justification for this, as previously discussed in Chapter 1 of this text, is that, despite their limitations, codes of ethics have an important role to play in the broader schema of professional nursing ethics insofar as they can provide a public statement on the kinds of moral standards and values that patients and the broader community can expect nurses to uphold, and against which nurses can be held publicly accountable. Second, they can also inform those contemplating entering the profession of the kinds of values and standards which they will be expected to uphold, and which, if not upheld, could result in some sort of professional censure. For example, *The ICN code of ethics for nurses* (ICN 2012a: 2) makes explicit that a nurse's 'primary responsibility is to people requiring nursing care', and that, in providing care, the nurse will promote 'an environment in which the human rights, values, customs and spiritual beliefs of the individual, family and community are respected'. If people contemplating entering the profession of nursing are informed of these prescriptions, and do not agree with them, they will be in a better position to make an informed choice about whether or not to enter the profession.

Another justification is that codes of ethics can help with the cultivation of moral character. They can do this by 'increasing the probability that people will behave in some ways rather than others' – specifically that they will behave in 'the right way' and, equally important, 'for the right reasons' (Lichtenberg 1996: 15). As already stated, although codes of ethics do not constitute a system of ethics (at best, they comprise only a list of rules that have been derived from systematic ethical thought), they nevertheless provide people with a reason to think and act ethically, not least by reminding them 'of the moral point of the sorts of activities they are involved in as members of the particular profession or group' (Coady 1996: 286). On this point, Lichtenberg (1996: 18) contends:

> *A code of ethics can increase the probability that people will think about it [what one is doing] – can make it more difficult to engage in self-deceptive practices – by explicitly describing behaviour that is undesirable or unacceptable.*

Crucial to the cultivation of moral character is self-conscious moral reflection. And, as Freckelton (1996: 130) contends, codes of ethics 'are a means to this end'. He states:

> *They [codes of ethics] have the potential to articulate the characteristics and ideals of a profession and to facilitate consciousness of and discourse about ethical issues. Through the process of moral deliberation thereby engendered, they may operate as the catalysts for ethical conduct both by heightening awareness of ethical priorities and by providing guidance from experienced professionals for the resolution of ethical conundra encountered at a practical level by practitioners … By articulating the parameters of a profession and of acceptable professional conduct by its practitioners, a code defines what a profession is and is not, as well as the limits of proper conduct.*

Self-conscious moral reflection and discussion about ethical issues are facilitated by codes of ethics in at least one other important way – namely by what Fullinwider (1996: 83) describes as supplying a vocabulary (which can be used for the purposes of stimulating 'moral self-understanding') and helping to 'create a community of users'. To put this another way, by expressing a given set of ethical values a code of ethics makes discussion and debate of ethical issues possible within a given professional group (community); it provides a (common) moral language, which can be used meaningfully by subscribers to a given code, to identify and discuss matters of moral importance and to advance the task of professional ethics generally in their milieu.

The point remains, however, as already argued, that codes of ethics have only prima-facie moral authority (i.e. they may be overridden by other, stronger moral considerations) and hence can only guide, not mandate, moral conduct in particular situations. Further, as Seedhouse (1988: 65) points out, it is important to understand that a code cannot inform a nurse about which principles to follow in a given situation, how to interpret chosen principles, how to choose between conflicting principles or 'how to decide when it is most ethical to disregard the rules and deliberate instead as a unique and independent individual' as is sometimes required. Accepting this, and as the examples given in the following chapters show, it can be seen that no code of professional nursing ethics should be regarded as an authoritative statement of universal action guides. Rather, it should be regarded only as a statement of prima-facie rules which may be helpful in guiding moral decision-making in nursing care contexts, but which can be justly overridden by other, stronger moral considerations (see also Biton & Tabak 2003; Meulenbergs et al 2004).

Codes of conduct

Codes of conduct (to be distinguished from codes of ethic), although designed to regulate professional conduct, are not ethics. Nor are they 'codes of ethics' (discussed above). This distinction has been clarified in the codes of conduct ratified by the respective nurse regulating authorities in New Zealand (NCNZ 2012a) and, more recently, Australia (NMBA 2018a). The NCNZ (2012a: 2), for example, describes its *Code of conduct for nurses* as 'a set of standards defined by the Council describing the behaviour or conduct that nurses are expected to uphold'. It goes on to clarify:

> This is not a Code of Ethics – *it does not seek to describe all the ethical values of the profession or to provide specific advice on ethical issues, ethical frameworks or ethical decision making. This type of advice is provided by professional organisations* [emphasis added] (NCNZ 2012a: 3).

Australia has recently taken a similar position. As noted in Chapter 1 of this book, the NMBA abandoned its *Code of ethics for nurses in Australia* (2008a) and adopted a code of conduct in its place, marking a significant shift towards a wholly regulatory (some might say managerial) approach to professional conduct. This is made clear in the Foreword to the Code, which states unequivocally: 'The *Code of conduct for nurses* (the code) sets out the *legal requirements* [emphasis added], professional behaviour and conduct expectations for nurses in all practice settings, in Australia (NMBA 2018a: 2). In a footnote, it is further clarified that:

> *The code does not address in detail the full range of legal and ethical obligations that apply to nurses. Examples of legal obligations include, but are not limited to, obligations arising in Acts and Regulations relating to privacy, the aged and disabled, child protection, bullying, anti-discrimination and workplace health and safety issues. Nurses should ensure they know all of their legal obligations relating to professional practice, and abide by them.* (NMBA 2018a: 6, §2)

These examples demonstrate that codes of conduct, unlike codes of ethics, tend to be *regulatory* (as opposed to aspirational) in nature – that is, they set minimal standards of practice against which nurses' conduct can be 'objectively' measured and breaches sanctioned (Snelling 2016). As minimum standards (unlike aspirational standards) tend to prescribe a lower standard of conduct, there is a risk, as Snelling (2016) contends, that merely 'just-good-enough' behaviour will result. Even though 'just-good-enough' behaviour might be higher than that otherwise expected of the general population (Snelling 2016: 230), it still may not be 'good enough' to justify public trust in the profession or indeed the profession's code.

Hospital or professional etiquette

Nothing could be more different from ethics than *etiquette*. Although both seek to guide behaviour and conduct, they do so in different ways and for different purposes. Ethics, for example, speaks to morally significant rights and wrongs, with behaviour being guided by critically reflective moral thought and the application of sound moral values that seek to maximise the moral interests of all people equally. Etiquette, in contrast, seeks more to maintain style and decorum, with behaviour being guided by the unreflective and arbitrary requirements of custom and convention. In application, etiquette paves the way for coordinated, consistent, predictable and, where possible, aesthetically pleasant practice and conduct, and serves only the interests of particular persons in particular circumstances (May 1975). As with legal law, what etiquette might demand in one situation, ethics might reject, and vice versa.

The extent to which the notions of ethics and etiquette can be confused in health care settings is illustrated by the following case – which demonstrates the reluctance by some health professionals (including nurses) to advise patients to seek a second medical opinion, in the mistaken belief that doing so would constitute a serious breach of ethics.

The case involves a middle-aged woman suffering moderately severe retrosternal chest pain and shortness of breath who presented to the emergency department (ED) of a large city hospital. The nursing staff admitted the woman into a cubicle equipped to deal with 'cardiac emergencies' and proceeded to perform an electrocardiograph (ECG). The ECG showed a number of cardiac arrhythmias, all of which were suggestive of an acute cardiac condition warranting immediate specialised medical and nursing care.

Upon further questioning, it was revealed that the woman was also suffering a mild pain in her left arm (a pain she had 'never had before'), which is characteristic of cardiac disease. The pain improved, however, while she rested in the ED. Her past medical history indicated no known heart disease or any previous incident of chest pain. This was the first time she had ever experienced such symptoms – symptoms that were indicative of significant underlying cardiac disease.

A junior first-year medical resident examined the woman and decided she should be admitted immediately into the coronary care unit for further cardiac monitoring and tests. As required by the hospital's admission policy, he contacted the registrar 'on call' to have his diagnosis confirmed and to arrange the woman's admission formally. Upon examining the patient, however, the registrar declined to admit her, since there were no 'cardiac beds' available in the hospital and he was not convinced that the ECG findings indicated a life-threatening cardiac condition. He discharged the woman, advising her to see her own general practitioner the following morning. He gave her a medical note and a prescription for an oral cardiac anti-arrhythmic agent.

The nursing staff members were very concerned, as was the first-year medical resident. All felt the patient should have been seen by another doctor for a 'second opinion', but could not decide whether to advise the woman to go immediately to another hospital. After some 20 minutes of deliberation, the attending nursing supervisor concluded it would be 'unethical' to advise the patient to go to another hospital for a second examination. The nursing staff and junior doctor involved agreed. The patient walked out of the door and was not informed that it would be in her interests to seek a second medical opinion. At this hospital, it was not 'decorum' to advise patients to obtain a second medical opinion.

What arguably was at issue here, however, was breaching hospital etiquette, not ethics. Advising the woman to seek a second medical opinion, in this case, would not have been unethical; indeed, the staff would have been both morally and professionally justified in taking appropriate action to ensure the patient received appropriate attention – which could have included contacting the cardiologist on call at the discharging hospital.

Etiquette obviously has its place in the professional and health care arena; it is not without limits, however. Unfortunately, as Blackburn (1984: 189) points out, people do 'often care more about etiquette, or reputation, or selfish advantage, than they do about morality'. The lesson to be learned here is that acting in accord with hospital or professional etiquette might sometimes be tantamount to engaging in substandard practice and ipso facto acting unethically. It is, therefore, important that nurses learn to distinguish between the demands of etiquette and those of ethics.

Hospital or institutional policy

Hospital policy or institutional policy is often appealed to in order to legitimise a worker's actions and, in some cases, to settle a conflict of opinion about what course of action should be taken in a particular situation. In this respect, institutional or hospital policy plays an important practical role – it helps to coordinate 'the running of the system' and to make institutional practices consistent and predictable; nevertheless, it also paves the way for uncompromising control. Like legal law and etiquette, institutional policy can be morally bad and in application can seriously conflict with the demands of ethics.

Research has suggested that, although the theorisation and practice of nursing ethics has developed substantially over the past 30 years, nurses continue to experience ethical conflict based on their disagreement with organisational values, policies and rules as well as the values and viewpoints of colleagues (Gaudine et al 2011; Idrees et al 2018; Johnstone 2012d; Kälvemark et al 2004; Leuter et al 2017; Pavlish et al 2014; Wlodarczyk & Lazarewicz 2011). A common example can be found in the case of a hospital's discharge planning policies which might require nurses to plan and implement the discharge or transfer of a patient who, in their professional opinion, is not yet ready to be either discharged home or transferred to another health care facility.

Public opinion, populism or the view of the majority[2]

The term 'public' originates from the Latin *pūblicus*, meaning 'of the people' (*Collins Australian dictionary* 2011: 1328). Just 'who' is *the public* and whether *publics* 'really exist', however, are moot points. Some suggest that, at best, 'publics' are more artefact than fact, and thus any political influence 'the public' might exert needs to be viewed with caution. At the very least, serious and probing questions need to be asked about who is 'this' public, and whose interests 'this public' is ultimately serving and to what ends?

Louw, an Australian-based political communications scholar, contends that publics are, in essence, 'media constructions' – that is, they are created by the mass circulation media. The mass circulation media create or 'assemble' publics by 'constructing and holding together public opinion' (Louw 2010: 24). And the means by which public opinion is created or constructed is via the intellectual exercise of conducting public opinion surveys (Louw 2010: 24). Thus, whereas 'publics' might not exist (they are artefacts), 'public opinions' (as measured by quantifiable surveys) do, even though these too are media constructions. Explaining the ethereal nature of 'the public' and 'public opinion', Louw writes:

> *These publics (containing millions of individuals) do not involve actual human interaction or communication between those incorporated into these 'publics'. The members of these publics do not know each other, or communicate with each other. They will never know each other, or communicate with each other. Yet publics can be 'brought together' by the mass media and can even be 'guided' (by the media) to carry out the same action (e.g. mourning the death of a celebrity they do not know, such as Princess Diana). Such 'publics' and 'public opinion' are the ultimate artificial 'hyper' construct. These publics have no real 'presence' because they are assembled in the ether of media representations. One cannot find 'a public', because it does not 'exist'. But one can find 'public opinion' by constructing it as an intellectual exercise (i.e. conducting public opinion surveys).* (Louw 2010: 24)

Louw goes on to explain that a major implication of the media creation of publics is that individuals within 'a public' become 'passive followers, "guided" by the limited agendas presented to them by the media' and, it should be added, the agenda setters manipulating it (Louw 2010: 24). Instead of being 'actively engaged citizens' who have a civic moral responsibility to question and call into question things as they are, individuals are held together as a 'media-ted passive public', vulnerable to manipulation and 'herding' towards a preferred political standpoint by agenda setters (Louw 2010: 24). While the individuals in this 'public' might feel they are purposefully interacting with other human beings, in reality they are situated as little more than isolated individuals who are experiencing only 'a form of manufactured "pseudo-interaction" received through mass media messages' (Louw 2010: 24).

Public opinion is often cited in defence of the 'ethics' of something such as the moral permissibility of abortion, euthanasia or the use of fetal tissue for research. For example, those in favour of the legalisation of euthanasia (discussed further in Chapter 10 of this book) will commonly cite public opinion polls favouring the legalisation of euthanasia to support their stance (Johnstone 2013a, 2014a).

Ethics is not something that can be determined or decided reliably by public opinion, however. If ethics were merely a matter of public opinion, all we would have to do is conduct an opinion poll and establish a 'majority view' on a matter to find out whether it was morally right or wrong. If ethics were determined by mere public opinion, our moral standards would be rendered unacceptably changeable, making it extremely difficult to practise ethically.

A public opinion or majority view of ethics is open to serious objection on a number of grounds. On a philosophical level, it violates a formal and necessary requirement for sound moral judgments, notably the requirement for internal consistency (Kuhse 1987: 25). Its findings are liable to reflect sudden and unpredictable changes in attitudes and opinions, and thus are morally unreliable and untrustworthy. More seriously, it lacks the justificatory power of sound moral theory. According to Beauchamp and

Childress (2013: 353–5) the criteria for assessing moral theories include the following: *clarity* (the theory and language used to articulate it must be unambiguous and avoid 'obscurity and vagueness'), *coherence* (there should be no conceptual inconsistencies), *comprehensiveness* (provides as full an account as is possible of justifiable norms and judgments), *simplicity* (in the sense of theoretical parsimony), *explanatory power* ('provides enough insight to help us understand morality'), *justificatory power* ('provides grounds for justified belief'), *output power* (it must 'generate more than a list of axioms already present in pretheoretic belief') and *practicability* (its demands must 'be able to be satisfied', i.e. 'a theory that presents utopian ideals or unfeasible recommendations fails the criterion of practicability'). Public opinion is frankly incapable of meeting these criteria.

Public opinion is problematic on a pragmatic level as well. As the ancient Greek philosopher Plato (c. 428–347 BC) explained in *The republic*, 'ordinary opinion' is comprised of *belief* and *illusion*, not *knowledge* (intelligence, pure thought and mathematical reasoning) (Plato 1955 edn: 274–5). Moreover, opinions are not fully thought through and, at best, can serve only as 'impressions' not knowledge. These views have contemporary application to the question of public opinion in our modern world.

In today's world there is always the troubling possibility that public opinion might be mistaken, wrong or misguided – particularly where it has been manipulated by pressure groups, politicians or by the media, as occurred in the much publicised 'Children overboard' incident that occurred in Australia in the lead-up to the 2001 Federal election. The incident involved the public misrepresentation of photographic images and false claims by Federal government politicians that asylum seekers, who were attempting to enter Australian territory 'illegally' by sea, had 'deliberately' thrown their children overboard from the boat they were on in order to force their rescue and subsequent entry into Australia via the HMAS Adelaide, a nearby naval ship. It was later revealed, however, and subsequently verified by a Senate Inquiry into the matter, that no children had, in fact, been thrown overboard (Senate Select Committee on a Certain Maritime Incident 2002). In the lead-up to the Federal election on 10 November, this incident was used along with other incidents (e.g. the Tampa rescue of Afghan refugees) to support the Federal government's 'hardline political response to unauthorised arrivals' and to sway public opinion against asylum seekers seeking refuge in Australia by portraying them (demonising them) as 'faceless, violent queue jumpers' (Australian Broadcasting Corporation (ABC) 2002), as 'illegal immigrants' and 'illegal refugees' (MacLennan 2002: 152) (rather than 'genuine' asylum seekers) and as people of poor moral character ('the kinds of people who would throw their children overboard' (Senate Select Committee on a Certain Maritime Incident 2002: xxi)). Post-election analyses indicated that the 'Children overboard' incident had influenced public opinion in favour of the Federal government's tough (some would say, inhumane) policies on the admission and detention of refugees and asylum seekers in Australia and contributed to the Federal government's re-election in 2001 (see also Hamilton & Maddison 2007; Manne 2005).

More recently, as voting in democratic elections and referenda around the world has shown (e.g. the USA presidential election in 2016, the UK 'Brexit' referendum in 2016), public opinion is extremely vulnerable to covert manipulation via the use of targeted political campaign advertising and the use of 'filter bubbles' (website algorithms that selectively manipulate information so users' access to contrary points of views is reduced), and 'fake news' bulletins like that which allegedly occurred via the activities of groups such as Cambridge Analytica (see Pariser 2011; Persily 2017; the ABC-TV Four Corners program 'Democracy, data and dirty tricks' – available at: http://www.abc.net.au/4corners/democracy-data-and-dirty-tricks:-cambridge/9642090). Adding to this, people rarely question the validity of opinion polls, accepting them instead at face value. Although pollsters often seek to qualify the accuracy of poll results by stating their margins of error, this does not mean they are immune to being wrong.

A public opinion view of ethics is problematic on another ground – *democracy*. Those who cite public opinion in defence of a stance on a moral issue will fervently argue that to ignore majority public opinion is an assault on democracy (the rule of the people). What is not always understood by those taking such a stance, however, is that democracy (a kind of political governance) has at its heart the promise that a nation's people will be kept free from tyrannical rules that would otherwise oppress them and place their lives in danger (Harrison 2005). Although the majority rules in a democracy, as long as the principles of democracy are operational the majority rule will be constrained so as not to deteriorate into *the ruling of a mob*. The threat of majority rule deteriorating into the rule of the mob has been increased in recent times owing to the rise of authoritarian populism in countries around the world. What is most worrying about authoritarian populism is its capacity to generate disturbing and disruptive forms of extremism which are now seriously threatening constitutional democracies (Solomon & Jennings 2017).

Democracy ensures the freedom and security of a nation's citizens by permitting diverse opinions and views to be expressed and debated freely within a system. Of necessity, this freedom must be balanced and measured by rational means as well as the rule of law based on democratic principles. Democracy does not support freedom that brings about destruction, however. Thus, although the majority rules by electing a preferred government, this does not mean that the majority views and opinions are required to be implemented without debate and rational decision-making. Although democracy allows freedom, it also protects the minority whose views and opinions are not congruent with the majority. A democracy should thus be considered first and foremost a device 'in which people discover their proper preferences through a process of mutual deliberation', rather than voting per se (Harrison 2005: 169).

Democracy has traditionally provided the justification of a whole variety of social and economic policies. However, when democracy is used to justify *moral policy* and government intervention, the moral judgments of individuals can be placed at risk of being substituted by what the state desires and thinks important. It is here that our greatest vigilance is required and why it is appropriate that procuring certain moral policy changes remains 'hard' and not governed by instruments of the state.

It is not being denied here that public opinion is an important and relevant consideration that warrants some attention especially when needing to identify, if not decide, ethical issues relevant to upholding the public interest. On the contrary: public opinion which reliably indicates a certain view on a given matter might well be a useful tool in guiding beneficial social policy and law reforms. However, public opinion is not infallible in matters of morality and mere common acceptance does not imply validity (Brandt 1959: 57). The moral rightness or wrongness of an act can be decided only by sound critical reflection and wise reasoning, not merely by public opinion, populism, 'collective desire' or 'collective preference'.

'Ethics by opinion' has long been criticised by philosophers (Salloch et al 2014). Despite this, public opinion polling and attitudinal research concerning ethical issues in a range of contexts has burgeoned in recent years (Jin & Hakkarinen 2017; Salloch et al 2014). Just how useful or warranted this work is in terms of informing normative deliberations in health care ethics and moral politics generally is a moot point.

Ethical judgments cannot be based on empirical research alone (Salloch et al 2014). While empirical data might be useful in identifying certain ethical issues in given contexts (e.g. health care), they are not sufficient to determine normative judgments concerning right and wrong. Given this, where empirical data are being sought, careful attention must first be given to determining:

- what kind of empirical data is needed
- how it will be collected and analysed
- what mechanisms will be in place to ensure their credibility, trustworthiness and reliability
- how the data once analysed will be used and to what ends or purpose
- how the data will be framed in discussions on ethical issues and theoretical perspectives
- whose interests will ultimately be served by the collection and use of the data
- what moral actions the data will inform.

Ideology

People who have a vested political interest in given ethical issues in health care (e.g. abortion, euthanasia, advance care planning, truth telling, etc.) often approach debates on these topics with their minds already made up and remain committed to their personal stance independently of credible evidence (Johnstone 2013a). In many instances, the basis of their arguments is not ethics, but rather *ideology* (a set of conscious and unconscious ideas) masquerading as ethics. When ideology masquerades as ethics the end result tends to be a deep polarisation of views, with an exacerbation rather than a remediation of the moral controversies and conflicts at stake.

A distinguishing feature of statements advocating an ideology (i.e. as opposed to an ethical stance) is that the statements indicate commitment to a social or ethical issue *without* requiring the backing of credible evidence or reasoned argument. In contrast, statements of ethics have as their basis ethical analyses that seek to 'defend a position by means of reasoned argument with reference to widely held ethical norms or principles' and, where available, empirical evidence (Campbell & Huxtable 2003: 182).

Ideologies often work by circumventing questions of ethics in the first place, such as by asserting an idea and then commending a related action without sound reasons justifying the relationship between the two. For example, those on the conservative side of politics are more likely than progressives to perceive poor people and the unemployed as being 'responsible for' and hence 'deserving' of their plight and ipso facto undeserving (and even 'never deserving') of welfare support (Appelbaum 2001; Larsen 2008; van Oorschot & Roosma 2015; van Oorschot et al 2017). This view is held irrespective of evidence to the contrary (e.g. that their plight is due largely to external factors beyond their control) or whether the poor fulfil established 'deservingness criteria' (Larsen 2008; Larsen & 2013; van Oorschot & Roosma 2015; van Oorschot et al 2017). Because they attribute individual rather than societal responsibility for people being poor or unemployed (e.g. 'people are poor/unemployed because they are lazy and lack willpower, not because of social structures'), conservatives are more likely to advocate a 'no-benefits' policy for the poor and to focus on 'undeserving groups' to justify the 'moral regulation' of welfare benefits via policies restricting public assistance, even in the case of dire need (Appelbaum 2001; Chunn & Gavigan 2004; Larsen 2008; Larsen & Dejgaard 2013; van Oorschot et al 2017). In some cases, by giving an inordinate amount of attention to so-called 'welfare cheats' (such as single parent mothers), conservatives have been successful in ideologically portraying welfare itself as fraud – one effect of which has been to criminalise poverty (Chunn & Gavigan 2004; Jørgensen 2012). As Chunn and Gavigan (2004: 219) contend:

> *The dismantling and restructuring of Keynesian social security programmes have impacted disproportionately on women, especially lone parent mothers, and shifted public discourse and social images from welfare fraud to* welfare as fraud, *thereby linking poverty, welfare and crime.* [emphasis added]

One reason why ideology has been successful in masquerading as ethics is that we live in a fundamentalist world, encompassing an 'age of ideology' (Davis 2004) – a period in which advocates on all sides of a public debate (in this instance on ethical issues in health care) tend to engage in 'rhetoric, not negotiation or compromise' (Davis 2004: 83) and are determined to crush all opposing ideas (Sim 2004). This situation is deeply problematic for several reasons. First, it allows ideology to triumph over ethics and, in doing so, contributes to a new dark age of dogma in a world that is already bereft of moral principles requiring recognition, respect and restitution for what is 'right'. Second, to borrow from Davis (2004: 94), it risks perpetuating 'polarization, gridlock and [policy] whiplash' in debates on important ethics issues rather than enabling cooperation and negotiation in the interests of promoting human welfare and wellbeing.

Nurses need to be aware of the insidious ways in which ideology can masquerade as ethics and, as such, can be used to reaffirm people's personal desires, beliefs, prejudices, fears, decisions and actions and to exaggerate threat – both real and imagined – to the welfare and wellbeing of the public.

Following the orders of a supervisor or manager

Following the moral commands of another is incompatible with the notion of ethics and the autonomous moral thinking that underpins it (for reasons that will be explained in Chapter 3). Moreover, it paves the way for the abdication of moral responsibility and accountability. Supervisors have supervisors, and these supervisors have still more supervisors. A hierarchical system of authority may mean in practice that, because everyone is accountable for a given action, it is difficult or impossible to decide who is to be held ultimately accountable.

The patient safety literature published over the past decade has highlighted some important lessons about the possible relationship between legal and moral responsibility and accountability – particularly in cases which have seen serious failures in clinical governance and the 'normalisation of deviance' (taking shortcuts) in health care (see, for example, Banja 2010; Casali & Day 2010; Driver et al 2014; Jones et al 2016; Wachter & Pronovost 2009). Nurses, like others, need to be aware that legal and moral responsibility and accountability travel a common path. Accordingly, it is not acceptable for nurses or other co-workers to justify their actions on the basis that they were simply 'working as directed' or 'following the orders of a superior'.

The intricate relationship between legal and moral responsibility and accountability was made evident long ago by the much noted Bormann defence, named after Martin Bormann, third deputy under the Nazi regime of World War II, who argued in defence of his involvement in wartime atrocities that he was 'just following orders' (Barry 1982: 13). This kind of defence may be regarded as a convenient 'moral cop-out' for those who have no sense of moral accountability, or a poorly developed sense, and who ordinarily try to justify their behaviour as Bormann did: 'I was told to do it', 'I was expected to do it', 'I was just doing my job', 'That's how things operate around here' and so forth (Barry 1982: 13). The outcome of the 1945–46 Nuremberg trials made it abundantly clear, however, that a plea of following the orders of one's superiors was not an acceptable or a legitimate defence in the eyes of the law.

Such a precedent had already been well established for nurses as early as 1929, however, with the successful prosecution in the Philippines of a newly graduated nurse by the name of Lorenza Somera, who was found guilty of manslaughter, sentenced to a year in prison and fined 1000 pesos because she had followed a physician's incorrect drug order (Grennan 1930). In court it was proved that the physician had ordered the drug, that Somera had verified it and that the physician had administered the injection. But, as Winslow (1984: 35) writes, 'the physician was acquitted and Somera found guilty because she failed to question the orders'. The case stunned nurses around the world. A campaign of protest was organised, and Somera was given a conditional pardon before serving a day of her sentence.

In an institutional setting, it is very easy to rationalise moral 'unaccountability'. As Barry (1982: 13) explains:

> So many people, even institutions, can get involved at so many levels that moral buck-passing can become the order of the day. The blind pursuit of prestige and profits also blurs moral accountability. And most important, the intense pressure to keep one's job and to secure promotions can be used to justify almost anything. The point is that working within an organisation provides easy excuses for abdicating personal moral accountability for decisions and actions.

One way of avoiding this abdication is to draw a firm distinction between ethics and following the orders of a supervisor or manager, and to recognise that moral demands are always the overriding consideration, irrespective of a supervisor's or a manager's orders.

The task of ethics, bioethics and nursing ethics

In considering what ethics is, and what it is not, it is also important to have some understanding of exactly what ethics, in its broadest sense, is attempting to achieve; in short, what is the task of ethics and to what extent do bioethics and nursing ethics respectively contribute to this task?

In identifying and exploring the task of ethics, it is necessary to give a brief historical overview of the development of Western moral thinking. The task of ethics has been the subject of rigorous philosophical debate for almost 3000 years. In the Platonic dialogues, for example, we are told that the ultimate task of morality is to find out 'how best to live' or, in other words, how to lead 'the good life' and enjoy supreme wellbeing (Allen 1966: 57–255). For the British philosopher Thomas Hobbes (1588–1679), the task of morality is a little different: notably, to find a device that will ensure mutual agreement and cooperation among all of society's members. It was Hobbes' view that if people were left to live in a 'state of nature' this would ultimately lead to 'a war of all against all'. Thus, unless such a device (i.e. a 'social contract' ensuring mutual agreement and cooperation among each of society's members) was adopted, the prospects of human survival would at best be slim (Hobbes 1968: 205).

Hobbes' concerns were echoed almost a century later by the Scottish philosopher David Hume (1711–76), who insisted, among other things, that morality was a subject of supreme interest since its decisions had the very peace of society firmly at stake (Hume 1888: 455). Like Hobbes, Hume recognised that the human mind was more than capable of courting the undesirable qualities of 'avarice, ambition, cruelty [and] selfishness' and, like Hobbes, he recognised that society's hope for peace depended very much on the formulation of certain rules of conduct (Hume 1888: 494–6). These rules of conduct need to be developed and enforced precisely because people fail to pursue the public interest 'naturally, and with a hearty affection' (p 496).

The influential German philosopher, Immanuel Kant (1724–1804) took a slightly different view from his predecessors. Unlike Hobbes and Hume, he saw the task of ethics (or rather, moral philosophy) as being 'to seek out and establish the supreme principle of morality' (Kant 1972: 57). Like those before him, Kant recognised that persons were vulnerable to being 'affected … by so many inclinations and lacked the power to conduct their life in accordance with practical reason'. Kant also argued that as long as the 'ultimate norm for correct moral judgment' is lacking, morals themselves will be vulnerable to corruption (p 55).

Kant's overall investigation succeeded in providing a supreme, although not uncontroversial, principle of morality for guiding human actions. Upholding the tenets of ethical rationalism (now regarded as a controversial thesis), this principle took the form of a categorical imperative which essentially commands that cognitively competent autonomous choosers should 'act only on that maxim through which you can at the same time will that it should become universal law' (Kant 1972: 84). In other words, act only on those moral rules and principles which you are prepared to accept apply to all other people as well. His final analysis made clear that the influences of self-interest and/or of individual 'feelings, impulses and inclinations' could have no place in a system of sound morality (p 84). If 'rational agents' are to act morally, they must act in strict accordance with the dictates of 'rational moral law'.

The moral law was seen by Kant as providing ultimate, overriding principles of conduct and ones which all cognitively competent people ought to respect. He was optimistic that if all 'rational' (cognitively competent) persons lived absolutely by the moral law then they could hope to live in a world (or rather 'a kingdom', as he called it) where cognitively competent persons would be respected as ends in themselves and not as the mere means to the ends of others (Kant 1972: 96).

The influential views of Plato, Hobbes, Hume and Kant concerning the task of ethics continue to have force in modern moral philosophy. For example, the Australian philosopher John Mackie (1917–81) argues that so-called 'limited sympathies' exist as a profound threat to what might otherwise be regarded as the 'good life' (Mackie 1977: 108).[3] Mackie echoes the view that if an all-enduring and decent (harmonious) life is to be secured, the problem of limited sympathies needs to be counteracted. The only way this can be done is by finding something which will coordinate and marry together individual and differing choices of action. In other words, what is needed is a device which could act as a kind of 'invisible chain' keeping together many sorts of 'useful agreements' (pp 116, 118).

The solution for Mackie (1977: 106) lies squarely at the feet of morality, which he interprets as:

a system of a particular sort of constraints on conduct — ones whose central task is to protect the interests of persons other than the agent and present themselves to an agent as checks on his [or her] natural inclinations or spontaneous tendencies to act.

Mackie (1977: 194) argues further that a morality applied appropriately is a morality which will help to facilitate the realisation of the overall wellbeing of people. In order for morality to work in this way, however, it must have at its core the vital component 'humane disposition'. A humane disposition in this instance is that which 'naturally manifests itself in hostility to and disgust at cruelty, and in sympathy with pain and suffering whenever they occur' (Mackie 1977: 194). People who are of humane disposition, suggests Mackie, 'cannot be callous and indifferent, let alone actively cruel either toward permanently defective [sic] human beings or toward non-human animals' (Mackie 1977: 194).

The English philosopher Richard Hare also views the task of ethics in terms of imposing stringent requirements on persons to act in morally just ways. On this, Hare argues that (1981: 228):

Morality compels us to accommodate ourselves to the preferences of others, and this has the effect that when we are thinking morally and doing it rationally we shall all prefer the same moral prescriptions about matters which affect other people …

Hare ultimately advocates morality as a form of compelling 'rational universal prescriptivism', and concludes that 'moral reason leaves us with our freedom, but constrains us to respect the freedom of others, and to combine with them in exercising it' (Hare 1981: 228).

The notion that the task of ethics is to supply a system of ultimate, overriding principles of conduct is also supported by the American philosopher Stephen Ross (1972: 283), who argues that the goal of morality is 'to reach a common set of moral ideals which everyone can follow' or, rather, to 'seek principles of conduct which everyone can live by'. According to Ross, moral principles are needed to regulate our moral decisions and to help settle competing alternatives. Moral principles remind us of our overriding duties to others and of the merits of morally principled action. Principles of morality also lend people 'tools' which can be used to deal appropriately and effectively with moral crises and dilemmas in both everyday and special (e.g. professional) worlds. They remind us that, without secure, ultimate and overriding rules of conduct, people may find it all too easy to abdicate their moral responsibilities and to commit atrocities — as contemporary examples in war-torn countries around the world constantly remind us.

Other American philosophers such as Tom Beauchamp and James Childress, David Gauthier and H. Tristram Engelhardt Jr have described the task of modern moral philosophy in similar terms again. Beauchamp and Childress, for example, suggest that the task of ethics is to supply an 'ideal code consisting of a set of rules that guide the members of a society to maximise intrinsic value' (1983: 40). Gauthier (1986: 6), in turn, describes the task of ethics as being concerned with validating the conception of morality 'as a set of rational, impartial constraints on the pursuit of individual interest'. Engelhardt (1986: 67–9) meanwhile sees the task of ethics as searching for common grounds to bind consenting individuals in a peaceable community — in short, to achieve peaceable bonds among persons without brute force. He also sees the task of ethics as being that which (p 26):

aspires to provide a logic for a pluralism of beliefs, a common view of a good life that can transcend particular communities, professions, legal jurisdictions, and religions, but whose grounds for authenticity are immanent to the secular world.

Both bioethics and nursing ethics share the task of ethics.

Conclusion

Advancing ethics, bioethics and nursing ethics inquiry and practice requires at least a working knowledge and understanding of the definitions and meanings of such terms as 'ethics', 'bioethics' and 'nursing ethics'. In this chapter, working definitions of these notions have been provided. (The definitions of other commonly used moral terms such as 'rights', 'duties' and 'obligations' will be given in Chapter 3.) In providing these working definitions, attention has also been given to demonstrating what ethics (bioethics and nursing ethics) is not. For example, ethics, bioethics and nursing ethics are not: legal law, codes of ethics, hospital or professional etiquette, hospital or institutional policy, public opinion or the view of the majority, ideology, or following the orders of a supervisor or manager.

A brief examination has also been made of the task of ethics: namely, to find a way to motivate moral behaviour, to settle disagreements and controversies between people, and to generally bind people together in a peaceable community. Both bioethics and nursing ethics share in this task, acknowledging, however, that such a task has been and remains a complex and complicated one. To help understand the complexity of this task and how it might be achieved, it is necessary first to gain some understanding of the theoretical underpinnings of Western ethics generally and of bioethics and nursing ethics, which have been strongly influenced by it. It is to examining these theoretical underpinnings and their influences on the development of contemporary bioethics and nursing ethics that the next chapter will now turn.

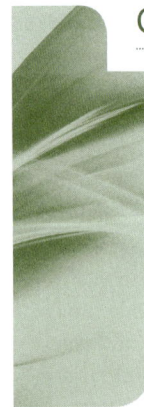

Case scenario 1

A second-year nursing student, who had recently completed a semester 1 unit on 'nursing ethics' as part of his undergraduate nursing program, was on clinical placement in a large metropolitan teaching hospital. During this placement he was assigned the care of a patient with an aggressive cancer-related illness. During a team meeting he learned that the team, in consultation with the patient's family, had agreed to withhold certain information about the patient's poor prognosis and the possible trajectory of her disease. Fresh from his classes on nursing ethics, the student decided that the team and family were 'morally wrong' to take this stance. Moreover, since he had just 'done ethics' and 'knew about patient autonomy', the student believed that he was in a better position than the team and family to judge what the 'morally right thing to do' was in this case. Accordingly, without consultation with the team members, the patient's family or his clinical teacher, he proceeded to inform the patient directly of the details of her poor prognosis and possible trajectory of her disease.

Case scenario 2

In 1996, reported to be the first case of its kind in Australia, a nurse was charged with murder after he turned off the life support machine sustaining the life of a 37-year-old woman (and mother of three) who was suffering from a rare and crippling brain disease. Although there was some suggestion that the woman was 'brain dead', she had not been 'formally declared dead' (Donovan 1996: 2). It was also alleged in media reports that 'the appropriate documents required to remove treatment from a comatose patient had not been signed at the time of the woman's death' (Walsh & Pirrie 1996: 1). Media reports also claimed that the nurse took the action he did on the grounds that he 'believed that he was acting in the patient's best interests' (Walsh & Pirrie 1996: 2) and that he also believed he had 'the permission of the woman's husband' (Das 1996: 7).

The case was reported to have focused 'national attention on the care and treatment of incompetent and severely brain damaged patients' and 'on hospital guidelines and regulations on the care of brain-damaged patients' (Walsh & Pirrie 1996: 2). Later media reports further suggested that the case had shown 'that there was a "demarcation dispute" about who had the right to disconnect life support machines' (Das 1996: 7).

CRITICAL QUESTIONS

1. What ethical issues are raised by each of these cases?
2. Were the decisions made and actions taken by the nursing student and registered nurse respectively 'morally competent' – that is, did they demonstrate the requisite moral knowledge, skill and attitude expected of a nurse? Give reasons for your answer.
3. If you had been in the situations in question, what would you have done?
4. Does the successful completion of a unit or subject on nursing ethics necessarily mean that a nurse has the moral competence necessary to make sound ethical decisions during the course of their practice? Give reasons for your answer.
5. To what extent do you believe that nurses 'really' understand the nature, content and requirements of nursing and health care ethics?

Endnotes

1. On Wednesday 29 November 2017 the State Parliament of Victoria passed its Voluntary Assisted Dying Bill (2017), due to come into effect mid 2019. Once in effect, in keeping with the legislation, there will be an 18-month implementation period so that any outstanding details and issues can be finalised. Assisted dying laws were similarly passed in Canada in 2016. In some Canadian jurisdictions, nurse practitioners may perform assisted dying via administering a lethal injection (https://www.crnbc.ca/crnbc/Announcements/2016/Pages/MAiD_NProle.aspx). The role of nurses in performing euthanasia will be considered further in Chapter 10 of this book.
2. Excerpts taken from Johnstone M-J (2013a) *Alzheimer's disease, media representations, and the politics of euthanasia: constructing risk and selling death in an aging society*, Ashgate, Farnham, Surrey, are reproduced by permission of Ashgate.
3. Quotations from J L Mackie (1977) *Ethics: inventing right and wrong*, Penguin Books, Harmondsworth, Middlesex, are reproduced by permission of Penguin Books Ltd.

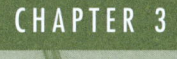

Moral theory and the ethical practice of nursing

KEYWORDS

autonomy
beneficence
deontology
ethic of care
ethical principles
ethical principlism
justice
moral duties
moral/ethical theory
moral justification
moral obligations
moral rights
non-maleficence
teleology
virtue ethics

LEARNING OBJECTIVES

Upon the completion of this chapter and with further self-directed learning you are expected to be able to:
- Explain moral justification.
- Discuss critically the importance of moral justification to moral decision-making and action.
- Outline the relationship between moral justification, moral theory and moral conduct.
- Define ethical principlism.
- Discuss critically how the moral principles of autonomy, non-maleficence, beneficence and justice might be used to guide decision-making in nursing and health care contexts.
- Discuss critically a moral rights theory of ethics and its application in nursing practice.
- Discuss critically the theory of virtue ethics.
- Examine the relationship between virtue theory, an ethic of care and nursing ethics.
- Distinguish between deontological and teleological ethics.
- Differentiate between a moral right and a moral duty.
- Discuss critically the limitations and weaknesses of contemporary moral theory.

Introduction

When encountering an ethical problem during the course of their work, nurses are confronted by at least three basic questions:

1. What should I do in this situation?
2. What is the 'right' thing to do?
3. How can I be sure (and be reassured) that my decisions and actions in the situation at hand are 'morally right', all things considered? In short, how can I be sure that I am behaving ethically and doing the 'right thing'?

In seeking answers to these questions, it would be natural for a nurse to incline towards and draw on his/her own personal values, beliefs, professional knowledge and life experience. Whether this would be sufficient to provide the moral warranties or 'moral authorisations' being sought is another matter, however. Deciding the 'morally right' thing to do in a situation and taking moral action accordingly is rarely a straightforward process. Among other things it requires a broadly informed, systematic, insightful and deeply experienced approach to thinking about the issues at stake and how best to resolve them. This, in turn, requires 'mastery' and 'not just surface competence' of relevant ethical concepts and principles as well as 'the skill to navigate them when they tangle together in concrete situations' (Little 2001: 35).

Most people have strong beliefs and opinions about the world. No matter how sincerely held, however, beliefs and opinions can sometimes be mistaken. For example, there was a period in history when people sincerely believed that the world was square and that if they sailed to the edge of it they would drop off. Although a sincere belief, the view that the world was square was obviously mistaken, as explorers and scientists later proved. People now hold very different beliefs about the shape and geology of the world and it is conceivable that these too may be challenged and changed in the future.

Most people also have strong beliefs and opinions about what constitutes 'right' (good) and 'wrong' (bad) conduct. Moral beliefs, like other kinds of beliefs, can be mistaken, however, as centuries of moral inquiry have shown. Indeed, the philosophical literature is full of examples demonstrating convincingly (and giving good reasons for accepting) that some moral decisions and actions are clearly better than others (e.g. acts of compassion are better than acts of cruelty), and that some moral beliefs and theories seem manifestly 'wrong' and ought to be rejected (e.g. women lack moral capacity, black people have no moral worth, gay and transgendered people are moral deviants, Nazis had a moral obligation to rid the German nation of its 'Jewish disease', and so on).

It is because moral beliefs and opinions can be misguided, misinformed and mistaken – and because people can make mistakes in their moral judgments – that those at the forefront of moral decision-making *must* provide strong 'warranties' (good reasons) for their decisions and actions. It is not acceptable for a person to claim that his/her point of view is more worthy and more moral than another's (is 'right') *just because* it is his/her point of view. For instance, I cannot claim that my point of view counts more or is more 'right' than your point of view just because it is my point of view. Much more is required – namely, there must be a *sound justification* for holding the point of view that is put forward. I must give good reasons why reasonable thinking and 'right minded' people should accept the point of view I am advancing. The question that arises here is: *What constitutes a 'sound justification'?*

In the discussion to follow, attention will be given to clarifying the nature and importance of justification to moral decision-making and the role of ethical theory (in particular, ethical principlism, moral rights theory and virtue ethics) in providing justification and warranties (moral reasons) for nurses' moral decisions and actions in the workplace.

Moral justification

Moral conflicts and disagreements occur frequently in health care contexts. This is not surprising given the 'value ladenness' of the health care practices that occur in health care domains. And given the complexity of the values that operate in health care domains, sometimes the choices we make will be 'problematic' insofar as they may express moral values, beliefs and evaluations that are not shared by others or which others do not agree with.

When experiencing situations involving moral disagreement and conflict, it is tempting to rely on our own ordinary moral experience and personal preferences to sustain the point of view we are advocating. As mentioned previously, however, sometimes our own 'ordinary moral experience' and personal preferences may not be reliable or worthy action guides because, as Kopelman (1995: 117) warns us, these can result from 'prejudice, self-interest or ignorance'. In light of this, we need to look elsewhere to strengthen the warranties of (in short, to justify) our moral choices and actions. Moral theory (which has as its focus showing *why* something is moral in addition to showing *that* it is moral) is commonly regarded as the definitive source from which such warranties (justifications) can be reliably sought.

Justifying a moral decision or action involves providing the *strongest moral reasons* behind them. However, as Beauchamp and Childress (2013) explain, merely providing a list of reasons will not suffice to justify a decision. This is because, 'Not all reasons are good reasons, and not all good reasons are sufficient for justification' (Beauchamp & Childress 2013: 390). For example, a majority public opinion supporting the legalisation of euthanasia may constitute a *good reason* for decriminalising euthanasia yet stop short of providing a *sufficient reason* for doing so. Other 'good and sufficient' reasons will need also to be put forward demonstrating why public opinion is not relevant or adequate to justify the legalisation of euthanasia, such as: majority opinion tells us only that a certain class of people hold a point of view, not whether that point of view is morally right (euthanasia could still be morally wrong despite a majority view to the contrary); public opinion is notoriously fickle and hence unreliable as a moral action guide – what is deemed 'right' by the majority today could equally be deemed 'wrong' tomorrow (violating the standards of consistency and coherency otherwise expected in the case of sound moral decision-making). Decision-makers thus need not only to provide 'strong reasons' for their decisions and actions, but also to distinguish:

> *a reason's relevance to a moral judgment from its sufficiency to support that judgment, [and also] to distinguish an* attempted *justification from a* successful *justification.* (Beauchamp & Childress 2013: 390 [emphasis original])

Here, *relevance* can be measured by the extent to which the reason (belief) has *direct bearing* on and makes a *material difference* to the evaluation made as part of the process aimed at making moral judgments and choices/decisions. *Adequacy* can, in turn, be measured by the extent to which it fulfils a need or requirement (in this instance to provide sufficient grounds for belief or action) without being outstanding or abundant. An *attempt* is simply to 'make an effort'; to *succeed* is 'to accomplish'.

Jaggar and Tobin (2013: 385) similarly argue that although our 'best available moral reasoning provides the most authoritative guide we have for morally appropriate action' it may still be insufficient particularly in contexts where people disagree on the methods, models and practices of justification. This problem may be compounded in situations where the disputants do not trust each other's knowledge claims (Tobin 2011). To help overcome this problem, they propose four conditions of adequacy that must be met:

- Plausibility – produce conclusions that have genuine moral force/weight (i.e. that are not arbitrary)
- Usability – disputants are able to participate in the reasoning practices being used to justify an act
- Non-abuse – the reasoning practices do not take wrongful advantage of power and vulnerability (i.e. misrepresent or distort evidence, use intimidation, fallacious logic ('dirty tricks' logic), ridicule or disregard disputants in order to discredit their views)
- Practical feasibility – reasoning must be intelligible and able to be followed apropos prescribing a course of action (adapted from Jaggar & Tobin 2013: 386–9).

Despite its importance to prescribing and proscribing human conduct, the notion of moral justification is not without difficulties. One reason for this is that there exist a number of different accounts of what constitutes a plausible model of moral justification, and even of how a given or 'agreed' model of justification might be interpreted and applied (Bauman 1993; Beauchamp & Childress 2013; Dancy 1993; Jaggar & Tobin 2013; Kopelman 1995; Nielsen 1989; Tobin 2011; Tobin & Jaggar 2013). Some even suggest, controversially, that there can be no adequate model of justification since there is always room to question the grounds that are put forward as 'good reasons' supporting a particular act or judgment (see, for example, Hughes 1995; Johnston 1989). The adequacy of conventional approaches to moral justification has particularly been called into question in contexts involving population diversity and inequality. Tobin and Jaggar (2013: 413), for example, contend that philosophers have tended to seriously underestimate the challenges that cultural diversity and socio-economic inequality can (and does) pose to achieving trustworthy moral justifications in real-world settings. One reason for this, they contend, is because there has been an 'invidious idealization' of privileged models of justification which, either wittingly or unwittingly, can be used as tools for domination and repression (Jaggar & Tobin 2013: 402, 404).

The problem of moral justification has long been recognised as a crucial one in moral philosophy. As Kai Nielsen reflects (1989: 53):

In ordinary non-philosophical moments, we sometimes wonder how (if at all) a deeply felt moral conviction can be justified. And, in our philosophical moments, we sometimes wonder if any moral judgments ever are in principle justified. Surely, we can find all sorts of reasons for taking one course of action rather than another. We find reasons readily enough for the appraisal we make of types of action and attitudes. We frequently make judgments about the moral code of our own culture as well as those of other cultures. But how do we decide if the reasons we offer for these appraisals are good reasons? And, what is the ground for our decision that some reasons are good reasons and others are not? When (if at all) can we say that these grounds are sufficient for our moral decisions? [emphasis original]

There are three possible answers to these questions raised by Nielsen – namely, that we can appeal to either: (1) moral rules, principles and theories; (2) lived experience and case examples of individual personal judgments and the moral insights gained by reflecting on these; or (3) a synthesis of both these (theoretical and experiential) approaches (see also Chappell 2009). This approach, unlike the other approaches, involves a strong synergy between theory and practice, with each informing the other and neither being immune to revision. This issue will be explored more fully in Chapter 5, Moral problems and moral decision-making in nursing and health care contexts.

Theoretical perspectives informing ethical practice

Western moral philosophy has given rise to many different and sometimes competing theoretical perspectives or viewpoints on the nature and justification of moral conduct. Having some knowledge and understanding of these different perspectives is crucial not just to enhancing our understanding of the complex nature of moral problems and the controversies and perplexities to which they so often give rise, but also to enhancing our abilities to provide satisfactory solutions to the moral problems we encounter in our everyday lives. Unfortunately it is beyond the scope of this book to give an in-depth account of the many ethical theories that have been and remain influential in Western moral philosophical thought. There are, however, three theoretical frameworks that warrant attention here – namely, those that involve respectively (and sometimes interdependently) an appeal to:

1. ethical principles (*ethical principlism*)
2. moral rights (*moral rights theory*)
3. moral virtues (*virtue ethics*).

These three approaches, each informed by the traditions of western moral philosophy, have emerged as having the most currency and credibility in contemporary health care contexts. Reasons for this include:
- they have largely emerged from and been refined by practice
- they are able to be readily applied to and in practice
- they are amendable so can be revised and refined in order to be more responsive to the lived realities of everyday practice.

Ethical principlism

One of the most popular theoretical perspectives used today when considering ethical issues in health care is the perspective called '*ethical principlism*'. Ethical principlism is the view that ethical decision-making and problem-solving are best undertaken by appealing to sound moral principles. The principles most commonly used are those of: autonomy, non-maleficence, beneficence and justice. These principles are generally accepted as providing sound moral reasons for taking moral action.

Although not free of difficulties, ethical principlism has become widely accepted as a reliable and practical framework for identifying and resolving moral problems in health care contexts. Given the dominance of ethical principlism in contemporary discussions on ethical issues in health care (largely because of the influential work on the topic by Beauchamp & Childress (2013)), it is important that nurses have some knowledge and understanding of this approach.

What are ethical principles?

Ethical principles are general standards of conduct that make up an ethical system. To say that a principle is 'ethical' or 'moral' is merely to assert that it is a behaviour guide which 'entails particular imperatives' (Harrison 1954: 115). In this instance the imperatives involve specification (in the form of prescriptions and proscriptions) that some type of action or conduct is prohibited, required, or permitted in certain circumstances (Solomon 1978: 408). By this view, an action or decision is generally considered morally right or good when it accords with a given relevant moral principle, and morally wrong or bad when it does not. To illustrate how this works, consider the action of making a measurement using a ruler. If the line you have drawn measures the desired length of, say, 12 cm – as measured against your ruler – you would judge the length as 'correct'. If, however, the line you have drawn is only 10 cm long – not the desired 12 cm – you would judge the length to be 'incorrect'. By analogy, principles also function like rulers, insofar as they provide a standard against which something (in this case, actions) can be measured. For example, if an action fails to 'measure up' to the ultimate standards set by a given principle, we would judge the action to be 'incorrect' or, more specifically, morally wrong. If, however, an action fully measures up to the ultimate standards set by a given principle, we would judge the action to be 'correct' or morally right. The next question is: What are these moral principles against which actions can be measured?

As stated earlier, moral principles commonly used in discussions on ethical issues in nursing and health care include the principles of autonomy, non-maleficence, beneficence and justice. It is to briefly examining the content, prescriptive force and application of these principles that this discussion now turns.

Autonomy

The term '*autonomy*' comes from the Greek *autos* (meaning 'self') and *nomos* (meaning 'rule', 'governance' or 'law'). When autonomy is used as a concept in moral discourse, what is commonly being referred to is a person's ability to make or to exercise self-determining choice – literally, to be 'self-governing'. Included here is the additional notion of 'respect for persons' – that is, of treating or respecting persons as ends in themselves, as dignified and autonomous choosers, and not as the mere means (objects or tools) to the ends of others (Benn 1971; Kant 1972). The *principle* of autonomy, however, is a little different, and is eloquently formulated by Beauchamp and Walters (1982: 27) as follows:

> *Insofar as an autonomous agent's actions* do not infringe on the autonomous actions of others, *that person should be free to perform whatever action he or she wishes (presumably even if it involves considerable risk to himself or herself and even if others consider the action to be foolish).* [emphasis added]

What this basically means is that people should be free to choose and are entitled to act on their preferences provided their decisions and actions do not stand to violate, or impinge on, the significant moral interests of others.

Both the concept and the principle of autonomy have important implications for nursing practice. For example, if autonomy is to be taken seriously by nurses, nursing practice must truly respect patients as dignified human beings capable of deciding what is to count as being in their own best interests – even if what they decide is considered by others (including nurses) to be 'foolish'. In short, nurses must allow patients to participate in decision-making concerning their care. Given this, it soon becomes clear that the whole practice of 'negotiated patient goals' and 'negotiated patient care' as advocated by contemporary nursing philosophy has its roots in the moral principle of autonomy and the derived duty to respect persons as autonomous moral choosers. It is not derived merely from a concept of 'acceptable professional nursing practice'.

In application, the principle of autonomy would judge as being morally objectionable and wrong any act which unjustly prevents autonomous persons from deciding what is to count as being in their own best interests. The kinds of act which might come in for criticism here include, for example:

- treating patients without their consent
- treating patients without giving them all the relevant information necessary for making an informed and intelligent choice
- withholding information from patients when they have expressed a considered choice to receive it
- imposing information upon patients when they have expressed a considered choice not to receive it
- forcing nurses to act against their reasoned moral judgments or conscience.

It should be noted, however, that while the moral principle of autonomy is helpful in guiding ethically just practices in health care contexts it is not entirely unproblematic. Indeed, its uncritical and culturally inappropriate application in some contexts may, in fact, inadvertently cause rather than prevent significant moral harms to patients, for reasons which are considered in Chapter 4.

Non-maleficence

The term '*non-maleficence*' comes from the Latin-derived *maleficent* – from *maleficus* (meaning 'wicked', 'prone to evil'), from *malum* (meaning 'evil'), and *male* (meaning 'ill'). As a moral principle, non-maleficence (literally 'refuse evil'), prescribes 'above all, do no harm' which entails a stringent obligation not to injure or harm others. This principle is sometimes equated with the moral principle of 'beneficence' (considered below under a separate subheading) which prescribes 'above all, do good'. Trying to conflate these two obviously distinct principles under one principle is, however, misleading. As Beauchamp and Childress (2013: 151) explain, not only are these two principles distinct (for instance, our obligation not to kill someone does seem qualitatively and quantitatively different from our obligation to rescue someone from a life-threatening situation), but it is important to distinguish between them so as not to obscure other critical moral distinctions which might be made in ordinary moral discourse. One instance in which 'other important distinctions might need to be made' is in the case of where both principles might apply to a given situation, but where the strength of the respective moral imperatives of each may nevertheless differ significantly and thus might prescribe different courses of action.

'Stringentness' thus stands as an important distinction that might be obscured if the principles of non-maleficence and beneficence were conflated into one single principle. Beauchamp and Childress (2013: 151) contend that generally 'obligations of non-maleficence are usually more stringent than obligations of beneficence', and, in some cases, may even override beneficence particularly in instances where beneficent acts (e.g. to help others and to provide benefits), paradoxically, are not morally defensible (e.g. depriving one's family of food for a week and risking eviction by failing to pay the rent because of donating the household's weekly budget to charity). However, Beauchamp and Childress (2013: 151) further contend that, while our obligations not to harm others might be more stringent in some situations than our obligations to help them, the reverse can also be true (e.g. the justified 'harm' of radical yet lifesaving and 'beneficial' surgery).

Applied in nursing contexts, the principle of non-maleficence would provide justification for condemning any act which unjustly injures a person or causes them to suffer an otherwise avoidable harm.

Before continuing, some commentary is warranted on the notion of 'harm' and how it might be interpreted (given that it is open to a variety of interpretations). For the purposes of this discussion, harm may be taken to involve the invasion, violation, thwarting or 'setting back' of a person's significant welfare interests to the detriment of that person's wellbeing (Beauchamp & Childress 2013: 153–4; Feinberg 1984: 34). Interests, in this instance, are taken to mean 'a miscellaneous collection, consist[ing] of all those things in which one has a stake' together with the 'harmonious advancement' of those interests (Feinberg 1984: 34). Interests are morally significant since they are fundamentally linked to human wellbeing; specifically, they stand as a *fundamental requisite* (although, granted, not the whole) of human wellbeing (Feinberg 1984: 37). Wellbeing, in turn, can include interests in:

> *continuance for a foreseeable interval of one's life, and the interests in one's own physical health and vigour, the integrity and normal functioning of one's body, the absence of absorbing pain and suffering or grotesque disfigurement, minimal intellectual acuity, emotional stability, the absence of groundless anxieties and resentments, the capacity to engage normally in social intercourse and to enjoy and maintain friendships, at least minimal income and financial security, a tolerable social and physical environment, and a certain amount of freedom from interference and coercion.* (Feinberg 1984: 37)

The test for whether a person's interests and wellbeing have been violated, 'set back', thwarted or invaded rests on 'whether that interest is in a worse condition than it would otherwise have been in had the invasion not occurred at all' (Feinberg 1984: 34). For instance, if a person (e.g. a patient) is left psychogenically distressed (e.g. in emotional pain, anxious, depressed and even suicidal) or in a state of needless physical pain and/or disability as a result of his/her experiences (e.g. as a patient in a given health care setting) our reflective commonsense tells us that this person's interests have been violated and the person him/herself 'harmed'. As the American philosopher Joel Feinberg (1984: 37) further explains, the violation of a person's welfare interests renders that person 'very seriously harmed indeed' since 'their ultimate aspirations are defeated too'.

Beneficence

The term 'beneficence' comes from the Latin *beneficus*, from *bene* (meaning 'well' or 'good') and *facere* (meaning 'to do'). The principle of *beneficence* prescribes 'above all, do good'; in practice, it entails a positive obligation to literally *act for the benefit of others, viz* contribute to the welfare and wellbeing of others (Beauchamp & Childress 2013). Acts of beneficence can include such virtuous actions as: care, compassion, empathy, sympathy, altruism, kindness, mercy, love, friendship and charity. It is recognised, however, that bestowing benefits on others is not always without cost to the benefactor. Thus there are some limits to the principle; that is, it is not 'free standing' and its application can be appropriately constrained by other moral (e.g. utilitarian) considerations. To put this another way, we are not obliged to act beneficently towards others when doing so could result in our own significant moral interests being seriously harmed or compromised in some way.

Although the notion of 'obligatory beneficence' remains a controversial one in moral philosophy (for instance, it is generally accepted that we are not morally required to benefit persons on all occasions, even if we are in a position to do so), there are nevertheless a number of conditions under which a person can indeed be said to have an obligation of beneficence and that this obligation might, sometimes, be overriding. An example of such conditions, devised by Beauchamp and Childress (2013: 207), is as follows:

> *a person X has a prima facie obligation of beneficence, in the form of a duty to rescue, toward person Y if and only if each of the following conditions is satisfied (assuming X is aware of the relevant facts):*
> 1. *Y is at risk of significant loss of or damage to life, health or some other basic interest.*
> 2. *X's action is needed (singly or in concert with others) to prevent this loss or damage.*
> 3. *X's action (singly or in concert with others) will probably prevent this loss or damage.*
> 4. *X's action would not present significant risks, costs, or burdens to X.*
> 5. *The benefit that Y can be expected to gain outweighs any harms, costs, or burdens that X is likely to incur.*

The principle and its prescribed obligation of beneficence stands to have an interesting and useful application in nursing practice. Consider the following hypothetical case. Mrs Jones, a Jehovah's Witness, is admitted to an intensive care unit in the final stages of life, suffering from advanced hepatitis B and severe liver failure. She has a slow internal haemorrhage and is only semiconscious. Before her alteration in consciousness she gives her doctors a written statement specifically requesting that she not be given a blood transfusion under any circumstances. Upon her arrival in the unit, however, the attending doctor prescribes a unit of blood and requests that it be given immediately. Mrs Jones' husband and children are all present and, upon overhearing the doctor's request, become very upset. Mr Jones approaches the doctor and asks that his wife not be given the blood transfusion. He reminds the doctor that Mrs Jones has made explicit her wish not to have a blood transfusion under any circumstances. Nurse Smith, the registered nurse caring for Mrs Jones, hears the discussion and is faced with deciding whether or not to intervene on her patient's behalf. In making her decision, Nurse Smith might appeal to the principle of beneficence in the following manner:

1. Mrs Jones, a Jehovah's Witness in the final stages of life, is at risk of suffering a significant loss (a violation of her spiritual values and beliefs) if she is given the medically prescribed blood transfusion.
2. Action by Nurse Smith, the attending nurse, is needed to prevent Mrs Jones from experiencing the loss in question.
3. Nurse Smith's action of refusing to administer the prescribed transfusion would probably prevent Mrs Jones' loss.
4. Nurse Smith's action will not present a significant risk to her (i.e. she will not lose her job).
5. The benefits gained by Mrs Jones outweigh any harms Nurse Smith is likely to suffer (given that Nurse Smith autonomously chooses to uphold Mrs Jones' interests, and does not stand to suffer any morally significant consequences of her actions).

Weighing up the benefits and burdens, Nurse Smith decides to refuse to give the transfusion which has been prescribed. The doctor, however, insists that it be given. In response to this, the nurse points out that the transfusion would probably be of no clinical benefit to Mrs Jones, as she was clearly in the end stages of her disease – to put it bluntly, 'she was dying'. Nurse Smith then suggests to the doctor that perhaps he would prefer to administer the transfusion himself. The doctor rejects this suggestion, and the transfusion is not given. Mrs Jones dies a short while later without having to experience a needless violation of her expressed wishes, values and beliefs.

In summary, by this principle, any act which fails to address an imbalance of harms over benefits where this can be done without sacrificing a benefactor's own significant moral interests warrants judgment as being morally unacceptable.

Justice

The principle of *justice* (its nature and content), unlike the principles above, is not so amenable to precise definition or quantification. Questions concerning what justice is and what its origins are have occupied the minds of philosophers for nearly 3000 years, and to this day remain the subject of philosophical debate (MacIntyre 1988; Nussbaum 2006; Powers & Faden 2006; Sen 2009; Solomon & Murphy 1990). Significantly, the end result of this protracted philosophical debate has not been the development of a singular and refined universal theory of justice, but rather that of a range of rival theories of justice – both traditional and recent (Beauchamp & Childress 2013; MacIntyre 1988). Different conceptions of justice (from the Latin *justus* meaning 'righteous') have included: *justice as revenge* (retributive justice – e.g. 'an eye for an eye'), *justice as mercy* (Christian ethics), *justice as harmony* in the soul and harmony in the state (Pythagorean ethics, 600 BC–1 AD), *justice as equity* (impartiality and fairness), *justice as avoiding parochialism and reducing (global) injustice*, *justice as equality* ('equals must be treated equally, and unequals unequally'), *justice as an equal distribution of benefits and burdens* (distributive justice and redistributive justice), *justice as what is deserved* ('each according to one's merit or worth'), and *justice as love* (Beauchamp & Childress 2013; MacIntyre 1988, 2007; Nozick 2007; Nussbaum 2006; Outka 1972; Powers & Faden 2006; Rawls 1971; Sen 2009; Singer 1991; Solomon & Murphy 1990; Waithe 1987). Over the past two decades, justice has also been conceptualised as *reconciliation and reparation* (restorative justice), a key purpose of which is to 'restore broken relationships' (Tutu 1999; see also Johnstone G 2002; Sullivan & Tifft 2006). Arguably one of the most novel conceptions of justice is that of *justice as a basic human need* that, like other basic human needs (notably those famously depicted in Maslow's hierarchy of human needs), is critical to producing the necessary conditions of life (Taylor 2003, 2006).

Given these different conceptions of justice, the problem arises of what, if any, conception of justice nurses should adopt? While it is beyond the scope of this book to answer this question in depth, there is nevertheless room to advocate at least three senses of justice which nurses might find helpful: (1) justice as fairness and impartiality (equity justice), (2) justice as the equal distribution of benefits and burdens (distributive and redistributive justice), and (3) justice as reconciliation and reparation (restorative justice). It is these three senses of justice which will now be considered.

Justice as fairness and impartiality (equity)

Justice as fairness finds interpretation in terms of 'what is owed or due' (Beauchamp & Childress 2013: 250). By this view, it can be said that one acts justly towards a person when that person has been given what is due or owed; an injustice, in turn, would involve withholding from that person what is otherwise due or owed.

If a person deserved something, justice is done when that person receives that particular something. Here, the 'something' may be either positive (a reward) or negative (a punishment). This view relies very heavily on an 'intuitive' sense of justice. For example, we may 'feel' it is unjust to punish or censure someone for a harm they did not cause, or not to punish someone for a harm they did deliberately cause. Likewise we may feel that it is unjust to reward someone for an accomplishment to which they contributed nothing, and yet not reward someone who contributed a great deal.

We do not need to look far in nursing practice to find sobering examples of where the principle of justice as fairness has been violated. Consider the notable historical cases where nurses have been subjected to severe legal and professional censure, held solely responsible and have even lost their jobs because of making an honest mistake (Johnstone 1994a; Johnstone & Kanitsaki 2006b).

Other examples involve cases where nurses have gained promotion or have secured employment on the basis of their claiming credit for the work of either their peers or their subordinates. At the other end of the continuum, some nurses have been denied promotion or employment because their superior has ignored, or refused for whatever reasons to recognise significant professional achievements the nurse applicant has in fact made.

How, then, might we make choices on this view of justice? One possible approach which has received widespread attention is that discussed by the contemporary American philosopher John Rawls. He argues, for example, that if parties are to exercise truly just or fair choices, they must choose from a hypothetically 'neutral' position, or from a position of what he describes as being 'behind the veil of ignorance' (Rawls 1971: 12). From such a position he argues:

> no-one knows his [sic] place in society, his [sic] class position or social status, nor does anyone know his [sic] fortune in the distribution of natural assets and abilities, his [sic] intelligence, strength, and the like ... [T]his ensures that no-one is advantaged or disadvantaged in the choice of principles by the outcome of natural chance or the contingency of social circumstances. Since all are similarly situated and no-one is able to design principles to favour his [sic] particular condition, the principles of justice are the result of a fair agreement or bargain. (Rawls 1971: 12)

While Rawls' view is problematic (it is open to serious question whether, in fact, all choosers are or could ever be 'similarly situated', as he assumes), it has nevertheless been extremely influential. A key reason for its influence relates to broader philosophical demands that are inherent in Western bioethics and which emphasise, among other things, that moral choice and judgment should be exercised from a position of *impartiality* and *objectivity*. However, whether in fact human beings are ever capable of exercising truly impartial and 'objective' choices – indeed, of choosing from behind that veil of ignorance – remains a matter of some controversy. Some critics also argue that Rawls' theory is too narrow, pointing out that it has failed to take a more responsive approach to *social cooperation* and the needs of people who are disabled, 'not equal', disadvantaged, and who belong to other non-human species (see Nussbaum 2006; Sen 2009). One reason for this is that it pays too much attention to patterns of distribution, rather than to the 'procedural issues of participation, deliberations and decision-making' (Young 2007: 600). Moreover, Rawls' theory fails to take into account that what is important is not just the *distribution* of benefits and burdens per se, but how various distributions came about (Nozick 2007).

Despite its weaknesses, Rawls' justice theory provides a useful catalyst for thinking about the notion of fairness and how it might be used in real-life situations. It also alerts us to some of the potential difficulties of trying to determine and apply an uncontentious view of justice.

Justice as an equal distribution of benefits and burdens

A second (and related) sense in which justice can be used is that pertaining to 'distributive justice' – that is, an equal distribution of benefits and harms. Benefits in this instance may be taken to mean 'primary goods' – things we can assume all reasonable people would want such as health, liberty, civil and political rights, income security, etc.; harms, in turn, may be taken to mean the untoward consequences of an unequal distribution of society's 'primary goods' and their associated benefits.

By this view of justice, all people are required to bear an equal share of their society's benefits and burdens. Such a view admits that all persons must have equal claims to liberty and opportunity, but in a way that is compatible with the claims of others. As well as this, there must be equal access (and opportunity to gain access) to positions of authority and power, and there must be an equal distribution of wealth and income (a point often missed in conservative constructions of justice as equity – such as outlined above). The only morally acceptable exception to this would be if an unequal distribution would work to everyone's advantage, or where an unequal distribution of benefits would be necessary so as to prevent unequal disadvantage. Simply put, inequalities in distributing benefits and primary goods is 'just' as long as this results in the least well-off (i.e. those who are already disadvantaged unfairly) achieving a decent minimum level of wellbeing (i.e. being advantaged by the benefits which have been conferred unequally).

As with the fairness sense of justice discussed earlier, we do not need to look far to find sobering examples in nursing where the principle of distributive justice has been violated. In many cases, nurses have had to (and continue to) bear unequal and intolerable burdens on account of certain inequities in the distribution of scarce health care resources. For example, historically nurses have had to endure poor and unsafe working conditions with a maximum of responsibility and a minimum of financial or personal reward (Johnstone M-J 1994a, 2002).

In calculating the balance or distribution of harms and benefits, notions of comparative and non-comparative justice are used. In the second edition of their foundational work, Beauchamp and Childress (1983: 185) explain that justice is 'comparative' when 'what one person deserves can be determined only by balancing the competing claims of others against his or her claims'. For example, whether a nurse qualifies for a job or a promotion will depend largely on the competing claims of the other applicants. If the other applicants are more qualified and more experienced, it seems reasonable to hold that they are more 'deserving' of the position being offered. Justice is 'non-comparative', on the other hand, when 'desert is judged by standards independent of the claims of others' (Beauchamp & Childress 1983: 185). For example, a nurse who is guilty of breaching acceptable professional standards of conduct deserves to be censured, or even deregistered, if the breach of conduct warrants such an action; a nurse who is innocent of professional misconduct, however, does not deserve to be censured or deregistered.

Justice as reconciliation and reparation

A third (and less well known) sense in which justice can be used is in a reconciliation and reparative sense, otherwise referred to as 'restorative justice'. In contradistinction to retributive justice (the primary aim of which is to assign blame and punish offenders), restorative justice has as its primary aim:

> *healing rather than hurting, moral learning, community participation and community caring, respectful dialogue, forgiveness, responsibility, apology and making amends.* (Braithwaite 1999: 6)

Historically, small societies have often used means other than retribution to 'resolve conflict and restore harmony' (Maxwell & Morris 2006: 72). Thus, instead of using punishment to redress a wrong, processes for promoting healing and restoration have been emphasised (Johnstone G 2002; Maxwell & Morris 2006; Sullivan & Tifft 2005, 2006). This approach has, however, also worked in large nations. A poignant example of this can be found in the extraordinary case of South Africa's Truth and Reconciliation Commission (TRC), which commenced in May 1996 following the collapse of the apartheid regime in that country. Based on the *Promotion of National Unity and Reconciliation Act, 1995* (available for viewing at: www.doj.gov.za/trc/), the TRC was conducted in the spirit of *ubuntu*, an African jurisprudence principle which emphasises 'the healing of breaches, the redressing of imbalances, the restoration of broken relationships' (Tutu 1999: 51). Although severely criticised by some for its 'religious components' (notably the promulgation of the assumptions that 'truth is a precursor to forgiveness' and 'forgiveness is necessary for healing') and the demonstrable negative impact it had on the mental health of some individuals and families (Swartz & Drennan 2000), the TRC is nonetheless credited with being an instrument of national healing. It has also been credited with providing a 'third way' for redressing the past and to enable the country to move forward and not descend into mayhem and civil war, as has happened so often in other countries where people have suffered years of oppression and brutality (Tutu 1999).

Over the past two decades, restorative values have also been translated and applied in practice as a form of 'therapeutic jurisprudence' in the cultural contexts of New Zealand, Canada, the United States (US) and Australia. Although primarily advanced as an Indigenous Justice Initiative aimed at assisting in the rehabilitation of young offenders from Indigenous communities and 'restoring' them to their communities (see Braithwaite 1999; Johnstone G 2002; Maxwell & Morris 2006; Sullivan & Tifft 2005, 2006), restorative justice has also been applied in broader contexts. Some notable examples include its use to improve compliance with regulatory standards in health care contexts (see Freckelton & Flynn 2004; Makkai & Braithwaite 1994), and to rehabilitate and restore community and population health (Ashworth 2002; Freudenberg 2001). As the negative health consequences of individual as well as institutional injustices become more apparent (see Herndon 1992; Taylor 2003, 2006), the need of a 'third way' to resolve conflict and restore harmony – to find out the truth, heal breaches, redress imbalances, restore broken relationships (after Tutu 1999: 51) and rehabilitate both victims and perpetrators injured by an offence without resorting to a system of retributive justice (Johnstone G 2002; Johnstone & Van Ness 2007) – will become more pressing, and the possible remedies offered by restorative justice compelling as both a 'moral measure' and a moral course of action.

Moral rules

Moral principles are not the only entities that make up an ethical system or ethical framework for guiding conduct. Moral rules also have a place in guiding and 'warranting' ethical conduct. Like moral principles, moral rules function by specifying that some type of action or conduct is either prohibited, required or permitted (Solomon 1978: 408–9). What distinguishes a moral rule from a moral principle in certain contexts is its structure and nature. Moral principles, for instance, tend to be regarded as providing the content of morality, and the bases or the 'parent' forms from which general moral truths (insofar as these can be determined) are derived. In application, moral principles incline more towards a general focus. Consider, for example, the broad moral principle of 'autonomy'. In general, the principle prescribes that persons should be respected as autonomous choosers, capable of judging what is in their own best interests. As such, people who have the capacity to make autonomous decisions should be free to act as they wish provided their actions do not violate the moral interests of others.

Moral rules, on the other hand, stand as being merely derivative of moral principles and theories and, in application, are much more particular in their focus. Although it is difficult to draw a firm distinction between moral rules and moral principles, it is generally recognised that moral rules have different force, sanctioning power, conditions of existence, scope of application and level of concreteness from moral principles (Solomon 1978). An example of a moral rule would be the demand, say, to 'always tell the truth' or 'never tell a lie'. Thus, if a patient asks an attending health care professional a question concerning a diagnosis and proposed treatment, the health care professional could be said to be obliged to give the information the patient has requested. The apparent 'obligation' here finds its force not just from the moral rule 'always tell the truth', but from the moral principle of autonomy which prescribes that people with the capacity to make self-interested decisions should be respected as autonomous choosers, and be given the information required to make an informed and intelligent choice.

Another example can be found in a set of rules that prescribe such things as 'do not kill others', 'do not cause pain and suffering to others', 'do not affect detrimentally the physical and mental health of others', and so forth. The apparent obligations here find their force not just from the rules stated, but also from the moral principle non-maleficence, which prescribes 'do no harm'.

In order for a particular moral rule (or set of moral rules) to be justified, it must be fully derived from and reducible to established parent principles of morality.

In summary, moral rules derive from moral principles, and as such have only prima-facie force (i.e. they can be overridden by stronger moral claims). Given their prima-facie nature, moral rules cannot override the moral principles from which they have been derived. To accept that they could, would be to suggest, somewhat paradoxically, that derived rules could meaningfully conflict with parent principles – which is absurd. The relationship between particular moral judgments, moral rules, moral principles and moral theories is shown in Fig. 3.1.

The question of moral rules is an important one for nurses, particularly as it relates to the broader issue of professional codes of conduct, an issue that will become clearer in the following chapters.

FIGURE 3.1
Moral justification and direction of appeal

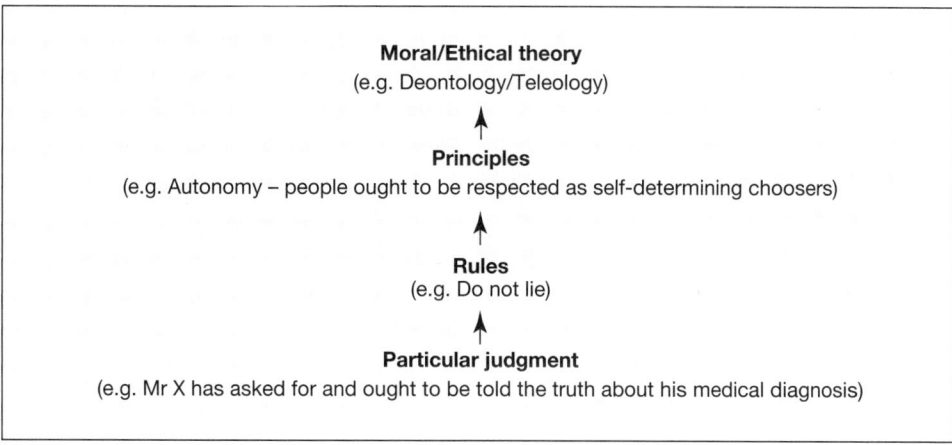

(Adapted from: Beauchamp T & Childress J (1994) Principles of biomedical ethics, 4th edn. Oxford University Press, New York: 15)

Problems with ethical principles

In considering ethical principlism it is important to be aware of a number of difficulties that can arise when appealing to the ethical principles described. For example, problems commonly associated with ethical principlism include:

- deciding correctly which principles apply in a given situation (e.g. 'Is it the principle of autonomy or beneficence that applies in this case, or both?')
- interpreting correctly the imperatives of the principles chosen to guide ethical decision-making in a given situation (e.g. 'What does the principle of autonomy require of me? Is it the case that the principle of autonomy ought always to be upheld?')
- deciding correctly the relative weights of given principles (e.g. 'Which principle has overriding consideration in this case – the principle of autonomy or the principle of non-maleficence?')
- balancing the demands of different principles in situations where their respective though equally weighted demands might conflict (e.g. 'How can I uphold the principle of autonomy without, at the same time, violating the principle of justice, which has an equal bearing in this case?')
- deciding whether ethical principles apply at all (e.g. 'This is a matter to be resolved by kindness and care – by being virtuous – not by appealing to ethical principles per se.')
- resolving disagreement with others regarding either of the above (e.g. 'I feel strongly that respecting the patient's autonomy in this case means withholding the information about his diagnosis as he has requested, but others in the team do not agree and are going to tell him, insisting he must be told so that he can make informed choices about his future treatment.').

The issue of moral uncertainty, moral dilemmas and moral disagreements in regard to the selection, interpretation and application of ethical principles will be explored further in the chapters to follow.

Moral rights theory

Of the moral theories that have been appealed to in the contemporary literature on ethics, a 'rights' view of ethics is probably the one that has the most currency among professional and lay communities alike. Certainly most people have a sense that they have 'rights', that their rights are 'justified' (Martin 2017) and that their rights, whatever these may be, 'ought to be respected'. Important questions to ask are: 'What are moral rights?', 'Who has them?' and 'To what extent are others obliged to respect them?'

Moral rights theory has emerged as an extremely influential theoretical perspective across the globe. Evidence of this can be found in the vast array of contexts in which moral rights discourse has been used. For example, we see moral rights discourse in: position statements and bills of clients'/patients' rights; professional codes of ethics and conduct (e.g. the International Council of Nurses' *Code for nurses* (ICN 1973, 2012a) and supporting position statements); statutory authorities (e.g. the various Australian state and territory Human Rights and Equal Opportunity Commissions); government inquiries (e.g. the *Report of the National Inquiry into the Human Rights of People with Mental Illness* by Burdekin et al 1993); and in international covenants, conventions and treaties (e.g. the *United Nations Universal Declaration of Human Rights* (United Nations 1949), and the ratification of *The International Bill of Human Rights* (United Nations 1978)). There is also an abundance of literature on the subject. If nurses are to participate effectively in discourses on moral rights, it is essential that they have some understanding of the theoretical underpinnings of a moral (and human) rights perspective on ethics. It is to providing a brief examination of moral rights theory that this section will now turn.

Moral rights

Moral rights (to be distinguished here from human rights, legal rights, institutional rights, civil rights, etc.) generally entail claims about some special entitlement or interest which ought, for moral reasons, to be protected. The kinds of interests for which protection might be sought include, for example, life, freedom, happiness, privacy, self-determination, fair treatment and bodily integrity. The language used in asserting rights typically involves expressions such as: 'I have a right to …', 'It's your right to …', 'They have a right to …', and so on. A rights claim is generally accepted as a sound moral reason for taking moral action.

There is no single thesis of moral rights. The following is a brief overview of some of the better-known classical and contemporary theories concerning the existence of moral rights and the conditions under which they can be validly claimed.

Moral rights based on natural law and divine command

Natural rights theory argues that certain entitlements are simply 'built into' the universe like the laws of gravity, and as such are neither the products of human invention nor the constructs of other moral theories (Martin & Nickel 1980). A variation of this thesis is that natural rights have been divinely ordained for all human beings. From both these points of view, since the laws of nature and the ordinances of God apply equally to all human beings, it follows that all human beings – young and old; male, female, transgender and intergendered (e.g. hermaphrodites); homosexual, heterosexual and bisexual; abled and disabled; black, white and coloured – unconditionally have natural rights.

Objections to this account of moral rights derive from those raised against a theological account of morality generally. For example, if it were shown that God did not exist, or that natural law did not exist, this account of moral rights would immediately collapse because its very foundation would be pulled out from underneath it. Another objection rests on the problem that natural rights essentially defy scientific verification.

Moral rights based on common humanity

Another popular natural rights thesis is that all human beings have rights simply by virtue of being 'human' and 'equal'. What is critical to this thesis is the notion that 'being human' is something over which we have no control; that is, we cannot choose to be either human or not human (Martin &

Nickel 1980). In this sense, then, we can be said to enjoy a 'common humanity'. This view of rights is vulnerable to the objection that not all human rights are *moral rights* per se. The human right to education, which is dependent on the availability of educational resources, is an example of a human right which is not a moral right per se.

Another more serious problem is that, given the recent advancements made in the field of genetic engineering, 'being human' may indeed be something over which we have control in the near future. Human genes have already been cloned onto animals (e.g. pigs and fish); it is not far-fetched to imagine that scientists will succeed (if they have not already done so) in cloning animal genes onto humans. Persons with a genetic makeup comprising both human and non-human genes could be said to be not 'fully human', at least, not in a 'speciesist' sense. Were someone to be not 'fully human', their claim to moral rights on the basis of a common humanity would be cast in doubt. Conversely, if a non-human nonetheless has human genes and/or human characteristics (e.g. chimpanzees that are capable of performing abstractions), it too might hold claim to what are otherwise upheld as being exclusively 'human rights' (see also Dershowitz 2004: 143).

Moral rights based on rationality

A Kantian thesis of natural rights (i.e. a thesis based on the philosophical views of the German philosopher Immanuel Kant circa 1724–1804) holds rationality as being the sole basis upon which a right's claim can be made. In other words, only those people who are capable of rational, autonomous thought are entitled to claim moral rights. One disturbing consequence of this thesis is that any human being (or non-human being, for that matter) who is unable to reason is not regarded as having moral status. Such a view clearly excludes infants, brain-dead and intellectually disabled persons, and others with severe organic brain states corrosive of their 'personhood' from having a just claim to moral rights. It might be tempting to dismiss this view as being merely an intellectual one, of interest only to moral philosophers. There is ample evidence, however, that this view is influential and has currency in the 'real world' of human affairs. (The most notable examples here can be found in the use of 'brain-dead' persons, fetuses and live-born anencephalics as organ donors (Bioethics Committee, Canadian Paediatric Society 2005; Fost 2004; Khan & Lea 2009; Meinke 1989; Siminoff 2004).)

Moral rights based on interests

The North American philosopher Joel Feinberg offers quite a different theory of moral rights. He argues that, in order for an entity to be able to claim rights meaningfully, that entity must have interests (Feinberg 1979). To have interests, the entity must be capable of being either benefited or harmed. In order to be either benefited or harmed, one must have the capacity to experience pleasure and pain – that is, have sentience. In short, unless one has sentience one cannot have interests, and thus cannot be either benefited or harmed, and therefore cannot make claims.

Some have taken this view even further contending that 'sentience is the bedrock of ethics', not just of moral rights (Balcombe 2016: 13). This is because it is fundamentally wrong to 'deliberately and maliciously cause another pain and suffering' because pain and suffering are in themselves fundamentally bad (Balcombe 2016: 13). This theory of moral rights can be expressed diagrammatically as shown in Fig. 3.2.

It can be seen that by this view it would be nonsense to assert, for example, that a rock has rights. Why? Because a rock does not have sentience and therefore cannot, strictly speaking, be benefited or harmed, and thus cannot meaningfully be said to have interests, and hence rights. Those who *value* rocks (e.g. conservationists, geologists, rock collectors) might be benefited or harmed by what happens to a rock, but it is not meaningful, philosophically speaking, to assert that a rock per se has rights. In contrast, any entity which can be shown to have sentience (i.e. the capacity to experience pleasure or suffer pain) would, by this view, be entitled to be respected as having rights. Given this, it is clear that we can, for

FIGURE 3.2
Feinberg's theory of moral rights

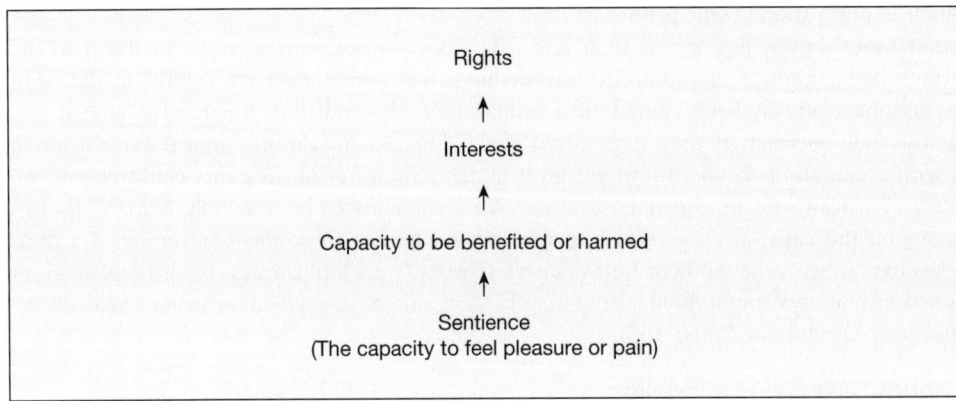

example, assert meaningfully that beings such as dolphins, puppies, kittens, horses, people who cannot think or reason or express their wishes because of an incapacitating brain injury or other debilitating brain disease, and babies have moral rights.

Like Bentham, the founding father of utilitarianism (to be discussed later in this chapter), Feinberg sees the *capacity to suffer*, not reason, as the ultimate basis upon which a person's interest claims become the focus of moral action.

One shortcoming of this view is that individuals must be able to represent their own interests. Feinberg (1979: 595) argues that, if individuals cannot represent their own interests, they have no more rights than 'redwood trees and rosebushes'. Unhappily, the 'human vegetable', it seems, is no better off under an interests-based thesis of moral rights than it is under a thesis based on reason.

Feinberg does not, however, offer an adequate account of why entities must be able to 'represent their own interests'. As contemporary theorists have recently shown, human beings (especially those who are vulnerable) do not necessarily 'have to be capable of making claims, or have the capacity to function as a moral agent in order to have rights' (Dyck 2005: 116). Feinberg also fails to account for why others (who are capable of making sound judgments about the moral interests of vulnerable persons and acting in a way to protect those interests) cannot speak for individuals, families and groups when they are unable or incapable of speaking on their own behalf. Moreover, there is considerable scope to suggest that an interests-based thesis of moral rights justifies and, in some contexts, even *demands* surrogate representation — particularly in the case of human beings who are vulnerable and unable (because of their age, impairment of cognitive function, physical confinement, political oppression, emotional distress, and so forth) to 'speak for themselves' and/or effectively represent their own best interests (Hoffmaster 2006; Kottow 2003, 2004; Purdy 2004).

Moral rights based on human experiences of grievous wrongs

Not all agree with the above theories of the origins of rights. Dershowitz, for example, a leading legal scholar from Harvard University, argues that human rights do not derive from God, nature, logic, or otherwise, but from 'particular human experiences' — notably of the 'worst injustices' and 'most grievous wrongs' and the ongoing quest by reasonable people to prevent their reoccurrence and to 'righting the wrongs' that have occurred (Dershowitz 2004: 81–2). With reference to some of the world's most potent historical examples of 'worst injustices' and 'most grievous wrongs' (genocide and slavery being two standout examples), Dershowitz (p 90) contends:

> *Where the majority does justice to the minority, there is little need for rights. But where injustice prevails, rights become essential. Wrongs provoke rights, as our checkered history confirms.*

Drawing on this observation, and advancing a thesis of 'nurtural rights' (to be distinguished from 'natural rights'), he concludes that *human rights* thus have their origin in *human wrongs*, and that, in essence, a theory of rights is ipso facto also a theory of wrongs (Dershowitz 2004: 81).

An important question to arise here is: *How are we to know what are 'most grievous wrongs'?* Dershowitz suggests, first, that 'if wrongs were not wrongs', then it is reasonable to ask why their perpetrators go to such lengths to hide or disguise them – pointing out that 'even Hitler and his henchmen tried to hide their genocidal actions behind euphemisms and evasive rhetoric' (Dershowitz 2004: 81). Second, there is likely to be more agreement than not among reasonable people as to what constitute 'most grievous wrongs'. On this point Dershowitz (2004: 83) argues:

> *Reasonable people will always disagree about the nature of the perfect good, but there will be less disagreement about the evils that experience has taught us to prevent.*

Finally, and arguably most propitiously, is the burgeoning of rights themselves immediately after a most grievous wrong has been acknowledged, as numerous examples in history can readily demonstrate (the formulation and ratification of the *United Nations Declaration of Human Rights* being just one example) (Dershowitz 2004: 94–5). Importantly, rights can also 'quickly contract' in the aftermath of wrongs 'believed to be caused by excessive rights' claims (Dershowitz 2004: 95) – an issue that is explored further under the subheading 'Rights and responsibilities' in this chapter.

Dershowitz (2004: 232) concludes that 'righting wrongs' is an ongoing process that will see rights in a constant state of flux as they adapt and counter each new injustice. Accordingly, those who believe in rights must 'take their case to the people' and must engage in the positive project of constantly proving that 'rights work', that 'they are necessary to prevent wrongs, and that they are worth the price we sometimes pay for them'.

Different types of rights

When speaking of moral rights, it is important to distinguish three different types which can be claimed, notably: inalienable, absolute and prima-facie rights.

Inalienable rights

An inalienable right is one which cannot be transferred under any circumstances. For example, if we accept the right to life as being an inalienable right, we are committed to accepting that it cannot be transferred to someone else or for some other cause under any circumstances. According to this view, sacrificing one's life in suicide, martyrdom, or in an act of supreme altruism (e.g. a mother sacrificing her life for her child) would be deemed as morally wrong. Of course, we may ask the question whether the right to life is an inalienable right.

Absolute rights

An absolute right, by contrast, is a right which cannot be overridden under any circumstances. For example, if we take the right to life as being absolute, we would be bound to respect it whatever the cost. By this view, any wilful taking of human life, whether through war, self-defence, abortion, capital punishment, or any other act, would be morally wrong. Here the question arises whether the right to life really is an absolute right.

Prima-facie rights

A prima-facie (from the Latin *primus*, meaning 'first', and *facies*, meaning 'face') right is a right which may be overridden by stronger moral claims. For example, a patient's right to privacy may be overridden by the right to life in a cardiac arrest situation where the patient's body is exposed during the resuscitation procedure. In such an emergency, it would be misguided for an ethicist to insist that the patient's right to privacy should take priority in the situation at hand.

Some argue against the notion of prima-facie rights by saying that if a right can be overridden it does not exist. Against such a criticism, Martin and Nickel (1980: 172–4) comment:

> *to describe a right as Prima Facie is to say something about its weight but not about its scope or conditions of possession … Overridence depends on whether the case of conflict is central to the values that the right serves to protect or whether it is a marginal case and thus can be expected in all cases without great loss to those values.*

Making rights claims

Having a right usually entails that another has a corresponding duty to respect that right (Martin 2017). As Feinberg (1978: 1508) explains, when people assert their moral rights, they assert a kind of 'moral power' over us which we feel constrained to respect. Where claims have a special convincing force they have a coercive effect on our judgments, which in turn make us feel driven to both acknowledge and support the interest claims being made as being genuine rights claims.

Rights which entail a corresponding duty are typically referred to as 'claims rights'. These rights can be either positive or negative, and can entail either a positive or a negative rights claim. Positive rights claims generally entail a correlative duty to act or to do, in contrast with negative rights claims, which generally entail a correlative duty to omit or to refrain (Feinberg 1978: 1509). For example, if a patient claims a right not to be harmed, this claim imposes a negative duty on an attending nurse to refrain from acts which may cause harm. On the other hand, if a patient claims a right to be benefited in some way, such as by having an intolerable pain state relieved, this imposes a duty on an attending nurse to perform the positive act of promptly administering an effective analgesic. If a person's rights claims are not upheld, or are infringed or violated in some way, that person generally feels wronged or feels a serious injustice has been done. In a rights view of ethics, if someone claims a right this is generally regarded as providing a 'moral reason' (a warranty) for taking moral action.

Rights and responsibilities

Any discussion on moral rights would not be complete without also considering the *responsibilities* that rights holders have when choosing to claim or exercise their rights in given contexts. The need to take into account the moral responsibilities associated with rights claims has become especially pressing in recent years on account of the rise-and-rise of 'unrestricted isolated individualism' (also called 'rampant individualism') in English-speaking democracies of the developed world (e.g. the United States, the United Kingdom (UK), Canada, Australia, New Zealand, and so forth) (see Dyck 2005; Glendon 1991; Nussbaum 2006; Young 1990). Paradoxically, this rampant individualism – sometimes decried in terms of 'people having all rights and no responsibilities' – is threatening to weaken and even nullify the very system of rights that, up until now, has served the significant moral interests of individuals, groups and even whole communities whose wellbeing has been at serious risk and even substantially harmed because of oppression, exploitation, violence and other harmful human behaviours perpetrated by more powerful and dominant others.

In recent years there has been increasing recognition (and criticism) of the tendency in classical moral rights theory to fail to take into account the fundamental connection between rights and responsibilities and, in particular, the responsibility that rights' holders have to exercise their rights in a *just and responsible manner*. This stance has given rise to a 'new' view of rights, notably, as a just expectation – that is, a state of being characterised by ties of mutually expected responsibilities to one another, as individuals and as members of groups and institutions (Dyck 2005: 117).

Referring to the classic works of the 19th century British philosopher John Stuart Mill, Dyck (2005: 115) contends that, since rights are fundamentally rooted in justice, then rights must themselves be exercised 'justly'. Quoting Mill ('Justice implies something which is not only right to do, and wrong not to do, but which some persons can claim from us as his [sic] moral right'), Dyck (p. 115) explains that, since justice is itself a 'moral responsibility', in the context of rights claims this imposes an obligation on people:

> *(1) to honour rights that justifiably claim one or another of our various moral responsibilities, and (2) to claim from other individuals, groups, or institutions only those actions for which they can be held morally responsible.*

Dyck goes on to caution that irresponsible rights claims stand to not only violate the principle of justice but also, in doing so, weaken the claims themselves. Irresponsible claims thus stand as 'violations' (i.e. of 'just expectations' that bona fide rights claims will be exercised responsibly) that, in turn, threaten to tear (and, as racial violence and civil war can readily attest, has torn) the moral fabric of communities apart. Dyck further cautions that unless individuals, groups and social institutions claiming rights 'are willing and able to act responsibly' – by which he means 'act to maintain the moral bonds of community' – then those rights 'are not and cannot be actualised' (Dyck 2005: 114). In other words, the failure to exercise rights claims *justly* and *responsibly* could nullify the rights claims altogether, something that could have serious consequences at both a practical and a theoretical level. In contrast, exercising given rights claims justly and responsibly actually *strengthens* the rights claims being made. Moreover, by recognising the responsibilities that come with rights, claimants help to form and maintain what Dyck (p 132) calls the 'inhibitions against causing evil', notably, 'destroying individuals and human relations' and the human wellbeing that is otherwise so dependent on these relations being maintained in a manner that is just and nurturing.

Problems with rights claims

In discussing rights it is important to keep in mind at least six central problems that can arise when dealing with rights claims. First, rights and interests can seriously compete and conflict with one another. For example, a patient's right to life could seriously compete or conflict with another patient's right to life in a situation involving scarce medical resources; or a nurse's conscientious refusal to assist with an abortion procedure could conflict with a patient's right to have an abortion and to receive care following the procedure. In such instances there may be no easy solution to the conflict of interests at hand.

Second, it may be difficult to establish the extent to which a person's rights claim entails a correlative duty. For example, if someone claims a right to life, who or what has the corresponding duty to respond to that claim? Does it fall to the health professional, or to family, friends, the hospital, the state or another entity? There may be no satisfactory answer to this question.

Third, there may be disagreement about which entities have rights. For example, some might argue that brain-dead people, anencephalic babies, the intellectually impaired and babies do not have moral rights, while others might argue that they do. Again there may be no satisfactory resolution to this type of disagreement.

Fourth, it may be very difficult to try and satisfy the rights claims of all people equally. For instance, if there is a genuine lack of resources, it may be impossible to satisfy all rights claims. Once again, we are left, unhappily, with an unresolved moral problem.

Fifth, it may be very difficult to determine what counts as a responsible or an irresponsible rights claim and the conditions under which an irresponsible rights claimant might forfeit his or her entitlements (have their rights claims nullified).

Sixth, and more seriously, is the controversial claim that moral rights theory is not a comprehensive moral theory at all as, among other things, it is unable to explain, account for or justify the significance and motives of people's actions (Beauchamp & Childress 2013: 374). At best, it is argued, rights theory amounts to little more than a 'statement of minimal and enforceable *rules* protective of individual interests that communities and individuals must observe' (Beauchamp & Childress 2013: 374).

On account of these and other difficulties, some have sought to avoid a moral rights perspective altogether, or at least to replace the language of rights. (For example, when referring to people's moral entitlements, instead of using 'rights' language some writers use such terms as 'interests', 'welfare', 'wellbeing', and so on.) Others, however, defend the use of rights language despite the theoretical weaknesses of a moral rights perspective. Beauchamp and Childress (2013), for example, point out that, for many scholars, political activists and others, rights theory is probably the 'most important type of theory for expressing the moral point of view' (p. 367). They go on to explain:

> *No part of the moral vocabulary has done more in recent years to protect the legitimate interests of citizens in political states than the language of rights. Predictably, injustice and inhumane treatment occur most frequently in states that fail to recognise human rights in their rhetoric, actions and documents. As much as any part of moral discourse, human rights language crosses international boundaries and enters into international law and statements by international agencies and associations.* (Beauchamp & Childress 2013: 374–5)

Others have taken a similar stance adding that rights discourse has a 'high reputation' and, for all its weaknesses, continues to enjoy 'pervasive popularity' in the world at large (Campbell 2006: 1, 5). Reasons for the success of rights discourse have been identified by Campbell (2006: 1, 5) as involving the strong association it has with the language of:

- *imperatives* ('To have a right is to have something that overrides other considerations in both moral and legal discourse')
- *individualism* ('A society based on rights is believed to manifest and affirm the dignity of each and every human life as something that is deserving of the highest respect')
- *remedies* ('Rights are not associated with simply aspiring to do what is good or desirable but demand restraint, redress and rectification of wrong done in violation of rights')
- *decisiveness* ('By establishing what it is right and just to do, rights in particular circumstances and excluding other considerations as being of lesser significance, rights promise clear answers to moral problems')
- *security* ('Having rights enables us not only to enjoy certain benefits but to have knowledge that they are ours "by right" and cannot therefore be taken away at the whim of others')
- *universality* ('The generality of rights offers protection to individuals against arbitrary treatment, a feature which is most evident when universal rights are ascribed to all persons irrespective of the race, religion, class or gender').

The issue of moral rights is an important one for nurses – particularly as the issue relates to patients' rights, to the People's Health Movement (PHM), and also to the relationship that exists between health and human rights – all of which have been receiving increasing attention in recent years. As these are substantial issues in their own right, they are considered separately in Chapters 6–9 and 13 of this book.

Virtue ethics

In recent times there has been a resurgence of virtue theory in ethics and a re-examination of the importance of 'characterological excellence' as an ingredient of authentic moral conduct (Athanassoulis 2013; Hursthouse 1999, 2007; van Hooft 2006; van Hooft et al 2013). Virtue ethics holds a particular relevance for nursing since virtuous conduct is intricately linked to therapeutic healing behaviours and the promotion of human wellbeing.

Virtue ethics (also known as character ethics) has an impressive history dating back to the ancient philosophical and theological texts of both Western and non-Western cultures (Beauchamp & Childress

2013; Hursthouse 1999, 2007; Kruschwitz & Roberts 1987; Pellegrino 1995; van Hooft et al 2013). As Pellegrino (1995: 254) writes, 'Virtue is the most ancient, durable, and ubiquitous concept in the history of ethical theory.'

Despite its durability, virtue theory has nonetheless been in various stages of decline over the past several centuries – particularly within the field of Western moral philosophy. This decline can be traced to the rise of scientism. By the late 17th and 18th centuries, for instance, the 'Enlightenment project of finding a rational justification for morality' saw moralists look away from the law of God 'to actual, observable human nature for a justification of traditional moral norms' (MacIntyre 2007: 39; Kruschwitz & Roberts 1987: 12–13). Although virtue ethics has retained its currency in some fields – for example the medical profession up until as late as the 1970s (Pellegrino 1995: 264), and the nursing profession up until the present time (Armstrong 2006, 2007; Begley 2006; McKie & Swinton 2000) – its importance to and in moral philosophy has long been lost, having been neglected by philosophers preoccupied with turning ethics into a science.

Significantly, since the 1980s, there has been a revival in virtue-based theories of ethics (Athanassoulis 2013; Hursthouse 1999, 2007; Pellegrino 1995; Pence 1984; van Hooft 2006; van Hooft et al 2013). This revival (which has included both religious and non-religious approaches to virtue theory) has been driven by an increasing dissatisfaction and frustration among some philosophers with the otherwise narrow, abstract, impersonal and at times oversimplified approach of traditional obligation-based theories of ethics, and the need to find an alternative approach that is more reflective of and responsive to the complexities of the moral life. Of particular concern has been the questionable neglect within mainstream moral philosophy of considerations relating to the moral character of moral agents (persons who engage in moral actions). One aspect of this concern is expressed eloquently by Pence (1991: 256), who, commenting on what he sees as 'a common defect in non-virtue theories', points out:

> On the theories of duty or principle, it is theoretically possible that a person could, robot-like, obey every moral rule and lead the perfectly moral life. In this scenario, one would be like a perfectly programmed computer (perhaps such people do exist, and are products of perfect moral educations).

The idea that persons could function as 'moral robots' is both disturbing and unsatisfactory to virtue theorists, and, it might be added, to others who feel at least an intuitive unease about the prospect of morality being merely a matter of following a set of rules. We do seem to think, as Clouser (1995: 231) reminds us, that morality 'also encourages us to act in ways that go beyond what is required' – beyond a robot-like obedience to rules.

There does seem to be something 'missing' in the traditional picture of 'the moral life'. For virtue theorists, this 'something' is character. As Pence (1991: 256) writes:

> we need to know much more about the outer shell of behaviour to make such [moral] judgments, i.e. we need to know what kind of person is involved, how the person thinks of other people, how he or she thinks of his or her own character, how the person feels about past actions, and also how the person feels about actions not done.

Furthermore, there is a sense in which virtue theory is inevitable. As Pellegrino (1995: 254) points out:

> One cannot completely separate the character of a moral agent from his or her acts, the nature of those acts, the circumstances under which they are performed, or their consequences. Virtue theories focus on the agent; on his or her intentions, dispositions and motives; and on the kind of person the moral agent becomes, wishes to become, or ought to become as a result of his or her habitual disposition to act in certain ways.

Virtue theory raises some important questions, namely: (1) What is virtue?, (2) What constitutes a virtuous person? and (3) Given virtue theory, does virtue ethics offer a plausible and viable alternative to traditional obligation-based theories of ethics and the decision procedures they supply?

The notion of virtue

The term 'virtue' (from the Latin *virtus* meaning 'manliness', courage from *vir* meaning 'man') denotes the quality or practice of moral excellence. As an ingredient of moral theory, it can be defined as:

> *a trait or character that disposes its possessor habitually to excellence of intent and performance with respect to the telos specific to a human activity. Virtue gives to reason the power to discern and to will the motivation asymptomatically to accomplish a moral end with perfection.* (Pellegrino 1995: 268)

There are many examples of 'the virtues' (see, for example, the 52 virtues listed by the Virtues Project at www.virtuesproject.com/, which are presented as core ingredients that people may use to 'create a culture of character'). Some examples of the better-known moral virtues include: altruism, caring, compassion, cooperation, courage, diligence, empathy, excellence, fairness (justice), forgiveness, friendship, generosity, kindness, love, loyalty, personal integrity, reliability, respectfulness, sympathy, trustworthiness and wisdom (Beauchamp & Childress 2013; Hursthouse 1999, 2007; Kruschwitz & Roberts 1987; Pellegrino 1995; van Hooft 2006; van Hooft et al 2013).

The virtuous person

The notions of 'virtue' and 'virtuous persons' are both universal constructs. As Pellegrino (1995: 255) points out:

> *Every culture has a notion of the virtuous person – i.e., a paradigm person, real or idealised, who sets standards of noble conduct for a culture and whose character traits exemplify the kind of person others in that culture ought to be or to emulate.*

Such paradigm persons include: Buddha, Confucius, Jesus Christ, the Prophet Mohammed and, in more recent history, the Catholic nun Mother Teresa (Vardey 1995), hailed for her charitable works in India. Buddha, for instance, is renowned for exemplifying such perfections of character as 'forbearance, self-restraint, contentment, compassion, generosity, mildness, courage, meditation, and wisdom' (Hursthouse 2007: 45). Confucianism, in turn, is renowned for its emphasis on 'character traits that typify the good or noble person', notably: humanity, benevolence, compassion, wisdom, righteousness, courage, trustworthiness, filial piety and propriety (Hursthouse 2007: 45). Islam, which takes a religious rather than a philosophical perspective on virtuous actions, places strong emphasis on doing 'good deeds' and upholding the key virtues taught in the *Qur'an*, notably of 'justice, benevolence, piety, honesty, integrity, gratitude and chastity' (Halstead 2007: 284).

The question remains: what is a virtuous person? In a purely virtue-based theory of ethics, morally exemplary (virtuous) persons (including moral heroes and moral saints) are generally distinguished from other persons who 'do their duty' in a somewhat impersonal, impartial, universalistic rule-bound sense (Blum 1988). In a purely virtue-based ethic, a virtuous person is taken to be 'the good person, the person upon whom one can rely habitually to be good and to do the good under all circumstances' (Pellegrino 1995: 254). A virtuous person may also be described as someone who is 'truly excellent' in action and feeling – who, as Hursthouse asserts (2007: 50), '"gets things right" in both action and feeling'.

Blum (1988) takes the notion of virtuous persons even further to include what he calls 'moral heroes' and 'moral saints'. A moral hero, by his view, is someone:

- who brings about a great good (or prevents a great evil)
- who acts to a great extent from morally worthy motives
- whose moral-worthy motives are substantially embedded in his or her own personal psychology
- who carries out his or her moral project in the face of risk or danger
- who is relatively 'faultless' or has an absence of unworthy desires, dispositions, sentiments, and attitudes (adapted from Blum 1988: 199, 203).

A moral saint, in contrast, is not altogether different from a moral hero, except for one feature. According to Blum (1988: 204), moral saints share three features in common with moral heroes:

they are animated by morally-worthy motives, their morally-excellent qualities exist at a deep level of their personality or character, and they meet the standard of relative absence of unworthy desires.

The salient feature which distinguishes a moral saint from a moral hero, however, is that the moral saint exhibits 'a higher standard of faultlessness' *viz* the absence of unworthy desires (Blum 1988: 204).

Virtue theory, an ethic of care and nursing ethics

A virtue theory of ethics holds a particular pertinence for nursing ethics in terms of providing a theoretical foundation and justificatory framework for nurses' moral decision-making and actions when providing nursing care. One reason for this can be found in the fundamental link between 'the virtues' and 'the right attitudes' or 'characterological traits' (e.g. of care, compassion, empathy, presence) that are generally recognised as being both essential to and constitutive of a healing health-professional–client relationship – the nurse–patient relationship included.

Conversely, the professional ethics of nurses and in particular nursing's *ethic of care* hold a promising prospect for virtue ethics – in that it provides a domain within which 'the virtues' can be shown to have both moral and practical clout. As Pellegrino (1995: 266) writes:

Unlike general ethics, professional ethics offers the possibility of some agreement on a telos – that is, an end and a good. In a healing relationship between a health care professional and a patient, most would agree that the primary end must be the good of the patient. The healing relationship, itself, provides a phenomenological grounding for professional ethics that applies to all healers by virtue of the kind of activity that healing entails. In general ethics, on the other hand, at least at present, the analogous possibility for agreement on something so fundamental as the telos, end, or good of human life is so remote as to be practically unattainable.

Pellegrino (1995: 268–70) goes on to articulate seven virtues which he believes will define 'the "good" physician, nurse or other health professional' and which can be supplemented by other virtues:

1 'fidelity to trust and promise' (encompassing a recognition of the importance of trust to healing)
2 'benevolence' (noting that people seek to be helped not harmed)
3 'effacement of self-interest' (to help protect patients against being exploited)
4 'compassion and caring' (so that patients can be assisted in their healing in the fullest sense)
5 'intellectual honesty' (to ensure competent practice)
6 'justice' ('removing the blindfold and adjusting what is owed to the specific needs of the patient, even if those needs do not fit the definition of what is strictly owed') and
7 'prudence' (encompassing the qualities of practical wisdom and the ability to deal effectively with complexity).

Pellegrino's views can be readily applied to and indeed overlap with the tenets of nursing ethics. The agreed end or *telos* of the profession and practice of 'good' nursing is the promotion of health, healing and wellbeing, together with the alleviation of suffering, in individuals, groups and communities for whom nurses care. This end is a moral end, and one that carries with it a strong moral action guiding force for nurses insofar as it requires nurses to engage in the behaviours necessary to promote health, healing and wellbeing in people, and, when manifest, to alleviate their suffering. In light of these ends, and the nature of the means necessary to achieve them (i.e. 'good' nursing care), nursing thus stands fundamentally as a benevolent (virtuous) activity or, more precisely, a 'moral practice' that aims to discover (through assessment), make explicit and accomplish (through cooperation and negotiation) whatever is 'good' for (read as 'conducive to the health, healing and wellbeing of') the individuals, groups and communities for whose care nurses share responsibility (Gastmans et al 1998: 58).

In speaking of 'good' nursing care, it is important to clarify that something much more than merely 'competent' nursing care is being referred to. Rather, it is competent care integrated with a 'virtuous attitude' of caring. As Gastmans and colleagues explain (1998: 45, 53):

> *It is only by integrating a virtuous attitude of caring with the competent performance of care activities* (caring behaviour) *that* good care *can be achieved … Morally virtuous attitudes are an integral part of nursing practice, since this practice takes place within a human relationship where the nurse and the patient are the main actors … This is in essence what is meant by caring behaviour:* the integration of virtue and expert activity. [emphasis added]

'Virtuous caring' is integral to 'good' (moral) nursing practice (and, by implication, nursing ethics) in at least two important ways. First, virtuous caring or 'right attitudes' (which include the behavioural orientations of compassion, empathy, concern, genuineness, warmth, trust, kindness, gentleness, nurturance, enablement, respect, mutuality, 'giving presence' [being there], attentive responsiveness, mindfulness, providing comfort, providing a sense of safety and security, and others) have all been thoroughly implicated as effective nursing healing behaviours in the alleviation of human suffering (hence the notions in nursing of caring as healing *and* nursing as informed caring for the wellbeing of others) (Armstrong 2006, 2007; Geary & Hawkins 1991; Leftwich 1993; McKie & Swinton 2000; Swanson 1993). Such behavioural orientations have been demonstrated as making a significant and positive difference not only to a patient's existential sense of – and actual – 'wellbeing', but also to the effectiveness of drugs, to wound healing, and even to survival itself (it is well known, for example, that premature newborns will 'fail to thrive' in the absence of attentive, 'high-touch' and informed nursing care and may even die; similarly, it is known that adults who are deprived of meaningful care will fail to heal and may even die prematurely from life-threatening diseases) (Ching 1993; Dossey 1993; Gastmans et al 1998; Gaut & Leininger 1991; Kanitsaki 2000; Moore & Komras 1993).

Second, 'virtuous caring' plays an important theoretical role in providing an account of moral motivation in nursing to act in beneficent ways. For instance, whereas in obligation-based theories the motivation to act morally is thought to be derived from a rationally appraised commitment to 'do one's duty', in the case of virtuous caring the motivation to be moral is derived from 'v-rules' (described in 'Problems with virtue ethics') informed by moral sentiment (for instance, caring about a thing in some way (Rachels 1988: 20)), and specifically a nurse's affective involvement in (i.e. caring about) the patient's wellbeing. The explanation of Gastmans and colleagues (1998: 54) is worth quoting at length; they write:

> *In addition to the collection and availability of relevant information [to plan and implement patient care], the caring nurse needs to be affectively involved in the patient's wellbeing. The caring nurse needs to be emotionally touched by what happens to the patient, both in a positive and a negative sense. The cognitive and affective dimensions of the virtue of care are not rightly understood as merely two separate components – a cognition and a feeling state – added together, rather they inform one another. The (altruistic) virtue of care is more than a passive feeling state that has a person in a state of woe as their object. The (altruistic) virtue of care involves an active, motivational aspect as well, relating to the promotion of beneficent acts aimed at helping the other person. In other words, the caring nurse must be motivated to respond to the appeal of the patient. Common to the altruistic virtue of care is a desire for, or regard for, the good of the other (for his or her own sake). This desire prompts (intended) beneficent action when the nurse is in a position to engage in it.*

The agreed ethical standards of nursing require nurses to promote the genuine welfare and wellbeing of people in need of help through nursing care, and to do so in a manner that is safe, competent, therapeutically effective, culturally relevant and just. These standards also recognise that in the ultimate analysis nurses 'can never escape the reality that they literally hold human wellbeing in their hands' (Taylor 1998: 74), and accordingly must act responsively and responsibly to protect it. These requirements are demonstrably consistent with a virtue theory account of ethics. Thus, as Armstrong (2006: 117) concludes, virtue ethics provides a distinct and credible theoretical basis for nursing ethics on account of its four central tenets:

1. It provides a detailed account of moral character.
2. It provides a rich account of moral goodness.
3. It provides a plausible account of moral education.
4. It provides a natural and convincing account of moral motivation.

Virtue ethics and an ethic of care in nursing – some further thoughts

Consistent with a virtue theory account of ethics is a nursing-specific articulation of an 'ethic of care' – long regarded by many nurse theorists as the moral foundation, essence, ideal and imperative of nursing (Benner & Wrubel 1989; Bowden 1994; Carper 1979; Cooper 1991; Fry 1989a; Gaut 1992; Leininger 1990a; Roach 1987; Watson 1985). Despite this, there has been mounting criticism over the past few decades about the place of 'care' in nursing ethics and also about the nursing profession's claim to be the exclusive guardians of care (Barker et al 1995). These criticisms have ranged from describing an ethic of care as being 'hopelessly vague' and as 'obscuring more than it promotes' (Allmark 1995: 20) to rejecting that care is a virtue at all (Curzer 1993). Still others denigrate care as an untenable form of 'subjugation' of women on account of its apparent 'sexist service orientation' that could see women (nurses) carrying a disproportionate 'burden of care' in a society (or a system) that is, for the most part, careless (Puka 1989: 21). A brief response to some of these criticisms is warranted here.

First, as just demonstrated, a reflective articulation of an ethic of care in relation to the moral ends of nursing helps to clarify the precise behaviours expected of a 'good' nurse. It not only prescribes 'do good', but also describes what those 'goods' are (the promotion of health, healing and wellbeing, and the alleviation of suffering), and how to achieve them (through an integration of expert and virtuous caring comprising a range of 'healing-promoting behaviours'). Second, given the mutually beneficial nature of 'virtuous caring' (it has demonstrable positive outcomes for both the receiver and the giver of authentic virtuous care), there is room to suggest that 'caring' that is unjustly burdensome is not only not 'virtuous caring' but also not ethical. Arguments against 'virtuous caring' are thus not correctly aligned at the right target; they are, as it were, 'attacking a straw man'. Third, the criticisms are not convincing. For instance, in the case of the criticism that an ethic of care could be unduly burdensome on women (nurses), it is not immediately clear why it would be any more burdensome than, say, an obligation-based theory of ethics. As the example of the Biblical story of Abraham demonstrates (Abraham came close to sacrificing his only son to fulfil his duty of obedience to God), 'doing one's duty' can, in some circumstances, be an extremely burdensome thing to do and further may not be able to be done without sacrificing something of moral importance. Further, to suggest that nurses might in some way become enslaved or 'subjugated' by an ethic of care seems to imply erroneously that (and, it must be added, to perpetuate the patriarchal myth that) nurses qua nurses lack the discretion and moral competence necessary to decide for themselves what moral standards they will adopt and uphold; in short it seems to suggest, incorrectly in my view, that nurses will just 'follow slavishly' an ethic of care. Finally, these criticisms seem to overlook that an ethic of care is, paradoxically, protective of its practitioners in that it rejects symbiotic (over)emotional involvement with 'the other', emphasising instead moral virtue (characterological excellence) as its foundation (Gastmans et al 1998: 54–7).

If there remain lingering doubts about the fidelity and force of an ethic of care in nursing, we do not need to look far for examples of the consequences of nurses failing to uphold such an ethic. The widespread publicity that has been given to what has been variously called 'a crisis of compassion' (Hehir 2013: 109) and 'crisis of care' (Darbyshire & McKenna 2013: 305) in nursing in the UK is such an example. Drawing on the findings of a series of damning reports on the British health care system (circa 2011–13), this crisis has involved the graphic public portrayal of nurses as being ambivalent, insensitive, uncompassionate, disengaged and, worse, of causing distress, danger and even death to patients (Darbyshire & McKenna 2013; Hehir 2013; Roberts & Ion 2014; Scott PA 2014). Scott is unequivocal in his supposition regarding what lies at the root of this crisis, namely: missing *qualities of character* or more specifically missing *virtues of character* (Scott PA 2014). Virtues of character, he contends, are essential to the nurse's ability to provide 'constructive care' – care that is patient oriented, committed, attentive, humanising and 'rooted in the needs of the individual patient' (p 177). To this end, the qualities of character (virtues) that nurses require need to be cultivated through education and role-modelling and, importantly, become embedded as 'enduring dispositions of character' approached from the perspective of 'habituated good nursing behaviour' vis-à-vis the excellences of nursing practice (Scott PA 2014: 177).

Problems with virtue ethics

Virtue ethics, like other theories of ethics, is not free of difficulties. Key among these are: the 'circularity of justification' in virtue theory (virtuous persons do what is good, the good is what virtuous persons do), the inability of virtue theory to explain adequately its force as a moral action guide (i.e. compared with other obligation-based theories that can rely on moral rules, principles and maxims to justify moral conduct), and the high expectations that virtue theory imposes on people to be 'good' (while a good many of us can be conscientious in our actions, few of us can be 'exemplary' (Pellegrino 1995: 262–3)). These difficulties, however, may be more a product of the adversarial nature of philosophical inquiry and its use to critically examine and raise objections to virtue theory, than a problem with virtue ethics itself. For instance, given the distinctive non-rational quality of the moral virtues, it seems odd to suggest that virtuous actions require 'justification'. (How does one 'justify' an inclination to be kind towards another, or to be fair? How does one 'justify' an act of saintliness or heroism?) Similarly, it seems odd to expect that virtue theory can be reduced to a set of justificatory rules, principles and maxims (noting that what makes the virtues what they are is their often spontaneous and unconditional expression beyond that otherwise required by rules, principles and maxims). There is room here to suggest that to 'justify' the virtues in a rational philosophical sense is to do violence to them and to all that they represent. Finally, it seems odd to suggest that expecting people to be 'decent' and 'morally excellent' human beings is 'too high an expectation'. Ethics is precisely about expecting people to strive to achieve the highest ideals of morality and to engage in morally excellent conduct. Virtue ethics is no different in this regard. That people may not achieve such an ideal is no reason to abandon ethics, and it is no reason to abandon virtue ethics either.

It is generally accepted that, although virtue theory cannot stand alone, it can be (and should be) 'related to other ethical theories in a more comprehensive moral philosophy than currently exists' (Pence 1984: 282; see also Pellegrino 1995: 254). Over the past two decades, scholars have shown that, contrary to the criticisms that have conventionally been directed against it, virtue ethics and 'the virtues' do provide an account of right action. Moreover, like other obligation-based theories, virtue ethics also includes rules – what Hursthouse (1999: 36) calls 'v-rules' (e.g. 'do what is honest', 'do what is kind', 'do what is charitable') – and thus is mostly compatible with traditional obligation-based theories (e.g. principles and rules). And where there exists a correspondence between virtue ethics (e.g. the virtues) and other moral theories (e.g. ethical principlism), even though 'rough and imperfect', they tend to be mutually reinforcing (Beauchamp & Childress 2013: 381). For example, respect for the principle of autonomy requires the virtue of respectfulness, commitment to and upholding the principle of beneficence requires the virtue of benevolence, and upholding the principle of non-maleficence requires the virtue of non-malevolence (Beauchamp & Childress 2013: 381).

Deontology and teleology

This discussion on moral theory would not be complete without reference being made to two main 'parent' theories of ethics, namely: *deontology* and *teleology* (also called consequentialism, of which utilitarian theory is a form).

Deontology

'Deontology' comes from the Greek *deon*, meaning 'duty', and *logos*, meaning 'word' or 'reasoned discourse'. According to deontological ethics, duty is the basis of all moral action. Taken at its most basic, the discourse of deontology asserts that some acts are obligatory (duty-bound) regardless of their consequences. For example, a deontologist might assert that one has a duty to always tell the truth. By this view, the deontologist is duty-bound to always tell the truth even when doing so might have horrible consequences. An important question to be asked here is: 'How do we know what our duty is?'

One possible answer to this question can be found in classical deontological theory that derives from religious ethics. According to this view, it is God's command that determines our moral duties. If, for example, God commands 'thou shalt not kill', 'thou shalt not steal' and the like, then conduct that accords with (obeys) these commands is morally praiseworthy (right and justified). This is 'because and only because it is commanded by God' (Frankena 1973: 28).

There are many examples of deontological ethics influencing decision-making in health care domains. For example, Jehovah's Witnesses are well known for their refusal of life-saving blood transfusions, on the grounds that to accept such treatment would be tantamount to violating God's command that, according to their beliefs, prohibits taking blood (Fry & Johnstone 2008). Another example can be found in a deontological adherence by some physicians and surgeons to the preservation of 'medically hopeless' human life whatever the costs (read consequences) resulting in the administration of 'futile' medical treatment to patients — sometimes even against their will (Schneiderman & Jecker 2011).

Another answer can be found in what is otherwise known as ethical rationalism. This view dates back to the work of the 18th century German philosopher Immanuel Kant, who held that the supreme principle of morality was reason, whose ultimate end is good will. According to a 1972 translation, Kant stated that reason is free (autonomous) to formulate moral law and to determine just what is to count as being an overriding moral duty. Kant held duty to be that which is done for its own sake, and 'not for the results it attains or seeks to attain' (Kant 1972: 20 ('The formal principle of duty', in original pp 13–14)). Kant further believed that moral considerations (duties) were always overriding in nature — in other words, should take precedence over other (non-moral) considerations.

In terms of determining what one's actual duty is, Kant suggested that this can be done by appealing to some formal (reasoned) principle or maxim. In choosing such a maxim, however, Kant warned that we must take care not to choose something that would privilege our interests over the interests of others. Kant's solution to this problem was to establish a universally valid law called the 'categorical imperative'. This law states: 'Act only on that maxim through which you can at the same time will that it should become universal law' (Kant 1972: 29 ('The formula of universal law', in original pp 51–2)). In other words, we should act only on maxims that we are prepared to accept as holding for everybody (including ourselves) throughout space and time. A variation of Kant's law can be found in what is popularly known as the Golden rule: 'Do unto others as you would have them do unto you'.

Teleology

'Teleology' comes from the Greek *telos*, meaning 'end', and *logos*, meaning 'word' or 'reasoned discourse'. According to teleological theory (also known as consequentialism) actions can be judged right and/or good only on the basis of the consequences they produce. In this respect, discourse on teleological ethics denies everything that deontological ethics asserts.

The most popularly known teleological theory of ethics is *utilitarianism*, which has as its central concern the general welfare of people as a whole, rather than individuals. In short, utilitarianism views the world not in terms of certain individual rights, which people may or may not claim, but rather in terms of people's collective and overall welfare and interests. The perspective of utilitarianism is persuasive in that it promotes a universal point of view – namely, that one person's interests cannot count as being superior to the interests of another, just because they are personal interests (Singer 1993; Smart & Williams 1973). To put this another way, I cannot claim that my interests are more deserving than your interests are, just because they are my interests.

Classical utilitarianism, first advanced by the English philosopher Jeremy Bentham (1748–1832) and later modified by the work of the British philosopher John Stuart Mill (1806–73), holds roughly that moral agents have a duty to 'maximise the greatest happiness / good for the greatest number' (Bentham 1962; Mill 1962). This view has resulted in classical utilitarianism being dubbed the 'greatest happiness principle'. Because of difficulties associated with calculating both individual and collective happiness and unhappiness, and the problem of individual interests being sacrificed for the collective whole, classical utilitarianism theory has been largely abandoned in favour of more recent utilitarian theories. Of particular note is preference utilitarianism, which views the maximisation of autonomy and individual preferences as being of intrinsic value rather than the maximisation of happiness per se. This is because, as Beauchamp and Childress (2013: 356) explain, what is intrinsically valuable is what individuals prefer to obtain, and utility is thus translated into maximising 'the overall satisfaction of the preferences of the individuals affected'.

Although not without difficulty, preference utilitarianism is also considered more plausible since it is relatively easy to calculate what people's preferences are: all we have to do is to ask people what it is they prefer. And where their preferences are at odds with ethical conduct, we have no obligation to respect them.

Moral duties and obligations

Common to all theoretical perspectives are the imperatives they impose for behaving in ways that respect the significant moral interests of others. It is generally accepted within moral philosophy that moral theories, moral principles and moral rights all provide sound moral reasons for deciding and acting (behaving) in certain ways towards others and for explaining why we should act morally. For example, the moral principle of autonomy and the moral right to informed consent both seem to provide strong reasons ('moral warrants') for giving information to patients / clients and why – that is, to enable them to make prudent and intelligent choices about their care and treatment. More than this, they impose a moral duty on us to do so. To understand what this means and how duties (and their counterparts, obligations) 'bind' us to be moral, it would be useful here to explain what duties and obligations are and how they work.

Moral duties

A moral duty (to be distinguished here from a legal duty, a civil duty, a professional duty and so on) is an action which a person is bound, for moral reasons, to perform. Language used in identifying duties typically involves expressions such as: 'I have a duty to …', 'You have a duty to …', 'They have a duty to …' and so on.

Duties are primarily concerned with avoiding intolerable results; they are thought to provide the basic requirements that may be demanded of everybody (i.e. universally) in an effort to achieve a 'tolerable basis of social life' (Urmson 1958, in Feinberg 1969: 73). They also work 'to secure reliability, a state of affairs in which people can reasonably expect others to behave in some ways and not in others' (Williams 1985: 187). If a duty fails to avoid an intolerable result, there is room for questioning whether in fact it was a duty in the first place (Urmson 1958). It might also be argued that if a duty can be overridden (e.g. where there appears to be a conflict of duties) it is not a duty at all; we have merely mistakenly thought that it was (Hare 1981: 26). On the other hand, it might be replied that just because a duty can be overridden this does not mean 'it was not a duty in the first place' but only that it was a 'prima-facie duty'. There is nothing philosophically wrong in holding that duties can be prima facie in nature (Ross 1930: 19).

As already stated, moral reasons binding people to act in certain ways can be provided from the following sources: a moral theory, a moral principle or a moral right. For example, from a teleological perspective, duties generally derive from the consideration of some predicted moral consequence that ought to be furthered or upheld. It might be argued, for instance, that one has a stringent moral duty to prevent otherwise-avoidable harmful consequences from occurring where this can be done without sacrificing other important moral interests. Given this 'teleological reason', if a person's action stands to prevent a particular harmful consequence from occurring, that person is duty-bound to perform that action, provided other important moral interests are not sacrificed in the process. An off-duty nurse, for example, could be said to be duty-bound to render life-saving care at the scene of a road accident, regardless of any inconvenience this might cause, since mere inconvenience is not generally regarded as a morally significant consideration. If the life of the nurse were put at risk, however, the moral duty to render assistance would not be so clear-cut.

Similarly in the case of ethical principlism – for example, the ethical principles of autonomy, non-maleficence, beneficence and justice all provide moral reasons binding people to act in certain ways towards others: the principle of autonomy, for instance, imposes on people a duty to respect the preferences and related decisions of others, the principle of non-maleficence imposes on people a duty not to harm others, the principle of beneficence imposes on people a duty to treat others well (beneficially), and the principle of justice imposes on people a duty to treat others fairly.

In a rights view of morality, and in contrast to the above approaches, a moral reason is supplied by a correlative rights claim. Thus if someone claims a right to be respected, this imposes on us a duty to respect that person; likewise, if someone claims a right to privacy, this imposes on us a duty not to disclose information of a private nature about that person, and so on.

The critical task for each of us is to decide just what our moral duties are. This, of course, is dependent on correctly determining what is to count as an overriding moral reason for doing something or, as in the case of rights, correctly determining whether a given rights claim is genuine and, further, whether we as moral agents do in fact have a duty correlative to the claim in question.

Moral obligations

A notion that is strongly related to the notion of 'moral duty' is that of 'moral obligation'. The language of obligations is very similar to the language of duties, and typically involves expressions such as: 'You have an obligation to ...', 'I have an obligation to ...', 'We have an obligation to ...', 'They have an obligation to ...' and so on. Although many philosophers treat the terms 'duties' and 'obligations' synonymously, an important and useful distinction can be drawn between them, which rests on the differing moral strengths each notion has rather than on a difference in their essential moral nature. Duties are regarded as having a stronger force than obligations, or, to put this another way, duties are more morally compelling than are obligations. Dworkin (1977: 48–9), an influential exponent of this distinction, gives the example that it is one thing to say a person has an obligation to give to a charity, but it is quite another to say that person has a duty to do so. Although it would be 'good' if someone made a charitable donation, it would be a mistake to suggest a moral compulsion to do so. To a limited extent, Dworkin's thesis helps to alleviate the tension created by the problem of supposed conflicting duties.

The concept of obligation and its distinctiveness from duty has interesting and important implications for nurses, particularly in relation to the issue of following a doctor's or a supervisor's directives. For instance, it may well be that nurses have an obligation to follow a doctor's or a supervisor's directives, but it is far from clear that they always have a *duty* to do so, either morally or legally. In fact, if a doctor's or a supervisor's directives are 'dubious', a nurse has both a legal and a moral duty to question such directives. In some cases, the nurse may even have a duty to refuse to follow a given directive if, for instance, it is 'unreasonable', 'unlawful' or 'unethical' – for example, likely to cause otherwise avoidable harm.

Clarifying the difference between rights and duties

Before concluding this discussion, the important task remains of clearing up some confusion which some nurses may have about their own rights and duties in relation to caring for patients. Consider, for example, a situation involving an abortion procedure. A nurse could reasonably claim either a right to refuse to participate in an abortion procedure or a duty to refuse to participate. What is important here is to distinguish the basis upon which each claim might rest and to remember that, whereas rights basically concern claims about one's own interests, duties basically concern claims about the interests of others. Thus, in an abortion case, if a nurse claims the right to refuse this is fundamentally a claim involving the protection of the nurse's own interests (as opposed to the interests of the patient). The nurse might, for instance, have a religious-based conscientious objection to abortion and assert an entitlement to practise the tenets of that faith. A refusal based on a duty claim is significantly different, however. In this instance, the refusal is based more on the consideration of another's interests – for example, the interests of the patient or the fetus. Here the duty to refuse would derive from the broader moral duty to, say, prevent harm or to preserve life.

By this brief account it can be seen that to use the terms 'rights' and 'duties' interchangeably is not only incorrect but misleading. When nurses speak of their right to, say, care for a patient in a certain way, or to practise their code of ethics, it is quite possible they are really asserting that they have a duty to care for the patient in that way or a duty to uphold their code of ethics.

Limitations and weaknesses of ethical theory

Over the past several decades, there has been mounting dissatisfaction among some moral philosophers in regard to the ability of commonly accepted moral theories to provide an adequate account of moral conduct and the 'moral life', and to provide practical guidance on how to deal with concrete everyday ethical problems. There has also been a related dissatisfaction with bioethics and its apparent (in)ability to deal effectively with ethical issues in health care and related domains and to guide practical solutions to the many complex ethical problems encountered in those domains. Feminist moral philosophers have been among the most ardent critics arguing that moral theory (particularly traditional or mainstream moral theory):

- is too abstract to be able to deal effectively with the concrete circumstances of life
- pays too much attention to upholding abstract rules and principles, rather than: (1) promoting quality relationships between people and (2) upholding the genuine welfare and wellbeing of people
- has tended to privilege dominant groups over marginalised groups (more specifically, it has tended to privilege the interests and concerns of white, middle-class, able-bodied, heterosexual, politically conservative males at the expense of those deemed 'other', and hence inferior – for example, women and children, people of non-English-speaking and culturally diverse backgrounds, people with disabilities, gay men and lesbians, people from lower socio-economic backgrounds, the uneducated and so on)
- places emphasis on rational argument that has tended to fuel rather than quell moral controversy, disagreement and distress

- has failed on account of its augmentative and adversarial approach tending to divide rather than unite and reconcile people in common bonds (see, for example, Card 1991; Code et al 1998; Cole & Coultrap-McQuin 1992; Gibson 1976; Gilligan 1982; Hekman 1995; Kittay & Meyers 1987; Little 1996; Noddings 1984; Porter 1991; Tronto 1993; Walker 1998; Wolf 1996).

In several respects the criticisms levelled at both traditional and contemporary moral theory have been warranted, especially those criticisms that have been advanced from the perspectives of feminist ethics. There is ample evidence to suggest that ethical theory, as it has been traditionally taught and considered, has been too far removed from the realities of practice and has failed too often to provide practical guidance on how to respond effectively to the complex moral questions of day-to-day living and practice. It is evident therefore that what has been called 'spaceship ethics' (i.e. a conception of ethics that operates from 'the secluded comfort of the arm chair' or from 'abstract apriori principles from which it hopes to derive answers to complicated, real-life practical problems') needs to change (Benjamin 2001: 29). Its opposite, however, 'subway ethics' – an approach 'that would have us focus on particular cases and contexts with little or no concern for theory' – is not the answer either (Benjamin 2001: 29). As Benjamin explains (p 29):

> *If spaceship ethics is too far removed from the concrete ethical problems that actually trouble us, subway ethics is too close to them.*

Where then lies the solution? For all the criticisms and controversies generated in response to ethical theory, one thing is clear: the solution is not to abandon it, but to enrich it. As Little explains (2001: 33):

> *whatever one thinks about them [the criticisms], they are clearly objections to* impoverished *moral theory, not to* moral theory *per se*. [emphasis added]

What is needed, therefore, is a richer moral theory (or, more to the point, moral theories) that is more responsive to the practical lived realities and complexities of everyday life. Whether we wish to admit it or not, ethical theory is 'essential to moral life' insofar as it provides useful generalisations that can be used to teach, to persuade others to accept, and to justify morally worthy points of view (Little 2001: 39).

With or without 'grand theories' of ethics, the fact remains that we all theorise about and try to make sense of our moral experiences. As Little (2001) contends, it is not enough to know *that*, we also need to know *why*, and we cannot know why without some kind of theoretical abstraction. In other words, the moral landscape simply cannot be understood without theoretical reasoning. But neither can the moral landscape or our moral experiences be understood simply by adopting or applying one or two 'master' concepts or principles or theories of ethics (Little 2001: 33). It is for this reason that we need to engage constantly in the positive project of constructing and developing alternative models, methods, procedures and discourses of ethics that are more responsive to the lived realities and experiences of people and the social–cultural contexts within which they live (Gross 1986). A key aim of this book is to assist nurses to engage in such a project.

Moral justification and moral theory – some further thoughts

The discussion in this chapter has shown that moral theory not only has an important role to play, but also is essential in terms of enabling people to give meaning and order to their everyday moral experiences. Moral / ethical theory does this by helping people to describe the moral world, devise meaningful moral standards and ideals, distinguish ethical issues from other sorts of issues, and provide a systematic justification of the actual practice of morality. When well developed, a moral / ethical theory 'provides a framework within which agents can reflect on the acceptability of actions and can evaluate moral judgments and character' (Beauchamp & Childress 1994: 44). It should be added, however, that 'good' ethical practice also provides a framework for evaluating and reflecting on what constitutes a well-developed mature ethical theory. In several respects, therefore, the relationship between moral theory and ethical practice is symbiotic; just as ethical practice cannot be evaluated independently of its theoretical underpinnings, neither can moral theory be evaluated independently of moral experience (see also Chappell 2009).

Ethical experience may, however, provide more than an evaluative framework for guiding theoretical reflections; in several respects it provides an important methodological starting point for developing moral theory (both 'ordinary' and 'formal'). Moreno (1995: 113), for example, defending what he calls 'ethical naturalism', persuasively argues that 'moral values emerge from *actual human experience* and are not superimposed on it by some transcendental reality' [emphasis added]. Clouser (1995: 228) takes a similar position. He states:

> Ordinary moral experience is our starting point. After all, morality cannot be invented. 'Look, here's my idea for a new morality … those with the most education get to say what happens to anyone with less education …!' We must begin with the moral system that is actually used by thoughtful people in making decisions and judgments about what to do in particular cases. Ordinary morality is generally expressed in what can be regarded as moral rules – e.g. don't cheat, don't kill, don't lie – and moral ideals – e.g. relieve pain, promote freedom, help the needy. If one were just initiating a study of morality as it is practiced, these rules and ideals would constitute the demarcations of the moral realm; they are the earmarks of morality at work; they are the phenomena on which the study would focus. [emphasis original]

The importance of moral experience in nursing and its relationship to the development and refinement of nursing ethics will be explored further in the chapters to follow.

Conclusion

In this chapter, attention has been given to clarifying the relationship between moral theory and ethical nursing practice. Particular attention has been given to examining the nature and importance of moral justification to moral decision-making and how various ethical theories (e.g. ethical principlism, moral rights theory, virtue ethics and an ethic of care) work to provide 'good reasons' for deciding and acting morally towards others. The notions of 'duties' and 'obligations' and the distinction between 'rights' and 'duties' have also been clarified. Having now considered what ethics is, and why nurses should be (i.e. have a duty to be) ethical, and having examined a number of different ethical frameworks within which nurses can operate to guide their moral decisions and conduct, there remains the task of exploring further some of the issues that nurses will encounter during the course of their work. Here it may be asked: 'What kinds of issues are nurses likely to encounter in health care contexts?', 'What "ethical competencies" do nurses need in order to address the issues they encounter?' and 'How should nurses respond to the ethical issues they encounter?' It is to examining these and related questions that the following chapters will now turn.

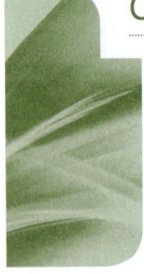

Case scenario 1

A 73-year-old woman is discharged from hospital following treatment for a leg ulcer and is referred to the local district nursing service for follow-up wound care. The district nurse arrives for the first scheduled visit only to discover that the woman is living in extreme squalor: almost every room of the house is cluttered with rubbish (newspapers, discarded clothing, crockery) and there seems to be hundreds of meals-on-wheels containers stacked in the fridge and freezer, as well as a number of open containers on the floor – most with rotting food inside. The toilet is broken and the kitchen barely useable. Worst of all, the house has an unbearable stench – which was detectable from the street. It later became apparent that this woman had 'flown under the radar'

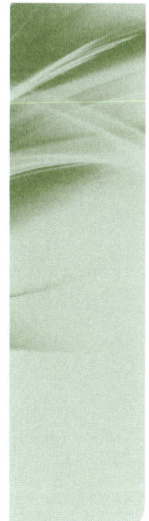

because she otherwise appeared 'normal and presentable' to those with whom she came into contact – including her neighbours. It was only when passers-by started to notice the stench emanating from the house that suspicions started to be aroused.

The nurse, shocked by what she had encountered, sought to discuss with the woman possible options for improving her living conditions and wellbeing – for example, having the house cleaned up by an approved provider, implementing support services, and the like. The woman, however, refused any hint of an intervention being made and stated emphatically that she 'does not want any help' and 'just wants to be left alone'. Deeply concerned about the woman's welfare the nurse immediately reports back to her team what she has found and the need to report the case to authorities. Not all members of her team agree, however, and argue that as it seems the woman has 'always lived in squalid conditions' she 'should be free to live the way she chooses' – that 'there was a duty to respect her autonomous wishes'. The nurse is perplexed by this response and raises the possibility that although appearing 'normal' the woman could nonetheless be suffering from Diogenes Syndrome (a distinct medical syndrome whereby people living in the community deviate from societal standards of hygiene and cleanliness) or some form of cognitive impairment. At the very least, the nurse argues, the woman should be referred to and properly assessed by the regional health service's psychogeriatric assessment team. She points out that the psychogeriatric assessment team not only provides comprehensive assessment of clients, but also has the capacity to provide supportive interventions and interim case management of those referred to it.

Case scenario 2

A school nurse is approached by a 13-year-old female student for information about having a human papilloma virus (HPV) vaccination. She has learned via social media that HPV vaccination is a safe and effective vaccine administered to prevent HPV infections – in particular, cervical cancer. She discloses to the nurse that her grandmother had cervical cancer and that she is afraid of also getting the disease 'when I am older'. She tells the nurse that she has accessed information on the internet recommending that HPV vaccination be administered to girls between the ages of 9 and 13 years, and that this will provide protection for between 5 and 10 years. She tells the nurse that 'her friends have had the vaccination without any dramas' and that she wants to have the vaccination too. She reveals that she has tried to discuss the matter with her parents and to obtain their permission for her to go to their GP and have the vaccination. They refused to discuss the matter, however, and would not give their consent for her to go to the family GP. She tells the nurse that her parents are 'very religious' and 'don't believe in vaccinations'. She further states that they were 'disgusted' with her wanting 'this particular vaccine' as only girls who were 'promiscuous' needed to have it.

CRITICAL QUESTIONS

1   What are the ethical issues raised by these cases?
2   What would you have done in the situations described?
3   Upon what basis would you have justified your decisions and actions?
4   What are the possible harms and benefits of the nurses intervening in these two cases?

Give reasons for your answers.

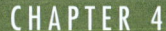
CHAPTER 4

Cross-cultural ethics and the ethical practice of nursing

KEYWORDS

cross-cultural ethics
cultural competency
cultural humility
cultural safety
culture
ethics
moral diversity
moral imperialism
moral pluralism
nocebo phenomenon
placebo effect

LEARNING OBJECTIVES

Upon the completion of this chapter and with further self-directed learning you are expected to be able to:
- Explain what is meant by the notion of 'culture'.
- Discuss the critical relationship between culture and ethics.
- Examine critically the nature and implications of applying cross-cultural ethics in nursing and health care contexts.
- Discuss the ways in which ignoring cultural considerations in nursing and health care contexts could adversely affect the significant moral interests of patients, families and communities from diverse cultural and language backgrounds.
- Discuss the relevance of cultural competency, cultural safety and cultural humility when dealing with ethical issues involving patients and families of diverse cultural and language backgrounds.
- Outline at least four questions that nurses should ask in order to assess their own cultural–moral competency to make moral decisions when caring for people of diverse cultural and language backgrounds.
- Discuss how nurses might cultivate the quality and ethos of cultural humility in nursing practice domains.

Introduction

The world in which we all live is characteristically multicultural in its nature and outlook. In 2004 the United Nations Development Programme (UNDP) estimated that more than 5000 different ethnic groups live in just 200 countries. The UNDP further estimated that in 'two out of every three countries there is at least one substantial ethnic or religious minority group, representing 10 percent of the population or more' (Fukuda-Parr 2004: 2). Today, due to the variety of criteria, characterisations and contexts that might be used to identify ethnic groups and nationalities, and the differing connotations that might be applied to these, accurately quantifying the ethnocultural characteristics of nations and the world is difficult (United Nations Statistics Division 2018). Likewise, quantifying countries – Worldometer, for example, states there are 195 countries in the world. This number, however, does not include a number of 'countries' which may fall under the jurisdictions of another 'recognised' country, for example, Taiwan, the Cook Islands, Niue, Dependences, and other countries not recognised by the United Nations as 'self-governing' (http://www.worldometers.info/geography/how-many-countries-are-there-in-the-world). Despite these difficulties, it is generally agreed that there are probably 'thousands' of different ethnic groups in the world and that most nations are composed of people from diverse cultural and language backgrounds (see, for example, https://www.infoplease.com/ethnicity-and-race-countries).

One of the greatest challenges facing nurses and allied health care professionals working in multicultural societies is caring effectively, appropriately and ethically for people from diverse cultural and language backgrounds (Degrie et al 2017). One reason why caring for people from diverse cultural backgrounds is challenging is that professional caregivers do not always know, understand or share the same cultural meanings, set of assumptions about the world of experience, ultimate beliefs and moral values held by those for whom they care. This lack of knowledge and understanding of the different cultural world views and life-ways of different people can make it difficult for professional caregivers to provide care that is culturally appropriate, meaningful, therapeutically effective and ethically just. This difficulty is compounded if professional caregivers also do not have appropriate knowledge and understanding of the complex relationship that exists between culture, health and healing (therapeutic) behaviours.

It is well documented that cultural–language incongruence between patient and health care provider can also be problematic. Such incongruence can result not only in disagreements between professional caregivers, and between professional caregivers and patients and their families, but also in wrong judgments being made and 'wrong care', or what Kanitsaki (2000, 2003) calls 'toxic service', being provided. This, in turn, can result in the undesirable moral consequences of patients' safety and quality care and even their lives being placed in jeopardy, as examples to be given in this and the following chapters will show (see also de Bruijne et al 2013; Divi et al 2007; Johnstone & Kanitsaki 2006a, 2007a, 2007b; Rodriguez et al 2013; Schwappach et al 2012; Shadmi 2013; Smedley et al 2003; Suurmond et al 2010, 2011; van Rosse et al 2016; Vermeulen 2015; Wilson-Stronks et al 2008). Of relevance to this present discussion is that cultural–language incongruence between patient, family and health care provider can also result in distressing moral disagreements about care and treatment options, particularly in contexts involving the provision of end-of-life care (Bullock 2011; Candib 2002; Chater & Tsai 2008; Gysels et al 2012; Johnstone 2012b; Johnstone & Kanitsaki 2009a; Sarafis et al 2014; Van Keer et al 2015).

In order to respond effectively to the challenges posed by caring for people from diverse cultural and language backgrounds, nurses and their co-workers need to have a robust understanding of the nature of *culture* and its relationship to *ethics*. What particularly needs to be understood is that *culture exists logically prior to ethics*, and not the other way around as has been classically contended in moral philosophy and other related disciplines (Cook 1999; Edel & Edel 2000; Moser & Carson 2001; Sikka 2011). In other words, ethics and the various systems of ethics that exist are every bit the products of the cultures and the times from which they have emerged and which have shaped, developed, refined and sustained them. They are '*always* culture specific' and are never 'culture free' in the sense that their:

> *validity, applicability and moral forces of persuasiveness is [sic] dependent upon the assumption of a plethora of cultural categories … [which] operate tacitly as background assumptions in the architecture of reasoning.* (Abimbola 2013: 31)

In short, ethics and its derivatives have been, and continue to be, 'culturally constructed' (Cortese 1990: 1) – that is, they are *human inventions* (not naturally occurring material facts that are interwoven into the fabric of the observable world), which are ultimately learned and developed by living with others. One observer argues even further, contending that so substantive is the relationship between culture and ethics that multiculturalism is itself 'a universal moral theory in its own right' (Durante 2018).

Arguably one of the most cogent explanations concerning the relationship that exists between culture and ethics has been advanced by Yetzer and colleagues (2018), who persuasively argue that 'Cultural worldviews provide the standards that moral behavior should reflect, and against which moral judgments are made' (p 244). Drawing on the tenets of terror management theory (TMT),[1] which they situate as being complementary to other contemporary theories of human ethics, they explain that the moral standards imbedded in people's cultural world views serve as powerful buffers against the anxieties that can be evoked when reminded of the inevitability of their own mortality – that is, that 'we are all fated to die'. Moral judgments and moral behaviour, they argue, are 'central components of this anxiety buffering system' as they play an important role in determining people's evaluations of themselves and others. Because of this, people are highly motivated to uphold morality in both themselves and others (Yetzer et al 2018: 246). They explain:

> *Those who violate the moral dictates of our culture challenge their validity. A person who fails to abide by moral principles is implicitly suggesting that these principles do not always apply; because these principles are essential for our [symbolic] victory over death, moral transgressors must be punished accordingly. And because our own immortality, both literal and symbolic, depends on being a valued participant in the meaningful reality provided by our culture, we are compelled to live up to the moral prescriptions that we have accepted as the fabric of our reality.* (Yetzer et al 2018: 246)

They conclude that a better understanding of the relationship that exists between TMT and ethics – and the role that human ethics/morality plays in managing people's death-related anxieties (see also Johnstone 2012b) – could yield important insights into the problems that societies locally and globally are facing.

Cross-cultural ethics and nursing

Leininger (1990b: 49), a noted American leader in transcultural nursing, has made the important claim that 'culture has been the critical and conspicuously missing dimension in the study and practice of ethical and moral [sic] dimensions of human care'. She has also criticised nurse ethicists for their failure to recognise the important and significant role that culture plays in guiding moral judgments and behaviour in human care contexts. She contends further that some nurse ethicists have even 'deliberately avoided' the concept of culture altogether, preferring instead to assume the universality of the ethical principles, codes and standards of human conduct that have become so prevalent in mainstream nursing ethics discourse (p 51). Leininger concludes that, if nurses are to provide appropriate ethical care to individuals, families and groups of different cultural backgrounds, they must have knowledge of and the ability to uphold sensitively and in an informed way the culturally based moral values and beliefs of the people for whom they care (p 52). On this point, she states:

> *most assuredly, the evolving discipline of nursing needs an epistemic ethical and moral [sic] knowledge base that takes into account cultural differences and similarities in order to provide knowledgeable and accurate judgments that are congruent with clients' values and life-ways.* (Leininger 1990b: 52–3)

Without this knowledge base, Leininger contends, it is not possible for nurses to make the 'right' decisions or to provide the 'right' (ethical) human care when planning and implementing nursing care (p 64).

Questions remain, however: 'What is culture?' and, further 'What is culture's relationship to and role in ethics generally, and nursing ethics in particular?' It is to briefly answering these questions that this discussion now turns.

Culture and its relationship to ethics

Culture is an extremely complex concept, and one that has over time been defined, interpreted and analysed from a variety of disciplinary perspectives (see, for example, Beals 1979; Boyd & Richerson 2005; Bullivant 1981, 1984; Chase 2006; Fieldhouse 1986; Handwerker 2009; Helman 1990; Kluckhohn 1962; Kroeber et al 1952; Leininger 1991; Mead 1955; Midgley 1991a; Prinz 2012; Sorokin 1957; Tyler 1871; Wuthnow et al 1984). Not surprisingly, this has seen the emergence of a number of rival theories and viewpoints on what culture is, and on what its relationship to and role in human affairs is or should be. Even anthropologists do not agree about how culture should be defined, interpreted and analysed. Nevertheless, there is some agreement among scholars that culture is a human invention and one which is critical for human survival and the development of human potential.

What then is culture? As already stated, culture has been defined, interpreted and analysed in a variety of ways. For example, Tyler (1871), who is credited with providing the discipline of anthropology with its first modern definition of culture, defined it (p 1) as:

> that complex whole which includes knowledge, belief, art, morals, law, custom, and any other capabilities and habits acquired by man [sic] as a member of society.

Eight decades later, after undertaking a comprehensive review of the way in which Tyler's definition had been used, Kroeber and colleagues (1952) famously published a refined narrower definition, notably that culture 'consists of patterns, explicit and implicit, of and for behaviour [...] including their embodiment in artifacts' (p 181). From that time scholars and researchers continued to review and revise their ideas of 'What is this "thing" called culture?' Drawing on these foundational definitions, contemporary answers have included a range of definitions such as the following.

Cohen, for example, argues that (1968: 1):

> culture is made up of the energy systems, the objective and specific artefacts, the organisations of social relations, the modes of thought, the ideologies, and the total range of customary behaviour that are transmitted from one generation to another by a social group and that enables it to maintain life in a particular habitat.

Bullivant argues along similar lines, adding to the description of culture that it is something which (1981: 19):

> can be thought of as the knowledge and conceptions embodied in symbolic and non-symbolic communication modes about the technology and skills, customary behaviours, values, beliefs, and attitudes a society has evolved from its historical past, and progressively modifies and augments to give meaning to and cope with the present and anticipated future problems of its existence.

Another description of culture, however, and one which is very helpful to this discussion, comes from an Australian nursing scholar and first Professor of Transcultural Nursing (circa 2000–2005, retired 2005), Olga Kanitsaki AM (Member in the Order of Australia). Kanitsaki describes culture as follows (1994: 95):

> Culture includes a particular people's beliefs, value orientations and value systems, which give meaning, logic, worth and significance to their existence and experience in relation to both the universe and other human beings. These value orientations, value systems and beliefs in turn shape customs and traditions, prescribe and proscribe behaviour, determine the structure of social institutions and power relations, and identify and

prescribe social relations, modes and rules of communication, moral order, and, indeed, the whole spirit and web of meaning and purpose of a given group in a particular place and time. Culture thus reflects the shared history, traditions, achievements, struggles for survival and lived experiences of a particular people. Its influence extends over politics, economics, the development and use of technology, the boundaries and meaning of class, the determination of gender roles, and so on. [emphasis added]

Kanitsaki further explains that (2002: 22):

Culture can be seen as an inherited 'lens' through which individuals perceive and understand the world that they inhabit, and learn how to live within. Growing up within any society is a form of enculturation, formal and informal, whereby the individual slowly acquires the cultural 'lens' of that society. Without a common consciousness and shared perceptions of the world, both the cohesion and the continuity of any human group would be impossible.

Unfortunately, it is beyond the scope of this text to discuss the concept of culture at the level and depth it warrants, and its consideration must be left for another time. Nevertheless, there is room to emphasise the point that, regardless of the competing theories on what culture is, there is general agreement that culture encompasses a:

(more-or-less) coherent set of patterned and coordinated activities rationalized by a shared set of norms, which are rationalized by a shared set of assumptions about the world of experience. (Handwerker 2009: 16)

As such, it also plays a fundamental and critical role in mediating people's values, beliefs, perceptions and knowledge about the world within which they live, influences people's behaviour and generally gives logic and meaning to a whole way of life in that world, and ultimately provides the 'blueprint' for their (human) survival in that world (Kanitsaki 2000). Given these considerations, it is clear that culture's relationship to and role in ethics (including its relationship to the theoretical underpinnings and practical application of ethics) cannot be plausibly denied.

Nearly all of us know that there are in the world many people whose moral values and beliefs are radically different from our own (Midgley 1991a: 72). And we also know that in any one society there is likely to be a diversity of valid moral viewpoints and approaches (*moral pluralism*), and that this has created the possibility for, and the actuality of, irreconcilable moral disagreements, examples of which are given throughout this text (Elliott 1992; Johnstone 2012b). Questions arising here include: 'What, if any, is the best way to respond to moral pluralism?' and, more specifically: 'How should nurses respond to the challenge of what can be appropriately referred to as cross-cultural ethics?' It is to briefly answering these questions that this discussion now turns.

The nature and implications of a cross-cultural approach to ethics

It is not the purpose of this text to advance a substantive theory of cross-cultural ethics or cultural relativism, or to provide an in-depth study of the ethical concepts, theories and practices of the world's different cultural groups. Such a task is beyond the scope of this present work and requires much more space than it is possible to provide here. (See, meanwhile, Cortese 1990; Coward & Ratanakul 1999; Edel & Edel 2000; Elliott 1992; Fry & Johnstone 2008; Leininger 1990b; Macklin 1998; Marshall 1992; Midgley 1991a; Moser & Carson 2001; Singer 1991.) Nevertheless, it is important to have some understanding of the nature and implications of cross-cultural ethics (a form of ethical pluralism), and of how nurses might respond better to the challenges it poses.

One crucial point requiring understanding is that, while all societies have some sort of moral system for guiding and evaluating the conduct of their members, the moral constructs of one culture (e.g. North American or English culture) cannot always be applied appropriately or reliably to another culture – at least not without some modification (Silberbauer 1991: 15). Further, language usage alone, and the difficulties encountered in reaching accurate culturally thick (rich) translations of accepted moral terms and concepts, may even make meaningful moral discourse across cultures impossible (Stout 1988). These points have, however, been largely overlooked by mainstream (Anglo-American) moral philosophers, who have tended to support an imperialist model of morality (termed '*moral imperialism*') – that is, that their way of moral knowing and thinking is not only superior but 'right', and is thus something to be applied (read imposed) universally on to others whose moral systems they have judged to be inferior (Jenkins 2011; Midgley 1991a).

This is an inadequate and misleading approach to ethical practice, however, and one which warrants being questioned. Nevertheless, this does not mean that mainstream Anglo-American moral philosophy itself should be abandoned. To the contrary – its rich traditions offer us important insights into our own culture-specific moral values and beliefs about how to be moral beings. We must, however, pay much greater attention to the influences of the primary organising principle of morality, namely *culture*. We also need to recognise that, although it is true that all cultures have some 'priority rules', or principles for arbitrating between conflicting obligations and duties, just what these rules and principles are, how they are defined and interpreted, which are emphasised and given priority, when and how they will be applied, and who ultimately applies them (and to what end) will, contrary to an imperialist model of ethics, vary across – and even within – different cultures (Midgley 1991b: 11; Tai & Lin 2001; Yetzer et al 2018). As Abimbola (quoted earlier) correctly points out: 'ethics are *always* culture specific' and as such will be expressed differently cross-culturally and intra-culturally (Abimbola 2013: 31).

An interesting example of the different ways in which morality can be expressed cross-culturally or even intra-culturally can be found in the case of small-scale and large-scale societies. In small-scale or traditional societies, for example, morality tends to be viewed as a process – as a means to an end – and is expressed through the *quality of relationships* (characterised by upholding values such as friendship, loyalty to kin, empathy, altruism, familial trust and so on) rather than a deontological adherence to abstract principles. Silberbauer explains (1991: 27):

> *Morality is less of an end in itself but is seen more clearly as a set of orientations for establishing and maintaining the health of relationships. Morality, then, is a means to a desired, enjoyed end.*

This view is in sharp contrast to that upheld by large-scale (non-traditional or industrialised) societies, in which relationships are less proximate, less intense and less significant, at both the individual and the societal level. Here morality is viewed as an end in itself rather than as a means to an end, and is expressed by adherence to rules (*viz* adjudicating the conduct between strangers) rather than by and in the quality of relationships per se. On this point, Silberbauer explains (1991: 27):

> *Morality certainly provides a set of orientations and thus helps to create and maintain coherent expectations of behaviour, but* operates impersonally *in that there is not the same capacity for negotiation. Morality thus tends to be valued more as an end in itself and less as a means to an end.* [emphasis added]

To illustrate the different ways in which small-scale and large-scale societies might each express their different moralities, Silberbauer (1991) uses the simple example of the relationship between a bus conductor and a passenger. He suggests that, in large-scale societies, where relationships tend to be 'single-purpose and impersonal', the relationship between a bus conductor and a passenger would be of limited importance, and would probably manifest itself quite differently than it would in a small-scale society, where relationships were more proximate, multi-purpose and personal. He points out (p 14):

> *how different it would be if the conductor were also my sister-in-law, near neighbour and the daughter of my father's golfing partner – I would never dare to tender anything other than the correct fare. In a small-scale society every fellow member whom I encounter in my day is likely to be connected to me by a comparable, or even more complex web of strands, each of which must be maintained in its appropriate alignment and*

tension lest all the others become tangled. My father's missed putts or my inconsiderate use of a motor-mower at daybreak will necessitate very diplomatic behaviour on the bus, or a long walk to work and a dismal dinner on my return.

A more relevant example here can be found in the comparison of nurses working in large city-based university teaching hospitals with those who work in small, close-knit rural 'outback' country communities. It has been my experience that nurses working in the small rural or remote ('outback') country communities (where 'everyone is known to everyone') are far more vulnerable to putting local community members 'off-side' by offending an individual member of that community than are nurses working in the large city-based university teaching hospitals. In this instance, we could speculate that nurses working in small country-based community nursing care settings might put more weight on *preserving the quality of relationships* in that community than on *upholding abstract moral principles*. Conversely, nurses working in the large and impersonal communities may put greater emphasis on upholding abstract principles of conduct than on preserving the quality of relationships with 'strangers' whom they are unlikely to encounter more than once during their working lives.

This is only an example, however, being used here to help clarify Silberbauer's point. In reality it is likely that nurses express morality both as a *process* (as a means to an end) and as an *end in itself*. Whether this is so, and the extent to which it is so (i.e. where the balance lies), may depend ultimately on the nature of the context they are in – whether it is characterised by personal or impersonal relationships. When it is considered that it is not contradictory to view the maintenance of quality relationships as an important moral end in itself (not just a means to an end), there is room to suggest that the distinction Silberbauer makes may, in the final analysis, be overstated.

Despite this observation, Silberbauer is correct to point out that abstract moral principles do not always have currency in some cultural or social groups, and that, even if there do exist some commonly accepted standards of moral conduct, we cannot assume that these standards will be expressed or applied uniformly across, or even within, different cultural groups. A good example of this can be found in the wide and popular acceptance of the moral principles of autonomy, non-maleficence, beneficence and justice, which were considered in Chapter 3. These principles are referred to and used widely in mainstream bioethics discourse (see in particular Beauchamp & Childress 2013), and are viewed popularly as 'self-standing conceptual systems by which we can impose some sort of order upon ethical problems' (Elliott 1992: 29; see also Abimbola 2013). But, as Elliott correctly points out, what proponents of this view tend to overlook is that, in reality, ethics does not stand apart. It is one thread in the fabric of a society, and it is intertwined with others. Ethical concepts are tied to a society's customs, manners, traditions, institutions – all of the concepts that structure and inform the ways in which a member of that society deals with the world (Elliott 1992: 29). He goes on to warn that, if people forget this inextricable link between ethics and culture (p 29):

> *we are in danger of leaving the world of genuine moral experience for the world of moral fiction – a simplified, hypothetical creation suited less for practical difficulties than for intellectual convenience.*

A helpful example of the inaccuracy of viewing ethical principles as self-standing conceptual systems rather than as ethical concepts tied to a particular tradition (culture) can be seen in the way in which the principle of autonomy tends to be interpreted and applied in professional health care contexts. As stated in Chapter 3, the concept of autonomy refers to an individual's *independent* and *self-contained* ability to decide. As a principle, autonomy prescribes that a *cognitively competent individual's preferences* ought to be respected even if we do not agree with them – and even if others consider them foolish – provided they do not interfere with or harm prejudicially the significant moral interests of others.

At first glance, this articulation of the concept and principle of autonomy appears unproblematic. And it is probably true that most nurses familiarising themselves with the moral nature and application of the principle of autonomy value the 'right' to make their own self-determining choices, and would probably feel a strong sense of outrage if their considered wishes were overridden arbitrarily by another. They may also share a strong conviction that patients should always be informed about their diagnoses, and about the details of their proposed treatment and care, and that it would be a gross violation of patient rights not to accept or facilitate patients' self-determining choices regarding their own care and treatment options. In most cases, this position would probably be a demonstrably justifiable one to take. It would, however, be a grave mistake to accept the concept and principle of autonomy (as articulated above) as holding *universally* — that is, without exception. Consider the following.

Earlier in this book, it was pointed out that definitions of ethical terms and concepts can be 'ethically loaded', and hence can themselves be an important influence on how a moral debate or analysis might be conducted and what the outcomes of a given debate or analysis might be. This is true even (or perhaps especially) in the case of moral principles — the moral principle of autonomy being a case in point. It will be noted, for example, that even the definition of the concept and principle of autonomy reflects the dominant cultural values of the highly individualised large-scale Western Anglo-American culture from which it has arisen (Abimbola 2013; Blackhall et al 1995; Candib 2002; Hanssen 2004; Jennings 2016; Johnstone & Kanitsaki 2009a; Kuczewski 1996; Marshall 1992; Neves 2004; Tai & Lin 2001). Of particular importance to this discussion are the following terms: *person, individual, independent, self, self-contained*. Here the ethical loading clearly rests on particular culturally constructed and culturally dependent (Western) ideas of 'personhood' and 'selfhood' and of respecting individualism, independence and isolation (insulation) from one's social 'connectedness'. (As a point of interest, in contemporary Italian culture the notion autonomy [*autonomia*] is often used synonymously for isolation (*isolamento*) (Surbone 1992: 1662).) For people who hold these values, this ethical loading is not a major problem. But for people who do not hold or share these values — who may, for instance, subscribe to the values of collectiveness, interdependence, and social connectedness (context) and whose idea of informed consent is informed by 'ontological beliefs about illness, words and the nature of causation' (Abimbola 2013: 36) — it is open to serious question whether the concept and principle of autonomy as popularly defined and applied in mainstream bioethics discourse could, or indeed should, be given any currency in mediating the relationships, and the responsibilities within those relationships, of people who do not subscribe to the values embraced by autonomy as described.

To illustrate the kinds of moral problems that can arise as a result of applying the principle of autonomy in an abstract, universal and context-independent way rather than in a substantive, context-dependent, culture-specific way, consider the case of Mr G (adapted from Johnstone & Kanitsaki 1991). Mr G, an elderly Greek man who spoke no English, was admitted to hospital for investigations, and was later diagnosed as having cancer of the lung. Mr G had a number of other health problems, including a mildly debilitating hemiplegia — although he could move about with assistance. Before his admission into hospital, Mr G was totally dependent on and cared for by his family.

When radiological and laboratory tests confirmed the provisional medical diagnosis of a malignant lung tumour, Mr G's physician arranged for an interpreter to come to the ward and through him informed Mr G directly that he had cancer of the lung. In this instance, it was the physician's personal policy to be candid with his patients, and inform them according to what he judged to be 'their right to know and be informed', as prescribed by the moral principle of autonomy. Unfortunately, in this case, although well intended, the physician's approach was culturally inappropriate, and had the undesirable moral consequence of causing the patient and his family otherwise avoidable suffering (Johnstone & Kanitsaki 1991).

A mainstream ethical analysis of the physician's actions in this case would probably support the view that informing the patient of his cancer diagnosis was a 'morally right' thing to do. And, interestingly, when I present this case to students (nursing and medical students alike), most contend that the physician's actions were not only morally correct but *praiseworthy*, given the reluctance by doctors in the past to be candid with their patients about diagnostic, care and treatment matters of this nature (see, for example, Candib 2002).

From a cultural perspective, however, the physician's actions can be shown to be not only mistaken but also morally harmful. In this case it would have been more culturally appropriate and morally beneficial had the physician communicated the cancer diagnosis to the patient's *family* rather than to the patient himself. This is because, as Johnstone and Kanitsaki point out (1991: 280), during a health crisis, patients like Mr G who are of a traditional (rural, small-scale societal) cultural background, who may have only partially acculturated to the mainstream culture of their host country and who have retained the core cultural values acquired in their country of origin tend to prefer:

> *the close involvement of their family and value the supportive, protective and therapeutic role that the family can and does play when one of its members is ill or suffering … Indeed, the involvement of the patient's family is an essential and integral part of the therapeutic relationship and of the process required to uphold the patient's best interests.*

By not recognising the protective authority of Mr G's family to decide '*if*, *when*, *how* and *by whom* the diagnoses should be disclosed to Mr G', the physician inadvertently 'pointed the bone' at his patient and thereby undermined rather than promoted Mr G's autonomy. The reasons for this are complicated, yet important. Kanitsaki (1989a) explains that for many rurally based Greeks who emigrated to Australia during the 1950s and 1960s the very word 'cancer' carries a whole range of negative connotations and thus is something never to be mentioned, since to do so would be to risk stimulating the nocebo phenomenon. The *nocebo phenomenon* or *nocebo effect* (from the Latin *noceo*, 'I hurt', and the Greek *nosis*, 'disease') is a phenomenon that is opposite to the *placebo effect* (Pilcher 2009). First described by Helman (1990) in his book *Culture, health and illness*, research over the past decade has increasingly shown that the nocebo phenomenon – sometimes described as 'placebo's evil twin' (Reid 2002) – comes into effect when negative health beliefs and expectations lead to a worsening of symptoms or general health (Barsky et al 2002; Benedetti et al 2007; Horsfall 2016; Liccardi et al 2004; Olshansky 2007; Planès et al 2016; Wells & Kaptchuk 2012).

The growing research-based evidence on the nocebo effect helps to explain why, in some cases, telling a patient 'you have got cancer' can be morally harmful. When such disclosures are made to patients whose cultural values and beliefs render such frank disclosures taboo it may inadvertently trigger deeply held negative beliefs and expectations about the disease and its pathway. This, in turn, may not only have a profoundly negative impact on the patient's will to live, but even shorten their life expectancy. In other words, truth telling in such cases may serve as a catalyst for a nocebo-induced premature death or at least an unexpected (and unexplained) worsening of the patient's medical condition. Although these risks have been contemplated in the literature, health professionals – including nurses – remain relatively unaware of the nocebo effect and unwittingly contribute to it in their day-to-day practice, for example, by refusing requests from family members not to disclose deadly cancer diagnoses to their relatives, such as occurred in the examples given in this chapter. The question remains, however, of why 'cancer' in particular has the potential to trigger a nocebo effect.

In response to the case of 'Mr G', Kanitsaki (1989a: 46) explains that, during the 1950s and 1960s, rural Greece had virtually no hospitals, and that if people required treatment for serious illness they would have to travel great distances to the nearest cities. She goes on to point out that, because of this, as well as because of scepticism about the ability of scientific medicine to treat diseases effectively, people from rural areas would seek hospital treatment only as a last resort. Kanitsaki explains (p 47):

> *the reluctance to frequent doctors and hospitals was exacerbated by a general dislike of hospitals, rumours about the lack of nursing care and unkind nursing staff, and a fear of cities generally. Pressures of local work*

demands, a lack of economic resources, and the probability of having to travel alone and thus without the protection, support, and physical presence of the family, also militated against scientific medical services being used by rural community members.

As a result of this reluctance – and, indeed, inability – to access credentialled medical services, many people suffering from cancer-related illness did not receive the optimal treatment available, and as a result frequently died painful and agonising deaths (Kanitsaki 1989a). It is the memories of these kinds of cancer-related deaths, and related beliefs and habits that have literally become frozen in times past (*viz* a 'fossilised' or 'frozen' culture), that many rural Greek immigrants have brought with them to Australia and which persist to this day (see Irwin 2007). Kanitsaki explains (personal communication) that many post WWII Greek immigrants of this background simply may not have any experiential knowledge of, or even a conception of, the kind of treatment and care that is currently available in Australia; thus even mentioning the word 'cancer' is sufficient to trigger in ill persons an overwhelming sense of hopelessness, which ultimately finds its expression in their losing their will to live. Under these circumstances, to tell such patients 'You've got cancer' – no matter how benevolent the intention in doing so – would probably be sufficient to trigger the nocebo phenomenon, resulting ultimately in the ill person's premature death (Johnstone & Kanitsaki 2009a; see also Zamanzadeh et al 2013 – reporting the experiences of cancer disclosures by Iranian patients, their families and physicians).

The way to avoid this disastrous situation is for the patient to be spared the information likely to stimulate the nocebo phenomenon, and for the patient's family to be respected as having the surrogate authority to decide – in the moral interests of and for the wellbeing of their sick loved one – *whether, when, where, how* and *by whom* information about the diagnosis of a serious illness and poor prognosis will be given (Johnstone & Kanitsaki 2009a). A major *moral* motivation for this is to avoid drastically and negatively altering the 'patient's view of his or her own future' (Kazdaglis et al 2010: 443) and thereby undermining their hope – that is, that they will be well cared for and supported, will live longer than expected, will be able to 'find meaning in their own life and worth' and the like (Clayton et al 2008: 655). By maintaining the patient's hope, his/her ability to continue making important life-interested choices is also maintained, thus ipso facto maximising their autonomy. In sum, maintaining hope is the linchpin to promoting autonomy (Johnstone & Kanitsaki 2009a). This is because without hope there is simply *nothing left to choose for.*

Interestingly, research has shown that, even in contemporary Greek society, truth-telling about a diagnosis of serious life-threatening illness (especially cancer-related illness) is still viewed by many Greeks (urban as well as rural) as being harmful and hence 'undesirable', on the grounds that it could undermine hope and the will to live (Dalla-Vorgia et al 1992; Georgaki et al 2002; Kazdaglis et al 2010; Mystakidou et al 1996).

It should be noted that this moral world view is not held exclusively by Greeks of rural or traditional cultural backgrounds. People of other traditional cultural backgrounds and cultural contexts (e.g. Iranian, Pakistani, Japanese, Italian, Korean, Chinese) also believe that, in some circumstances, patients should not be told that they have a serious life-threatening illness (especially cancer) and that to do so would be harmful (see, for example, Grassi et al 2000; Irwin 2007; Jafarey & Farooqui 2005; Karim 2002; Kwak & Haley 2005; Lee & Wu 2002; Locatelli et al 2013; Macklin 1998; Mo et al 2012; Pellegrino 1992; Sato et al 2012; Seyedrasooly et al 2014; Surbone 1992; Tai & Lin 2001; Zamanzadeh et al 2013). The following anecdote shows this.

The case concerns an elderly non-English-speaking Italian man who, like Mr G, had emigrated to Australia in the 1950s. He was admitted to hospital for tests, which later confirmed a cancer diagnosis. Although the man's family explicitly requested that their father not be given any information about the test results if they were positive, an interpreter was called in their absence and the man was told of his cancer diagnosis and poor prognosis. This information caused the man to become extremely distressed and, as his son commented later, 'The life just went out of his eyes and we knew he would die very soon.' The son, who was Australian born and a qualified pharmacist, decided in consultation with the rest of his family to remedy the situation. This he did by contacting Italian-Australian friends who worked as doctors at the hospital where his father was a patient and arranging for all his father's tests to be repeated. His friends agreed to explain to his father that the tests needed to be repeated because 'there had been a terrible mistake' and that 'his earlier test results had got mixed up with someone else's'. They later returned to tell the man that his tests showed he in fact did *not* have cancer. The son explained that his father was told he still needed medical treatment, but that he would 'be all right'. Ultimately, the family took their father home and cared for him. He continued to live well beyond the time limit suggested by his poor prognosis and, in fact, was still alive at the time the anecdote was being shared – 18 months after being told that he would not live very long. The son attributed this to the fact that they were able to convince their father all was not hopeless, which in turn had the effect of restoring his will to live. In short, the son's actions reversed his father's sense of hopelessness, and thus promoted rather than undermined his father's autonomy.

Interestingly, when I have shared this anecdote with students, many are appalled at the blatant deception that was employed in this case. Others, however, notably those whose parents are from rural Greece or Italy, have expressed enormous relief at the insights this and other cases like it have given them. One postgraduate nursing student, for example, commented (personal communication):

> *I've always felt that if either of my parents should get cancer they should be told their diagnosis. But when speaking of this issue, my mother – who is Italian – has always insisted, 'No! you must not allow that to happen'. My Australian side of me tells me it is wrong not to tell them. But now I can see it would be wrong to tell them, and that my mother is right. I can live with this now. It is such an enormous relief. I am no longer in a dilemma. Thank you.*

The comments of this student are included here because, among other things, they demonstrate the very practical help that adopting a cross-cultural view of ethics can offer; of particular note, they help to support the view that, by tying ethical views to the cultural traditions that inform them, we will be in a much better position to embrace morality as an experience rather than as an abstraction (Marshall 1992: 53–7), and that, by embracing morality as an experience rather than an abstraction, we can avoid falling prey to the unhelpful, idle fantasies of moral fiction which, as Elliott (1992: 2) suggests, are suited more to the purposes of intellectual convenience than to resolving genuine practical difficulties in the concrete circumstances of life. The student's comments and, indeed, the anecdotes themselves also show, to borrow from Cortese (1990: 157), that 'relationships … are the essence of life and morality', and that to view morality simply as conceptions of abstract reified rational principles is 'to remove us from the real world in which we live, and separate us from real people whom we love'. The lesson to be learned here is that, unless we embrace morality as an experience rather than as an abstraction, what we will end up with is only a concept of morality and not morality itself. Also, borrowing again from Cortese (1990: 158), unless we have a 'deep sense of relationship, we may have a conceptualisation of the highest level of justice, but we will not be moral'. The point is that, without relationships, justice – morality – 'contains no system of checks and balances. It becomes primarily an end in itself without regard to the purpose of morality' (Cortese 1990: 158).

Although only the principle of autonomy has been considered here, the other principles considered in Chapter 3 (non-maleficence, beneficence and justice) could all be examined along similar lines. We could, for example, ask in regard to each of these principles: 'From whose perspective are these principles to be meaningfully and appropriately defined, interpreted, analysed and applied?' In the case of non-maleficence, for instance, meaningful questions can be asked about what constitutes a 'harm' in a given culturally constructed clinical context. By whose standards and cultural perspectives is the notion of harm to be measured and evaluated? It is likewise for the principles of beneficence and justice.

Where then does this leave the role of moral principles and culturally different moral viewpoints and approaches in our nursing ethics discourse? In answering this question, it might be useful at this point to consider the nature and implications of diversity or pluralism in moral values and moral worldviews.

Moral diversity and the challenge of moral pluralism

The multicultural nature of the world (described in the opening paragraph to this chapter) has brought with it a diversity or pluralism of moral values and beliefs. Some fear that this diversity or pluralism of values may be 'the barrier to agreement' (Elliott 1992: 32) and, hence, the catalyst to producing a world hopelessly divided by radical and destructive moral disagreement. Others reject moral pluralism outright on the grounds that, in their view, it is 'just another name for confusion' (Stout 1988: 1). Moral diversity need not lead to destructive disagreement, however, nor to blinding confusion. Indeed, as is well recognised within the discipline of moral philosophy, moral disagreement has historically been the beginning and has seen the development of moral thinking, not its end or disintegration (see also Benhabib & Dallmayr 1990; Stout 1988). Further, as Mary Midgley correctly points out, 'nobody is infallible; and for that reason many different points of view are needed' (Midgley 1991a: 83).

What must also be recognised and understood here is that, just as diversity is the key to survival in other areas (e.g. market diversity, agricultural diversity, artistic diversity, etc. (Lakoff & Rockridge Institute 2006)), a diversity of values and beliefs is the key to a morality's survival and development; it prompts critical reflection, rather than uncritical acceptance, and in so doing invites constant revision and creative refinement. Moral diversity also helps to ensure that no one moral point of view dominates; in short, it helps to prevent what might otherwise be termed 'moral fascism'. Meanwhile, its emphasis on *understanding difference* rather than *striving for uniformity* will help to ensure that the moral systems we end up embracing will be of a nature that is truly responsive to the lived realities and experiences of all human beings, not merely those of a select few whose positions of power have enabled them to manipulate morality into a tool for repressing unwanted truths and legitimating further the authority of moral imperialists who would impose their values on others as a means of maintaining rather than challenging the domination of their world views.

Adopting a cross-cultural approach to ethics can be beneficial in a range of ways. Among other things, at a global level it can enable cross-cultural interactions that 'build bridges of understanding between persons and cultures that make cooperation possible and conquest unnecessary' (Fasching 1993: 6). It can also help to avoid the perils of 'moral suprematism' such as those that have been amply exemplified during wartime (see, for example, Fasching 1993). For instance, during WWII, the world bore witness to Nazis believing in 'their own moral superiority (supported by ultimate justification)' and the consequential rendering as mute 'all opposing views' (Gergen 1994: 113). As Gergen (1994: 113) points out in relation to this historical period:

> Had the means been available much earlier for an unobstructed interpretation of meaning systems – Nazi, Jewish, Christian, Marxist, feminist, and the like – one must imagine that the consequences would have been far less disastrous.

We thus stand warned that what is sometimes presented as *the* 'superior morality' might well prove to be little more than 'the morality of the superior' – meaning the extremely powerful and the dominant – who, convinced that they are 'right', justify their right to harm others (as happened during the Nazi era and was epitomised by Nazi characterisations and brutal treatment of the Jews) (Bauman 1993: 228).

At a more local level, a cross-cultural approach to ethics can enrich greatly our moral view of the world and the various relationships (including nurse–patient relationships) we experience within it. In the case of the nurse–patient relationship, however, a cross-cultural approach to ethics may enhance not only the moral quality but also the therapeutic effectiveness of that relationship (most notably through avoiding the harmful consequences of the nocebo phenomenon (Johnstone 2012b; Johnstone & Kanitsaki 2009a)) and hence the moral ends of nursing itself (referred to in Chapter 3).

An important lesson for nurses here is that moral diversity is not something to be feared, but something to be embraced as a means of challenging our complacent thinking about the moral world we live in, and of improving our understanding of and ability to experience both ourselves and others as moral beings who have a mutual interest in living a worthwhile and meaningful life. Further, whether we wish to admit it or not, as Elliott points out (1992: 35):

> *Moral disagreement will be with us as long as there is disagreement about what way of life is best for human beings. It is not at all obvious that this is a question that is answerable, even in principle. There may be no best life, only better and worse lives. And if morality is tied to a form of life, then it is a mistake to think that we can eliminate moral differences without eliminating the differences in cultures, and in individuals, to which morality is tied.*

Elliott (p 35) goes on to make the additional point that:

> *Though the biological characteristics humans share will mean that some lives, and some features of lives, are necessarily good or bad for human beings, there is no compelling reason, universally applicable, for adopting any one particular sort of life over all others – even if we had the choice, which we do not. For this reason, we should expect diversity in the sort of lives that people live, as well as the moral differences that inevitably follow.*

Dealing with problems associated with a cross-cultural approach to ethics in health care

Before concluding this discussion, it is important to acknowledge that upholding a cross-cultural view of ethics can sometimes be extremely difficult, and may give rise to serious ethical dilemmas for health care professionals – nurses included. For instance, it is not uncommon for nurses to encounter a situation in which a patient requests one thing and his or her family requests another. A typical scenario is as follows.

A patient from a traditional cultural background (e.g. Greek, Italian or Chinese) discloses to an attending nurse: 'If my test results come back positive and I have cancer, I want to be told. I know my family has told you not to tell me, but I must ask you not to take notice of them. I want to know. And that is the end of the matter.' The family, meanwhile, may request: 'If our father's test results come back positive and he has cancer, under no circumstances is he to be told. We know him. Such news will kill him. You must give us the information and we will deal with it. This is family business and that is the end of the matter.' Usually, the attendant nurses in these kinds of situations are desperate to do what is best for all concerned, but are troubled about how to decide what, in fact, *is best* for all concerned. Typically, the questions they ask include: 'Who do I listen to – the patient, or the family?', 'How best can I serve the patient's interests given that the family just might be right – that is, the information might "kill him"?' and 'What should I do?'

Just what attending nurses ought to do, however, might not be as problematic as at first it appears to be. Consider the following.

In responding to the kind of scenario just outlined, it is vitally important that nurses do not *stereotype* people of different cultural backgrounds and assume that 'all immigrants' ipso facto practise traditional life-ways, or that 'all immigrants' ipso facto practise a family-centred (versus an individualistic) model of informed decision-making in health care contexts. Many immigrants to a host country assimilate to the mainstream culture of their new country, and have internalised very effectively the core cultural values of the (new) mainstream culture. Immigrants to Australia, New Zealand and other countries are no exception in this regard. For example, when a 'new Australian' (as immigrants to Australia have been known in the past) makes an explicit request to the effect 'If my test results come back positive and I have cancer, I want to be told', it is highly probable that not only does he/she mean it, but will also be able to deal with it in a culturally adapted way. In such instances, there is no question that the nurse's primary responsibility is to initiate steps to ensure that the patient's request for information is honoured. Where then does this leave the family's request?

Giving primacy to the patient's request for information does not mean that the family's request has no bearing on the matter or should be ignored altogether (Kuczewski 1996). On the contrary: the family's request is just as deserving of consideration as is the patient's — not least because *they too* are experiencing the health crisis of their loved one. What differs, however, is the way in which nursing and medical staff might respond to a family's requests. Kanitsaki, for example, advises (personal communication) that, after securing consent from the patient, the following actions might alleviate the situation considerably:

- Inform the family that the patient has explicitly requested to be told the details of a diagnosis, and that the doctors and nurses have a legal and moral obligation to honour this request.
- Express understanding of the pain of the situation, and acknowledge that the family is only trying to do what is 'good and right' for their loved one.
- Invite the family to be present when the information is to be given to their loved one.
- Negotiate a plan of care that, in the event of a 'bad' diagnosis, all parties can be mutually supported, for example:
    - it might be necessary to arrange for the family to meet with the attending physician on a regular basis in order to obtain and discuss details of their loved one's health status and progress
    - it might be necessary to organise culturally relevant help (e.g. counselling — noting, however, that it might be necessary not to call it 'counselling' for cultural reasons) to assist family members and their sick loved one to re-establish communication patterns that the 'telling/not telling' scenario has possibly disrupted, and consequently left family members feeling alienated from one other.

In most instances, a 'commonsense' approach to managing individuals and families experiencing grief crises will result in satisfactory outcomes and a 'therapeutic partnership' between lay and professional (nursing) carers.

Another kind of problem that is not uncommon in nursing care domains involves extended-family members visiting in contravention of hospital visiting rules — for example, visiting outside of a hospital's regulated visiting hours and/or in numbers in excess of a unit's visiting rules. In regard to the latter, this is regarded as problematic by nurses since it is sometimes perceived as compromising the entitlements of other patients — especially when the presence of a large number of extended-family members creates a level of 'noise' that is intrusive and disruptive to the ambience of the environment for other patients. It is also seen as problematic by nurses since it is not uncommon, over the duration of their visit and/or the patient's hospital stay, for different family members to ask the same nurse the same question about the health condition of their loved one. Nurses not infrequently cite being frustrated at repeatedly being asked the same question by different family members as, among other things, this is commonly seen by nurses to stretch even further their already strained 'time resources' to attend other patients. All things considered, however, this problem is not as problematic as at first it might appear to be.

First, research is increasingly showing that, rather than being a 'problem', the presence and participation of family members in a patient's care can be very protective. Because of a family's (and friends') prime position as informants of the patient's condition and personal circumstances, constant bedside vigilance, capacity to mediate important information between the patient and health care team, and capacity to help modulate a patient's illness / injury experience and support the patient's decision-making (including, where necessary, acting as a surrogate decision-maker), families can substantially contribute to achieving positive health and patient safety outcomes in their loved ones (Åstedt-Kurki et al 2001; Berwick & Kotagal 2004; Carr & Clarke 1997; Carr & Fogarty 1999; Chang 2001; Dudley & Carr 2004; Johnstone & Kanitsaki 2006a, 2009b; Jubb & Shanley 2002; Koutantji et al 2005; Levine & Zuckerman 2000; Meyers et al 2004; Weingart et al 2005).

Second, and related to the above, it is important for nurses to understand that 'presencing' by extended-family members is a crucial component of the lay–therapeutic relationship (Johnstone & Kanitsaki 2009a; Johnstone et al 2016; Kanitsaki 1994, 2000). By being 'present', family members believe they are contributing to the healing process by 'giving strength' to their loved one. Significantly, it is not uncommon, especially in the case of seriously ill patients, to see family members strategically placed around the bed of a sick person, for example, with one family member touching the head, another the left hand, another the right hand, another the left foot, and another the right foot of the ill person. This 'touching' (often manifest as massage of a given part of the body or the sprinkling of healing waters over the part) is an important component of the process of giving 'healing energy' to the ill person so as to assist them to 'get well'. The loved one, meanwhile, generally regards the presence of his/her family members as an indication of their caring. To ask family members to leave under these circumstances thus stands as a violation of the lay–therapeutic relationship, and it is understandable that extended-family members might react 'badly' to a nurse's directives to 'be considerate' of other patients and to observe a 'two-visitors-per-patient' rule. The question to arise here is: 'How can nurses best manage the situation?'

Key to the effective management of extended-family visiting is for nurses themselves to understand the lay–therapeutic (healing) nature of this visiting, as well as the crucial role it also plays as a 'quality assurance' check of the care a loved one might be receiving. For instance, the repeated questioning of nursing staff by family members is an attempt to secure as much information as possible about the care of their loved one, which can subsequently be interrogated by family members for its consistency, accuracy and hence reliability (Kanitsaki 1994, 2000). Obviously, if six family members ask the same nurse the same question, yet receive six different answers, they would have grounds to be suspicious about whether their loved one was, in fact, receiving optimal care. Similarly, if their repeated requests for information are met with annoyance or hostility by nurses, this could be construed as meaning that the nurses 'do not care' and, again, that their loved one is not receiving optimal care. This, in turn, could result in the family removing the loved one from a given location of care and taking them elsewhere for care – even overseas (Kanitsaki 1994, 2000).

There are a number of strategies which nurses might use to help remedy a situation such as this. These include (adapted from Kanitsaki, personal communication):

- asking the family to nominate a spokesperson for the family and for a primary nurse to agree to meet with this person, as required, to answer any questions the family might have
- advising the family (in non-serious cases) of the constraints under which nurses are forced to operate and explain the need for considering the interests of other patients
- in the case of seriously ill patients, moving the patient to a single room so that the lay–therapeutic relationship can be expressed as fully as is possible under the circumstances.

Feedback from nurses over the years has indicated that the implementation of these and related kinds of strategies have been very effective in maximising the quality of care experienced by patients (and their chosen carers) of culturally diverse backgrounds, and improving nurses' job satisfaction when involved in the care of such patients.

The third and final kind of problem to be considered here, and which nurses not infrequently have to deal with, concerns the codified demand on nurses to respect certain religious and traditional practices of patients. The nature of the problem is as follows.

The ICN code of ethics for nurses (ICN 2012a: 2) prescribes that 'in providing care, the nurse promotes an environment in which the human rights, values, customs and spiritual beliefs of the individual, family and community are respected'. The Nursing and Midwifery Board of Australia's *Code of conduct for nurses* (NMBA 2018), which includes a specific standard for 'Cultural practice and respectful relationships' (Principle 3), similarly prescribes that, when caring for people from diverse cultural and language backgrounds, nurses have a responsibility to ensure that they engage with people in a 'culturally safe and respectful manner', and 'adopt practices that respect diversity and avoid bias, discrimination and racism' and challenge assumptions they may make about a person's gender, race, ethnicity, religious beliefs, and the like (p 8). Likewise the Nursing Council of New Zealand's *Code of conduct*, which also contains the specific standard 'Respect the cultural needs and values of health consumers' (NCNZ 2016, Principle 2, pp 11–12). The nursing ethics codes of other countries carry similar provisions. The problem for nurses, however, is that some religious and traditional practices either pose a threat or are actually harmful to patients – the case of female genital mutilation (called 'traditional cutting' by its proponents) is an instructive example here (see Affara 2000, 2002; James 1994; Macklin 2016; Reyners 2004; World Health Organization (WHO) 2018a). In such instances, nurses are troubled by what appears to be two conflicting demands: on the one hand to respect the patient's cultural values and beliefs, and yet on the other hand to protect the patient from harm. This dilemma is compounded by postmodernist theoretical requirements to explain: 'harm' by *whose standards*? and 'harm' by *whose world view*?, and to demonstrate that the apparent moral dilemma at issue is not merely a creation of 'moral ethnocentrism' or 'cultural (moral) imperialism' (James 1994).

Most nurses would probably agree that they have at least a prima-facie obligation to respect the cultural practices of their patients. More specifically, they would probably accept that:

> *Intolerance of another's religious or traditional practices that pose no threat of harm is, at least, discourteous and at worst, a prejudicial attitude. And it does fail to show respect for persons and their diverse religious and cultural practices.* (Macklin 1998: 7)

This does not mean, however, that nurses are obliged – either on the basis of the above view or on that of the nursing profession's formally adopted code of ethics – to tolerate, *without reflective judgment*, all religious and cultural practices of their patients. There are a number of reasons for this. First, to borrow from Macklin (1998: 17), we can 'be respectful of cultural difference and *at the same time acknowledge that there are limits*' [emphasis added]. Second, the 'limits' to our obligation of respect can be discerned by a critical examination of: (1) the internal cultural justifications and considerations raised in support of a given 'harmful' religious or traditional practice, and (2) external viewpoints (i.e. from other cultural groups) about the 'harmfulness' of the practice (recognising here that culture is not static and can change in positive ways when exposed to relevant influences). Third, we are not obliged to be respectful of practices which, when examined comparatively from an intra-cultural and cross-cultural perspective, are themselves disrespectful and oppressive of persons (see also the United Nations Development Programme *Human development report 2004: cultural liberty in today's diverse world* (Fukuda-Parr 2004)).

Ethics, cultural competency, cultural safety and cultural humility

Families of diverse cultural backgrounds, whose cultural values and beliefs are at odds with an autonomy-based ethical decision-making process, will go to great lengths to protect their loved ones from a system they see as being hostile to their loved one's wellbeing and interests (Johnstone & Kanitsaki 2009a, 2009b). This is particularly so in instances where well-intended but misguided processes are imposed by a health care system which family members know, through direct experience, will have a profoundly negative impact on the life and wellbeing of their loved one.

In keeping with the standards of practice expected of registered nurses (see, for example, NCNZ 2016; NMBA 2016), all nurses are required to be responsive to patients' needs and to think critically and reflect on their practice, feelings and beliefs and the consequences of these for the individuals, families and groups they care for. This includes searching out and applying research and evidence for practice. Although this requirement is generally interpreted as applying to clinical practice (evidence-based practice), it also applies to the practice of ethics (evidence-based ethics). As examples given in this chapter have shown, truth-telling about a cancer diagnosis is a 'practice' that warrants deep consideration from an evidential, not just a values basis. This is because truth-telling about cancer diagnoses is a *value,* which is informed by strong cultural beliefs that are not universally shared (Johnstone 2012b; Johnstone & Kanitsaki 2009a; Kazdaglis et al 2010; Mollarahimi-Maleki et al 2016). This underscores the point that, if members of the nursing profession are to fulfill their responsibilities in regard to upholding reflective, evidence-based and ethical practice, the ethical issues encountered in practice need to be considered in a more culturally competent, culturally humble and culturally responsive way. How these capacities might be developed is briefly considered below.

Cultural competency

Over the past several decades there has been an emerging international consensus about the nature and importance of practitioners developing cultural competence 'as an essential component of accessible, responsive, and high quality care' (Lewin Group 2002: 1). In more recent years this idea has been transferred to the realm of ethical decision-making in health care as scholars, researchers, practitioners and policy-makers alike have come to recognise the critical (missing) link between culture and ethics, and the profound influence that cultural world views (ultimate beliefs and values) have on ethical decision-making and behaviour across the entire health care system.

The notion of 'cultural competence' is believed to have been derived from the field of medical anthropology (especially work pioneered by Kleinman et al 1978), with the first published use of the term appearing in Cross and colleagues' (1989) influential work: *Towards a culturally competent system of care: a monograph on effective services for minority children who are severally emotionally disturbed* (American Institutes of Research 2004: 7). Predicated on theories that 'language and culture affect health care beliefs, choices, and treatment', the notion of cultural competence has been described as an 'explicit statement that one-size-fits-all health care cannot meet the needs of an increasingly diverse population' in a given country (Brach & Fraserirector 2000: 183). Cultural competence is also described as going beyond mere 'cultural awareness and sensitivity' to include:

> not only possession of cultural knowledge and respect for different cultural perspectives but also having skills and being able to use them effectively in cross-cultural situations. (Brach & Fraserirector 2000: 183)

Most definitions of cultural competence contain elements of or are a variation of Cross and colleagues' (1989) original foundational definition and explanatory notes, notably:

> *A set of congruent behaviours, attitudes, and policies that come together in a system, agency, or amongst professionals and enables that system, agency, or those professionals to work effectively in cross-cultural situations. The word culture is used because it implies the integrated pattern of human behaviour that includes thoughts, communications, actions, customs, beliefs, values, and institutions of a racial, ethnic, religious, or social group. The word competence is used because it implies having the capacity to function effectively. A cultural competent system of care acknowledges and incorporates – at all levels – the importance of culture, the assessment of cross-cultural relations, vigilance towards the dynamics that result from cultural differences, the expansions of cultural knowledge, and the adaptation of services to meet culturally-unique needs.* (Cross et al 1989: iv–v)

Despite the development and operationalisation of the above and other working definitions of cultural competence and related standards for health care systems, there is currently no consensus across the different health care professions on what *specifically* constitutes individual cultural competence or how it might best be measured. Nonetheless there is general recognition of the essential nature and importance of the complex interrelationship that exists between having the 'right attitude', 'right knowledge', 'right skills' and 'right assessment processes' (*viz* competence) in a given cultural context. As can be readily demonstrated, it is not sufficient to have *only* the 'right attitude', *or* the 'right knowledge', *or* the 'right skills' and so forth. For example, a practitioner might have the 'right attitude' (e.g. be well intended, be empathic) but not have the appropriate cultural knowledge and skill, and, as a result, inadvertently 'do the wrong thing'. Thus, simply having the 'right attitude' is not sufficient to ensure culturally competent practice; health care providers need to have the right attitude *and* the right knowledge *and* the right skills *and* the right assessment processes in place. This encompasses the need for also giving careful attention not only to *what* should be known (content) but also to *when, where, how* and *by whom* knowledge and information pertinent to the development of the necessary attitudes, knowledge and skills comprising cultural competence are shared, taught and assessed (Sue 2001a, 2001b).

Some have worried that the cultural competence model for improving the quality, safety and ethics of health care delivery to culturally and linguistically diverse populations might inadvertently undermine the very goals that the model has been devised to progress (Gregg & Saha 2006). For example, rather than foster attitudes of respect for cultural differences and the importance of culture in people's lives, the cultural competence model might foster a 'check list' approach that risks stereotyping patients and stigmatising their cultural differences. In an attempt to mitigate this undesirable risk a complementary approach has been proposed, namely 'cultural humility' (Austerlic 2009; Hook et al 2013; Tervalon & Murray-García 1998), to be discussed later in this chapter.

Cultural safety

In response to the need to be mindful of and responsive to the culturally mediated knowledge, values, beliefs and practices of indigenous peoples, some have advocated that a process called '*cultural safety*' be adopted. The notion of cultural safety, or *Kawa Whakaruruhau*, is credited with having originated in the work of New Zealand Māori nurse educators during the late 1980s and was principally constructed as a political response to the long-term negative impact and effects of colonisation on the health of Māori people of Aotearoa/New Zealand (for a helpful account of the negative impact of colonisation and Eurocentric nursing care on Māori health see McKillop et al 2013). As Johnstone and Kanitsaki (2007b) and Gerlach (2012) have each respectively noted, cultural safety was thus not so much about fostering cultural care practices as it was about fostering recognition of the social, economic and political position of Māori (and other First Nations peoples) and the continuing impact of these processes on Māori/indigenous health.

Despite its original political orientation and intent, the concept of cultural safety was nonetheless adopted by the New Zealand nursing profession as a framework and mechanism for 'improving the health status of all people in New Zealand through the relationship between Māori and the Crown' (Ellison-Loschmann 2001; Richardson 2003). In 1991, under the leadership of the late New Zealand nurse academic Irihapeti Ramsden, cultural safety guidelines were developed and, in 1992, approved by the Nursing Council of New Zealand (NCNZ 2011).

A distinctive and distinguishing feature of the New Zealand cultural safety model is its characterisation of having originated in an *uniquely indigenous response* (notably of Māori) to difficulties perceived and experienced in the provision of mainstream health care services (Ramsden 2002; Wepa 2005). This is in contradistinction to a more formalised anthropological view of ethnocentric health service delivery and the problem of ethnic disparities in access to, receipt of and health outcomes of mainstream health care services (Johnstone & Kanitsaki 2007b). Another distinctive feature of the New Zealand cultural safety model is its emphasis on the provision of culturally safe health care services *as defined by the end-users of those services* (notably, the Māori people of Aotearoa / New Zealand), and not by non-Māori providers of health care irrespective of its evidence base (Clarke 2005; Papps 2005).

It is notable that, since its inception, the notion of cultural safety has not been without controversy. A particularly controversial feature of the cultural safety model was that, despite New Zealand being a multicultural country, it was situated as a *bicultural* construct encompassing just two cultures: *Māori* and *non-Māori 'immigrant others'* (Johnstone & Kanitsaki 2007b). Also problematic were the unresolved conceptual and theoretical weaknesses and a lack of empirical evidence supporting its practice (Gerlach 2012; Johnstone & Kanitsaki 2007b). Arguably one of the most controversial consequences of what might be termed here the 'cultural safety movement' was its original ideological adoption in nursing curricula and its questionable, and at times punitive, application when assessing students undertaking nursing programs. In July 1995, following public concerns being raised about the way in which cultural safety was being applied in practice, the cultural safety component of nursing curricula was made the subject of an inquiry by a Select Committee of the New Zealand Parliament (Papps & Ramsden 1996). Coinciding with this inquiry, the New Zealand Nursing Council also conducted a review, the outcome of which was a revised definition of the term (NCNZ 2011).

Today cultural safety stands as a uniquely New Zealand nursing construct. Adopted as a core standard of practice it is defined as:

> *Cultural safety is the effective nursing practice of a person or family/whānau from another culture, and is determined by that person or family. Culture includes, but is not restricted to, age or generation; gender; sexual orientation; occupation and socio-economic status; ethnic origin or migrant experience; religious or spiritual beliefs; and disability. The nurse delivering the nursing care will have undertaken a process of reflection on their own cultural identity and will recognise the impact their personal culture has on their professional practice. Unsafe cultural practice comprises any action which diminishes, demeans or disempowers the cultural identity and well-being of an individual.* (NCNZ 2011: 13)

The notion of cultural safety has been adopted by other countries (e.g. Australia, Canada) grappling with the problem of indigenous health disparities, although also not without controversy (see Gerlach 2012; Johnstone & Kanitsaki 2007b). It has also been adopted and expanded to redress the perceived inadequacies of conventional patient safety processes in hospital contexts generally (Walker et al 2009). To this end, a cross-cultural model of 'cultural patient safety' has since been proposed. Building on the ideas and constructs constitutive of the broader global patient safety and cultural competency movements, cross-cultural patient safety takes a distinctive patient-centred approach to health care safety. Among the core risk factors it aims to address in the interests of promoting patient safety among Indigenous peoples are: *linguistic issues* (e.g. the potential for miscommunication), *cultural issues* (e.g. the potential for cultural misunderstanding), *medical literacy* (e.g. taking into account that native languages do not always include conventional medical or related terminology; the inability of patients to navigate the health care system), *practice issues* (e.g. where conventional services may contrast or clash with traditional healing practices), *contextual issues* (e.g. the potential for misunderstanding due to differences in cultural knowledge or cultural habits), *systemic issues* (e.g. access and availability issues), *genetics* (e.g. failure to take into account issues specific to certain racial / ethnic populations) and *racism / discrimination* (e.g. manifest as prejudice, indifference, intolerance, or unjust differential provision of health services) (Walker et al 2009).

In keeping with its origins in an indigenous response to the harmful impact of colonisation on the health of an indigenous people, cultural safety has been promoted in some contexts as a 'basic right' of indigenous peoples *everywhere* (Williams 1999).

Cultural humility

The notion of 'cultural humility', referred to earlier, has its origins in the work of Tervalon and Murray-García (1998). In keeping with the moral underpinnings of cultural competence education, Tervalon and Murray-García (1998: 118) recognised that, when working with people of diverse cultural and language backgrounds, practitioners require humility. Specifically, they need to 'continually engage in self-reflection and self-critique as lifelong learners and reflective practitioners' (Tervalon & Murray-Garcia 1998: 118) and, via these processes, to redress the power imbalance that otherwise exists in the professional–patient relationship. To this end Tervalon and Murray-Garcia (1998) describe cultural humility as incorporating 'a lifelong commitment to self-evaluation and critique, to redressing the power imbalances in the physician–patient dynamic, and to developing mutually beneficial and non-paternalistic partnerships with communities on behalf of individuals and defined populations' (p. 123).

A beginning first step to developing cultural humility is for practitioners to reflect on their own 'ill-defined and multidimensional cultural identities and backgrounds' (Tervalon & Murray-García 1998: 119). Tervalon and Murray-García (1998: 119) believe that the lessons learned from this reflection will enable practitioners to become:

> *flexible and humble enough to say that they do not know when they truly do not know and to search for and access resources that might enhance immeasurably the care of the patient as well as their future clinical practice.*

In short, cultural humility invites health care providers:

1. *to engage in self-reflection and self-critique*
2. *to bring into check the power imbalance, by using patient-focused interviewing and care*
3. *to assess anew the cultural dimensions of the experiences of each patient*
4. *to relinquish the role of expert to the patient, becoming the student of the patient*
5. *to see the patient's potential to be a capable and full partner in the therapeutic alliance.*
   (Austerlic 2009: 2)

By engaging in these processes, it is anticipated that the moral ideals of culturally competent and safe care will ultimately be realised (see also Foronda et al 2016; Yeager & Bauer-Wu 2013).

Conclusion

Cross-cultural ethics recognises the inherent difficulties associated with genuine moral problems in human life being 'confronted as abstraction rather than experiential realities' (Marshall 1992: 52) and affirms that, if moral abstractions are to count for anything, they must be brought 'back to earth' (Stout 1988: 8). It also recognises the inability of abstract and decontextualised moral thinking to provide concrete answers to complex questions concerning a range of human experiences. Key among these experiences are: human pain and suffering, intense and sometimes conflicting human emotions, ambivalent and ambiguous human relationships and, not least, differing cultural world views about the value and meaning of life – all of which often (too often) have to be dealt with in the face of overwhelming uncertainty, the unpredictability of probable outcomes (positive and negative), fallible modes of communication and the fallibilities of decision-makers (Cortese 1990; Elliott 1992; Johnstone 2014b; Marshall 1992; Stout 1988).

Unlike other moral critiques, however, cross-cultural ethics offers an optimistic outlook. Its suggestion that acceptance of – and achieving a harmony of – co-existing moral diversity offers the key to sustaining the existence and purpose of morality; it also provides an important basis upon which we can all develop not just our moral thinking and sensibilities, but also our ability to *actually be moral* in a world characterised by diverse and competing valid world views. This is not merely compromise, as some might believe, or even tolerance – the blinded eye of an indiscriminate mind (see Midgley 1991a; Wolff et al 1969). Nor is it confusion. Rather, it is celebration. In particular, it is the celebration of the 'other' as different, but not inferior, fallacious or superstitious — as having something worthwhile to share, and not as being something worthless to be marginalised, trivialised and ignored. If we accept this, we will all be in a much better position to judge what is really unethical as opposed to being merely disliked, what is truly wrong as opposed to being merely unfamiliar and strange, and what is really confusion as opposed to simple misunderstanding of another's moral language with which we are not familiar (Stout 1988). This insight is, among other things, what we stand to gain by embracing a diversity of moral values and beliefs as being the beginning of morality and not its end.

In conclusion, there are a number of questions which nurses can ask when making moral decisions about the nursing care of people from diverse cultural backgrounds, and which will assist them to check that they are 'on the right track'. Borrowing from Kanitsaki (1989b: 70) these questions are:

- *Is my understanding of this person's values and value systems such that it entitles me to override her or his family's requests or instructions?*
- *Can I by way of a third party (such as an interpreter) really ensure that my interventions will result in benefits not harms to that person?*
- *Are my values and frame of reference the only ones which warrant overriding consideration in this relationship?*
- *How do I know my judgments in this relationship are morally and culturally appropriate? In short, how do I know I am right?*

By asking these and similar questions, by embracing cultural humility, and by seeking the 'right' answers to them, nurses will demonstrate successfully that they are able to embrace morality as something more than a set of abstract self-standing principles. They will also demonstrate that, in the ultimate analysis, it is people and relationships that count – not a blind deference to rules which, when stripped of their cultural content, context and hence meaning become little more than intellectual curiosities empowered by arbitrary will, incapable of responding to the lived realities and needs of human beings who have been born into circumstances which are very often beyond their control. Embracing this approach will also remind us that:

> *any theory of ethics is, in the end, only as plausible as the complete picture of the world of which it forms a part.* (McNaughton 1988: 41)

Case scenario 1

A 69-year-old Greek-born man, who had grown up in a village and who spoke little English, was admitted to a major metropolitan hospital in Melbourne for follow-up assessment and tests for a cancer-related illness that had been diagnosed and treated some years earlier. Initially, when first diagnosed and treated, the man's prognosis was thought to be 'good' and his disease 'under control'. Unfortunately, his condition changed unexpectedly and his test results revealed that his cancer had spread and that only palliative care could now be offered for his condition. He was in no pain, however, and although tired was eager to return home. Meanwhile, his treating doctor decided that before being discharged the man had a right to be told about the change in his prognosis and of what lay ahead. The man's Australian-born daughter, however, took a different view and insisted that 'under no circumstances was her father to be told his poor prognosis' since this would 'destroy his hope' and affect his quality of life.[2] When the doctor objected to her request, the daughter explained that, in their (Greek) culture, it was wrong to tell someone they had terminal cancer; she then begged the doctor not to tell her father his test results or that 'they [the doctors] were not going to do anything [medically] for him, other than to provide palliative care'.[2] The doctor again objected to the daughter's request, arguing that the matter was 'not about culture, but about ethics' and that her father 'had a right to know'.

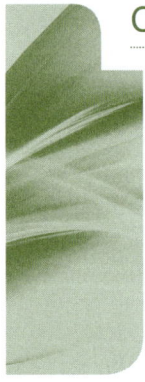

Case scenario 2[3]

An elderly English man suffering 'shortness of breath' was admitted to hospital for observations and further investigations. A few days later, a CT scan revealed what seemed to be a 'sizeable, aggressive tumour' on his right lung. A later bronchoscopy examination, however, revealed this initial diagnosis to be wrong and that the lump was in fact a 'pea' that he had swallowed but which had 'gone down the wrong way' (Hough 2013). Ten days later the man died of pneumonia despite being given active treatment for this condition. Although the man was informed that the initial diagnosis had been wrong, according to his widow her husband 'would still be alive if doctors had diagnosed him correctly […] The doctors told [him] he had got a tumour on his lung. He was scared rigid and basically worried himself to death […] [He] was told the news [of his misdiagnosis] but it was too late, his body had already given up and the treatment didn't make any difference' (Hough 2013).

CRITICAL QUESTIONS

1 If you were a nurse assigned to the care of this elderly Greek-born man and you came across the doctor and the man's daughter arguing about his 'right to know', how would you respond to the situation? In the case of the elderly English man, should he have been told that he had a tumour on his lung – particularly given that the provisional diagnosis had not yet been confirmed by a bronchoscopy examination?

2 What ultimate values and beliefs would you draw on to inform your thoughts, decisions and actions?

3 What assistance would *The ICN code of ethics for nurses* (ICN 2012a) or your own national nurses association's code of ethics provide in helping you to decide what to do?

4 What might be the consequences to the Greek man and his family if the doctor ignores the daughter's requests, calls an interpreter and tells the patient that his prognosis is poor and that only palliative care can now be offered to him?

5 What might be the consequences to the English man and his family if the doctors had decided to *withhold* the initial CT scan results? Is this case an example of the 'nocebo phenomenon', which perhaps could have been averted?

6 Upon what basis, if at all, is imposing unwanted information (e.g. a poor prognosis) on a patient morally justified?

Endnotes

1 TMT was first proposed in 1986 by social psychologists Jeff Greenberg, Tom Pyszczynski, and Sheldon Solomon (Greenberg et al 1986) and has since been validated by over 500 studies in 30 countries (Yetzer et al 2018: 246). Informed by the work of cultural anthropologist, Ernest Becker (1971, 1973, 1975), the premise of TMT is that human beings are painfully aware of the inevitability of their own future death. This awareness has the potential to cause paralysing terror, since it clashes with our instinctual desire for continued life. The terror of death is, however, largely suppressed by human culture or 'cultural worldviews' (Becker 1973; Pyszczynski et al 1996). By suppressing the terror of death, culture thus 'makes human life possible' by imbuing it with meaning and significance (Becker 1973: 265) (see also the discussion on 'Bioethics, cultural differences and the problem of moral disagreements in health care: a terror management theory' (Johnstone 2012b)).

2 Personal communication, identifying details altered.

3 Taken from Hough A (2013) Grandfather dies after doctors 'misdiagnosed pea on lung for cancer'. *The Telegraph* 22 April. Online. Available: https://www.telegraph.co.uk/news/health/news/10009756/Grandfather-dies-after-doctors-misdiagnosed-pea-on-lung-for-cancer.html.

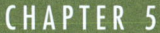

Moral problems and moral decision-making in nursing and health care contexts

KEYWORDS

everyday ethical issues
moral decision-making
moral differences
moral disputes
moral problems
needs
quantum morality
wants

LEARNING OBJECTIVES

Upon the completion of this chapter and with further self-directed learning you are expected to be able to:

- Discuss the three distinguishing features of a moral problem.
- Explain why moral problems are different from other kinds of (non-moral) problems.
- Distinguish the moral difference between 'wants' and 'needs'.
- Discuss the nature of the moral problems listed below and their possible implications in regard to the ethical practice of nursing:
  – moral unpreparedness / incompetence
  – moral blindness
  – moral insensitivity
  – moral indifference
  – moral disengagement
  – moral fading
  – amoralism
  – immoralism
  – moral complacency
  – moral dumbfounding / stupefaction
  – moral fanaticism
  – moral disagreement
  – moral conflict
  – moral dilemmas
  – 'moral distress'.
- Define moral decision-making.
- Discuss critically the role that reason, emotion, intuition and life experience might play in moral decision-making.
- Discuss processes for dealing effectively with moral disputes.
- Explore a range of 'everyday' ethical issues that nurses might face in the course of providing nursing care to patients.

Introduction

Nurses at all levels and in all areas of practice encounter *moral problems* during the course of their everyday professional practice. A *moral problem* (to be distinguished from a non-moral or 'ordinary' problem) is defined for the purposes of this discussion as a moral matter or issue that is difficult to deal with, solve or overcome and which stands in need of a moral solution.

Moral problems can range from the relatively 'simple' to the extraordinarily complex, and can cause varying degrees of perplexity and emotional reactions (e.g. disgust, anger, distress, guilt) in those who encounter them. In either case, nurses, like other health professionals, have a stringent moral responsibility to be able to identify and respond effectively to the moral problems they encounter (whether 'simple' or 'complex') and, where able, to employ strategies to prevent them from occurring in the first place. In order to be able to do this, however, nurses must first be able to distinguish moral problems from other sorts of (non-moral) problems (e.g. legal and clinical problems), and to be able to distinguish different types of moral problems from each other. It is in advancing knowledge and understanding of the different kinds of moral problems that nurses might encounter in the course of their day-to-day practice – and how best to deal with them – that provides the focus for this chapter.

Distinguishing moral problems from other sorts of problems

All health professionals encounter a variety of problems in the course of their everyday practice, and nurses are no exception. Significantly, most of these problems probably have a moral dimension to them. It is important to clarify, however, that not all problems that have a moral dimension are *moral problems* per se. This raises the question: How are we to distinguish a bona fide moral problem from other kinds of (non-moral) problems? One clue to answering this question lies in the degree to which the moral dimensions of a given problem might be deemed 'weightier' and thus prima facie as 'overriding' of the other dimensions of the problem, and the kinds of solutions that might be fruitfully employed to resolve the problem. Consider the following example.

A patient is in severe and intolerable pain due to not receiving pain medication. Nevertheless, while this is a problem and one which clearly has a moral dimension, it is not immediately evident that the problem is a 'full-blown' moral problem requiring moral analysis, debate and possibly the intervention of an 'ethics expert' or clinical ethics committee. Further analysis is required. It might be, for instance, that the patient's pain management has, for some reason, been neglected. What is required in this instance is a competent and compassionate clinical assessment of the patient and the swift administration of needed analgesia. The problem may thus be correctly characterised as a 'technical or practical problem' requiring, and resolvable by, a 'clinical solution'. It might also be, however, that the patient is in pain owing to her refusing pain relief on religious grounds. In such an instance even the most competent and compassionate of clinical assessments will not necessarily result in the identification of a satisfactory solution to the problem of the patient's pain since the obvious 'clinical solution' (i.e. of giving analgesia) is precluded by the moral demand to respect the patient's autonomous wishes. The problem may thus be correctly characterised as a *moral problem* (not merely a clinical problem) since:

- the patient's moral interest and wellbeing are at risk (if her autonomous wishes are respected, she will suffer the harm of otherwise preventable intolerable pain; conversely, if her pain is alleviated by the administration of analgesia, she will suffer the harm of having her autonomous wishes violated),

- the nurses' moral interests and wellbeing are at risk on account of the emotional distress they may experience at their genuine inability to maximise the patient's moral interests in not suffering unnecessarily, and, finally,
- assistance is required to help attendant nurses to answer the question: What should we do?

To help clarify the basis upon which the above distinction has been made, the following framework is offered. It is generally accepted that something involves a (human) moral/ethical problem where it has as its central concern:

- the promotion and protection of people's genuine wellbeing and welfare (including their interests in not suffering unnecessarily)
- responding justly to the genuine needs and significant interests of different people
- determining and justifying what constitutes right and wrong conduct in a given situation (Amato 1990; Beauchamp & Childress 2013; Frankena 1973).

In adopting this framework it is important to understand that a '*need*' (to be distinguished from a mere '*want*') is something which is essential – necessary – for human survival and which a human being must have fulfilled in order to live a recognisably human life. Needs are also strongly related to moral interests. For example, health is a basic human need. Thus it is reasonable to claim that people have a strong moral interest in being healthy and receiving good health care.

A '*want*', in contrast, pertains more to desires and preferences. For instance, people can desire and prefer things that they do not need and that might even be contrary to their survival interests (e.g. smoking cigarettes). The reverse is also true – people may not desire or prefer things they do need (e.g. a weight reduction diet).

Unlike 'wants' and 'preferences' (which generally pertain to things that are inessential, optional and even trivial), other people's needs suggest a degree of urgency and seem to exert a kind of moral force over us which we feel compelled to respect. When having a special convincing force, a needs claim can have a powerful effect on our judgments, which in turn makes us feel driven to acknowledge and support the needs claim as genuine and commanding our attention.

The nursing profession is fundamentally concerned with the promotion and protection of people's genuine wellbeing and welfare and, in achieving these ends, responding justly to the genuine needs and the significant moral interests of different people. The nursing profession is, therefore, fundamentally concerned with 'moral problems' as well as other kinds of problems (e.g. technical, clinical, legal, and so forth). In order to deal with moral problems appropriately and effectively it is evident that nurses need to know, first, what form a moral problem might take and how to recognise it and, second, how best to decide when dealing with them. It is to answering these questions that this discussion now turns.

Identifying different kinds of moral problems

The nursing literature has, to date, tended to give prominence to one type of moral problem: namely, the *moral dilemma* (also referred to as an *ethical dilemma*) and the assumed 'moral distress' that moral dilemmas give rise to. While it is true that the moral/ethical dilemma is an important moral problem in nursing and health care domains, it needs to be clarified that it is by no means the only, or even the most common, moral problem that nurses (or others) will encounter when planning and implementing care. Moreover, it is important to place in context that what is generally known today as 'quandary ethics' (involving situations in which people find it difficult to decide *what they should do*) is a relative 'new comer' to the field of bioethics (see Pincoffs 1971: 553) and one that has not necessarily been amendable to advancing nursing ethics discourse (Johnstone & Hutchinson, 2015).

In all, there are at least 14 different kinds of moral problems that can and do arise in nursing and health care contexts; these are:

1. moral unpreparedness and incompetence
2. moral blindness
3. moral indifference and insensitivity
4. moral disengagement
5. moral fading/ethical fading
6. amoralism
7. immoralism
8. moral complacency
9. moral dumbfounding/stupefaction
10. moral fanaticism
11. moral disagreements
12. moral conflicts
13. moral dilemmas
14. 'moral distress'.

If nurses are to respond effectively to the moral problems encountered in nursing and health care contexts, it is important that they understand the nature and implications of the different kinds of moral problems that can arise. It is to examining this issue further that the following discussion now turns.

Moral unpreparedness/moral incompetence

The first type of moral problem to be considered here is that of general 'unpreparedness' to deal appropriately and effectively with morally troubling situations. What sometimes happens is that a nurse (or other health professional) enters into a situation without being sufficiently prepared or without the moral competencies necessary to deal with the ethical issues at hand (Johnstone 2015a). The nurse (or other health professional) may, for instance, lack the requisite moral knowledge (e.g. of moral theories, codes and guidelines), skills and experience (e.g. of ethical reasoning and decision-making, how to interpret and apply ethical principles and standards of conduct), 'right attitude' (e.g. 'excellence in character', virtue), and moral wisdom (e.g. moral awareness, insight, perception, astuteness) otherwise necessary to be able to deal with the complexities of the ethical issues in the situation at hand (this could also count as moral incompetence or moral impairment, discussed in Chapter 1 of this book). When eventually faced with a particular moral problem, the nurse acts in bad faith by pretending that the situation at hand is one which can be handled 'with one's given moral apparatus' (Lemmon 1987: 112). The risks of 'poorly reflected and inconsistent ethical decisions' (Eriksson et al 2007: 213) and moral error ('getting it wrong') in such instances are considerable.

To illustrate the seriousness of moral unpreparedness, consider the analogous situation of clinical unpreparedness. A nurse who is not educated in the complexities of, say, intensive care nursing, but who is nevertheless sent to 'help out' and care for a ventilated patient in intensive care, would not only be inadequate in this role, but could even be dangerous. Such a nurse might not have the learned skills necessary to detect the subtle changes in a sedated patient's condition – changes indicating, for example, the need for more sedation, or the need to perform tracheal suctioning, or the need to increase the tidal volume of air flow or oxygen administration. Neither might this nurse be able to distinguish the many different alarms that can go off on the high-tech equipment being used to give full life support to the patient, or to detect any malfunctioning of this sophisticated equipment. Without these skills, a nurse working in intensive care would be likely to place the life and wellbeing of the patient at serious risk.

The argument of the seriousness of unpreparedness also applies to the complexities of sound ethical reasoning and ethical health care practice generally. Such a nurse, left to deal with a morally troubling situation, would not only be inadequate in that role but, as the intensive care example shows, his or her practice could be potentially hazardous. Without the learned moral skills necessary to detect moral problems and to resolve them in a sound, reliable and justifiable manner, an unprepared nurse, no matter how well intentioned, could fail to correctly detect moral hazards and the risk of moral injuries occurring in the workplace, and therefore fail to act or respond in a way that would prevent adverse moral outcomes from occurring.

The kinds of preventable adverse moral outcomes or 'near misses' that can occur as a result of nurses' (and other allied health professionals') moral unpreparedness to deal appropriately and effectively with moral problems in health care contexts are well documented in the nursing, bioethical, legal and other related literature. To give just one stand-out example, consider the notorious case of the Chelmsford Private Hospital in Sydney, Australia. In this case, many people were left permanently damaged and scarred – some even died – as a result of receiving deep sleep therapy (DST) prescribed by Dr Harry Bailey, a consultant psychiatrist, who later committed suicide in connection with the scandal that was eventually uncovered (Bromberger & Fife-Yeomans 1991; Rice 1988). It is now known that approximately one thousand patients were 'treated' with DST at this hospital. It is also known, as revealed as early as 1977 by the current affairs television program *60 Minutes*, that many of these patients did not receive the standard of care and treatment they were entitled to receive. Among other things – including the deaths of seven people between 1974 and 1977 – the *60 Minutes* program revealed that 'recognised standard precautions for the safety of patients were not taken; and that patients received the treatment without their consent' (Bromberger & Fife-Yeomans 1991: 142). In the Chelmsford Royal Commission that was eventually established in 1988 to 'examine the provision of Deep Sleep Therapy and the administration of Chelmsford Private Hospital', it was confirmed that:

> *The signature of some [consent] forms was obtained by fraud and deceit. Some were signed by people whose judgment was compromised by drugs. Some patients were even woken up from their DST [Deep Sleep Therapy] treatment to complete their authorisation. Other patients were treated contrary to their express wishes and some were treated despite the fact they had specifically refused the treatment.* (Commissioner Slattery, cited in Bromberger & Fife-Yeomans 1991: 171)

Nursing care was also seriously substandard. In one notable case, the nursing care had been so negligent that a patient developed severe decubitus ulcers between her knees, which became 'glued' together as though they had been skin grafted. The former patient recalled:

> *I was having hallucinations about a lot of coloured ribbons and trying to climb out through them finding the world again. I woke up in a bath tub and two nurses were bathing me. I felt really dirty. One of the nurses said, 'My God, look at her knees.' I looked down and they were joined together. The nurses gently pulled them apart.* (Bromberger & Fife-Yeomans 1991: 94)

Another example of the substandard nursing care that was provided can be found in the experiences of another patient, Barry Hart, outlined in the following statement read to the New South Wales Parliament in 1984:

> *Basic, commonsense nursing practice was ignored. Patients were sedated for ten days and given no exercise during this period. They were incontinent of faeces and urine most of the time and were left lying incontinent of faeces until they woke up.*
>
> *There was no attempt to maintain a fluid balance. Patients wet the bed and remained lying in the urine until the sheets were changed. The staff made an approximation of whether the patients were actually passing urine (i.e. a fluid output) by seeing how wet the bed was.* (cited in Rice 1988: 47)

One of the troubling things about the whole Chelmsford scandal is that rumours about Dr Bailey's unscrupulous practices had been circulating for years, yet nothing was done about it (Bromberger & Fife-Yeomans 1991: 176). Equally disturbing is the fact that it was not until 1988 – 24 years after the investigated death of the first 'deep sleep' patient, and only after 'treatment' had led to the deaths of 24 patients – that a Royal Commission was set up to investigate the allegations concerning the patient abuse that was subsequently proved to have occurred at Chelmsford Private Hospital (Bromberger & Fife-Yeomans 1991: 162). Significantly, in the Royal Commission of Inquiry that was conducted, and in the report on its findings, it was revealed that between 1963 and 1979 only two nurses took action in an attempt to expose the unscrupulous practices they had observed (Report of the Royal Commission into Deep Sleep Therapy 1990: 127). There is room to suggest here that, had the nursing staff been better prepared to recognise and respond effectively to violations of professional ethical standards, the trauma and suffering experienced by the patients at Chelmsford could have been prevented.

Not all adverse moral outcomes occurring in health care contexts are as ethically dramatic as those that occurred in the Chelmsford Private Hospital case, however. Preventable adverse moral outcomes can and do occur on a much more commonplace level in the health care arena, as examples to be given in the following chapters of this book will show.

Moral blindness

A second type of problem nurses sometimes encounter is what might be termed 'moral blindness' (also called 'ethical blindness'). A morally blind nurse (or other health professional) is someone who, upon encountering a moral problem, simply does not see it as a moral problem. There are four possible explanations for this. First, the nurse may perceive the problem confronting her as either a clinical or a technical problem only. A tendency by health professionals to sometimes 'translate ethical issues into technical problems which have clinical solutions' was first recognised over four decades ago (Carlton 1978: 10), and persists in various forms to this day. A second (and possibly related) explanation relates to a phenomenon termed 'inattentional blindness'. First described by Neisser (1979) and later popularised by US researchers Chabris and Simons (2010) in their now famous 'invisible gorilla' experiment (this can be viewed at http://www.theinvisiblegorilla.com/gorilla_experiment.html), inattentional blindness fundamentally involves 'failing to see things that are in plain sight' on account of the observer *not expecting to see them*. Just as inattentional blindness has implications for patient safety in clinical settings (Jones & Johnstone 2017), so too does it have implications for moral safety in healthcare contexts. Onlookers may, for instance, 'not see' the ethical dimension of an issue because, quite simply, they are not expecting to see it and are not looking for it. A third explanation may lie in the moral psychology of individuals who, lacking moral insight and awareness (and some may argue, intrinsic moral character and moral will as well), are 'ethically blind' to their previous behaviours involving ethical failures. Similar in nature to the problems of moral disengagement and moral fading (both discussed below), instead of reflecting on their previous questionable conduct and lack of moral sensibilities, they normalise them (Chugh & Kern 2016; Mortensen 2002). Borrowing from the patient safety literature, this outcome may be referred to as 'the normalisation of deviance' (Banja 2010; Price & Williams 2018) – in this case of morally questionable acts. The normalisation of deviance involves a process of insensitivity occurring imperceptibly – sometimes over years – until a point is reached where a deviant practice 'no longer feels wrong' (Price & Williams 2018: 1).

A fourth and final explanation may relate to the phenomenon of what Margaret Heffernan (2011) has influentially described as 'willful blindness'. Willful blindness is a legal concept that dates back to the 19th century and holds that a person is responsible for something that they 'could have known, and should have known' but instead 'strove not to see' (Heffernan 2011: 2). Heffernan (2011: 1) explains that, in practice, willful blindness involves the denial of truths that are too painful or too frightening to confront even though these truths 'cry out for acknowledgment, debate, action and change'. One of the insidious effects of willful blindness is that 'bad acts' are not committed in some dark and hidden way so that people cannot see them, but rather in the plain view of people who 'simply [choose] not to look and not to question' (Heffernan 2011: 1).

Moral blindness can be likened, in an analogous way, to colour blindness. Just as a colour-blind person fails to distinguish certain colours in the world, a morally blind person fails to distinguish certain 'moral properties' in the world. In short, they have a 'moral blind spot'. Perhaps a better example can be found by appealing to a set of imageries commonly associated with Gestalt psychology and theories on the nature of perception. Consider the two following drawings, which are popularly presented in psychology texts to demonstrate certain perceptual phenomena, including perceptual organisation and the influence of context on the way in which an object is perceived.

The first of these drawings (Fig. 5.1) depicts what initially appears to be a white vase or goblet against a black background; after a more sustained glance, the drawing changes (or rather, one's perception 'shifts') and what is perceived instead are two black facial profiles separated by a white space. Some people see the alternating vase–face images relatively quickly and easily, while others struggle to shake off what for them remains the dominant image (i.e. either the vase or the faces).

The second ambiguous drawing (Fig. 5.2) depicts what can be seen as either a duck or a rabbit. As with the vase–face drawing, some people see the alternating duck–rabbit images relatively easily, while others literally get 'stuck' with a dominant perception of either the duck or the rabbit.

Psychologists claim, however, that people's perceptions can be altered by context – in this instance, by showing photographs before the ambiguous drawings are viewed. They claim that, on an initial viewing of an ambiguous drawing, a majority will report seeing one dominant image first – for example, the duck. If subjects are shown photographs of the alternative image before seeing the drawing, however, almost all see the alternative image (e.g. the rabbit) first. The same 'reversals' can be achieved by conditioning subjects with photographs to see the alternative image (e.g. the duck/rabbit) first (see also Atkinson et al 1983: 147).

It is not the purpose of this analogy to advance a theory of moral perception but rather to highlight the possible risks of impaired moral perception in health care contexts. Drawing on this analogy, there

FIGURE 5.1
Reversible figure and background

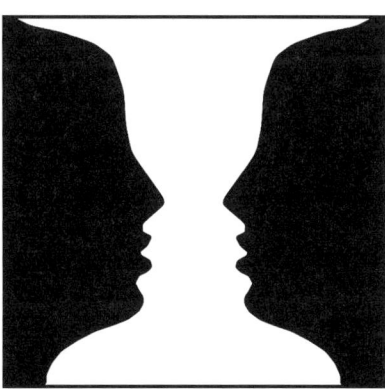

(Source: John Smithson 2007/commons.wikimedia.org/wiki/File:Rubin2.jpg)

FIGURE 5.2
Ambiguous stimulus

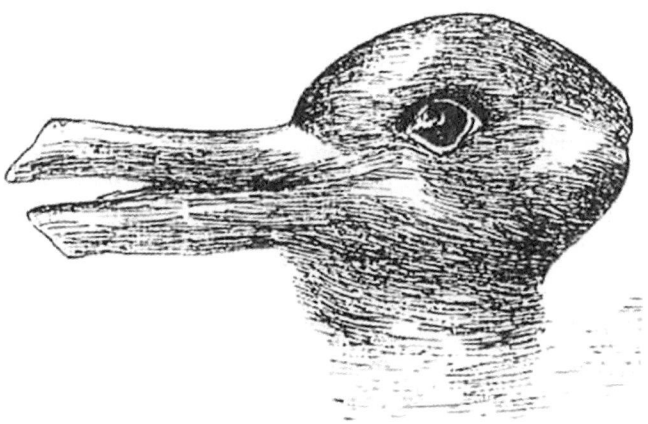

(Jastrow, J. (1899). The mind's eye. Popular Science Monthly, 54, 299–312)

is room to suggest that health professionals (including nurses) are sometimes so conditioned by the 'clinical imagery' (context) around them that, when they do encounter a bona fide moral problem, it tends to be perceived not as a *moral* problem, but as a *clinical* or a *technical* problem and, as such, one requiring a clinical solution, not a moral solution. Some health professionals have a healthy perception of the alternating moral–clinical images depicted by a given scenario; others, however, remain stuck with a dominant *clinical image* and do not see the alternative *moral image*, which for them is less discernible. One unfortunate consequence of this is that *technically correct* decisions are sometimes made at the expense of *morally correct* decisions.

The extent to which clinical perceptions and judgments can dominate over moral perceptions and judgments can be illustrated by the once-common practice of defending 'Do Not Resuscitate' (DNR) directives (also called 'Not For Resuscitation' or NFR directives) on hopelessly or chronically ill patients on medical grounds ('medical indications') alone. In the past many doctors and nurses perceived DNR directives as involving a *clinical issue*, not a *moral issue*, and, as such, one to be decided by doctors, not ethicists. The clinical–moral Gestalt problem became apparent at an Australian nursing law and ethics conference in 1988. After presenting a paper on the nature and moral implications of DNR / NFR directives, a keynote speaker was approached by several registered nurses with what, at the time, became a familiar and distressing comment: 'My God! I had never thought about it [DNR / NFR] as a moral issue before … What have I done?'; other nurses wanted to challenge or attack the view that DNR / NFR directives involved moral considerations and moral decisions. The then state president (in Victoria) of the Australian Medical Association, Dr Bill McCubbery, was prompted to respond to the issue, and is reported as saying that 'NFR decisions had to depend on professional judgment' (Schumpeter 1988: 21).

Today there is a much greater recognition of the moral dimensions of DNR / NFR directives and the degree to which such directives are informed by moral considerations (see the discussion on DNR in Chapter 9 of this book). The once common view that DNR / NFR decisions are based 'simply' on medical concerns / indications (not ethical concerns) and are more a matter of 'good medical judgment' (rather than – or as well as – sound moral judgment) is rarely advanced in contemporary debate, at least not credibly. Nevertheless, this kind of thinking persists in regard to other issues. For example, in 2001, in a highly publicised surgery ban imposed on smokers by doctors in the Australian state of Victoria, surgeons were reported as defending their stance by arguing that:

> *Medical concerns, not moral judgments, were the bottom line in banning smokers from a range of life-saving treatments.* (Chandler 2001: 9)

The specific treatments banned, in this instance, were reported to include artery by-passes, coronary artery grafts, lung reduction surgery and lung and heart transplants (Taylor 2001: 4). Over a decade later, the issue of clinical judgments versus moral judgments in regard to treating smokers (and other patients with 'lifestyle' diseases) captured national headlines in the UK, after that country's National Health Service (NHS) reportedly banned general practitioners (GPs) from performing minor surgeries on patients who were smokers or who were obese (Adams 2013; Campbell 2012; Palmer 2012). The authorities and GPs supporting this stance denied this was a case of making moral judgment about people's 'lifestyle choices' or about how valuable they thought the patients' lives were, or whether they thought such patients did not 'deserve treatment' because of having brought their health problems on themselves (Adams 2013; Campbell 2012; Palmer 2012). Rather, it was contended, their stance involved a 'purely medical decision', based 'on the fact' that evidence shows people who smoke or who are overweight are at 'greater risk of developing serious complications and recover more slowly from surgery' (Palmer 2012).

The issue of 'moral blindness' among nurses is an important one since, as with the problem of moral unpreparedness, it can result in 'wrong decisions' being made and otherwise preventable moral harms occurring. This problem is not insurmountable, however. Just as people can be 'conditioned' to see the white goblet rather than the two black faces in the ambiguous drawing shown in Fig. 5.1, or of the rabbit rather than the duck in the ambiguous drawing shown in Fig. 5.2, so too can nurses be 'conditioned' (or rather educated) to see the moral dimension of an ambiguous scenario which can be perceived as involving either a moral problem or a clinical or technical problem. Arguably, the best way to achieve such a Gestalt moral shift in perception is by appropriate ethics education and reflective ethical practice.

Moral indifference and insensitivity

A third type of problem which nurses may encounter is that of 'moral indifference' and 'moral insensitivity'. Moral indifference is characterised by an unconcerned or uninterested attitude towards demands to be moral; in short, it assumes the attitude of: 'Why bother to be moral?' The morally indifferent person is someone who typically refrains from expressing any desire that certain acts should or should not be done in all comparable circumstances (Hare 1981: 185). Moral insensitivity, in turn, similarly reveals itself in the everyday failure to respond to the suffering of others, in refusing to understand others, and in 'the casual turning away of one's ethical gaze' (Bauman & Donskis 2013: 9) – in other words, assuming the stance of a morally passive bystander. Moral insensitivity in this instance is compounded by what Bauman and Donskis (2013: 11) describe as the 'non-perception of early signals that something threatens to be or is already wrong with human togetherness and the viability of human community', and that if nothing is done 'things will get still worse'. Moral indifference is different to moral blindness in that the individual 'sees' a moral issue but is indifferent to it.

An example of a morally indifferent and morally insensitive nurse would be a nurse who failed in his or her everyday practice to respond to the suffering of patients, refused to understand them, and blithely turned away from promoting and protecting their moral interests. Such a nurse may, for example, be unconcerned about and uninterested in alleviating a patient's pain, or be unconcerned about or uninterested in the fact that a DNR directive or a directive to perform electroconvulsive therapy (ECT) has been given on a non-consenting patient, or be unconcerned about and uninterested in any form of violation of patients' rights. As well as this, a morally indifferent and insensitive nurse would refrain from expressing a desire that anything should be done about such situations.

The problem of moral indifference and moral insensitivity in nursing was first captured by Mila Aroskar (1986) in her classic article 'Are nurses' mind sets compatible with ethical practice?' Aroskar (1986: 72) cites the findings of a study undertaken in the late 1970s which showed that nurses tended to defer to institutional norms 'even when patients' rights were being violated'. She also points out that, despite the North American nursing profession's formal commitment to ethical practice (as manifested, among other things, by its formal adoption of various codes and standards of practice), arguments were still widely heard among nurses that 'ethical practice is too risky and requires a certain amount of heroism on the part of nurses' (Aroskar 1986: 69). Although written over two decades ago, Aroskar's words still apply today. For example, the former secretary of the Australian Nursing Federation (ANF), Jill Iliffe, had cause to reflect (2002: 1):

> *What do you do when something happens that you know to be wrong, unethical or inappropriate? [...] A colleague behaves unprofessionally; health care is provided that you know to be inappropriate; a decision is made that is ethically questionable; there is an adverse outcome that could have been avoided, or was perhaps even the result of negligence. What do you do? It is often a difficult decision to make, particularly when the other person or persons are more senior to you and in a position of power and authority.*

More recently, a much cited review of the literature on nurses' ethical reasoning and behaviour found that nurses still tend to be 'conformist' in their practice and feel hindered by 'dominance within the medical profession, a stressful work environment, insufficient resources, time and workload pressures' (Goethals et al 2010: 644; see also Dierckx de Casterlé et al 2008).

The retreat by nurses into moral indifference and insensitivity (moral blunting), while not condonable, is understandable. There are many examples that demonstrate the kinds of difficulties that nurses might find themselves in when attempting to uphold morally responsible professional practice, and the ultimate price that can be paid for taking an independent moral stand on a matter. Many nurses know (and have possibly personally experienced) the forces that can be brought to bear when taking a moral position which conflicts with established hospital norms and etiquette. It is, then, perhaps understandable (even though inexcusable) that nurses become morally indifferent to breaches of ethical standards and unjust practices in health care domains. Compounding this situation, institutional and legal constraints can sometimes make it difficult for nurses to uphold the agreed ethical standards of the profession (Johnstone 1994b, 2002). The price paid for acting morally or for taking a moral stand can be high, as other examples to be given in the chapters to follow will show. What this signifies, however, is not that nurses should abandon the demands of morality; rather, they should seek ways in which they can uphold morality's demands safely and effectively. This issue will be considered in more depth in Chapter 11 of this book.

Moral disengagement

A fourth problem that may be encountered is that of moral disengagement. The notion of 'moral disengagement' (like moral fading, which will be considered under the following subheading) was first articulated by Canadian-born psychologist Albert Bandura (1986, 1990, 1999; Bandura et al 1996) and is broadly defined as a process whereby an individual convinces himself/herself through a process of elaborate self-serving rationalisations that ethical standards do not apply to them in given situations and thus they do not need to self-censure. Bandura contends that moral disengagement may centre on one or all of the following:

> *(a) The reconstrual of the conduct itself so it is not viewed as immoral, (b) the operation of the agency of action so that the perpetrators can minimize their role in causing harm, (c) the [distortion of] consequences*

that flow from actions, (d) how the victims of maltreatment are regarded by devaluing them as human beings [dehumanization] and blaming them for what is being done to them. (Bandura 1999: 194)

Moral disengagement from self-censure is thought to be a gradual process (i.e. it occurs over time) with people often not even recognising that they are changing. As Bandura (1999: 203) explains, 'Disengagement practices will not instantly transform considerate people into cruel ones'. He goes on to use the example of a prison guard who assists with the executions of prisoners on death row. Over time, the guard became 'less bothered' by his role, ultimately seeing it as 'just another job' (Bandura 1999: 204).

More recent work on the subject has revealed the problem of moral disengagement to be a significant and growing problem worldwide at all individual, collective and institutional levels. Today there is a plethora of research (too numerous to cite here) on the subject of how, when, where and why people selectively disengage their moral self-regulation without feeling guilt or shame. Significantly this research has been conducted from a range of disciplines and domains including business, organisational behaviour, sports psychology, criminology, military psychology, insurgent terrorism, child and adolescent development, by-stander effect, refugee aid, police repression and cyberbullying, to name some of them (see, for example, Antony 2017; Enemark 2017; Hindriks 2015; Kavussanu & Stanger 2017; Meter & Bauman 2018; Moore 2008, 2015; Moore et al 2012; Neal & Crammer 2017; Soares et al 2018; Thornberg et al 2016; Wang C et al 2017; Zapolski et al 2018).

The problem of moral disengagement, as described above, has only recently been considered in the nursing literature (Fida et al 2016; Hyatt 2017). Although limited, this work has highlighted the risks of moral disengagement in nursing – in particular, its role in enabling nurses to rationalise their non-compliance with the profession's ethical standards and hindering the conscientious and civic behaviour otherwise expected of them. Examples of morally disengaged behaviours by nurses include academic dishonesty, cheating in both classroom and clinical settings, workplace bullying, theft from patients, the misappropriation of pharmaceutical products from work, discrimination, and rude and uncompassionate behaviour towards patients (Johnstone 2016b, 2016c, 2017; Lipscomb 2016; see also the 2016 special issue of *Nursing Philosophy* on 'Dishonesty and deception in nursing' at https://onlinelibrary.wiley.com/toc/1466769x/17/3). Of particular concern, however, are the risks that moral disengagement poses to patient safety and the organisational culture of health care institutions (Hyatt 2017). Whether moral disengagement can be effectively remedied by targeted interventions designed to prevent or counteract its incidence and harmful impact is not clear. Research suggests, however, that those with a strong moral identity tend to be strongly motivated to be ethical and thus are less prone to moral disengagement, in contrast with those whose moral identity is weak (Hindriks 2015).

Moral fading/ethical fading

A fifth problem, which in several respects stands as both a consequence of and a component of moral disengagement, is 'moral fading' (also termed 'ethical fading'). Ethical fading fundamentally involves self-deception (encompassing 'language euphemisms, the slippery-slope of decision-making, errors in perceptual causation, and constraints induced by representations of the self'). This self-deception, in turn, plays a fundamental role in people overestimating their disposition towards being ethical and underestimating their capacity to engage in unethical behaviour (Tenbrunsel & Messick 2004).

Research on moral fading (like research on moral disengagement) has shown that people are often not as ethical as they think they are. Explaining this observation, Tenbrunsel and colleagues (2010: 154) write:

People believe they will behave ethically in a given situation, but they don't. They then believe they behaved ethically when they didn't. It's no surprise, then, that most individuals erroneously believe they are more ethical than the majority of their peers.

Research also suggests that when people are faced with extreme situations (e.g. public health emergencies, unjust organisational cultures), they will abandon 'the illusion that certain values are infinitely important' and make moral compromises (Tetlock 2003: 322) – in short, their otherwise ordinary ethical standpoints 'fade'.

The problem with moral fading is that even 'good' and well-intentioned people can find themselves crossing ethical boundaries and being 'ethically faded' and 'ethically adrift' without even realising it (Moore & Gino 2013: 55). Powerful and subtle influences can, for example, misdirect an individual's inner sense of right and wrong and (mis)lead them to believe that they are being ethical when they are not (Moore & Gino 2013; Tenbrunsel & Messick 2004).

Contributing to and facilitating ethical fading are what Moore and Gino (2013) have termed in another context *moral neglect*, *(faulty) moral justification* (manifesting as self-verification), and ultimately *moral inaction*. In the case of moral neglect, individuals succumb to the social norms of the day, eager to 'fit in' and to behave in socially approved ways, and lose sight of the possible moral consequences of their behaviour. Wanting to retain membership (and the approval) of the 'in-group', the grounds are set for moral disengagement, moral hypocrisy, moral fading and ultimately moral inaction. In addition, there is the problem of what Moore and Gino (2013) describe as 'organisational aggravators', which include organisational socialisation and identification, role expectations, goal orientation and group loyalty – all of which can, in various ways, be morally degrading and corrupting. Taken together, these processes can create a powerful barrier to 'doing the right thing'. In the case of nurses, they can also work to accustom individuals to 'tolerating behaviors that are outside the realm of considerate conduct', often without their even being aware of it (Felblinger 2008: 238).

Amoralism

A sixth type of moral problem which nurses might encounter is that of 'amoralism', which is characterised by an absence of moral concern and a rejection of morality altogether (a position significantly different from *immoralism*, discussed below, which accepts that morality exists, but violates its demands). An amoral person is someone who refrains from making moral judgments and who typically rejects being bound by any of morality's behavioural prescriptions and proscriptions. If an amoralist were to ask: 'Why should I be moral?' it is likely that no answer would be satisfactory.

A nurse who is an amoralist would reject any imperative to behave morally as a professional. For example, the amoral nurse might reject that he or she has a moral duty to uphold a patient's rights. The amoral nurse would also probably claim that it does not make any sense even to speak of things like a patient's 'rights' since moral language itself has no meaning. The amoralist's position in this respect is analogous to the atheist's rejection of certain religious terms. The atheist, for example, would argue against uttering the word 'God', since it refers to nothing and therefore has no meaning. Such an atheist might also claim that there is no point in engaging in a religious debate on the existence of God, since there is just nothing there to debate. The amoralist may argue in a similar way in relation to the issue of morality.

It can be seen that the amoralist's position is an extreme one, and one which is very difficult to sustain. (Even thieves, who may appear amoral, act on the 'moral' assumption that it is 'good / right' to steal.) Perhaps the most approximate example that can be given here is that of psychopaths or frontal-lobe-damaged persons who simply lack all capacity to be moral – an issue that has been comprehensively explored in the neuroethics literature (see, for example, Damasio 1994, 2007; Gazzaniga 2011; Gellene 2007; Koenigs et al 2007; Lehrer 2009; Strueber et al 2007). If amoralism is encountered in health care contexts, it is likely that very little can be done, morally speaking, to deal with it. The only recourse in dealing with the amoral health professional would be to appeal to non-moral censuring mechanisms such as legal and / or professional disciplinary measures.

Immoralism

A seventh type of problem that might be encountered by nurses is 'immoralism' or immoral conduct. At its most basic, immoral conduct (also termed *unethical conduct*) can be defined as any act involving a deliberate violation of accepted or agreed ethical standards. As previously discussed in Chapter 1 of this book, immoralism can encompass both *moral turpitude* and *moral delinquency*. Moral turpitude may be more specifically defined as:

> *anything done knowingly contrary to justice, honesty, principle, or good morals … [or] an act of baseness, vileness or depravity in the private or social duties which a man [sic] owes to his fellow man [sic] or to society in general. The term implies something immoral in itself.* (*Seary v State Bar of Texas* 1980, cited in Freckelton 1996: 142)

Moral delinquency, it will be recalled, refers to any act involving moral negligence or a dereliction of moral duty. As discussed in Chapter 1, moral delinquency in professional contexts entails a deliberate or careless violation of agreed standards of ethical professional conduct.

Accepting the above definitions, an immoral nurse can thus be described as someone who knowingly and willfully violates the agreed norms of ethical professional conduct or general ethical standards of conduct towards others. Judging immoral conduct, by this view, would require a demonstration that the accepted ethical standards of the profession were both (1) known by an offending nurse, and (2) deliberately and recklessly violated by that nurse. There are many 'obvious' examples of immoral conduct by nurses. These include: the deliberate theft of patients' and/or clients' money for personal use; the sexual, verbal and physical abuse of patients/clients; xenophobic behaviours (including racism, sexism, ageism, homophobia and a range of other unjust discriminatory behaviours); participation in unscrupulous research practices; and other morally unacceptable behaviours, examples of which are given throughout this book.

It should be noted that, regardless of whether an act involving the violation of agreed professional or general ethical standards results in a significant moral harm to another, it would still stand as an instance of immoral or unethical conduct. For example, a nurse who knowingly and recklessly breaches a patient's confidentiality would have committed an unethical act even if the breach in question did not result in any significant moral harm to the patient.

Moral complacency

An eighth type of moral problem nurses can encounter is that of 'moral complacency', defined by Unwin (1985: 205) as 'a general unwillingness to accept that one's moral opinions may be mistaken'. It could also be described as a general unwillingness to 'let go' the primacy of one's own point of view, or to regard one's own point of view as just one of many to be compared, contrasted and considered. Again, we do not need to look far to find examples of moral complacency in health care contexts. Nurses and others who are 'true believers' in advance care planning in contexts where patients and their families have indicated they do not want to engage in such a process and do not accept the assumed value of such plans is an example (Johnstone 2012b; Johnstone & Kanitsaki 2009a).

Like moral unpreparedness and moral blindness, moral complacency is something which can be remedied by moral education, moral consciousness raising and reflective practice in an ethical environment that has organisational support. The objective of taking this action would be to produce in the morally complacent person the attitude that nobody can afford to be complacent in the way he or she ordinarily views the world – least of all the moral world. This is particularly so in instances where other people's moral interests are at stake. It is a 'thinking error' and also arrogant to assume that our moral opinions are 'right' just because they are our own opinions.

As ethical professionals, our stringent moral responsibility is to question our taken-for-granted assumptions about the world – and about bioethics discourse generally – and not to presume that they are always well founded and unable to be challenged. It also requires going beyond mere values clarification and embracing what Garrett (2014: 1) refers to as 'two more ambitious agendas' for bioethical thinking. The first of these agendas involves 'critique, unmasking, interrogating and challenging the presuppositions that underlie bioethical discourse'; the second agenda involves 'integration' and adopting a transcendent stance which encompasses 'honoring and unifying what is right in competing values' (Garrett 2014: 1).

Moral dumbfounding / stupefaction

The ninth problem to be considered here is that of 'moral dumbfounding' – also called 'moral stupefaction'. Although there is no single agreed definition of moral dumbfounding, it is generally held to occur when people stubbornly maintain a moral judgment despite not having reasons to either support or defend the judgments they have made (McHugh et al 2017). When pressed to supply reasons for their stance, people typically become 'dumbfounded' or 'stupefied' (left with a 'mental blank') and resort to making unsupported declarations such as 'It is just wrong' as a justification (McHugh et al 2017). Examples classically used in the literature are generally taken from Haidt's foundational work (Haidt 2001; Haidt et al 2000) on the subject and include acts such as (i) consensual protected sex between adult siblings; (ii) cannibalism of a body that is already dead and soon to be incinerated; and (iii) eating one's pet dog after it has just died from an accident. When asked about their views on these and similar examples, research participants typically declare that the acts in question 'are wrong'. When pressed to ultimately provide sound reasons and justifications for their negative verdicts on these examples, participants have tended to become 'dumbfounded' admitting either that 'they don't know', 'they can't explain', or that it (incest, cannibalism, eating your pet) is 'just wrong' (seemingly based on a misattribution of these acts being harmful) – or 'just disgusting' (an emotional response) (Haidt 2001; Haidt & Björklund 2008; Haidt et al 2000; Hindriks 2015; McHugh et al 2017).

Not all agree that the phenomenon of moral dumbfounding / stupefaction exists and to date it remains the subject of controversy. Gray and colleagues (2014: 1600), for example, contend that 'perceiving harm in immorality is intuitive and does not require effortful rationalization'. This accounts for why people are not always able to provide *reasons* for their negative verdicts of perceived morally harmful acts – that is, their 'reasons' are normative moral *intuitions* which cannot be rationalised.

Royzman and colleagues (2015), meanwhile, contend that where the thesis fails is the assumption that the acts in question are 'harmless'. They argue that research participants may have 'excellent reasons' to disapprove of the acts – that is, they may not believe that incest, cannibalism, and eating your pet are 'truly' harmless and, accordingly, that they are indeed 'wrong'; they may later recant their previous 'dumbfounding' statements and give a reason; and once the cultural standards of normative evaluation are factored in their responses are, all things considered, 'reasonable' (Royzman et al 2015).

A search of the literature has found that, apart from works addressing intuitionism in nursing, the existence, relevance and possible implications of moral dumbfounding / stupefaction in nursing and health care contexts have not yet been considered. This stands as an area that would benefit from future inquiry.

Moral fanaticism

A tenth type of moral problem which may be encountered by nurses, and which is similar in many respects to moral complacency, is that of 'moral fanaticism'. The moral fanatic is someone who is thoroughly 'wedded to certain ideals' and uncritically and unreflectingly makes moral judgments according to them (Hare 1981: 170). Richard Hare's classic case of the fanatical Nazi is a good example here (Hare 1963: Chapter 9). The fanatical Nazi in this case stringently clings to the ideal of a pure Aryan German race and the need to exterminate all Jews as a means of purging the German race of its impurities. The Nazi falls into the category of being a 'fanatic' when he/she insists that, if any Nazis discover themselves to be of Jewish descent, then they too should be exterminated along with the rest of the Jews (Hare 1963: 161–2).

Examples of moral fanaticism exist in health care contexts. The maintenance of absolute confidentiality, even though harm might be caused as a result, is an example. So, too, is the example of a doctor or a nurse forcing unwanted information on a patient in the fanatical belief that all patients '*must* be told the truth' – even if the patient in question has specifically requested not to receive the information, and the imposition of the unwanted information on the patient can be shown to be a 'gratuitous and harmful misinterpretation of the moral foundations for respect for autonomy' (Pellegrino 1992: 1735).

In the case of moral fanatics, an appeal to overriding considerations or principles of conduct would not be helpful (Hare 1981: 178). As with the amoralist, the problem of the moral fanatic in health care contexts is likely to have disappointing outcomes. In the final analysis, it may be that other (non-moral) mechanisms will have to be appealed to in order to resolve the moral problems caused by moral fanaticism; for example, it may be necessary to seek the involvement of a public advocate, a court of law or a disciplinary body to arbitrate the matter.

Moral disagreements

An eleventh type of moral problem nurses will very often encounter is that involving 'moral disagreement' – concerning, for example, the selection, interpretation, application and evaluation of moral standards. In his classic article 'Moral deadlock', Milo (1986) identifies two fundamental types of moral disagreement: internal moral disagreement and radical moral disagreement.

Internal moral disagreement

Three forms of internal moral disagreement can occur. The first of these involves a fundamental conflict about the force or priority of accepted moral standards. For example, two people may agree to common moral standards but disagree about what to do when these standards come into conflict. Milo (1986: 455) argues that the disagreement here is not necessarily attributable to 'any disagreement in factual beliefs or to bad reasoning', but rather to a disagreement in *attitude* (see also McNaughton 1988: 17, 29). Consider the following hypothetical example to illustrate Milo's point.

Two nurses might both accept a moral standard which generally requires truth telling, but may disagree on when this standard should apply. Nurse A, for instance, might favour (i.e. have a 'pro-attitude') towards) telling the truth to patient X about a pessimistic medical diagnosis and prognosis. Nurse B, on the other hand, might not favour (i.e. might have a 'con-attitude' towards) telling the truth to patient X about this diagnosis and prognosis, and prefer a pro-attitude to avoiding unnecessary suffering (e.g. as a result of a nocebo effect (see Chapter 4) that might be inadvertently stimulated in the patient upon his learning about the diagnosis and poor prognosis). It is not that these two nurses have different criteria of relevance, as such, but rather have *different principles of priority* (Milo 1986: 457).

A second type of internal disagreement centres on what are to count as acceptable exceptions and limitations to otherwise mutually agreed moral standards. As Milo explains, we generally accept that moral standards are limited by other moral standards, as well as by the competing claims of self-interest. (Morality does not usually expect us to risk our own lives or our own important moral interest in morally troubling situations.) People might agree that, as a general rule, we should all make certain modest sacrifices in terms of our own interests (a minimal requirement of justice), but may disagree 'about what constitutes a modest sacrifice' (Milo 1986: 459). In many respects this type of disagreement could be loosely described as a disagreement in *interpretation* of an accepted moral standard. Consider another example.

Two nurses might agree that patients' rights should not be violated. Nurse A might further hold that, in situations involving violations of patients' rights, a nurse should act – even if this means threatening the nurse's job security (which Nurse A views as a modest sacrifice). Nurse B, on the other hand, might agree that nurses should in principle act to prevent a patient's rights from being violated, but disagree that nurses should do so if they stand to lose their jobs as a result (something which Nurse B views as an unacceptable and extreme sacrifice). What these two nurses are essentially disagreeing about is not the moral standard per se (that nurses should act to prevent violations of patients' rights), but about when morally relevant considerations can be and cannot be overridden by self-interest. In disagreements like this, and where the disagreement is based on preferences rather than attitude, there may well be no satisfactory solution, a situation which Milo calls a 'moral deadlock' (1986: 461).

A third and final type of internal moral disagreement centres on the selection and applicability of accepted ethical standards. This kind of disagreement has nothing to do with whether a standard can be overridden by other considerations, but concerns whether it should have been selected or appealed to in the first place. For example, two nurses may agree that killing an innocent human being is wrong. They may disagree, however, that abortion is wrong. Nurse A, for example, might argue that, since the fetus is not a human being, abortion does not entail the killing of an innocent human being and therefore is not wrong. Appealing to a moral standard prohibiting the killing of innocent human life would then, for Nurse A, be quite irrelevant. Nurse B, on the other hand, may argue that the fetus is a human being, and therefore abortion, since it entails killing an innocent human being, is absolutely morally wrong. Appealing to a moral standard prohibiting the killing of innocent human life would then, for Nurse B, be supremely relevant. The disagreement between these two nurses hinges very much on a disagreement about the *moral relevance* of the facts on what constitutes a human being.

Radical moral disagreement

Milo (1986) identifies two types of radical moral disagreement; the first type he calls 'partial radical moral disagreement', and the second type 'total radical moral disagreement'.

In cases of *partial radical moral disagreement*, dissenting parties might agree on some criteria of relevance but not all. For example, a nurse might argue that directly killing terminally and chronically ill patients with a lethal injection is morally wrong, whereas merely 'letting nature take its course' or 'letting patients die' is not morally wrong. Another nurse might agree that directly killing terminally and chronically ill patients is wrong, but thoroughly disagree that merely 'letting patients die' is less morally offensive. Here there may be no court of appeal to reconcile the distinction between direct 'killing' and merely 'letting die'. In this case, partial radical disagreement is very similar to internal moral disagreement. It may be very difficult to distinguish between the two – a point which Milo reluctantly concedes.

In cases of *total radical moral disagreement*, disputants do not agree on any criteria of relevance, and do not share any basic moral principles. For Milo (1986: 469), this is 'the most extreme kind of moral disagreement that one can imagine'.

An example of total radical moral disagreement would be where two theatre nurses radically disagree with each other about the moral acceptability of organ transplantations. Nurse A argues that retrieving or harvesting organs from so-called 'cadavers' is an unmitigated act of murder, since the person whose organs are being retrieved is not yet fully dead. (Nurse A, in this instance, rejects brain-death criteria as indicative of death.) Nurse A also argues that, even if the potential cadaver is restored to nothing more than a persistent vegetative state, and even if another person may die as a result of not getting a life-saving organ transplant operation, this does not justify violating the sanctity of life of the potential organ donor. The death of another person through not receiving a new organ, while 'unfortunate', cannot be helped. Such are the tragic twists and tradeoffs of life.

Nurse B, on the other hand, argues that retrieving organs is nothing like murder since, among other things, the person is already dead. (Nurse B, in this instance, totally accepts brain-death criteria as indicative of death.) Nurse B also totally rejects a 'sanctity of life' view, arguing that it has no substance;

only quality-of-life considerations have ethical meaning. Nurse B further argues that, even conceding the unreliability of brain-death criteria as indicative of death, retrieving the organs is still morally permissible, since the donating person can at best look forward only to a 'vegetative existence' and one devoid of any 'quality of life' (which is cruel and immoral), whereas an organ recipient could look forward to a renewed quality of life and indeed to life itself.

In the dispute between Nurse A and Nurse B, resolution is unlikely. As Milo points out, in total radical disagreement the disputants reach a total and irreconcilable impasse. The possibility of this situation occurring in health care contexts is something which needs to be taken seriously, and which has important implications for conscientious objection claims (an issue that is given separate consideration in Chapter 11 of this book).

It should be clarified here that, while moral disagreements can certainly be problematic (particularly if a person's life and wellbeing are hanging in the balance, and an immediate decision is needed about what should be done), these need not be taken as constituting grounds upon which ethics as such should be viewed with scepticism or, worse, rejected. As Stout (1988: 14) argues persuasively, the facts of moral disagreement 'don't compel us to become nihilists or sceptics, to abandon the notions of moral truth and justified moral belief'. One reason for this, he explains, is that moral disagreement is, in essence, just a kind of moral diversity or, as he calls it, 'conceptual diversity' (Stout 1988: 15, 61). While moral disagreement may rightly challenge us to 'meticulously disentangle' diverse and conflicting moral points of view, it does not preclude or threaten the possibility of moral judgment per se, either within a particular culture or across many cultures (Stout 1988: 15).

As argued previously, moral disagreement has historically been the beginning of critical moral thinking, not its end. Given this, there is room to suggest that we should be very cautious in accepting Milo's pessimistic conclusions about the irreconcilability of radical moral disagreement. Instead, we should look towards a more optimistic solution, and view such disagreements as an important and necessary opportunity for 'enriching [our] conceptions of morality through comparative inquiry' (Stout 1988: 70), and thereby augment our collective wisdom about what morality is, and what it really means to be moral in a world characterised by individual and collective (cultural) diversity. In the ultimate analysis, the solution to the problem of moral disagreement may not be to engage in adversarial dialogue (fight / litigate), or even to negotiate a happy medium between conflicting views (compromise). Rather, the solution may be, to borrow from Edward de Bono (1985), to engage in 'triangular thinking', to engage in moral disagreement not as a judge or as a negotiator but as a 'creative designer' who is able to escape the imprisonment of the positivist logic and language that is so characteristic of mainstream Western moral discourse, and to engage in moral disagreement as someone who is able ultimately to resolve the conflicts and disagreements which others have long since abandoned as hopeless and irreconcilable impasses. Such an approach, however, requires not just an ability to think about new things but, as Catharine MacKinnon (1987: 9) puts it, to engage in 'a new way of thinking'. Possible approaches to dealing effectively with moral disagreements and disputes will be considered later in this chapter under the subheading 'Dealing with moral disagreements and disputes'.

Moral conflict

The twelfth type of problem to be considered here is that of a 'moral conflict'. Moral conflict (to be distinguished from conflicting principles and obligations that underpin moral dilemmas, as discussed above) fundamentally involves a clash of opposing ideas and interests of different agents (e.g. members of the health care team, family members and the like). In several respects, moral conflict is the logical extension of intractable moral disagreement. Matters commonly identified as being the source of moral conflicts are: goals of patient care and treatments, quality of care, preventing and alleviating patient suffering, poor communication, and resource allocation (Edelstein et al 2009; Gaudine et al 2011;

Leuter et al 2017; Pavlish et al 2013, 2014). Conflicts can manifest as contentious moral arguments, emotional outbursts and other disruptive behaviours (Danjoux et al 2009; Pavlish et al 2014). Unresolved they can have a significant negative impact on relationships, patient care and the culture of the organisations – specifically they can weaken an organisation's ethical climate (Pavlish et al 2013).

It is difficult to assess the incidence and impact of moral conflict in nursing domains. One reason for this is that it has not been comprehensively studied. Instead the problem of moral conflict has tended controversially to be positioned as the 'cause' of moral distress in nursing, with attention focusing more on the nature and impact of 'moral distress' than on moral conflict per se. What has been misunderstood by those who have conflated the issue of moral conflict and moral distress is that, whereas moral distress concerns *conflict within oneself*, moral conflict concerns *conflict with others*. The problem of moral conflict is considered further in Chapter 11 of this text.

Moral dilemmas

Another significant moral problem (the thirteenth) to be considered here (and one which has been widely discussed in both nursing and bioethical literature) is that of the proverbial 'moral dilemma' (also called 'ethical dilemma'). Broadly speaking, a dilemma may be defined as a situation requiring choice between what seem to be two equally desirable or undesirable alternatives; it may also be described as an 'awful feeling of being stuck'. A moral dilemma, however, is a little different, and can occur in one of several forms.

First, a moral dilemma can occur in the form of *logical incompatibility* between two different moral principles. For example, two different moral principles might apply equally in a given situation, and neither principle can be chosen without violating the other. Even so, a choice has to be made. Consider the case of a nurse who accepts a moral principle which demands respect for the sanctity of life, and who also accepts another moral principle (non-maleficence) which demands that persons should be spared the harm of intolerable suffering. In the context of caring for a patient with intractable pain, it may not be possible to uphold both principles where, for example, a medical prescription for palliative sedation has been prescribed (the issue of palliative sedation is discussed in Chapter 10 of this book). The ultimate question posed for the nurse in this situation is: Which principle should I choose? The options open to the nurse are:

- to modify the principles in question so that they do not conflict (i.e. by adding 'riders' to them)
- to abandon one principle in favour of the other
- to abandon both principles in favour of a third (e.g. autonomy and respect for the patient's wishes).

It should be noted that none of these options is free of moral risk.

A second type of moral dilemma is that involving *competing moral duties*. Consider the following case. A nurse working in a specialised unit is assigned a patient with a known history of drug addiction, and is instructed to chaperone the patient when there are visitors to make sure that illicit drugs are not 'slipped in'. The nurse, however, believes that the duty to protect this patient from harm (such as might occur from receiving illicit drugs) competes with the duty to respect the patient's privacy. The question for the nurse in this scenario is: Which duty should I fulfil?

In another case, a nurse is assigned a patient of traditional Greek background who has recently been diagnosed with metastatic cancer. The doctor has ordered that the patient not be told his diagnosis. The patient, however, keeps asking the nurse and his family for information about his diagnosis. The family knows the diagnosis, but wants the doctor to tell the patient. Here the nurse is caught between a duty to tell the truth to the patient, and a duty to respect the wishes of the family. The nurse is also obliged to follow the doctor's directives. The question for the nurse in this scenario is, again: Which duty should I fulfil — my duty to the patient, or to the family, or to the doctor, or to whom?

Philosophical answers to questions raised by a conflict of duty are varied and controversial. In the classic work *The right and the good*, Ross (1930) argues that duties are prima facie or 'conditional' in nature. Thus, when two duties conflict, we must 'study the situation' as fully as we can until we are able to reach a 'considered opinion (it is never more) that in the circumstances one of them [the duties] is more incumbent than any other' (Ross 1930: 19). Once we have worked out which of the conflicting duties is the more 'incumbent' on us, we are bound to consider it our prima-facie duty in that situation. Richard Hare (1981: 26), however, takes a different view. He argues that, if we find ourselves caught between what appear to be two conflicting duties, we need to look again. For it is likely that, in the case of an apparent conflict in duties, one of our so-called 'duties' is not our duty at all; we have only mistakenly thought that it was. In other words, what happens here is that one of the two apparently conflicting duties is eventually 'cancelled out'.

Williams (1973) disagrees. While he believes that one of the conflicting *duties* has to be rejected (but only in the sense that both conflicting duties/oughts cannot be acted upon), he does not agree that this means that the duties or oughts in question do not apply equally in the situation at hand, or that one of the conflicting duties must inevitably be 'cancelled out'. To the contrary: our reasoning may assist us to deal with a conflict of duty and may assist us to find a 'best' way to act, but this does not mean that we abandon one or other of the duties in question. How do we know? Even after making a choice between two conflicting duties, we are still left with a lingering feeling of 'regret'. And it is this very feeling of regret which tells us that we have not altogether abandoned or 'cancelled out' the duty we decided could not, in that situation, be also acted upon.

In the drug addict case, we might well side with Richard Hare and unanimously agree that the nurse is mistaken in a belief that there is an overriding duty to respect the patient's privacy, and that clearly the primary duty is to prevent the patient from suffering the harms likely to be incurred by the administration of illicit drugs. But here the question arises: Is it really a nurse's duty to act as a kind of police warden? What if the patient is not receiving any form of therapy for the immediate drug addiction problem, and is at risk of developing severe and life-threatening withdrawal symptoms? How is the nurse's duty to 'prevent harm' to be regarded in this instance? Does cancelling out one of the conflicting duties here relieve the moral tension created in this scenario? Or is there more to be achieved by exploring ways in which they can be reconciled with each other?

In the cancer diagnosis case, it might be unanimously agreed that the nurse's primary duty is to the patient, and that any apparent duty owed to the family is not a bona fide one. Placed in a cultural context, however, the scenario takes on a whole new dimension. As was considered in Chapter 4 of this book, families from a traditional cultural background often play a fundamental and highly protective role in mediating the flow of information to a sick loved one. To ignore a family's request in such a situation could be to risk a violation of the wellbeing of the patient. Where this is likely, it is imperative that the nurse works closely with the family and ensures that the transfer of information to the patient is handled in a *culturally appropriate manner*. While the family may be perceived as 'interfering', in reality it may be providing an important link in ensuring that the patient's wellbeing and moral interests are fully upheld.

Cancelling out one of the duties in this scenario is unlikely to relieve the moral tension generated by the patient's request for and the doctor's refusal to give the medical information on the patient's diagnosis. Had the only criterion for action been what superficially appeared to be a primary duty to the patient, the nurse may have unwittingly facilitated the flow of information in a *culturally inappropriate* and thus harmful manner. By reconciling the apparent conflict in duties, and by working closely with the family, however, the nurse is able to facilitate the flow of information to the patient in a culturally appropriate and thus less harmful manner. In this instance, by fulfilling the duty owed to the family, the nurse could also succeed in fulfilling the duty owed to the patient.

It might be objected that the examples given here do not involve difficult cases, and that the required choices are relatively easy to make. But even if we admit 'hard cases', Hare's position is somehow unsatisfactory, as is his argument that when there is an apparent conflict in duties it is likely that one of the duties involved is not our duty at all. There is always room to question how we can ever be really sure that a 'cancelled' duty was not our duty in the first place. The cancer diagnosis case, I think, illustrates this point well. Ross's (1930) and Williams' (1973) positions, on the other hand, remind us that matters of moral duty are never clear-cut and, further, that we always have to be careful in our appraisal of given situations and in the choices we make regarding to whom our moral duties are owed and what our moral duties actually are.

A third kind of moral dilemma, and one closely related to a dilemma concerning competing duties, is that entailing *competing and conflicting interests*. Here the question raised for the moral observer is: Whose interests ought I to uphold?

Consider the following case. A clinical teacher on clinical placement at a residential care home is informed by a student that an elderly demented resident has been physically and verbally abused by one of the ward's permanent staff members, as witnessed by the student. The clinical teacher is temporarily undecided about what to do. It is a very serious matter – and, indeed, a very serious accusation – but it will be difficult to prove. If the incident is not reported to the home's nursing administrator, the staff member concerned will probably continue to abuse the home's residents. If the incident is reported, there is a risk that the interests of both students and the school of nursing could be undermined. (The home's administrator might, for example, refuse to continue allowing students to be placed at the home for the purposes of gaining clinical experience.) The dilemma for the clinical teacher is whether to not report the matter and thereby protect both the students' and the school's interests in having continued clinical placements, or to report the matter fully, whatever the consequences to the school and the students, and thereby protect the residents' interests.

The teacher and the student mutually agree that the matter is too serious to ignore and decide they would risk the consequences of reporting the incident. The exercise, as feared, proves extremely distressing and painful for both the student concerned and the clinical teacher. The accused staff member denies having abused the elderly resident, and in turn accuses the student of lying and of being the one who has really committed the abuses. The opinion of the patient cannot be sought, as the elderly resident concerned is suffering from advanced dementia. Fortunately, the matter is eventually resolved to everyone's satisfaction. The administrator takes the allegation seriously and, later, takes the initiative to emphasise to all staff the importance of protecting and upholding residents' rights. The student is reassured that she has done the 'right thing', and that she has fulfilled her professional and moral obligations both (1) in *reporting* the incident and (2) in the *manner* in which she had reported it (i.e. she has followed proper processes). The clinical supervisor and administrator reach an agreement that any matters of concern discussed during clinical teaching placements be referred directly and immediately to the administrator for action. The staff member who was the subject of the unsubstantiated allegation is counselled in confidence by the administrator.

A fourth type of dilemma is taken from a feminist moral perspective, and is described by Gilligan (1982) in terms of being caught between attachments to people and trying to decide upon ways that will avoid 'hurting' each of these 'attached people'. Gilligan uses the example of a woman contemplating an abortion; she argues that generally a woman faced with having to make a choice in this situation 'contemplates a decision that affects both self and others and engages directly the critical moral issue of hurting' (Gilligan 1982: 71). Here the question to be raised in contemplating a difficult choice is: How can I avoid hurting the people to whom I am attached?

It might be objected here that Gilligan's sense of 'hurt' and 'avoiding hurt' is not very different from the general moral principle of non-maleficence and its demand to avoid or prevent 'harm'. While it might be conceded that 'hurt' is a type of harm, there is a subtle distinction between 'hurt' in the sense that Gilligan seems to be using it and 'harm' in an abstract sense as used by philosophers. It is important to draw a distinction between these two notions so as not to obscure other important distinctions which can be drawn in moral discourse. Let us examine this point a little more fully.

The sense in which 'hurt' is being used here is not simply 'physical', but rather existential. There is even room to make the radical claim that the notion of 'avoiding hurt' is not being asserted as a *principle* as such, but more as an *attitude*, and one which reminds us that we need to take very special care in our selection, interpretation and application of general moral principles in our everyday personal and professional lives. In short, it is an attitude which serves to *mediate* the use of more general moral principles. Consider, for example, the demand to 'avoid hurt' in a situation involving a patient who has yet to be told an unfavourable medical diagnosis. The demand to 'avoid hurt' reminds us that it is not enough just to *give* the patient the diagnosis (as may otherwise be required by the moral principle of autonomy), but that it must also be given in a caring, compassionate and culturally appropriate manner. Furthermore, it is not clear that, in this instance, the principle of non-maleficence fully captures the demand to be caring, compassionate and culturally appropriate in manner when performing such an unpleasant task as giving someone an unfavourable medical diagnosis. And in some instances, taken to its extreme, the principle of non-maleficence might even instruct that the diagnosis should not be given at all. 'Avoiding hurt', on the other hand, recognises that the information that needs to be given could be 'harmful' and is probably 'hurtful', but that there is a way of *lessening* if not *avoiding* this harm and hurt. To illustrate this point, consider the following case.

A newly graduated doctor walks into a patient's room, stands at the end of the bed and, in full view and hearing distance of other patients in the room and without greeting the patient or smiling, states abruptly: 'We've looked at your throat and the lump you have there is cancer.' Without another word, the doctor then briskly walks off. The patient has previously expressed a desire to know the diagnosis when it was available, so in several respects it could be concluded that the doctor acted 'ethically' in that the patient's wishes have been respected and the requested information has been relayed to the patient. What is evident in this case is that the doctor has not considered ways to give the information less 'hurtfully' – or, if such ways have been considered, they were not heeded. For example, the doctor might have at least greeted the patient, used a compassionate tone of voice, drawn the curtains around the patient before speaking, sat down on a chair to be at the same level as the patient, and stayed long enough to allow the patient to ask questions, which the patient later confides she wanted to do. If the doctor felt inadequate to deal with this situation, it would have been advisable to wait until a medical colleague or a nurse was available to accompany him. Or, more simply, the doctor should have deferred to someone else who was more experienced and better prepared to deal with the situation. By using such an abrupt manner, the doctor not only failed to 'avoid hurt', but exacerbated it.

Nurses have likewise failed to avoid or to lessen the hurt of a given situation. An example of this can be found in the tragic case of a middle-aged man who was dying from advanced cancer. A close friend and members of his family were greatly distressed about his deteriorating condition, and even accused the nursing staff of 'trying to kill' their loved one by giving him morphine for his pain. On one occasion the nursing staff observed the family friend clutching his friend and pleading with him not to accept the morphine injections, telling him: 'Don't you see, they are killing you! They are killing you! You don't have to have them …' The nursing staff tried to get the friend to leave, but he refused to go. When he became abusive, the nursing staff contacted a hospital security officer, and he was forcibly removed. There is room to speculate about this case: had the friend's behaviour been recognised as a grief response (which it was), had his grief been properly addressed by the nursing staff, and had the dynamics and benefits of effective pain management been fully explained to him, then he, the patient, the patient's family and the attending nursing staff would have been spared the 'hurt' that this awful situation caused.

These two cases demonstrate that 'avoiding hurt' is not something that can be fully directed or achieved by an abstract moral principle. Rather, it requires that we draw on our past experience, knowledge, intuition, awareness, insight, feelings and interpersonal skills, as well as on a thorough and systematic analysis of the facts of the situation at hand.

'Moral distress'[1]

The fourteenth and final type of moral problem to be considered here is that of 'moral distress'. During the course of their day-to-day practice, nurses will invariably encounter situations in which they may be required to make a moral decision. In some instances, despite deciding what they believe is the 'right thing to do', nurses may nonetheless feel constrained in acting on their moral judgments and, in the end, either *do nothing* or *do what they believe is the wrong thing to do* (Jameton 1984). This situation has been hypothesised in the nursing ethics literature as giving rise to what has been controversially termed 'moral distress'.

The notion of moral distress dates back to the foundational work of US philosopher Andrew Jameton and may take one of two forms:

- *initial moral distress*, which is characterised by feelings of frustration, anger, anxiety and guilt when faced with perceived institutional obstacles and interpersonal conflict about values, and
- *reactive moral distress* (also called *moral residue*), which occurs when an individual fails to act on their initial moral distress and is left with 'residue' or lingering distress (Jameton 1984, 1993; see also Epstein & Hamric 2009).

The 'root cause' of moral distress in nursing has been attributed to three key domains: *clinical situations* (e.g. controversial end-of-life decisions; inadequate informed consent; working with incompetent practitioners); *internal constraints* (e.g. nurses' lack of moral competencies; perceived lack of autonomy and powerlessness to act; lack of knowledge and understanding of the full situation); and *external constraints* (e.g. hierarchies within the health care system; inadequate communication among team members; hospital policies and priorities that conflict with patient care needs) (Hamric et al 2012). Of these domains, clinical situations involving 'prolonged, aggressive treatment that the professional believes is unlikely to have a positive outcome' are regarded as being the most common cause of moral distress in nurses (Epstein & Hamric 2009: 2).

In recent years, moral distress has been portrayed as a 'major problem in the nursing profession, affecting nurses in all health care systems' (Corley 2002: 636; see also Musto & Rodney 2018).[2] It is depicted as threatening the integrity of nurses and, in turn, the quality of patient care. It has also been implicated in the problem of nurse retention, with some scholars suggesting that unresolved moral distress can lead to nurses experiencing job dissatisfaction, burnout, and ultimately abandoning their positions and even their profession altogether. More recently, it has been cited as 'the cause' of moral disengagement by nurses (Hyatt 2017). Even so, as Johnstone and Hutchinson (2015) argue, the notion of moral distress is not without controversy and may even be misguided. Moreover, without further inquiry into the psychological underpinnings and ethical components of nurses' responses to moral issues in the workplace, there is a risk that continuing nursing narratives on 'moral distress' might serve more to confuse rather than clarify the ethical dimensions and challenges of nursing work.

Linchpin to the theory of moral distress is the idea that 'nurses *know* what is the right thing to do, but are unable to carry it out'. This idea is highly questionable, however, since it assumes without supporting evidence the unequivocal correctness of nurses' moral judgments in given situations. It also underestimates the capacity of nurses to take remedial action even in difficult environments (Johnstone & Hutchinson 2015).

Research has shown that different people can make quite different yet equally valid moral judgments about the same situation. Even when presented with 'the facts', decision-makers rarely change their minds (see also moral dumbfounding/stupefaction, discussed as problem nine in this section). Instead they will search for and accept only information that reaffirms their initial intuitions (Sonenshein 2007). One reason for this is that people approach situations with their own individual system of ethics and a pre-determined stance on what they value and believe is right and wrong. In keeping with their own 'bounded personal ethics' individuals will construct, interpret and respond to issues 'based on their own personal motivations and expectations' (Sonenshein 2007: 1026) as well as past behaviours including 'blind spots' that have obscured their previous moral failures (Chugh & Kern 2016).

Nurses are no exception in this regard. Even in contexts plagued by uncertainty and complexity (of which clinical environments are a prime example) nurses are just as vulnerable as are others to constructing idiosyncratic 'subjective interpretations of issues beyond their objective features' (Sonenshein 2007: 1026). It is thus inevitable that they will encounter moral disagreements in the workplace and that some of these disagreements might engender an intense emotional reaction.

Essential to the theory of moral distress is the assumption that such a state *in fact* exists. Much of what has been written about moral distress, however, involves little more than an appropriation of 'ordinary' psychological and emotional reactions (e.g. frustration, anger) that nurses may justifiably feel when encountering moral issues and disagreements in the workplace. Whether these reactions necessarily constitute 'moral distress', however, is another matter.

Research ostensibly identifying nurses' moral distress and exploring its incidence and impact in the workplace is also problematic. First, the scenarios used in survey research instruments (see Corley 2002) tend to depict situations that lack equivocality and uncertainty than is likely in the clinical settings in which nurses' work. These instruments thus minimise the role of 'issues construction' by nurses and erroneously frame the scenarios as involving a clear choice between right and wrong (see Jones 1991). Second, the very presentation of given issues in the moral distress scales used by researchers already pre-code and interpret the situations presented as involving 'moral distress' thus priming respondents to accept both the existence and incidence of moral distress as a 'reality' in their practice.

In order to better understand the foundations of moral disagreements in the workplace and nurses' reactions to them, more needs to be known about nurses' taxonomy of ethical ideologies – that is, what their personal ethical standpoints are, the extent to which their personal views frame their ethical decision-making and behaviours in professional contexts, and the bases upon which they justify their conduct. Until further inquiries are made, the assumed credibility of 'moral distress' as a bona fide problem in nursing will remain dubious.

Making moral decisions

When encountering a moral problem, there comes a point at which nurses have to decide *what* to do about it and *how* best to go about doing what they have decided – that is, how best to address the problem (or problems) they have encountered. Before engaging in moral decision-making, however, an individual must first perceive that the problem at hand has a morally salient dimension, that the situation involves choice alternatives of 'right' and 'wrong', and that they have the motivation to 'do the right thing' – *viz* they have the will to be moral (Chorus 2015).

When encountering a moral problem, questions invariably arise of: 'How do I decide what to do?', 'How, if at all, should I act on what I have decided?', and 'How do I know whether my ethical decision-making is "good", all things considered?' Before considering these questions, it would be useful first to clarify what a moral decision is and the various processes that might be used for making moral decisions. Following this, attention will then be given to examining briefly how to deal with moral disagreements and disputes in workplace contexts.

Moral decision-making – a working definition

The word 'decision' may be defined as 'a judgment, conclusion or resolution reached or given'; it may also be defined as 'the act of making up one's mind' (*Collins Australian dictionary* 2011: 437). A moral decision may be similarly defined – that is, as a moral judgment, moral conclusion or moral resolution reached or given, notably, about what constitutes 'right' and 'wrong' conduct. *Moral decision-making* may be further defined as that which is fundamentally concerned with reconciling moral disagreements between disputing parties, each of whom may hold equally valid moral viewpoints and may reach different yet reasonable conclusions on what constitutes 'right' and 'wrong' conduct in a given context (Wong 1992).

An essential and distinguishing feature of moral decisions is that they are based on and informed by moral considerations, which are regarded as paramount to the moral decision-making process. Another distinguishing feature of moral decisions is that they provide a definitive starting point from which moral action can be taken in order to prevent moral harms from occurring and to promote morally desirable or at least tolerable outcomes.

In terms of determining whether a person has made 'good moral decisions', this can be ascertained by taking into account and assessing what Callahan (1995: 254) has posited as the 'three essential elements' of good individual decision-making:

- *self-knowledge* – noting that this is fundamental since 'feelings, motives, inclinations and interests both enlighten and obscure moral understanding'
- *knowledge of moral theories and traditions* – noting that, while not easy to achieve and that moral theory is unlikely to give 'all the ingredients needed for an informed, thoughtful moral judgment', it can nonetheless be successfully applied when complemented by 'self-understanding and reflectiveness about the societal and cultural contexts of our decisions'
- *cultural perception* – noting that none of the above elements is sufficient on their own to foster good moral judgment; rather what is required is a 'toing and froing' among all three elements: 'the reflective self, the interpreted culture, and the contributions of moral theory' together with an individual and collective (culturally constructed) vision of 'human good'.

Processes for making moral decisions

Moral decisions can be made either by an individual (e.g. a nurse, doctor, and so on) or by a collective entity (e.g. a health care team, a stakeholder group or a committee). In either case, the decision-making process needs to be approached with the utmost diligence, vigilance and wisdom. Decision-makers need to take particular care in ensuring that a careful appraisal is made of the relevant facts of the matter as well as of the values that are operating in the given context at hand. One reason for this is that facts/values can each exert considerable influence on the other and, as a consequence, may even lead to profound changes in our conceptions of them and hence the moral decisions we ultimately make. This is because, as Benjamin (2001: 25) explains:

> *What counts as relevant factual considerations may change as exploration of an ethical issue progresses. In some cases, facts considered important at the outset fade into the background as others, barely noticed at first, come to the fore. In others [...] we not merely replace one set of factual considerations with another, but the facts either alter our ethical values and principles or we revise factual consideration in the light of values and principles.*

One way of ensuring that moral decision-making is approached in a wise, diligent and vigilant way is to use a systematic step-by-step decision-making process, much like the five-step decision-making process that has become universally associated with the clinical reasoning process used in nursing. Such a five-step process requires moral decision-makers to:

1. assess the situation (including making a diligent appraisal of the salient moral cues and dimensions of the situation as well as the relevant facts of the matter and operating values in the situation at issue)
2. diagnose or identify the moral problem(s) at hand
3. set moral goals and plan an appropriate moral course of action to address the moral problems identified
4. implement the plan of moral action
5. evaluate the moral outcomes of the action implemented.

(Note: In the event that a morally desirable outcome has not been achieved, this process will need to be repeated.)

This model may be expressed diagrammatically as shown in Fig. 5.3. It needs to be clarified at this point that, when using a systematic moral decision-making process, deliberations during each of the steps identified involve appeals to reason, emotion and intuition, with each of these, in turn, being informed or 'fine-tuned' by the awareness and insights gained through life experience.

Moral decision-making also requires moral insight and imagination – that is, an ability to reflect and imagine possible moral 'futures' (options) and solutions to problems, and possible ways of progressing these even in situations that are hostile to moral considerations and which may also involve a 'moral deadlock'. Since the role of reason, emotion, intuition and life experience in moral decision-making is not always understood and, ironically, has itself been the subject of moral dispute, some further discussion of it is warranted here. Consider the following.

FIGURE 5.3
Moral decision-making model

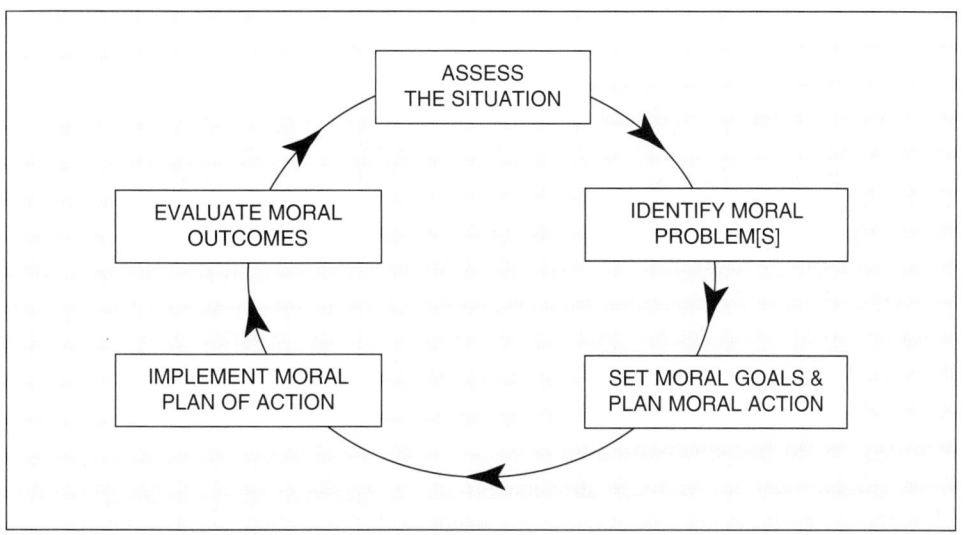

Reason and moral decision-making

Throughout history, dating back to the days of the Ancient Greek philosophers, it has been popularly assumed (and argued) by moral philosophers that, in order for a moral decision to be 'sound', it must be based on rational or 'reasoned' (abstract) moral principles of conduct. The thinking behind this view (which dates back to the works of the Ancient Greek philosophers) is that, unlike *feelings* (e.g. emotion and intuition, which are, by their nature, value laden and subjective), *reason* is value neutral and objective, and therefore more reliable and hence supreme as an enlightened authority on how best to conduct one's behaviour in the world of competing self-interest. By this view, to be rational is to be moral since, by upholding rationality as the supreme principle of morality, decision-makers will be able to avoid the 'corrupting influences of the passions' and thereby avoid falling prey to deciding in favour of their own self-interests.

An influential advocate of this view was the German philosopher, Immanuel Kant (1724–1804). Kant contended that what distinguished human beings from other (non-human) beings was their capacity to reason. His reasoning behind this view was that *reason is free* (i.e. autonomous) to *formulate moral law* (something that animals, for example, cannot do) and to determine just what is to count as being an overriding moral duty — the basis of all moral actions. A duty, according to Kant, is that which is *done for its own sake* — for its own intrinsic moral worth — and 'not for the results it attains or seeks to attain' (Kant 1972: 20). What is to count as one's duty, in turn, is determined by appealing to some formal (reasoned) principle or 'maxim'. In choosing such a principle or maxim, however, decision-makers must take care not to choose something which serves merely to uphold their own individual interests or to satisfy their own unruly desires. Indeed, Kant went on to assert that it is precisely because of our human weaknesses (especially our inclinations towards satisfying our own desires and interests) that the maxim we adopt must have the characteristics of being a universally valid 'law' — that is, something which 'commands or compels obedience' and which is binding on all persons equally (Kant 1972: 21).

Kant believed that moral considerations are always overriding ones. Thus, in situations where a number of considerations are competing (for instance, between practical, social, economic, political, moral and cultural considerations), it is always the moral considerations which should 'win out'. For example, if a nurse is in the position of having to decide whether to risk losing his or her job (a practical consideration) by exposing the unethical conduct of a supervisor (a moral consideration), it is the moral consideration which is, according to Kant's view, the weightier of the two; the nurse, by this analysis, should expose the supervisor.

As well as holding that moral considerations should always override non-moral considerations, Kant maintained that moral imperatives (as based on universal moral law) are by their very nature unconditional, absolute and inescapable. This means that moral imperatives, or duties in this instance, are both overriding and binding regardless of their consequences. Therefore we, as rational autonomous moral choosers, cannot escape the demands which a moral imperative may place upon us; the bottom line, according to Kant, is that we are absolutely required and therefore compelled to fulfil our moral duties. By this view, morally decent persons are those who fulfil their duties and who are not distracted by self-interested or practical considerations; morally indecent persons, on the other hand, are those who shirk or abandon their moral duties — probably in favour of other considerations such as the pursuit of material self-interest and pleasure. How do we know this? According to Kant, because reason tells us it is so. This viewpoint remains influential today.

Emotion and moral decision-making

Not everyone agrees that reason is the supreme authority governing ethics or that reason provides a more reliable guide to moral decision-making and action than other human faculties such as emotion or intuition. The Scottish philosopher David Hume (1711–76), for example, maintained that 'reason is, and ought only to be, the slave of the passions and can never pretend to any other office than to serve and obey them' (Hume 1888: 415).

Hume rejected reason or science as having ultimate moral authority, arguing that these things are nothing more than the 'comparing of ideas and the discovery of their relations' (Hume 1888: 466). He regarded reason as 'utterly impotent' (p 457) in moral domains and said that it is 'perfectly inert, and can never either prevent or produce any action or affection' (p 458). The only power reason has, in Hume's conceptual framework, is to shape beliefs – and, even then, beliefs cannot be relied upon to move one to action, unless they are relevant to the satisfaction of some passion, desire or need (Harmon 1977: 5).

The question remains, how do Hume's views capture the making of moral judgments and decisions? In essence, Hume's morality is something to be 'properly felt' rather than 'rationally judged', with goods and evils being known simply by particular sensations of pleasure and pain (Hume 1888: 470). He argued (p 469):

> *Nothing can be more real, or concern us more, than our own sentiments of pleasure and uneasiness; and if these be favourable to virtue, and unfavourable to vice, no more can be requisite to the regulation of our conduct and behaviour.*

In summary, Hume's account of morality sees the sensations of pleasure (moral sentiments) as distinguishing that which is virtuous, and the sensations of pain or uneasiness as distinguishing that which is vicious. If something appears either virtuous or vicious, there is no reason to doubt that appearance or to resist an inclination to act in response to them. On this point, Hume argued famously that ''Tis not contrary to reason to prefer the destruction of the whole world to the scratching of my finger' (Hume 1888: 416). In other words, it is perfectly 'reasonable', paradoxically, to respond to and act upon a sentiment or sensation.

Hume has not been alone in his critique of reason as a moral action guide. The supremacy and role of rationality and 'pure practical reason' in moral decision-making has also been challenged more recently both by moral philosophers (particularly feminist philosophers) and by biomedical scientists. The British philosopher, Alasdair MacIntyre, for example, raises the provocative question: 'What is it about rational argument which is so important that it is the nearly universal appearance assumed by those who engage in moral conflict?' (MacIntyre 1985: 9). His short answer to this is that there is nothing compelling or important about it at all. If anything, the rational paradigm of moral argument is uncomfortably aligned with a 'disquieting private arbitrariness' (MacIntyre 1985: 8). What appears to be a 'rational' approach is not a rational approach at all, at least not in the genuine 'critically reflective' sense. Philosophical opponents enter into moral debates with their minds already firmly made up. Their lack of irrefutable criteria to convince their opponents inevitably sees what should be an instructive and enlightening debate reduced to nothing more than a battleground characterised by dogmatic assertions and counter-assertions. Small wonder, MacIntyre ponders, that 'we become defensive and therefore shrill' in our public arguments.

Feminist moral philosophers have also been extremely critical of reason being regarded as the supreme authority governing morality. In their critiques of this assertion, they have resoundingly rejected the view that reason (1) is 'value neutral' (they assert that reason is no more objective than the subjectivity that prefers and values it (Gatens 1986: 25)), and (2) is a reliable guide to sound moral decision-making and action (Addelson 1994; Card 1991; Code et al 1988; Cole & Coultrap-McQuin 1992; Gatens 1986; Harding & Hintikka 1983; Kittay & Meyers 1987; Noddings 1984; Tronto 1993; Walker 1998). They have also raised serious questions as to why reason should be regarded as having any more authority in moral thinking and decision-making than the moral sentiments of, for example, empathy, compassion, sympathy, kindness, friendliness or caring. The short answer to this question is, that it does not and any assertion to the contrary is utterly baseless and contrary to life experience.

Neuroscientists have also argued persuasively that sound and effective moral decision-making requires an appeal to emotion and intuition as well as to reason. In a classic work on the subject, entitled *Descartes' error: emotion, reason, and the human brain*, the renowned neurologist Antonio Damasio (1994) presents a compelling account of the crucial role of emotion in moral decision-making. In this book, Damasio examines a number of case studies involving people who have suffered serious brain injuries. Significantly, his research has found that, under certain circumstances, just as *too much* emotion can disrupt reason, so too can *too little* emotion. Calling into question traditional accounts of the relationship between reason and emotion, Damasio (p 53) suggests that a reduction in emotion may, paradoxically, 'constitute an equally important source of irrational behaviour'. It can also give rise to annihilistic decision-making. On the basis of observations made of people with 'defective emotional modulation' (in particular, those who could be described as being 'flat' in emotion and feeling), Damasio concludes that there is a significant 'interaction of the systems underlying the normal processes of emotion, feeling, reason, and decision-making'; where the emotion centres of the brain are affected adversely, so too is a person's capacity to make important life-sustaining (moral) judgments (pp 40, 54). Significantly, this is so even in the case of where a brain-injured person's basic intellect, language ability, attention, perception, memory and language remain intact. In sum, to borrow from Damasio, a decline in the emotions can and does result in serious 'decision-making failures'.

Drawing on his scientific findings, Damasio (1994) goes on to warn of the inherent dangers to personal and interpersonal human relationships, and to human survival, of adopting a purely rationalistic and rule-bound approach to moral decision-making. He writes (p 171):

> The 'high-reason' view, which is none other than the commonsense view, assumes that when we are at our decision-making best, we are the pride and joy of Plato, Descartes and Kant. Formal logic will, by itself, get us to the best available solution for any problem. An important aspect of the rationalist conception is that to obtain the best results, emotions must be kept out. Rational processing must be unencumbered by passion.

After outlining a step-by-step approach to 'pure' rational decision-making, Damasio continues (p 72):

> Now, let me submit that if this strategy is the only one you have available, rationality, as described above, is not going to work. At best, your decision will take an inordinately long time, far more than acceptable if you are to get anything done that day. At worst, you may not even end up with a decision at all because you will get lost in the byways of your calculations. [...] You will lose track. Attention and working memory have a limited capacity. In the end, if purely rational calculations is how your mind normally operates, you might choose incorrectly and live to regret the error, or simply give up trying, in frustration.

He concludes that experience with brain-damaged patients such as those considered in his book suggest that 'the cool strategy advocated by Kant, among others, has far more to do with the way patients with prefrontal damage go about deciding than with how normals [sic] usually operate' (p 172). In contrast, 'integrated' decision-makers will fare much better. This is because somatic markers ('gut feelings' / emotions) help improve both the accuracy and efficiency of the decision-making process. Damasio explains (p 173):

> [The somatic marker] focuses attention on the negative outcome to which a given action may lead, and functions as an automated alarm signal which says: Beware of danger ahead if you choose the option which leads to this outcome. The signal may lead you to reject, immediately, the negative course of action and thus make you choose among other alternatives. The automated signal protects you against future losses, without further ado, and then allows you to choose from among fewer alternatives. There is still room for using a cost / benefit analysis and proper deductive competence, but only after the automated step drastically reduces the number of options.

Given the findings of Damasio's research, there is considerable room to suggest, contrary to the rationality thesis, that sound moral decision-making requires a collaboration between *reason* and *emotion*. Anything less could risk the practice of a defeatist and life-destructive ethic – that is, an ethical perspective that justifies annihilation rather than survival. Later work in neuroethics further validates Damasio's conclusions (Damasio 2007; Gellene 2007; Northoff 2006; Strueber et al 2007).

Intuition and moral decision-making

Intuition, like emotion, also has an important role to play in moral decision-making. Underpinning this idea is the theory of *moral intuitionism*, which holds that certain moral principles and moral judgments are 'self-evident' and known to be true by a cognition process akin to perception (Haidt 2001, 2012).

Proponents of moral intuitionism reject the view that reason has ultimate moral authority in ethical decision-making (Frankena 1973: 102–5). As suggested in the previous section, rationalism and moral reasoning have long been positioned as the most plausible model of moral judgment and decision-making in Western moral thinking. Defined as a conscious mental process that is 'intentional, effortful, and controllable' and which transforms 'given information about people in order to reach a moral judgment' (Haidt 2001: 818), moral reasoning has historically been portrayed as the very antithesis of moral intuition.

Moral intuition, in contrast, may be defined as:

> *the sudden appearance in consciousness of a moral judgment, including an affective valence (good–bad, like–dislike), without any conscious awareness of having gone through steps of searching, weighing evidence, of inferring a conclusion.* (Haidt 2001: 818)

Going on to claim that *intuition comes first*, proponents of this view contend that the reasoning process which has been so revered in Western moral philosophy has been overemphasised and that it is *reasoning* which is in the service of rationalising and justifying our moral intuitions, not the other way round (Haidt 2001, 2013; see also Brockman 2013; Gazzaniga 2005, 2011; Lehrer 2009).

The question remains, how does intuitionism actually determine the moral rightness or wrongness of a particular act?

Moral intuitionism is based on a meta-theory about the character of moral knowledge and the moral properties of things – notably that it is possible to know some moral facts in the world *non-inferentially* (i.e. not reasoned from evidence), for example that harming others is prima facie morally wrong (Tropman 2009, 2011). By this view, the intrinsic good or bad nature of a given act derives from the properties of that act – that is, whether the act in question is intrinsically good or bad. For example, an intuitionist might claim that the willful act of leaving a road accident victim to die on the side of the road when his life could have been saved has the *self-evident property* of 'wrongness', whereas the thoughtful act of assisting and resuscitating a road accident victim and thereby preventing an untimely death has the *self-evident property* of 'goodness'.

The process of knowing by intuition the rightness or wrongness of an action goes something like this: first, properties making the act in question right or wrong must be determined. These properties in turn are classified as being either 'prima-facie right' (i.e. the 'rightness' of the properties may be overridden by stronger moral properties) or 'wrong, all things considered' (i.e. in light of other morally significant considerations, and when these considerations have been weighed up against each other, the act is wrong) (Baier 1978a: 415). For example, resuscitating a road accident victim may be regarded as 'prima-facie right' where other stronger moral considerations do not impinge (e.g. the rescuer may risk her or his own life in the attempt to resuscitate or save the victim), whereas leaving the road accident victim to die needlessly might be regarded as 'wrong, all things considered' (e.g. when the rescuer is regarded as well qualified to instigate life-saving measures, and would be likely to succeed in the attempt, but is in too much of a hurry to stop, having promised to meet friends for a social dinner).

The second step involves determining the relative weight of given properties and deciding which imposes the more stringent of duties on a person to act. Once it has been decided which of the duties in question is the more stringent, the 'final duty' or 'duty, all things considered' can be established (Baier 1978a: 415). For example, once it is determined that the duty to save a road accident victim's life is more stringent than the duty to fulfil one's promise to friends to share a social meal with them, so too is it established that saving the life of the road accident victim is the 'final duty' or 'duty, all things considered'. How do we know this is our final duty, it might be asked? The answer is: we 'just know', it is 'self-evident' and that is all there is to say on the matter.

Moral intuitionism fell out of favour in the 1950s and is still considered by many philosophers to be implausible (Tropman 2009). Since this time, philosophers have criticised intuitionism on the grounds that it is misleading, that it fails to answer important moral questions, that it is unable to define and analyse the properties to which ethical terms refer, that it lacks objectivity, that it fails to provide a theory of moral motivation (i.e. what motivates people to do morally good acts), that it fails to provide a convincing theory of moral justification, and, more seriously, that it cannot be relied upon to resolve moral conflict (Baier 1978a; Frankena 1973; Rawls 1971; Swanton 1987; Warnock 1967). More recently, however, these criticisms have been found wanting and challenged from an unexpected source: contemporary work in the field of cognitive sciences (including the 'new science of decision-making'), which is consistently demonstrating the nature of intuition and its practical importance to and in decision-making (see, for example, Brockman 2013; Davis-Floyd & Arvidson 1997; Haidt 2001, 2013).

It is also important to note that not all moral philosophers have agreed that intuition has no place in our moral schemes. For example, in *Moral thinking: its levels, method and point*, Richard Hare (1981) concedes the role of intuition in moral thinking. Although Hare completely rejects intuition as the basis of moral thinking, and rejects its independent ability to resolve moral conflict, he nevertheless accepts that (Hare 1981: 210):

> *the intuitive level of moral thinking certainly exists and is (humanly speaking) an essential part of the whole structure.*

Hare basically argues that neither intuition nor reason is adequate on its own to deal effectively with moral problems. A sounder or more complete approach to moral thinking and decision-making, he suggests, would be to admit a kind of 'collaborative relationship' between these two faculties and to cease viewing them as being necessary opponents (p 44):

> *Let us be clear, first of all, that critical and intuitive moral thinking are not rival procedures, as much of the dispute between utilitarians and intuitionists seem to suppose. They are elements in a common structure, each with its parts to play.*

Psychologists also stress the importance of intuition in our everyday practical and working lives, and the need to enhance it if we are to make better rational decisions. Goldberg (1983: 33) argues that intuition is very much a part of reason, and in fact plays a crucial role in aiding the reasoning process itself. Intuition does this by feeding and stimulating rational thought and then by evaluating its products. If a reason or a thought does not 'feel' right, the reasoner or thinker simply switches tracks. Contending that 'reason is merely slow intuition' (Goldberg 1983: 37), Goldberg (p 23) goes on to assert that intuition has a particularly important role to play when dealing with problems which are too complex to be solved by rational analysis. What is needed, concludes Goldberg (p 28), is:

> *a balance and a recognition of the intricate, mutually enhancing relationship between intuition and rationality. We need not just more intuition but better intuition. We need not only to trust it but to make it more trustworthy. And at the same time we need sharp, discriminating rationality.*

Although there has been a renewed interest in moral intuitionism in recent years (see, for example, Stratton-Lake 2002; Tropman 2009, 2011), objections remain. Regardless of the objections that continue to be raised against it, the role of intuition in our moral thinking and in our everyday lives cannot be credibly denied. As Haidt (2001: 820) posits with reference to what he terms the 'social intuitionist solution':

> *The intuitive process is the default process, handling everyday moral judgments in a rapid, easy and holistic way. It is primarily when intuitions conflict, or when the social situation demands thorough examination of all facets of a scenario, that the reasoning process is called upon.*

Life experience and moral decision-making

It is becoming increasingly accepted that *life experience* and the awareness and insights gained from it are critical to the process of moral decision-making on account of their practical effects (both positive and negative) on the capacity of people to make sound moral choices in their daily lives and to take appropriate action based on those choices (Benjamin 2001; Beauchamp & Childress 2013; Little 2001; Moreno 1995; Walker 1998). It is also becoming increasingly recognised that moral viewpoints and the theoretical stances underpinning them are not set in stone, and that they can and do change (and sometimes ought to change) in the light of life experience and the new insights and knowledge(s) gained in the process. As W T Anderson (1990: 258) points out, many have come to accept 'morality, and moral discourse, as a living and central element in human existence'. He explains (pp 258–9):

> *We see our interpersonal relationships as collaborative efforts in constructing values. We see education as, among other things, a training in the skills of moral reasoning – morality not merely handed down but learned and created and re-created out of experience. And when there is conflict about that, as there inevitably will be, we accept the conflict also as an arena for expressing and creating values … Morals are not being handed down from the mountaintop on graven tablets; they are being created by people out of the challenges of the times. The morals of today are not the morals of yesterday, and they will not be the morals of tomorrow.*

It is this possibility for creating and re-creating (changing) our moral viewpoints and refining the moral values that inform them that makes the project of reconciling disputes about moral matters possible, feasible, viable, hopeful and sustainable. Consider the following.

As discussed in Chapter 3 of this book, we seem to recognise and accept that some moral decisions and actions are better than others (e.g. acts of kindness are better, morally speaking, than acts of cruelty). It is also evident that when some moral beliefs are shown to be 'wrong' or 'mistaken', people can and do change them. For instance, as Benjamin (2001: 26) explains:

> *Some of us may have been raised to believe that black people, gay people, poor people, or rich people don't have the same basic hopes, fears, wishes, and values as we do, or that there can be no morality without God, but what we read and experience for ourselves makes these [beliefs] seem doubtful.*

Benjamin goes on to explain that when our beliefs are found to be at 'odds' with our life experiences we subsequently revise our beliefs to ensure a better (more coherent) 'fit' between them and our lived experiences. In instances where our background beliefs seem 'wrong' and lacking 'fit' with the world, Benjamin writes (2001: 26) that:

> *we revise our overall outlook to achieve a better overall fit among its elements. None of them is basic or sacrosanct. Each may be modified in the interests of the outlook's achieving greater overall breadth and coherence. Sometimes we'll revise an increasingly dubious particular judgment in the interests of coherence with some more secure values or principles or background beliefs and theories. At other times, we'll revise an obsolete value or principle to fit with a particular moral judgment and background belief and theory. In some*

cases ... we'll even revise a background belief or theory – our understanding of what the world is like – to square with particular judgments and values and principles.

Benjamin further contends that if we are to succeed in our quest to develop a practical and plausible approach to ethics – and one that will be successful in improving, if not resolving, 'concrete practical problems' – then sometimes our moral viewpoints *have* to change; he contends (2001: 25):

Values and principles, in the light of experience, sometimes have *to be revised, modified, or replaced. Moreover, in some cases, a commitment to certain ethical values and principles will* require *that we revise our understanding of the world, the facts.* [emphasis added]

Reason, emotion, intuition and life experience – some further thoughts

Reason, emotion, intuition and life experience all have an important role to play in guiding our moral judgments and ethical decision-making. Acting in 'collaboration', these processes can work effectively as 'mutually correcting resources in moral reflection' (Callahan 1988: 9) and tutor, test and fine-tune our perceptions of and responses to moral problems in the workplace and elsewhere.

Dealing with moral disagreements and disputes

As pointed out in Chapter 1, moral problems and disagreements constitute an inevitable and unavoidable aspect of both our personal and our professional lives. Wong (1992: 763) suggests that we might even expect serious conflict to feature regularly in our ethical lives, 'involving people with whom continuing relationships are both necessary and desirable'. One reason for this is that 'informed, thoughtful individuals will not always agree about complex moral and political issues' and 'a number of important conflicts will have no clear resolution' (Benjamin 2001: 27). This is because (as already alluded to in this chapter, in the discussion on moral disagreement):

- different individuals can interpret the same evidence differently and draw quite different yet reasonable conclusions from that evidence
- the evidence itself may be contradictory, leading reasonable people to draw reasonably different conclusions
- even when individuals agree about what the relevant facts or considerations of a given matter are, they may nevertheless reasonably disagree about the weightings that should be given to the facts and considerations, and arrive at quite different conclusions (e.g. the debate about the moral permissibility of abortion and euthanasia rests more on disagreement about the weightings of relevant moral principles than about the applicability of the moral principles per se)
- moral concepts are often ambiguous and open to a variety of interpretations; individuals may make different reasonable interpretations of these, which, in turn, may lead to different though reasonable conclusions (adapted from Benjamin 2001: 27 – citing Rawls 1971, 1993).

Compounding the problem of moral disagreements is that there are 'no neutral criteria for determining that one reasonable world view and way of life is in all respects superior to the others' (Benjamin 2001: 28). The question that arises here is: How are we to respond to disagreements about moral matters and the conflicts that they sometimes give rise to? It is to briefly answering this question that the remainder of this chapter now turns.

Being accepting of different points of view

There is a variety of ways in which the task of moral decision-making in the face of moral disagreement might be approached. One approach that is particularly promising for dealing with serious conflict is the little-known approach called '*quantum morality*' (Zohar 1991; Zohar & Marshall 1993, 2000). Quantum morality uses a model of thinking and reasoning associated with quantum physics or the 'new physics' as it is sometimes called (Heisenberg 1990). Unlike the *either/or* divisionary way of thinking commonly associated with the classical physics of Isaac Newton (and from which Western moral philosophy has borrowed heavily), this new perspective rests on a *both/and* approach to moral thinking and moral decision-making. Whereas the classical model of Western moral thinking advocates an adversarial approach to interrogating ideas and discovering 'the moral truth', quantum morality advocates a cooperative and creative approach that accepts many different moral viewpoints as having the potential to be right, rather than assuming there is only one single correct view that *must* be defended even if this means destroying other points of view.

Underpinning a 'quantum morality' approach is the recognition that without difference there is no real choice – no real opportunity to develop, to grow, to evolve – no opportunity to sharpen and refine our moral thinking, and no opportunity to learn to understand another's point of view and to discover the 'creative unity in our differences' (Zohar & Marshall 1993: 273). Here, quantum morality takes as its starting point the view that being open to different viewpoints expands the potential of a situation, allows for more questions to be asked and more to be learned, and ultimately allows for common ground to be found.

Moral decision-making, by this view, is seen as involving a shared and cooperative venture, where people have time and can take time to talk, to really listen to other people's points of view (and thereby give recognition to others by listening), and to negotiate choices that strike 'a creative balance between more fixed attitudes of control at the one extreme or total receptiveness at the other' (Zohar & Marshall 1993: 102). For this approach to work, however, participants must come to the moral deliberating process with a willingness to: (1) 'let go' of their own point of view as the *only* point of view, and (2) put their own views alongside others 'as one of many to be compared, contrasted and considered' (Zohar & Marshall 1993: 235). Through cooperative and creative dialogue, the differing viewpoints of all participants can evolve into a new 'synthesised' complex whole. In so far as evaluating whether the 'correct' choices have been made, the following applies: if the values and meanings of the choices break down 'and the moral equivalent of physical chaos sets in', the participants may conclude that 'everything has fallen apart' and that a morally good outcome has not been achieved (Zohar 1991: 182). Conversely, if the values and meanings of the choices made do not break down, and the moral equivalent of physical order and unity sets in, the participants may conclude that everything has stayed together as a harmonious whole evolving towards a viable and sustainable future, and that a morally good outcome has been achieved.

Benjamin (2001), Moreno (1995), Wong (1992) and Jennings (1991), among others, argue along similar lines. These authors contend that, at the very least, moral decision-making in the face of moral disagreement must be approached in a consensual rather than a conflictive (adversarial) manner; democratically rather than dictatorially; with a genuine interest in and commitment to learning about *moral differences* and bridging the gap between them, instead of denigrating and dismissing differences as 'other' and hence deviant and wrong; and with a willingness to reciprocate rather than reproach attempts to create (new) common ground even – and, perhaps, especially – in instances where it may appear that none exists. In defence of a consensual and democratic approach to moral problem solving, Benjamin (2001: 28) argues:

> *Balancing personal conviction with respect for reasonable differences, the democratic temperament combines the standpoints of agent and spectator. The trick – and part of being human – is being able to retain both standpoints while judiciously tacking between them.*

Wong (1992: 780), however, contends that in the case of serious moral conflict much more than 'democratic discussion' is required. He explains:

> *An openness to be influenced by others, to bridge differences, may also take the form of a preparedness to expand one's conception of the good and the right upon further understanding and appreciation of other ways*

of life. This sort of preparedness goes beyond what could be required by the ideal of fair and democratic discussion — beyond, for example, the passive virtue of being prepared to change one's views in the face of undermining evidence. Learning from others often requires instead an active willingness *to gain a more vivid and detailed appreciation of what it is like to live their ways of life, an appreciation that can only be achieved through significant interaction with them.* [emphasis added]

Unfortunately, not all are willing to engage in a quantum moral approach to moral disagreements or to cultivate an 'active willingness to gain a more vivid and detailed appreciation of what it is like to live [other] ways of life'. Tragically, this unwillingness to consider other points of view has sometimes led to *moral disputes* being expressed via extraordinary acts of violence, resulting in serious injuries to and even the deaths of people whose viewpoints moral dissidents do not share. For example, in 1993, Dr David Gunn, a medical practitioner engaged in abortion work at the Pensacola Women's Medical Services clinic in the United States, was fatally wounded by an anti-abortion demonstrator engaged in a pro-life protest outside the clinic (Rohter 1993: 7). Described by authorities as the first slaying of its kind in the US, the incident exemplified the increasing violence against abortion clinics and workers across the nation, which is still happening today. With regards the death of Dr Gunn, Rescue America (a pro-life group) was reported as commenting that 'while Gunn's death is unfortunate, it's also true that quite a number of babies' lives will be saved' (Sharkey 1994: 3). Just over a year later, again in the US, a second doctor was killed outside an abortion clinic by a pro-life protester; at the time, a British commentator on anti-abortion protests in the US was reported as saying that the slaying was 'the start of the new Pro-Life movement, the new activism' (Sharkey 1994: 3). This new 'pro-life activism' has involved bombing and arson attacks against clinics, and the murder and injury of health workers. It has been reported that 'one hundred per cent of the bombers, arsonists and now murderers are Christian fundamentalists' (Sharkey 1994: 4).

The US is not, of course, the only country troubled by the increasingly public and sometimes violent manifestations of radical moral disagreements about bioethical issues. Australia has encountered its own problems. For example, in 1995 the Brisbane *Courier-Mail* reported that a member of the group called Christians Speaking Out stated that 'it is a Christian's duty to stop abortionists by any means' (13 May 1995). The member was also reported as condoning the killing of abortionists, arguing that it was 'justifiable homicide' (*Courier-Mail* 13 May 1995). In 2002, Peter Knight, an anti-abortion crusader, was sentenced to life imprisonment for the murder of a security guard outside an East Melbourne abortion clinic. Knight is reported to have arrived at the clinic with two bags — one containing a high-powered Winchester rifle and the other '16 litres of kerosene, spare rounds of ammunition, cigarette lighters, torches that could be soaked in kerosene, ropes and gags' (Berry & Munro 2002). It was evident that Knight intended to massacre the 15 staff and 26 patients at the clinic, but was overpowered by two men (one the boyfriend of a patient) before he could do so.

In light of these and other examples, perhaps one of the greatest challenges ahead may not be how to devise new ways of thinking about ethics or about developing better models of moral decision-making for dealing with moral conflict. Rather, the challenge may be to find new ways of motivating moral behaviour and to foster among those who hold differing moral values and beliefs a genuine interest in approaching moral disagreement in a consensual rather than a conflictive and adversarial manner, and in a manner that seeks first to understand before seeking to be understood.

Everyday moral problems in nursing

Before concluding this chapter, some comment is required on the less 'exotic' issue of 'everyday' moral problems in nursing practice. As already stated, nurses have to deal with ethical issues *every day*. The nursing ethics literature does not, however, always represent or reflect the reality of the kinds of 'everyday' problems that nurses face. Instead, this literature has borrowed heavily from mainstream bioethics to shape nursing ethics discourse and in a way that has sometimes been at the expense of nurses' own experiential wisdom.

In Chapter 2 of this book, under the discussion on nursing ethics, it was suggested that the actual lived experiences of nurses and the lived realities of nursing practice provide a more reliable methodological starting point to nursing ethics inquiry than do the 'top-down' theories of Western moral philosophy and the field of bioethics which is derivative of it. This is because an examination of nurses' lived experiences and lived realities of practice yields important knowledge about and insights into the actual *everyday ethical issues* and moral problems with which nurses have to deal. Examples include problems concerning the:

- moral boundaries of nursing (e.g. nurses as carers being 'in relationship' with others, as opposed to being what the North American philosopher, John Rawls, advocates, the 'detached observers choosing from behind a veil of ignorance' (Rawls 1971))
- catalysts to moral action in nursing (e.g. 'experiential triggers' such as 'the look of suffering in a patient's eyes', as opposed to abstract moral rules and principles)
- operating moral values in nursing (e.g. sympathy, empathy, compassion, human understanding and a desire 'to do the best we can', rather than an obsession to 'do one's duty')
- ethical decision-making processes in nursing (e.g. which tend to be collaborative, communicative, communal and contextualised, rather than independent, private, individual, solo and decontextualised)
- barriers to ethical practice in nursing (e.g. structural as well as knowledge based – for example, the power and authority of doctors to determine patient care, organisational norms forcing compliance with the status quo, and negative attitudes and a lack of support from co-workers and managers, lack of moral competency in decision-makers)
- need for cathartic moral talking in nursing care domains (e.g. 'talking through' moral concerns in a safe and supportive environment to help relieve the emotional distress that so often arises as a result of trying to be moral in a world that appears to be becoming increasingly amoral).

What talking with nurses so often reveals is that it is *not* the so-called paramount ('exotic') bioethical issues (e.g. abortion and euthanasia) that trouble them, but rather the more fundamental issues of:

- how to help a patient in distress in the 'here and now'
- how to stop 'things going bad for a patient'
- how best to support relatives or chosen carers during times of distress and when the 'system' appears to be against them
- how to make things 'less traumatic' for someone who is suffering
- how to reduce the anxiety and vulnerability of the people being cared for
- where to get help with their (the nurses') own emotional distress
- how to make a difference in contexts which have become manifestly indifferent to the moral interests of others.

The above and other related concerns are all issues worthy of attention and consideration both within and outside of the nursing profession. They are also issues that deserve to be recognised as 'moral problems in nursing' just as the other 'paramount' issues of bioethics are.

Conclusion

Nurses will encounter many complex moral problems in the course of their work. To be effective in dealing with these problems and preventing the kinds of moral harms that can follow as a consequence of them, it is imperative that nurses have an informed knowledge and understanding of the nature of moral problems, the various forms in which they can manifest, and the kinds of processes that can be used for dealing with them effectively. This chapter has sought to provide such knowledge and understanding. Other processes, for example, conscientious objection and whistleblowing, will be considered in Chapter 11 of this book.

In the past, when confronted by the moral problems of life, it has been 'too easy to reach solutions that fail to do justice to the difficulty of the problem' (Nagel 1991: xi). We do not have to look far to see that many of the answers gained and the solutions reached in contemporary bioethics have been found inadequate when applied to and in the concrete circumstances of life. Arguably, what is required to help remedy this situation is a mindset that not only seeks to ask questions, but seeks to also *call into question* things as they are (Freire 1970, 1972). There also needs to be the recognition that when faced with morally perplexing issues:

- we need to think better and harder about the issues in question (Boyle 1994)
- we need to remember that moral ambiguity, uncertainty, controversy and disagreement can and do have many causes, both practical and theoretical (McCullough 1995)
- we need to accept that addressing moral problems in a sound and effective manner requires an appeal to a moral approach that recognises a multiplicity of possible solutions to a given problem, and that a moral approach which insists on there being just one single correct answer (a 'final solution') to a given moral problem may compound rather than remedy that problem (Fasching 1993).

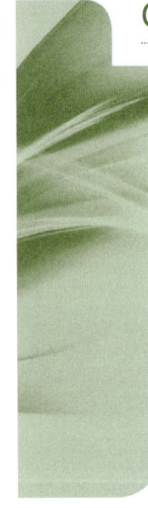

Case scenario 1[3]

An intensive care nurse of several years' experience was assigned the care of a man who had been estranged from his identical twin brother for several years. The man's condition was serious and it was evident that he was dying. Despite being aware of his deteriorating condition, the man was adamant that 'he did not want any contact with his twin brother' and that 'his twin brother was not to be contacted and told about his condition'. Having had personal experience of the relationship dynamics between twins in her own family, and having an 'intuition' that the man was not making the 'right choice' in the circumstances at hand, the nurse decided to 'respectfully disagree' with her patient's request and to go against his expressed wishes. Recognising that time was running out (the man was not expected to live very long), she immediately set in motion a chain of events that resulted in the estranged brothers being reunited and reconciled before the ill brother died. Prior to the ill twin's death, both brothers were adamant that the nurse had 'done the right thing' and expressed their deep appreciation for her insights, sensitivity and actions – especially her decision to 'go against the ill twin's expressed wishes'. Other staff in the unit, however, had reservations about the way in which the nurse had handled the situation. They were especially concerned about her decision to go against the patient's expressed wishes, which they perceived as a violation of his right to decide.

Case scenario 2

A newly appointed lecturer in a School of Nursing approaches a professor in the school seeking advice. In keeping with his new academic position and expected performance goals, he has prepared three manuscripts for publication based on work completed in his area of expertise and early career research projects. He was shocked, however, to receive a message from his academic supervisor insisting that she be named as first author on all three papers even though she did not meet the authorship attribution guidelines as prescribed by International Committee of Medical Journal Editors (ICMJE) guideline *Recommendations for the conduct,*

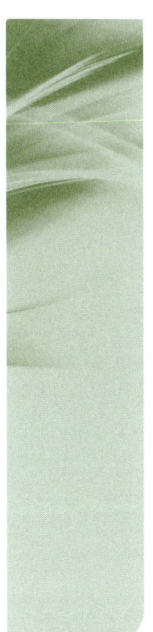

reporting, editing, and publication of scholarly work in medical journals (www.icmje.org). Not only had she not made any substantial contribution to the conception or design of the work, or to the acquisition, analysis and interpretation of data being reported in the manuscripts, but she had not contributed in any way to either drafting the manuscripts or revising them critically for important intellectual content. In short, she had contributed nothing to the manuscripts other than to read them and approve their submission for review and publication. The lecturer confided that he had tried unsuccessfully to discuss the matter with the supervisor. Her response was to tell him in a very curt tone that 'it was his perception only that she hadn't contributed to the manuscripts' and that 'as the most senior person in the research centre to which he was affiliated, he was obliged to name her as first author on the papers'. Moreover, if he did not name her as first author, 'there would be consequences'. He confided that he felt too intimidated to ask what she meant by 'there will be consequences' and reflected that he was soon due to undergo his probationary performance review and that his employment contract was also up for renewal at the end of the following year. He expressed deep concern that the supervisor might sabotage his career progression as rumoured she had done with other research staff under her supervision. He also indicated that he felt he 'could not go to the Head of School as she was in a very "cliquey" relationship with the supervisor' and doubted he would get her support. The professor responded that she understood his situation, but that 'there was nothing she could do' as she was not in a managerial role. She also explained that it was 'common practice in the school for colleagues to "free-load" on the work of others and be cited as co-authors, even if they had not made a substantial contribution to a given manuscript'. This was because of the enormous pressure academic staff were under to 'publish or perish'. She agreed that this practice was neither fair nor ethical, but 'everyone did it'.

CRITICAL QUESTIONS

1 What are the moral problems demonstrated by these cases?
2 If you were the nurse who had been assigned to care for the patient depicted in the first case scenario, or were a bystander observing the involvement of another nurse, what would you have done in the situation at hand?
3 What processes would you have used in order to address the moral problems raised in the two case scenarios presented?
4 Do you think your 'ordinary' moral values, beliefs, knowledge and experiences (e.g. such as those acquired before you entered into nursing or studied ethics) would have been adequate to guide you on how to act in the case scenarios given?

Endnotes

1 Section taken from Johnstone M-J (2013b) Moral distress. *Australian Nursing Journal* 20(12): 25. Reproduced with permission.
2 At the time of writing, a word search of contents published in the international journal *Nursing Ethics* alone located 571 articles published between 2002 and 2018.
3 Taken from Johnstone M-J (2004a) *Effective writing for health professionals*. Allen & Unwin, Sydney, pp 3–4.

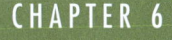

Ethics, dehumanisation and vulnerable populations

KEYWORDS
dehumanisation
delegitimisation
disadvantage
discrimination
humanness
moral disengagement
moral exclusion
moral inclusion
prejudice
stigma
vulnerability
vulnerable populations

LEARNING OBJECTIVES
Upon the completion of this chapter and with further self-directed learning you are expected to be able to:
- Discuss critically the notion of vulnerability.
- Define dehumanisation and critically examine the different forms it can take.
- Examine the possible relationship between human vulnerability and dehumanisation.
- Discuss critically the notion and possible impact of delegitimisation.
- Explore the processes of 'moral inclusion' and 'moral exclusion'.
- Discuss critically the relationship between dehumanisation, delegitimisation and moral disengagement.
- Identify vulnerable individuals and groups for whom nurses may have special responsibilities.
- Discuss critically the definitions and differentiating characteristics of a: refugee, asylum seeker, internally displaced person, stateless person, returnee, migrant and immigrant.
- Explore the role and responsibilities of nurses in mitigating the morally harmful consequences of the dehumanisation of vulnerable individuals and groups in health care and society.

Introduction

National and international nursing standards, position statements, codes of conduct and related scholarship are replete with references to the role and responsibility of nurses: to consider the needs of the 'most' or 'especially vulnerable', to give 'special attention' to vulnerable groups and populations, and to 'emphasise vulnerable groups' when applying human rights protection. Just what is meant by the notion 'vulnerability', who counts as being '*the* most vulnerable', who should determine this and how the notion might be operationalised as an action guiding principle in nursing ethics discourse are, however, not well understood. Thus questions remain of:

- What is vulnerability?
- When is it appropriate to describe a person or group as 'especially vulnerable', all things considered?

- How, if at all, might the notion of 'human vulnerability' function as a guide to moral action?
- What special responsibilities and remedial measures should considerations of human vulnerability inspire and require of nurses in the course of their everyday practice?

It is to answering these questions that the discussion in this chapter will now turn.

Vulnerability[1]

The idea of *vulnerability* (from the Latin *vulnerāre* to wound) has many meanings and applications. As such it may be described as a 'contested' notion. Nonetheless, there is general agreement that the notion of vulnerability entails an entity (e.g. a sentient being) having the capacity to be wounded or hurt physically and emotionally, and/or who is susceptible to being harmed through being exploited, or exposed to disaster, in morally significant ways (Hoffmaster 2006; Masferrer & García-Sánchez 2016; Ruof 2004). It is also recognised that using vulnerability as a conceptual frame is 'an important way to capture disadvantage' – particularly of those who have been, or who are at risk of being, marginalised by mainstream society (Blacksher & Stone 2002: 421).

In his classic work *Protecting the vulnerable*, Goodin (1985: xi) clarifies that some vulnerabilities (and the responsibilities that emerge in response to them) are 'natural, inevitable, and immutable', whereas others are 'created, shaped, or sustained by current social arrangements'. Given this, there is scope to hold that 'vulnerability is a human condition from which we all suffer' and from which 'we all deserve equal protection' (Kottow 2003: 461; see also Andorno 2016; Cortina & Conill 2016; Masferrer & García-Sánchez 2016). To put this another way: 'None of us is invincible; all of us are vulnerable' and, as such, vulnerability needs to be addressed as a moral concern (Hoffmaster 2006: 43).

Identifying vulnerable populations

Human vulnerability may indeed be a universal condition and a state from which we all deserve equal protection (Kottow 2003; Masferrer & García-Sánchez 2016). Even so, as can be readily demonstrated, there are some people who are more vulnerable than others and who, for various reasons, are less able to protect their own interests when these are at risk of being harmed. Correct identification of these people is essential if the special protective responsibilities that others have towards them are to be realised in policy and practice.

Vulnerability can be *individual* (individual vulnerability) or *aggregate* ('vulnerable groups', 'vulnerable populations', 'social vulnerability') (de Chesnay & Anderson 2012; Masferrer & García-Sánchez 2016; Mastroianni 2009). In the case of individual vulnerability, entities commonly identified (particularly in national research guidelines) include people who:

- are very young and lack maturity (e.g. infants, children and young adolescents)
- are highly dependent on medical care (and who may be unable to give consent)
- have a cognitive impairment or who have an intellectual disability
- have a mental health problem or illness
- have a physical disability (and who are dependent on others for their daily care)
- are very old, frail and isolated (e.g. the dependent elderly)
- are of low socioeconomic status (e.g. the poor, homeless, and/or unemployed)
- are serving a prison sentence for criminal offences (prison inmates)
- are members of an ethnic minority group or population
- are refugees, asylum seekers, displaced persons or stateless persons

- (in Australia) identify as being Aboriginal or Torres Strait Islanders
- (in New Zealand) identify as being Māori.

In the case of *aggregate vulnerability*, entire groups, populations and even countries can be characterised as being vulnerable – for example, groups and populations that are at risk of premature mortality or morbidity (Purdy 2004), and poorer nations or countries that are at risk of exploitation by researchers (see examples given in Liamputtong 2007; Macklin 2003), drug companies, fast food companies, mining magnates and the like.

Vulnerability as a guide to action

Not all agree that vulnerability is a useful concept or even that it has a place as a guide to ethical conduct. Some critics argue that labelling individuals and groups as vulnerable may have the undesirable consequence of paradoxically stigmatising them and also risk their being marginalised on the basis of the very characteristics for which they have been deemed to be vulnerable (e.g. old age, disability, decisional incapacity). Thus, individuals and groups labelled vulnerable may find themselves also carrying the burden of what Martha Minow (1990: 20) calls the 'stigma of difference' and the 'moral pathology of prejudice' that underpins it. (According to Minow, the stigma of difference is so potent that it 'may be created both by ignoring it and by focusing on it'.)

Other critics, meanwhile, object to identifying people as vulnerable on grounds that it could seem patronising and condescending. Danis and Patrick (2002: 320), for example, argue that 'Labeling individuals as "vulnerable" risks viewing vulnerable individuals as "others" worthy of pity', a view rarely appreciated (e.g. a healthy and active octogenarian may not appreciate being categorised as 'vulnerable' simply on the basis of his or her old age; likewise a pregnant woman, consenting to be interviewed for a research project, may not appreciate being categorised as 'vulnerable' simply because of being pregnant).

It is not clear that these and similar criticisms are sustainable, however. This is especially so when considered in relation to the possible link that exists between vulnerability and dehumanisation (to be considered shortly). Moreover, new and emerging works are increasingly suggesting that the notion of vulnerability not only gives functional structure to the moral obligations that people have towards others, but also inspires and requires them to engage in actions that respect, protect and remediate breaches of people's human rights and social justice violations (Andorno 2016; Masferrer & García-Sánchez 2016). The identification of vulnerability as a 'missing feature' of contemporary moral philosophy (Hoffmaster 2006) and as an understated source of our 'special responsibilities' to protect others (Goodin 1985: 109) further challenges the criticisms raised by its detractors.

In light of these developments it can be seen that, despite the criticisms which have been labelled against it, the concept of vulnerability remains essential to contemporary bioethics (Andorno 2016; Cortina & Conill 2016; Goodin 1985; Hoffmaster 2006; Masferrer & García-Sánchez 2016). It also stands as an extremely useful reminder to practitioners, policy makers and researchers alike that all human beings have the capacity to be 'hurt or wounded', that this capacity to be hurt needs constantly to be taken into consideration in their day-to-day practices and proceedings, and that attempts to define and protect '*vulnerable populations*' through codes, standards and institutional regulations are not necessarily a case of 'bureaucratic overreach' (Blacksher & Stone 2002; Goodin 1985). In short, contrary to the views of its detractors, the concept of vulnerability may, in practice, be *the* key to the prevention of ethics and social justice violations in both health and social care contexts.

Vulnerability and nursing ethics

Vulnerability has been identified as an 'understated foundation' of ethical sensibility in nursing (Nortvedt 2003) and as a construct that ought to have an important, if not pre-eminent, place in nursing ethics.

There is a need, however, for nurses not only to *learn* about vulnerability and its importance as a foundational ethical concept, but also to *feel* it. This is because, as examples to be given in this and the following chapters of this book make plain, unless we *feel* our own vulnerability we will not be able to affirm either our own or others' humanity. And unless we 'recognise the depth and the breadth of our vulnerability' we will not realise 'how much we need the help of others to protect us from our weaknesses and our infirmities' (Hoffmaster 2006: 44) or, conversely, how much others may need us to assist *them* when weak and unable to help themselves.

Until nurses recognise both the universal and particular vulnerability of people and the related moral obligations we all share to help and protect those who have become unable to protect their own interests, the risk of 'vulnerability tragedies' occurring and also being repeated will remain high. So too will the risk of nurses being left unnecessarily as 'guilty bystanders' to the plight of vulnerable people in hostile care environments (Fitzgerald et al 2016). To help further explain why this risk exists, an exploration of the notion of dehumanisation and its underrecognised link to human vulnerability is warranted.

Humanness, dehumanisation and vulnerability

An understated cause and consequence of human vulnerability is *dehumanisation* and the unfair ways in which this can *disadvantage* people. Dehumanisation is a recognised predictor of prejudice, discrimination, marginalisation and extreme violence against people deemed 'other', notably by those who have a social dominance orientation (to be explained shortly) and who view those they have 'othered' as being less morally worthy and hence less morally deserving than themselves or their 'in-group'. In order to understand the possible relationship between vulnerability and dehumanisation, some understanding of the nature of dehumanisation and its capacity to have a devastating impact on the moral interests and the humanity of all people is warranted. To this end, in the discussion to follow, consideration will be given to the interrelated notions of humanness, dehumanisation, delegitimisation, moral exclusion, moral inclusion, stigma, prejudice, discrimination and disadvantage.

Humanness

In order to make sense of what dehumanisation is (commonly taken to mean the denial of humanness) an account of *what* is being denied – that is, what constitutes *humanness* – is first required (Haslam et al 2008). 'Humanness' and what it means to be human are 'slippery' notions and have occupied the attention of philosophers for centuries. More recently it has been the subject of a growing body of research and scholarship in the field of social psychology, which is giving rise to new and important insights into the phenomena of humanness and dehumanisation, although this work has by no means settled ongoing debates about the subject (Bain et al 2013; Kaufmann et al 2011a). As Haslam (2013: 36) notes, 'one of the key developments in recent research and theory is that humanness is not a unitary idea'.

Conventional philosophical debates on what it means to be a human being have typically focused on drawing a distinction between an entity being *genetically human* and having *personhood*. Meeting the criteria of personhood has been quintessential to determining whether or not an entity ought to be categorised as 'human' and accorded moral status (Bastian et al 2011). This distinction has had particular resonance in the abortion debate, whereby the human fetus has been characterised as genetically human, yet not necessarily as having personhood (this issue will be discussed in more depth in Chapter 10), and likewise debates about the use of anencephalic infants for organ donation to help overcome organ shortages for transplantation in infants (Glasson et al 1995; John & Bailey 2018; Khan & Lea 2009; Nagakawa et al 2017; Shewmon et al 1989). On account of not having personhood, human fetuses and anencephalic infants have tended to be positioned as beings without moral status and thus without any of the moral rights that might otherwise be commensurate with an entity having moral status.

Debate surrounding the issues of abortion and the use of anencephalic infants as organ donors are just two examples that may help to explain why addressing the question of humanness is important. Specifically, it highlights the normative belief that the 'qualities that make us human are also those that give us moral status' (Bastian et al 2011: 469). This, in turn, highlights the moral problem that there is a relatively short step between denying people their humanness and denying them their moral status. As Opotow (1993) has observed, when people are portrayed as being outside of the category 'human' they lose all the protections that being human entails. This is because the denial of humanness places people 'outside the boundary in which moral values, rules, and considerations of fairness apply' and renders them 'nonentities, expendable and as morally undeserving' (Opotow 1990a: 1). Moreover, if they are harmed as a result of their moral exclusion, it is likely the harms experienced would be construed by its perpetrators as being not only acceptable, but also appropriate and just (Opotow 1990a; see also Bar-Tal 1990).

The questions remain: 'What is humanness?' and 'Is it something that one person or group can credibly deny another?'

Social psychologists suggest that, notwithstanding the difficulties in achieving a consensual definition of humanness, there are two senses in which humanness tends to be viewed, both of which serve the purpose of distinguishing humans from other entities (Haslam 2006; Haslam et al 2008). The first sense, which contrasts humans with animals, is *human uniqueness* – meaning properties that are uniquely human and not shared by other beings (Haslam 2013: 36). An example would be the human capacity for *complex emotions* (such as disillusionment, felicity, embarrassment, optimism, admiration), which is in contrast to the *basic emotions* (such as anger, fear, sadness, surprise, pleasure) that other animals also share (Leyens et al 2000). Other *uniquely human* characteristics that have been suggested include the properties of 'civility [culture], refinement, moral sensibility, rationality, logic and maturity' – properties which other species are presumed to lack (Haslam 2006: 257).

The second sense of humanness, which contrasts humans with inanimate objects (e.g. machines, robots and automatons), encompasses what is regarded to be *typically human* in that it reflects *human nature* (Haslam 2006; Haslam et al 2008). *Human nature*, in this instance, may manifest as 'emotional responsiveness, interpersonal warmth, cognitive openness, agency and individuality, depth [of character]' (Haslam 2006: 257) – properties that robots and machines simply do not have.

Dehumanisation

Dehumanisation fundamentally entails denying the humanness of others. Such denial can take several forms, can be expressed in different ways and can result in extremely harmful consequences (e.g. ethnocide). If the effects of dehumanisation are to be mitigated then the phenomenon itself needs to be understood. Specifically, the different forms that dehumanisation can take, the different ways it can be expressed in everyday life, why it occurs, what its consequences are and how if at all it might be deterred all require examination. It is to examining these issues that this discussion now turns.

Forms of dehumanisation

Research suggests that dehumanisation corresponds in varying ways to the two senses of humanness outlined in the previous section – that is, that which is *uniquely human* and that which reflects *human nature* or is *typically human* (Haslam 2006; Haslam et al 2008). Accordingly, dehumanisation may take one or more of the following forms:

- *animalistic dehumanisation* – whereby people are deemed to be more 'animal-like' than other categories of people, or summarily demoted to animal status (e.g. characterised as 'rats', 'pigs', 'dogs', 'cows', 'asses', 'monkeys', 'spiders', 'snakes', 'parasites', 'cockroaches' and other vermin)

- *mechanistic dehumanisation* – whereby people are reduced or demoted to inert, unfeeling automatons (e.g. the biomedical characterisation of the human body as a 'machine' with 'parts' that require fixing, replacing, or removal; employees on an assembly line treated 'as if' they are robots)
- *superhumanisation* – whereby people are either elevated to the status of and/or idealised as gods and angels; or derogated as satans, devils and demons (e.g. a philanthropist characterised as a 'saint' or 'angel', a fiend characterised as 'the devil incarnate', a murderer portrayed as a 'monster') (Bain et al 2013; Bar-Tal 1989, 1990; Haslam et al 2008; Hodson et al 2013).

Underpinning each of these forms of dehumanisation is a psychological process that Bar-Tal (1990: 65) has termed '*delegitimisation*', which he defines as the:

> *categorization of a group or groups into extreme negative social categories that are excluded from the realm of acceptable norms and/or values.*

He explains that delegitimisation (also a type of stereotyping and of prejudice) has the following distinguishing characteristics (p 66):

1. it utilizes extremely negative, salient, and atypical bases for categorizations;
2. it denies the humanity of the delegitimized group;
3. it is accompanied by intense, negative emotions of rejection, such as hatred, anger, contempt, fear, or disgust;
4. it implies that the delegitimized group has the potential to endanger one's own group; and
5. it implies that the delegitimized group does not deserve human treatment and therefore harming is justified.

The processes of dehumanisation and delegitimisation, in turn, rest on what Bandura (1999: 193) has termed '*moral disengagement*' (discussed earlier in Chapter 5 of this text). In this instance, moral disengagement sees perpetrators of dehumanisation cognitively restructure their inhumane conduct as being 'benign and worthy' via a complex interplay of the following processes:

> *moral justification, sanitizing language, and advantageous comparisons; disavowal of a sense of personal agency by diffusion or displacement of responsibility; disregarding or minimizing the injurious effects of one's actions; and attribution of blame to, and dehumanization of, those who are victimized.*

As will be considered shortly, because these processes operate and can be advanced in extremely subtle ways, they can often be difficult to detect and thus difficult to deter and remedy.

Explicit and subtle expressions of dehumanisation

Research suggests that dehumanisation can be expressed in various ways, ranging from the 'obvious', overt and explicit expressions of dehumanisation (the kind that has tended to receive the most attention up until recently) to the less obvious, covert and subtle expressions – the everyday expressions that often go unnoticed. In the case of overt and explicit expressions of dehumanisation, 'othered' people are *consciously and deliberately* described as 'non-human'. There are many examples of this throughout recorded history, some of the most notorious modern examples being: the Nazi characterisations of Jews and Gypsies as 'rats' and 'vermin'; the Hutu characterisation of Tutsis as 'cockroaches' during the Rwandan civil conflict, which saw the genocidal mass slaughter of between 500 000 and 1 million Rwandans (70% of whom were Tutsis); Africans being called 'apes'; and indigenous Australians being called 'monkeys' (Bain et al 2013; Bar-Tal 1990; Costello & Hodson 2009; Haslam 2013).

In the case of subtle or covert expressions of dehumanisation, people subtly downplay or attribute fewer 'uniquely human' qualities to others – usually members of an 'out-group' – that is, they portray them as being more 'animal like' than themselves. Also called 'infrahumanisation' (Haslam & Loughnan

2014; Leyens et al 2000, 2007), a distinguishing feature of subtle or covert dehumanisation (compared with its more explicit form) is that it tends not to be reported directly and is expressed by perpetrators without conscious awareness that their expressions are dehumanising (Bastian et al 2011). Examples can be found in cases of stereotyping 'people of difference' (Bastian et al 2011).

A stand-out example of the infrahumanisation of people is the dehumanising, stereotypical depiction, by the media and politicians, of refugees and asylum seekers as 'queue jumpers' and 'cheats not willing to follow fair procedures' (Esses et al 2008: 5). They are relentlessly portrayed as having 'less capacity' for complex emotions and moral values ('be like us'), and as being primarily motivated by only the 'basic emotions' that animals share (e.g. fear and pleasure). The subliminal message here is that 'these people' ostensibly lack the moral motivations and personal control that a more 'civilised' and 'cultured' people ('us') would otherwise exhibit. Recall the 'Children overboard' incident discussed in Chapter 2. This incident involved the public misrepresentation of photographic images and false claims by Federal government politicians that asylum seekers who were attempting to enter Australian territory 'illegally' by sea had 'deliberately' thrown their children overboard from the boat they were on so they would be rescued. It was later revealed and subsequently verified by a Senate Inquiry into the matter that no children had, in fact, been thrown overboard. This, however, did not stop politicians or the media from portraying them ('demonising them') as 'faceless, violent queue jumpers' and as people of poor moral character, as was widely quipped at the time 'the kinds of people who would throw their children overboard' (Senate Select Committee on a Certain Maritime Incident 2002: xxi).

In addition to being either explicit or subtle, researchers contend that expressions of dehumanisation may also be relative or absolute, a feature that must also be assessed when attempting to mitigate its effects. In the case of *relative expressions*, the target individual or group (usually an *out-group* or individual) is portrayed as being less than human 'relative' to another (usually the *in-group* or individual) (Haslam 2013). In contrast, *absolute expressions* of dehumanisation are explicit: the target individuals or groups are characterised unequivocally as *being* animalistic, or devilish, or monstrous in and of themselves *independent of comparisons that might otherwise be made with other beings or entities* (Haslam 2013).

It is important to clarify that, although the various ways in which dehumanisation can be expressed have been described in dichotomous terms (e.g. humanness/non-humanness, object/animal, explicit/subtle, conscious/unconscious, relative/absolute), as Haslam (2013) concedes, in practice its expression probably occurs along a continuum that encompasses subtle variations of all the dimensions identified. What these categorisations enable, however, is a better understanding of the phenomena at issue and whether the diverse forms that human denial can take are to qualify as cases of 'dehumanisation' (Haslam 2013: 42).

Why dehumanisation occurs

The causes of dehumanisation, the possible neural mechanisms involved and the psychological motivations for people to engage in harmful dehumanising behaviours are extremely complex, with some suggesting that the human brain has been 'hard wired' through evolutionary processes to favour in-groups ('us') over out-groups ('them') (Greene 2013; Lee & Harris 2013). Although research on the subject is inconclusive, one thing is clear: *everyone* has the capacity to dehumanise others – especially those identified as being outliers to one's own 'in-group' and hence labelled (often unconsciously) as 'other'. Research also strongly suggests that when an in-group perceives that its resources and/or identity are threatened by an out-group, this often leads to a 'rejection response' and the dehumanisation of those deemed to pose the 'resource threat' or the 'identity threat' to members of the in-group (Costello & Hodson 2009; Hodson & Costello 2007; Leyens et al 2000). Given this, it would be a grave mistake to assume that it is only the ignorant, the misguided, or the manifestly psychopathic individuals who are capable of denying 'others' their humanness and the moral protections and entitlements that come with this status. This is not to deny, however, that some people are more predisposed than others to perpetrate acts of dehumanisation, or that some are more motivated than others to expose and mitigate this predisposition.

Research to date suggests that people who see animals as inferior to humans, who have a 'social dominance orientation' and who subscribe to 'right-wing authoritarianism' are more likely to engage in the dehumanisation of people outside of their in-group than are those who do not have such ideological orientations (Haslam 2013; Hodson & Costello 2007; Leyens et al 2000). This is because people who hold these ideologies tend to see themselves as 'superior' to others and to value social hierarchies and group dominance. The world is seen as a competitive jungle, with 'intergroup interactions perceived as zero-sum competitions over finite resources' (Haslam 2013: 6) and over their social and political identities (Bar-Tal 1990; Tajfel & Turner 1979). When out-groups are perceived as a threat, depending on the severity of the threat (whether real or imagined) this perception tends to be accompanied by fear, stress and feelings of uncertainty and vulnerability by the in-group (Bar-Tal 1990; see also Becker 1973; Crimston et al 2018). This helps to explain why people with these orientations and dispositions tend to be associated with 'prejudice towards a variety of outgroups, particularly subordinate and competitor outgroups' (Haslam 2013: 6), for example immigrants and asylum seekers (Esses et al 2008; Hodson & Costello 2007).

In contrast, people who have 'inter-species' empathy and concern (e.g. value and even anthropomorphise animals, and encourage perceptions of the similarities between animals and human beings), who emphasise inter-group similarities, and who have a low preference for and tolerance of social hierarchies and dominance tend to be less associated with prejudice and intolerance of out-groups and people otherwise deemed 'different to us'.

In sum, there seems to be a link between a perception that 'humans are different from and superior to animals' and a disposition to dehumanise others, and especially people who are perceived as belonging to out-groups and as posing a threat to the in-group's resources, identity and social–political standing. Conversely, those who hold beliefs about animal–human similarities are less predisposed towards and are less likely to dehumanise others – and indeed may actually foster *out-group humanisation* and the *rehumanisation* of those who have already been dehumanised – for example, immigrants (termed 'immigrant humanisation') (Costello & Hodson 2009: 17).

Consequences of dehumanisation

Some researchers contend controversially that not all instances of dehumanisation are harmful and, indeed, may even be adaptive and necessary (Lee & Harris 2013). For example, a surgeon may not be able to perform effectively unless focused on the 'mechanics' of the human body and its constitutive parts that lay beneath his scalpel blade. Such instances tend to be the exception not the norm, however. Although unlikely to exacerbate an entity's vulnerability per se, such instances of 'benevolent' mechanistic dehumanisation may nonetheless result in what some have termed 'human dignity violations', a form of dehumanisation that encompasses the humiliation and degradation of human beings (Kaufmann et al 2011b). Thus, the diligent surgeon may well have performed a perfect surgical procedure and prolonged the life of his patient, yet may still have committed a dignity violation – albeit one that was unintended: the patient, stripped of her body part (a limb, a breast, a sex organ, the side of her face), although grateful for her life-prolonging treatment, may nonetheless feel degraded and 'less than human' on account of losing the part that has been amputated and the function it once afforded.

Putting aside what might be termed 'benevolent mechanistic dehumanisation', dehumanisation remains morally problematic. The main reason for this, as suggested in the opening paragraphs to this discussion, is that it justifies what Staub (1990) and Opotow (1990a, 1990b) call '*moral exclusion*' and the related moral harms that would otherwise be considered unconscionable. As noted earlier, moral exclusion occurs when:

individuals or groups are perceived as outside the boundary in which moral values, rules, and considerations of fairness apply. *Those who are morally excluded are perceived as nonentities, expendable, or undeserving; consequently harming them appears acceptable, appropriate, or just.* [emphasis original] (Opotow 1990a: 1)

Opotow (1990b: 174) explains that moral exclusion emerges when '*group differences* (or "we–they" distinctions) are salient and when *difficult life conditions* (such as harsh social circumstances, destructive conflict, or threat) exist' [emphasis original]. It can also emerge where there are perceived *conflicts of interests* that give rise to *group categorisations*, which in turn 'contribute to *moral justifications* for *unjust procedures*, which can themselves be injurious and which permit other *harmful outcomes* to ensue' [emphasis original] (p 174).

Opotow concludes that what primarily makes moral exclusion problematic is not only that it enables the unjust and even brutal treatment of others considered 'less than human' and inferior, but also that it is insidious and difficult to detect. This is because its justifications are largely unspoken on account of being based on shared social perceptions that are 'institutionalized, invisible, and accepted as if inevitable' (Fine 1990: 111). Opotow (1990a: 13) cautions, however, that:

> *moral exclusion is neither an isolated nor inexplicable event, but occurs with great frequency, depends on ordinary social and psychological processes to license previously unacceptable attitudes and behaviour, and can cause great harm, from personal suffering to widespread atrocities.*

Deterring dehumanisation

Dehumanisation is a malevolent process: it unjustifiably denies the humanness of 'others' and, by virtue of this denial, justifies harming or at least failing to protect the significant moral interests of those targeted. Targeted individuals and groups are not the only 'victims', however. Research has shown that when people dehumanise others they also dehumanise themselves (Bastian et al 2011, 2012); likewise, in harming others, perpetrators harm themselves (Rodriguez 2017). Thus denial of humanness is a double-edged sword that cuts both ways: not only does it risk the self-perpetuation of the *dehumanisation–delegitimisation–moral exclusion cycle* that ultimately will harm the moral interests of us all, but it also risks the corruption and decline of our moral systems generally and their capacity to cultivate peaceable bonds between people in the interests of promoting human welfare and wellbeing.

As examples to be given in this chapter and the following chapters will demonstrate, dehumanisation and the moral exclusion it justifies needs to be detected and deterred (Opotow 1990b). This is particularly so in health care domains where the processes of dehumanisation and moral exclusion have resulted in disparities in access to and the beneficial outcomes of quality health care. The question remains, however, how might dehumanisation be detected and deterred, if at all? In attempting to answer this question, attention will be given to the following four strategies:

- addressing the root causes of dehumanisation
- fostering the moral inclusion of 'out-groups' and individuals
- detecting and exposing instances of dehumanisation
- energising dissent.

Addressing the root causes of dehumanisation

Little is known about the mechanisms that might help to reduce and deter dehumanisation, with some authors acknowledging that the problem is 'a knotty one' owing to the interrelated complexities that drive it (Haslam & Loughnan 2014: 417). Even so, evidence is growing that various mechanisms can be used to help reduce the incidence and negative impact of dehumanisation (Haslam & Loughnan 2014: 417–18) and that addressing the 'root cause' of dehumanisation is an important starting point. Endeavours could begin, first, by redressing the 'hierarchal divide between humans and animals', which has enabled the 'justified' oppression and subjugation of people deemed to be 'animal-like' (Costello & Hodson 2009: 5). Processes by which this hierarchy could be redressed might include emphasising empathic attitudes towards the similarities (e.g. sentience, cognitive abilities and relative moral intelligence) as opposed to the differences between humans and animals. Research has revealed, for instance, that some social mammals (e.g. gorillas, elephants, wolves, rats, bats and others) exhibit a range of cooperative 'moral' behaviours akin to those exhibited by humans – for example, justice, empathy, forgiveness, care, trust and reciprocity (including helping each other when in trouble) (Balcombe 2016; Bekoff & Pierce 2009). Far from being a case of anthropomorphising animals, scholars in the field remind us that 'humans are animals too', so it should not come as any surprise that animals and humans exhibit a similar range of moral behaviours. They have gone on to conclude that many animals have moral intelligence and are in essence 'moral beings', which means that human beings 'are not alone in the moral arena' (Bekoff & Pierce 2009: 152; see also Balcombe 2016).

In light of the above insights and observations, there is room to conclude that the moral gap between humans and other species – if it exists at all – has been overstated. By emphasising animal-to-human similarities, a humanisation process can be activated and engaged, which, as one Canadian study has found, can prompt heightened empathy and stronger inclinations to perceive members of both an in-group and an out-group (e.g. immigrants) 'as belonging to the same inclusive ingroup' (Costello & Hodson 2009: 17).

Fostering moral inclusion

Commensurate with the above, a second strategy to deter dehumanisation is to consciously and actively foster *moral inclusion* and the *rehumanisation* of dehumanised individuals and groups. According to Opotow (1990a: 4) moral inclusion may be taken as comprising the following 'coherent cluster of attitudes':

1. *believing that considerations of fairness apply to another*
2. *willingness to allocate a share of community resources to another, and*
3. *willingness to make sacrifices to foster another's wellbeing.*

How best to cultivate these and related attitudes, however, remains the subject of ongoing debate. Even so, there are a number of processes that are germane to fostering in people a disposition towards the virtue of moral inclusion and to expanding people's 'moral circles' to be more inclusive of entities that otherwise lie outside their 'in-group' (Crimston et al 2016, 2018); these include:

- making a commitment and actively seeking opportunities to become more familiar with the life-ways and world views of those who have been 'othered' (see, for example, the Australian television series 'Go back to where you came from', which sought to give Australians from various walks of life an opportunity to challenge their preconceived notions about refugees and to gain insight into what it is 'really' like to be a refugee or asylum seeker fleeing a troubled land; this series can be viewed via http://www.sbs.com.au/goback/. (See also Ai Weiwei's 2018 epic film 'Human Flow', which documents the plight of the world's 65 million people displaced since World War II; this film provides an opportunity to challenge the prejudices and biases held against refugees and asylum seekers, and the cruel and spiteful treatment they are too often exposed to. Information about this film can be viewed at https://www.humanflow.com/.)
- searching for similarities and shared human experiences
- adopting a pluralistic perspective (see Opotow 1990b: 176–7)
- engaging in mindful practice aimed at fostering a sense of compassion for those who are vulnerable to dehumanisation (see, for example, the Compassion Cultivation Training (CCT)

program founded in 2008 and developed by the Center for Compassion and Altruism Research and Education (CCARE) at Stanford University School of Medicine; this can be viewed at: http://ccare.stanford.edu/education/about-compassion-cultivation-training-cct/; see also the use of mindfulness to cultivate compassion (DeValve & Adkinson 2008) and to reduce stress and anger (Bergman et al 2016) in members of the US Police force).

Detecting and exposing instances of dehumanisation and moral exclusion

As suggested earlier in this discussion, dehumanisation (especially its subtle form) can be very difficult to detect. Even those who have been the targets of dehumanising processes may not always recognise it as such and, instead, through a process of internalised dehumanisation (whereby they internalise the very norms and beliefs systems that victimise them), *blame themselves* for the way they are treated (Opotow 1990b: 176). Because of this and also because of their felt vulnerability at the hands of the perpetrators, victims of dehumanisation might not always be able and/or willing to give voice to and expose their plight. For example, asylum seekers and detainees awaiting the outcome of their visa applications to stay in a host country, or charitable organisations supporting marginalised people that are dependent on government funding, may understandably be reluctant to speak out and expose their situation. There is, however, another category of persons who can take a proactive stance in detecting and exposing instances of dehumanisation and moral exclusion, notably *bystanders*.

A 'bystander' may be defined as any member of society who is neither a victim nor a perpetrator, and who witnesses the injustice of dehumanisation and moral exclusion but is not directly affected by it (Opotow 1990b). Bystanders can be individuals, groups, professions and even whole nations. Opotow (1990b: 176) argues that among the actions that bystanders can (and ought) to take is: first and foremost to *detect the problem, define it* and provide an *early response* to it (this is crucial to the process of 'reinstating victims in the moral realm'). Following this, bystanders then need to 'call attention' to the injustices witnessed and assert the inhumanity of the actions promulgated by the perpetrators – whether these are individuals, groups, governments or entire nations.

According to Opotow (1990b) bystanders are in an ideal position to take such a proactive stance as, from their vantage point, the injustice that victims of dehumanisation and moral exclusion experience 'is less personally threatening to them' and hence more easy to recognise (Opotow 1990b: 176). Bystanders, however, must do more than just 'passively observe', recognise, and expose the injustices of dehumanisation and moral exclusion; they also need to actively combat it. This is because merely exposing dehumanisation might not be sufficient to generate the public outrage otherwise necessary to demand reform of the societal and political structures and processes that otherwise enable and sustain the whole sophisticated dynamic of dehumanisation and moral exclusion of 'othered' people.

Energising dissent

Those who do not agree with conventional ideologies that underpin the dehumanisation and moral exclusion of 'othered' people need to 'energise dissent' (Martin 2007) and strategically resist pressures to conform to the status quo (Opotow 1990b). This can be done by dissenters using unofficial channels to share with likeminded people the information they have and their interpretations of 'what is going on', something that is now relatively easy to achieve via the use of social media. As their actions and views gain traction, it will become increasingly difficult for them to be credibly ignored, notwithstanding the tactics that might otherwise be used by opponents intent on spreading misinformation ('fake news') and disrupting and discrediting them.

Information sharing, exposing injustices to the public, and providing credible explanations for 'what is going on here' will not, however, be sufficient to energise dissent. This is because perpetrators of injustice use powerful methods to reduce and even suppress public outrage (Hamilton & Maddison 2007; Martin 2007) or, conversely, provoke extreme right wing authoritarian populism to energise dissent in the 'wrong direction', as has occurred via the activities of groups such as Cambridge Analytica (see Persily 2017). As Martin (2007: 63) reveals:

> *They cover up evidence and information about the event, devalue the target, reinterpret what happened, use official channels to give an appearance of fairness, and intimidate or bribe participants and observers.*

Martin (2007) goes on to argue that dissenters must combat these powerful methods, which are cleverly used by perpetrators to reduce public outrage (refer back to the 'children overboard' incident, cited earlier and, more recently, see the ABC-TV Four Corners program 'Democracy, data and dirty tricks' regarding the tactics used by Cambridge Analytica – available at: http://www.abc.net.au/4corners/democracy,-data-and-dirty-tricks:-cambridge/9642090). To this end, he proposes the following five corresponding approaches (Martin 2007: 63):

- 'expose the actions' (this is essential to enable people to be as well informed as is possible)
- 'affirm the value of the targets' (this is essential to counter the denigration of targets)
- 'interpret the situation as unfair' (the damaging consequences of what has been done and the vested self-interests and denial of responsibility, ultimately, cannot be kept hidden – 'truth will out')
- 'mobilise support and avoid or discredit official channels' (be aware that 'official channels' can be cumbersome, take time and can distort the issues in favour of maintaining the status quo)
- 'resist and expose intimidation and bribery' (every time a progressive bystander speaks out, it makes it easier for others to do the same).

These and other strategies will be considered further later when discussing specific individuals and groups whose dehumanisation and moral exclusion give rise to special responsibilities for members of the nursing profession.

Stigma

Stigma (from Latin via Greek meaning 'brand' or 'bodily sign') is literally a distinguishing mark of social disgrace. It presupposes the acquisition of an attribute or attributes that others (usually those who are dominant members of a mainstream culture or group) find or regard as deeply discrediting (personally, socially and morally) and, importantly, who have the power to discredit those deemed 'marked' as socially disgraced (Goffman 1963; Link et al 2004; Link & Phelan 2006). What is regarded as a 'distinguishing mark of social disgrace', however, and what impact it will ultimately have on people, will depend on the culture from which it has originated and what that culture deems as being 'deviant' (Link et al 2004).

According to Jones and colleagues (1984) the incidence and impact of a given stigmatised 'characteristic' or 'condition' will depend on the following five dimensions:

- '*concealability*' – refers to how obvious a characteristic is and the degree to which it can be concealed from others
- '*disruptiveness*' – refers to 'the extent to which a mark strains or obstructs interpersonal interactions'
- '*aesthetics*' – refers to the extent to which a mark elicits an 'affective reaction of disgust'
- '*origin*' – refers to 'how the condition came into being' and particularly whether the marked person was responsible for the condition (e.g. whether genetic, accidental or self-caused)
- '*peril*' – refers to 'feelings of danger or threat that the mark indicates in others' (cited in Link et al 2004: 512).

The process of stigmatisation becomes problematic when it evolves into a situation in which an individual is disqualified from full social and cultural acceptance on the basis of his/her carrying a given 'distinguishing mark of social disgrace' (e.g. being immigrant, disabled, homosexual, mentally ill, old, etc.) (Goffman 1963). Inevitably this means that stigma almost always carries with it commensurate processes of discrimination – that is, the unfair treatment of persons on the basis of their 'distinguishing mark(s)'. This treatment is unfair since judgments are made on the somewhat arbitrary basis of morally irrelevant distinguishing marks, rather than on moral considerations per se, hence the notion that stigma and stigmatisation are unjustly discriminatory. This outcome is unethical since, by focusing on one (or more) arbitrary characteristic(s) of a person (e.g. the marks that may 'distinguish them'), stigma and discrimination undermine the moral worth (dignity) of a person (results in them 'losing face', if you will) and thus dehumanises the person. The stigmatising and (negative) discriminatory treatment of persons thus stands in contradistinction to the respectful treatment of persons – that is, responses to persons that are guided by moral considerations, not merely arbitrary ones.

It is important to note that stigma can involve both 'public' (public-stigma) and 'self' (self-stigma) reactions. *Public stigma* has been described as comprising 'reactions of the general public towards a group based on stigma about that group', and as consisting of three elements – stereotypes, prejudice and discrimination – that occur in 'the context of power differences and leads to reactions of the general public towards the stigmatized groups as a result of stigma' (Rüsch et al 2005: 530, 531). *Self-stigma*, in contrast, refers to 'reactions of individuals who belong to a stigmatized group and turn the stigmatizing attitudes against themselves' (Rüsch et al 2005: 531). Like public stigma, self-stigma also consists of three elements: stereotypes, prejudice and discrimination, but with the notable distinction that all three tend to be strongly aligned with public stigmatisation, with individuals internalising the negative public attitudes against themselves; for example 'That's right; I am weak and unable to care for myself' (Rüsch et al 2005: 531).

Prejudice and discrimination

The term *prejudice* (literally to 'prejudge' without adequate facts) may be defined as 'any belief (especially an unfavourable one), whether correct or incorrect, held without proper consideration of, or sometimes in defiance of, the evidence' (Flew & Priest 2002: 326). The counterpart of prejudice is *discrimination*. Discrimination, in turn, may be broadly defined as 'the unfair treatment of a person, racial group, minority, etc., based on prejudice' (*Collins Australian dictionary* 2011: 478).

Within the concept of discrimination, two forms are distinguished: direct discrimination and indirect discrimination, which may be either intentional or unintentional. In Australian and New Zealand jurisdictions (as well as in others, e.g. Canada, EU, Hong Kong(China), South Africa, USA), *direct discrimination* may be held to have occurred when a person (or group of people) with certain characteristics protected by law (e.g. their race, sex, pregnancy, marital status, family responsibilities, breastfeeding, age, disability, sexual orientation, gender identity or intersex status) is 'treated less favourably than another person or group' based on their personal characteristics – noting that some limited exceptions and exemptions may apply (Australian Human Rights Commission nda; New Zealand Human Rights Commission nd). It needs to be understood that one does not have to have acted intentionally or to believe that one's actions were not discriminatory for a complaint of discrimination to be upheld. *Indirect discrimination* (which is controversial in some jurisdictions) may be held to have occurred 'when there is an unreasonable rule or policy that is the same for everyone but has an unfair effect on people who share a particular attribute' (e.g. a public building that has only stairway access will disadvantage those who are wheelchair dependent for their mobility) (Australian Human Rights Commission ndb; New Zealand Human Rights Commission nd). In short, although seemingly neutral, a policy or practice (e.g. stairway-only entry to a public building) may nonetheless indirectly discriminate against a person insofar as it has a 'disparate impact' on and causes 'disproportionate disadvantage' to that person compared with other cognate groups (Collins & Khaitan 2018; Khaitan 2018). As in the case of direct discrimination, indirect discrimination can be established without reference to whether it was intentional or known; instead it is established by demonstrating a 'disparate adverse impact' (Collins & Khaitan 2018) – for example, a wheelchair-dependent person being unable to access a public building because it has only stairway access.

Disadvantage

Before concluding this section, a brief comment about the notion of *disadvantage* is warranted. Disadvantage, in its most basic sense, may be taken to mean a deprivation that is unfavourable or detrimental to a person's interests. The notions of vulnerability, dehumanisation, delegitimisation, moral exclusion, stigma, prejudice and discrimination as discussed in this chapter are all correlated in important ways with the notion of disadvantage. In this instance, disadvantage correlates with the notion of equal opportunity and the ways and extent to which this is denied when people are dehumanised, marginalised and excluded from the moral community. Disadvantage, in this case, can result regardless of whether the processes of dehumanisation, delegitimisation and moral exclusion are covert or overt. This is because these processes disrupt what would otherwise be a level playing field and result in privileged groups (i.e. those with a social dominance orientation) accruing unearned advantages over those they have subordinated.

People who are subjected to dehumanisation, delegitimisation, moral exclusion, stigma, discrimination and prejudice are all vulnerable to being disadvantaged in terms of realising the health benefits commonly associated with having equitable access to the social, cultural and political conditions that promote safe and high-quality health care. It is for this reason that identification of and emphasis on the special responsibilities that others might have towards vulnerable populations are warranted.

Identifying vulnerable individuals and groups

It is well established locally and internationally that people who are old (especially those who are frail, cognitively impaired and socially isolated), or who suffer from a mental illness or are disabled, are among the most stigmatised, discriminated against and marginalised in society. Also vulnerable to be treated in prejudicial and discriminatory ways are: indigenous peoples (i.e. peoples of the world's first nations); ethnic minorities; refugees, asylum seekers, displaced people and stateless people; the unemployed, 'deserving' poor and homeless people; and those who are perceived to have deviated from or breached society's accepted norms – illicit drug users and addicts, sex workers, people living with sexually transmitted disease (e.g. HIV/AIDS) and people imprisoned for criminal offences. If sharing membership of more than one of these demographic groups (e.g. if old, disabled and suffering from a mental illness), an individual may face a 'double jeopardy' or even 'triple jeopardy' of being stigmatised, discriminated against and ultimately abandoned by society and left languishing on its margins.

The issue of vulnerability and dehumanisation has particular resonance for nurses, particularly when encountering people who are disadvantaged by their vulnerability and who may require the intervention of nurses (individually and collectively) to rehumanise and destigmatise them and foster their re-inclusion in the moral realm of health care. Of particular note, some of whom are also the subject of position statements by the International Council of Nurses, are:

- older people
- people with mental health problems and illnesses
- immigrants and ethnic minorities
- refugees, asylum seekers, displaced people and stateless people
- people with disabilities
- indigenous peoples
- prisoners and detainees

- homeless people
- sexual minorities (lesbian, gay, bisexual, transgender, intersex, queer/questioning (LGBTIQ) people).

People who require and are dependent on medical treatment and nursing care might also be characterised as being vulnerable and hence as giving rise to 'special responsibilities' in the moral realm. Since the ethical issues associated with this population group are extensive and also inclusive of the vulnerable population groups identified above, they will be considered separately in Chapter 7.

Older people[2]

The world's population is ageing in an unprecedented manner. According to the United Nations Department of Economic and Social Affairs (UN DESA 2017a, 2017b) and WHO (2017a), by the year 2050, 2.1 billion people (representing almost a quarter of the world's population) will be over the age of 60 years, most of whom will be living in low- and middle-income countries. It has been further estimated that around 46% of older people will be living with disability as a consequence of 'accumulated health risks across the lifespan of disease, injury and chronic illness' (UNFPA and HelpAge International 2012: 61). The top three causes of old-age disability are visual impairment, hearing loss and osteoarthritis, followed by ischaemic heart disease, chronic obstructive pulmonary disease, dementia, cerebral vascular disease and depression (UNFPA and HelpAge International 2012: 61). In light of these estimates, it is envisaged that the world's projected population ageing will have a profound impact on societies across the globe socially, economically, culturally and politically, requiring significant adaptions in each of these areas (Biggs 2014).

For many, the world's ageing population is a triumph of human and social development and one that deserves to be celebrated (UNFPA and HelpAge International 2012). For others, however, a more circumspect view is required – particularly when consideration is given to the significant 'social, economic and cultural challenges to individuals, families, societies and the global community' that population ageing poses (UNFPA and HelpAge International 2012: 11).

One particular challenge confronting all societies globally is the problem of *ageism*. The notion of 'ageism' was first coined in 1968 by Dr Robert Butler, founding director of the US National Institute on Ageing, who originally defined the term as a:

> *systematic stereotyping of and discrimination against people because they are old, just as racism and sexism accomplish this with skin color and gender. Old people are categorized as senile, rigid in thought and manner, old-fashioned in morality and skills [...] Ageism allows the younger generation to see older people as different from themselves; thus they subtly cease to identify with their elders as human beings.* (Butler 1989: 139)

Contemporary definitions reflect the elements of this original definition. For example, the World Health Organization (WHO) (2018b) defines ageism as 'the stereotyping, prejudice and discrimination towards people on the basis of their age' (http://www.who.int/ageing/ageism/en/).

Older people today are amongst the most discriminated against, marginalised and vulnerable groups of people in the world. As HelpAge International (HAI) has observed:

> *all societies discriminate against people on grounds of age. Ageism and stereotyping influence attitudes, which in turn affect the way decisions are taken and resources are allocated at household, community, national and international levels.* (HAI 2001: 1)

Although there is now a much greater awareness about the nature and negative impact of ageism, it remains highly prevalent and insidious, with the WHO (2018b) contending that it is 'the most "normalised" of any prejudice' and as such, unlike other forms of discrimination (e.g. sexism, racism), is rarely challenged (see also Officer & de la Fuente-Núñez 2018).

Ageism can occur in any socio-cultural context including health care, which can be hostile to the needs and interests of older people. Ageism in health care (also called medical ageism) can be expressed in a variety of ways, including 'stereotypes about the recuperative abilities of elderly patients, or value judgments about the quality or worth of elderly lives, or misconceptions about the desires of elderly people for certain forms of treatments' (Williams 2009: 11). The use of chronological age as decisional criteria (irrespective of a patient's medical condition) and dehumanising age-based language (e.g. 'bed blockers', 'train wrecks', 'disaster waiting to happen', 'nightmare on a stretcher', etc.) to refer to elderly patients is also an example of ageism in health care.

Arguably one of the most insidious forms of ageism can be found in the scapegoating of older people in public debates on the public affordability of pensions and health care. These debates (which tend to emphasise 'demographic crisis thinking', 'apocalyptic demography' and 'apocalyptic economics') are primarily shaped by *prejudice, politics, ideology and social organisation*, and not by demography as the public is often led to believe (Ebrahim 2002; Evans 2002; Fine 2014; Howe & Healy 2005; Spies-Butcher & Stebbing 2018). What the 'crisisisation' of population ageing does is promulgate a spurious portrayal of older people as a perpetual 'costly burden on society' and a threat to the social wellbeing of future generations (commonly framed as 'threatening generational equity' and ipso facto causing 'intergenerational conflict') (Fine 2014; Spies-Butcher & Stebbing 2018). This portrayal is spurious for at least three key reasons: first, it arbitrarily ignores that older people throughout the world (including those who are disadvantaged and poor) actually make positive and substantial contributions to society (in economic, social capital and cultural capital terms) as paid and unpaid workers, as consumers, as volunteers and as contributors to the wellbeing of their children and grandchildren (noting that analyses across the globe have shown that private wealth tends to flow more strongly downwards – i.e. from old to young) (Fine 2014; Spies-Butcher & Stebbing 2018; WHO 2000); second, it overlooks the inadequacies of current inter-generational frameworks in terms of their capacity to provide 'a reliable picture of the future economic costs and benefits of population ageing' (Fine 2014: 224); finally, it ignores the fact that the future burdensome costs of health care are more probably due to changes in *technology* and not demography per se (Spies-Butcher & Stebbing 2018).

In keeping with their advocacy role and responsibilities, nurses and their professional associations have an obligation to safeguard the safety of older people. This includes influencing debates on global ageing and policies addressing the problems of ageism, stigma, dehumanisation and the moral exclusion of the elderly, and the possible harmful impact these processes can have on the health and wellbeing of older people. How nurses might best mitigate the prejudice, discrimination and stigma that germinate from these processes will require considered attention as well as close and coordinated collaboration with other organisations and groups committed to combating ageism locally and globally (see, for example, Officer & de la Fuente-Núñez 2018). If nurses are to be able to uphold their professional obligations to safeguard vulnerable older people, they first need to understand what ageism is and how it works to dehumanise older people and ultimately lead to their being 'soft targets' for the 'understandable' and 'justified' exclusion from some of society's limited health resources.

Protection of the safety, welfare and wellbeing of older people is going to require more than knowledge and understanding of the impact of ageism, however. Nurses must also actively engage in a campaign of 'detection and deterrence' of ageism and its negative impact on older people in health care. This includes their engaging in what Butler has termed the 'New Ageism', which seeks to: foster respect for age diversity, debunk the gerontophobic 'decline and failure' model of ageing (Whitton 1997), dispel the myths around the costs of caring for the elderly and dying (as Butler correctly notes, an honest accounting of the 'cost of life' would examine *all sources of expenditure* for *all people* – young and old – not just health care and the elderly), and counter negative ageist attitudes generally in the interests of promoting intergenerational solidarity – of generations working together – in recognition that 'there is a continuity and unity to human life' (Butler 1989: 145). By taking such a stance nurses will help restore the boundaries of moral inclusion and reinstate older people as moral entities deserving our respect and recognition as fellow human beings.

Older people remain vulnerable to abuse, abandonment and neglect. According to a 2017 systematic review of 52 studies conducted across geographically diverse countries ($n=28$), it was estimated that approximately 1 in 6 older people (around 141 million) experience some form of abuse annually (Yon et al 2017). In light of these figures, the authors conclude that elder abuse stands as a 'neglected global public health priority' especially when compared with other types of violence (Yon et al 2017: e147). (As the issue of elder abuse warrants discrete attention in its own right, it will be considered separately in Chapter 12.) Older people are also vulnerable to not having their health rights recognised. Moreover, there is growing recognition that the current system of health rights is not sufficient to protect the rights and interests of older people. In response to this situation, in 2011 a Global Alliance for the Rights of Older People was established (http://www.rightsofolderpeople.org/). The Alliance is using its global network of more than 120 organisations in over 75 countries to spearhead a global movement for recognising the rights of older people (http://www.helpage.org/who-we-are/our-affiliates-/). Together with a growing number of other campaigners, including non-government organisations (NGOs), academics, lawyers and UN member states and individuals, HelpAge International and the Global Alliance for the Rights of Older People (GAROP) are calling for the development of a *Convention on the rights of older people* together with the creation of 'a new special rapporteur on older people's rights' who would report to the Human Rights Council (http://www.helpage.org/what-we-do/rights/towards-a-convention-on-the-rights-of-older-people/?keywords=convention). HelpAge International suggests that, in addition to enabling the rights of older people to be protected under international law, such a convention is necessary to:

- establish legal standards that challenge and replace stigmatising and dehumanising ageist attitudes and behaviour
- clarify how human rights apply in older age
- ensure that states understand their human rights obligations to us in our older age
- better understand and assert our rights in our older age
- improve accountability of states for their human rights obligations towards us in older age
- provide a framework for policy and decision-making (http://www.helpage.org/what-we-do/rights/towards-a-convention-on-the-rights-of-older-people/?keywords=convention).

Insofar as what *specific human rights* are relevant to the experience of ageing and should be protected for older people, GAROP and HelpAge International have respectively identified the following general principles:

- non-discrimination
- respect
- dignity
- autonomy
- equality
- self-fulfilment and personal development
- full and effective participation and inclusion in society
- respect for difference and diversity
- accessibility
- inter-generational solidarity

- recognition of intrinsic value and worth as a human being (GAROP 2015: 6; HelpAge International 2015: 3).

Nurses are in a good position to actively engage with the processes of championing the development and adoption of a *Convention on the rights of older people* and the creation of new special rapporteur on older people's rights. A first step to engage in these processes would be for nurses to join the Global Alliance for the Rights of Older People (http://www.rightsofolderpeople.org/) and to encourage eligible organisations to also sign the HelpAge International petition to support a convention on older people's rights (available at http://www.helpage.org/get-involved/).

People with mental health problems and mental illness

It is well documented that people suffering from mental illness (including severe and complex mental illnesses)[3] are among the most stigmatised, discriminated against, marginalised, disadvantaged and hence vulnerable individuals in the world. As the World Health Organization (WHO) noted in its 2012 background paper for the development of a comprehensive mental health action plan:

> *Persons with a mental disorder have their own set of vulnerabilities and risks, including an increased likelihood of experiencing disability and premature mortality, stigma and discrimination, social exclusion and impoverishment.* (WHO 2012a: 2)

Moreover, despite the efforts of mental health consumer groups and other mental health activists across the globe, people with mental and psychosocial disabilities continue to experience the violation of many of their basic human rights. One of the main reasons for this, as explained by the WHO, is that:

> *There is a commonly held, yet false, assumption that people with mental health conditions lack the capacity to assume responsibility, manage their affairs and make decisions about their lives. These misconceptions contribute to the ongoing marginalization, disenfranchisement and invisibility of this group of people in their communities.* (WHO 2012a: 2)

WHO (2012a) has characterised the continual stigmatisation of the mentally ill as 'a hidden human rights emergency'. In an attempt to readdress this emergency, in 2011, WHO initiated the QualityRights initiative, the aim of which is to 'unite and empower people to improve the quality of care and promote human rights in mental health and social care facilities' (WHO 2012b: 2). It is anticipated that this project (visit: http://www.who.int/mental_health/policy/quality_rights/en/) will leave a 'lasting legacy of respect for human rights' (WHO 2012b: 2).

In the past it has been difficult to provide reliable national and global estimates of the prevalence, incidence, remission and mortality in mental illness (Baxter et al 2013). Today, however, a more reliable picture is available. Comparative epidemiological studies of the incidence and impact of mental illness in different countries have now been undertaken, enabling improved understanding of the prevalence and impact of mental illness across the globe (WHO 2017b). These studies have affirmed earlier estimates that high-prevalence illnesses and conditions (e.g. depression, anxiety) and low-prevalence illnesses (e.g. bipolar disorder, schizophrenia, eating disorders) occur to varying degrees in all societies and contribute significantly to the global burden of disease (Baxter et al 2013; WHO 2013a, 2017b).

Mental health problems and illnesses also have a significant economic impact. According to one study, the estimated cumulative global impact of mental illness in terms of lost economic output will amount to US$ 16.3 trillion between 2011 and 2030 (WHO 2013a, 2013b). A 2017 systematic review of the economic impact of mental illness has further estimated that the accumulative costs associated with mental illness (including the direct costs of health care, lost productivity in the workplace, and welfare pensions) will increase sixfold within the next 30 years (Doran & Kinchin 2017).

In many countries there is a substantial gap 'between the burden caused by mental disorders [sic] and the resources available to prevent and treat them', especially in low-income countries (WHO 2011a: 5). According to the WHO's most up-to-date figures, public expenditure on mental health is 'very low' in low- and middle-income countries (LMIC) (WHO 2015). According to Rathod and colleagues (2017), the expenditure on mental health globally is less than US$2 per year per person across all LMIC countries; in low-income countries it is less than 25 cents per year per person (in contrast, in Australia for the period 2015–16, $373 per person was spent). The medium number of mental health workers is similarly 'very low' in low-income countries (e.g. 1 per 100 000 compared with more than 50 per 100 000 in high-income countries (WHO 2017b)). This means that 4 out of 5 people with serious mental illness living in LMIC do not receive the evidence-based mental health services they need (WHO 2011a; Rathod et al 2017); many receive no treatment at all (Thornicroft et al 2016).

People caught up in conflict zones, disasters and humanitarian emergencies are especially vulnerable to developing mental illness owing to their traumatic experiences and uncertainty about the future (Priebe et al 2016). Although the prevalence of psychotic, mood and substance use in refugee and migrant groups is similar to that found in a host nation, rates of post-traumatic stress disorder and depression (after 5 years of settlement) are significantly higher in this population (Priebe et al 2016). People belonging to other vulnerable groupings in society (e.g. ethnic minorities, older people, women and young people, LGBTIQ youth) are also vulnerable (WHO 2012a, 2013a, 2013b).

In Australia it has been estimated that around 8.5 million people aged between 16 and 85 years (45%) will experience a common mental health-related problem in their lifetime (Australian Institute of Health and Welfare (AIHW) 2017a: 2). It is further estimated that, each year, 1 in 5 Australians will experience the symptoms of a mental health problem or illness; of these, the most common problems are: affective (mood) disorders (e.g. anxiety disorders such as post-traumatic stress disorder and social phobia, and depression) and substance use disorders – e.g. alcohol dependence (AIHW 2017a). Of this population, an estimated 64 000 people have a psychotic illness (with schizophrenia being the most common psychotic illness experienced) and are in contact with public specialised mental health services each year (AIHW 2017a: 3).

According to some international authorities, the singularly most significant barrier to the effective treatment of mental illness is *stigmatisation*. A notable proponent of this view is Professor Norman Sartorius, former director of the WHO's Division of Mental Health and a former president of the World Psychiatric Association. Sartorius (who has been described as one of the most prominent and influential psychiatrists of his generation) contends that stigmatisation is 'often buried deep within governments, public health agencies, health services and the general public' (Sartorius 2014: 2). Stigma, in turn, leads to discrimination against the mentally ill as well as their families and others who provide them with care. Discrimination, as indicated earlier, can take several forms – not least the failure to develop appropriate policies and allocate appropriate resources to ensure the delivery of quality mental health care to those who need it. On this point, Sartorius asks rhetorically, 'Who wants to help a person with schizophrenia? If he dies sooner, that's a decrease in cost' (Sartorius 2014: 8).

Taken together, stigmatisation and discrimination can lead to an insidious and generally under-recognised form of the dehumanisation of people with mental health-related problems.

In order to redress this problem, people who work in the field of mental health promotion have to be 'indefatigable' (change can sometimes take decades) and need to embark on a strategy of what Sartorius calls 'enlightened opportunism'. By this he means that people must keep themselves:

> *in a state of watchful preparation and look for opportunities. Understand [their] local surroundings and their needs, and stand ready with the best tools. Opportunities will arise; luck will come. And then … you pounce [on that opportunity]!* (Sartorius 2014: 9)

Mental health is everybody's business. Accordingly, nurses share with others the collective responsibility to promote mental health, to promote the prevention of mental illness, to challenge the stigmatisation and dehumanisation of people with mental health problems and to champion improved access to mental health care and services for all who need it.

More specific ethical issues arising in the context of mental health, such as the capacity to decide, advance psychiatric directives, and preventing the moral harms of suicide, will be considered separately in Chapter 8.

Immigrants and ethnic minorities

Culture and ethnicity are recognised predictors of disparities in the safety and quality of health care and related health outcomes. In its landmark report *Unequal treatment: confronting racial and ethnic disparities in health care*, the US Institute of Medicine (IOM) (Smedley et al 2003) presented evidence suggesting that immigrants and ethnic minorities[4] tended to receive a lower quality of health care than did their non-minority counterparts, and experienced greater morbidity and mortality rates (Smedley et al 2003: 1). The IOM also found that, with few exceptions, the ethnic disparities noted were 'remarkably consistent across a range of illnesses and health care services' (Smedley et al 2003: 5).

It was further noted that some of the ethnic disparities revealed were associated with socio-economic differences and that these diminished significantly when socio-economic factors were controlled. It was also observed, however, that the vast majority of the disparities noted remained even after adjustments had been made for socio-economic differences and other health care access-related factors. Defining *disparities* in health care as 'racial or ethnic differences in the quality of health care that are *not* due to access-related factors or clinical needs, preferences, and the appropriateness of interventions' [emphasis added], the IOM concluded that the disparities revealed were 'not acceptable' and that action needed to be taken to address this situation (Smedley et al 2003: 4–5).

Although originating in the USA, the IOM report had relevance for health services around the world and provided an important catalyst for health service providers and policy makers alike to reflect on ethnic disparities in their own local health care services and what must be done to redress the inequities that are found to exist. Since this report was published there have been a plethora of articles published on the subject (too numerous to list here) and the implications of racial and ethnic disparities for patient safety in general (see, for example, Baehr et al 2015; Fiscella & Sanders 2016; Okoroh et al 2017). Arguably one of the most important developments in the field has been the establishment in 2014 of the *Journal of Racial and Ethnic Health Disparities*, described by the publisher as 'the first journal of its kind dedicated to examining and eliminating racial and ethnic [health] disparities' (https://www.springer.com/medicine/journal/40615).

As noted previously in Chapter 4, there are probably thousands of different ethnic groups in the world and that most nations are comprised of people from diverse cultural and language backgrounds.

In order to ensure that people of immigrant and ethnic minority backgrounds get equal access to the safe and high-quality care otherwise enjoyed by non-minority patients, some governments (e.g. in Australia, Canada, New Zealand, UK, USA) have initiated what might be termed 'cultural diversity plans' for their respective health care services. Some notable examples are: the landmark US Health and Human Services Office of Minority Health (2013) *The national standards for culturally and linguistically appropriate services in health and health care* (the *National CLAS standards*) (available: https://www.thinkculturalhealth.hhs.gov/clas), Wilson-Stronks and colleagues (2008) *One size does not fit all: meeting the health care needs of diverse populations* (available: http://www.jointcommission.org/assets/1/6/HLCOneSizeFinal.pdf), and the Department of Health, Victoria (2016) *Delivering for diversity – cultural diversity plan 2016–2019* (available: https://www2.health.vic.gov.au/about/publications/policiesandguidelines/dhhs-delivering-for-diversity-cultural-diversity-plan-2016-19). In New Zealand (NZ) culturally responsive health care is guided primarily by the principles imbedded in the Treaty of Waitangi[5] and which underpin the relationship between Government and Māori (https://www.health.govt.nz/); the NZ Ministry of Health has not, however, developed cultural diversity plans as such, although individual health boards have (see, for example, the Waitemata District Health Board (2013) *Best practice principles: CALD competency standards and framework* – available at http://www.comprehensivecare.co.nz/wp-content/uploads/2013/03/Best-Practice-CALD-Cultural-Competency-Standards-Framework-Jun13.pdf). These and similar plans require health care services to have in place processes that will ensure and increase their capacity to be appropriately responsive to the needs of their culturally and linguistically diverse communities, and to provide 'culturally competent' care.

Despite the initiatives taken by governments and other bodies (e.g. health professional associations), patients of diverse cultural and language backgrounds ('ethnic minorities') nonetheless continue to suffer discrimination based on their personal characteristics such as race, ethnicity and culture (encompassing forms of 'old' and 'new' racism (Johnstone & Kanitsaki 2008a)). Underpinning what Came and Griffith (2018) have termed this '"wicked" public health problem' is a reluctance by those in the field (practitioners, researchers, and policy makers alike) to specifically name and redress the problem of racism in health care (Bailey et al 2017; Bastos et al 2018; Came et al 2018; Feagin & Bennefield 2014; Fiscella & Sanders 2016; Hicken et al 2018; Johnstone & Kanitsaki 2008a, 2010). This reticence to 'talk openly about racism' in health care has also been identified in nursing (Hilario et al 2018; Thorne 2017).

Although racism is recognised internationally as a modifiable determinant of health (Came et al 2018), its preventable and unjust harmful impact on the health and wellbeing of 'racialised others' continues. Even so, as Came and Griffith (2018) point out, systems can and do change. If efforts to eradicate racism and remedy the unjust harms it causes are to succeed, attention must first be given to understanding the complex nature of racism, the various levels on which it operates and the concerted and cumulative negative impact it has on those affected. To this end, Came and Griffith (2018) contend that much more than mere 'consciousness raising' is required; rather, what is required is working with allies and operationalising a substantive 'anti-racism praxis' encompassing the following five core elements:

- reflexive relational praxis
- structural power analysis
- socio-political education
- monitoring and evaluation
- system change approaches (Came and Griffith 2018).

The International Council of Nurses has made explicit in a position statement that both it and its affiliated national nurses' associations (NNAs) have particular responsibilities for the immediate and long-term health and nursing care needs of immigrants, refugees and displaced people (ICN 2018). To this end the ICN encourages NNAs to examine the extent of the problem in their countries and to undertake cooperative action to ensure the provision of safe and appropriate health services for immigrants and ethnic minority groups. The ICN has also taken the stance that NNAs and their members have a responsibility, through collaborative action, to 'strengthen public awareness of the health vulnerabilities and healthcare-related challenges' faced by this cognate group (ICN 2018: 3).

It is important to note that, although the ICN has merged consideration of 'migrants' with 'refugees and displaced people', these entities are not synonymous, as the United Nations High Commission for Refugees (UNHCR) working definitions of these entities (discussed in the following subsection) clarifies. Moreover, while each of these entities face similar issues, there are also significant differences in the kind and degree of experiences that refugees, asylum seekers, displaced people and stateless people have compared with migrants. For example, the plight of a stateless person or a refugee forced to live for years in a resource-depleted refugee camp cannot be meaningfully compared with an immigrant who has moved to a new host country by choice or a person who is a second-generation citizen (i.e. born of migrant / immigrant parents) even though both these entities might experience the hardships and health consequences of being vilified or discriminated against by their fellow citizens on the basis of their race, ethnicity or culture.

Refugees, asylum seekers, displaced people, stateless people and returnees

In its *Global report 2016*, the United Nations High Commission for Refugees (UNHCR) confirmed that, at the end of the year, the global number of people of concern to the agency was 67.7 million people (3.8 million more than in 2015) (UNHCR 2016: 6); the UNHCR further estimated that these figures represented an equivalent of 20 new displacements every minute (UNHCR 2017). Significantly, as the UNHCR points out, the forced displacement of people in recent years 'has reached unprecedented levels, with 2016 seeing the highest level of people displaced by violence and persecution since the Second World War' (UNHCR 2016: 174). The report goes on to point out that, while many countries have generously hosted millions of displaced people, the sheer scale and scope of the problem 'has compelled the international community to revisit traditional approaches' to addressing the problem (UNHCR 2016: 174).

Of those displaced, approximately 22.5 million are refugees, 40.3 million are internally displaced, and 2.8 million are registered asylum seekers and, although exact figures have been almost impossible to calculate, around 10 million people are stateless (UNHCR 2017: 2). In 2016, 51% of refugees were children (under 18 years of age), the highest ratio in a decade. In 2016, resource-poor low- and middle-income countries disproportionately hosted the vast majority (84%) of forcibly displaced people, who remain living close to conflict zones (UNHCR 2017: 20).

Throughout recorded human history, people have been forced to leave their homes, become displaced and/or have been forced to seek refuge within and outside the borders of their own countries. What is unprecedented today are the drivers of displacement, the sheer number of people seeking refuge and the sometimes-brutal dehumanisation of asylum seekers by politicians perpetrated solely for political gain.

The world's troubled history of 'forced migration' has given rise to the following various categorisations of people deemed to be of concern to the UNHCR: *refugees, asylum seekers, stateless persons, internally displaced people, and returnees*. Sometimes the terms 'refugee' and 'asylum seeker' are used interchangeably. The terms 'migrants', 'refugees' and 'displaced people' are also sometimes conflated as referring to the same or at least comparable thing in organisational policy and position statements. This usage is, however, incorrect and care should be taken not to confuse the terms at issue. To help clarify what each of these categorisations refers to, the UNHCR (2014a, 2014b) has proposed the following working definitions:

- *Refugees* – described in the 1951 Refugee Convention as someone who 'owing to a well-founded fear of being persecuted for reasons of race, religion, nationality, membership of particular social group or political opinion, is outside the country of his [sic] nationality, and is unable to, or owing to such fear, is unwilling to avail himself [sic] of the protection of that country'.
- *Asylum seeker* – is someone who says he or she is a refugee, but whose claim has not yet been definitely assessed. The term contains no presumption either way – it simply describes the fact that someone has made a claim. Some asylum seekers will be judged to be refugees and others will not. Those whose claims are rejected can be sent back to their home countries.
- *Internally displaced person* – someone who has been forced to move from his or her home because of conflict, persecution (i.e. refugee-like reasons) or because of a natural disaster or some other unusual circumstance of this type. Unlike refugees, internally displaced people remain in their own country – that is, they have not crossed an international border.
- *Stateless person* – is an individual who is not considered to be a national by any state under the operation of its law. Although some stateless people are also refugees, the two states are

regarded as being distinct. Because they do not 'officially exist', stateless people virtually have no legal rights at all.
- *Returnees* – are individuals who were of concern to the UNHCR when outside his/her country of origin, and who remain so for a limited period (usually 2 years), after returning to their country of origin.
- *Migrant* (to be distinguished from a refugee, displaced persons and an immigrant) – is an individual who chooses to move not because of a direct threat of persecution or death but mainly to improve their lives by finding work, or in some cases for education, family reunion and other reasons. Their move is for a certain length of time (usually a minimum of 1 year, so as not to include temporary visitors, such as tourists, people on business trips, students on education visas, etc.). Accordingly, migrants are different and should be treated as being different to refugees, asylum seekers and displaced people. Unlike refugees and displaced people, who cannot return home safely, migrants face no impediments to return to their country of origin.
- *Immigrant* (to be distinguished from a migrant) – someone who takes up permanent residence in a country other than his or her original homeland.

As examples already given in this chapter have shown, refugees and asylum seekers are extremely vulnerable to being vilified and dehumanised and, accordingly, denied the moral protections and entitlements that would otherwise be owed them (see also the penetrating analyses by Every & Augoustinos (2007) and Leach (2003) respectively, which reveal the disturbing vilification and racist practices supported by Australian politicians and which were squarely aimed at dehumanising refugees and asylum seekers in Australia; see also Antony 2017; Canetti 2016; Pedersen & Hartley 2015). Stateless people are especially vulnerable in this regard since, unlike the other categories of people described above, they have *no rights whatsoever* and thus are at risk of being left not only without any residence status but, worse, in prolonged detention (UNHCR 2014b: 2).

During the past century the international community has worked together to assemble various guidelines, laws and conventions aimed at protecting the human rights of refugees and also for ensuring that those who have refugee status receive 'adequate treatment' by their hosts. Notable among the works progressed has been the development and adoption of *The Convention and Protocol relating to the Status of Refugees* ('*1951 Convention*'). Initiated by the League of Nations in 1921, the Convention was later adopted by a diplomatic conference in Geneva and later amended by the 1967 Protocol (UNHCR 2011a: 1). These landmark documents (which can be viewed at: http://www.unhcr.org/protect/PROTECTION/3b66c2aa10.pdf) defined who qualified for refugee status, the legal protections they were entitled to receive upon being deemed refugees, and who were not entitled to qualify for refugee status (e.g. war criminals) (UNHCR 2011a: 2). The Convention also clarified the obligations that refugees had towards their host country, which rested on its cornerstone principle of non-refoulement contained in Article 33. According to this principle,

> *a refugee should not be returned to a country where he or she faces serious threats to his or her life or freedom. This protection may not be claimed by refugees who are reasonably regarded as a danger to the security of the country, or having been convicted of a particularly serious crime, are considered a danger to the community.* (UNHCR 2011a: 2)

Other rights contained in the *1951 Convention* include:

- the right not to be expelled, except under certain, strictly defined conditions (Article 32)
- the right not to be punished for illegal entry into the territory of a contracting State (Article 31)

- the right to work (Articles 17 to 19)
- the right to housing (Article 21)
- the right to education (Article 22)
- the right to public relief and assistance (Article 23)
- the right to freedom of religion (Article 4)
- the right to access the courts (Article 16)
- the right to freedom of movement within the territory (Article 26), and
- the right to be issued identity and travel documents (Articles 27 and 28)

(these can be viewed in detail via the following web-link: http://www.unhcr.org/protect/PROTECTION/3b66c2aa10.pdf).

As indicated previously, the above rights and protection do not apply to stateless persons who, as explained, while stateless have no rights at all. This status is, however, in contravention of Article 15 of the *Universal Declaration of Human Rights* (United Nations (UN) 1949), which affirms that 'everyone has the right to a nationality'. While this might not seem a priority right, in the context of displacement, nationality is important because it:

> *provides people with a sense of identity but, more importantly,* enables them to exercise a wide range of rights. *The lack of any nationality, statelessness, can therefore, be harmful, in some cases devastating to the lives of the individuals concerned.* [emphasis added] (UNHCR 2014c: 1)

Although it is generally understood by governments that statelessness should be avoided, the UNHCR has noted that many states 'have yet to take action to ensure that everyone enjoys the right to a nationality' and, because of the various approaches taken to this issue, 'some individuals continue to "fall through the cracks" and become stateless' (UNHCR 2014c: 2).

An often-overlooked issue for the above populations is their precarious health status, which is often poor and frequently aggravated by deprivation, physical hardship, stress, human rights violations and a lack of resources by host countries to adequately meet even their fundamental needs for food, shelter and clean water. Nurses have a moral responsibility and an important role to play in ensuring that the health and human rights of refugees, asylum seekers, displaced people and stateless people do not 'fly under the radar' (Carrigan 2014). One way to ensure this is to join with others in 'energising dissent' and rehumanising this highly vilified and dehumanised population.

People with disabilities

People with disabilities may be described as persons:

> *with long-term physical, mental, intellectual or sensory impairments which in interaction with various barriers may hinder their full and effective participation in society on an equal basis with others.* (UN 2006a: Article 1)

The WHO estimates that more than 1 billion people (or around 15% of the world's population) live with some form of disability. Of these, almost 200 million experience 'considerable difficulties with functioning' (WHO 2011b: 5). Although not all people with disabilities are vulnerable, research suggests that some people with disabilities are more vulnerable than others on account of being at a higher risk of abuse because of being dependent on a high number of caregivers and difficulties in communication (WHO 2011b: 147).

In its first (and now much cited) *World report on disability*, the WHO highlights that people with disabilities tend to have 'poorer health outcomes, lower education achievements, less economic participation, and higher rates of poverty than do people without disabilities' (WHO 2011b: 5). One reason for this is that people with disabilities experience many barriers to accessing services (including health care) that people without disabilities often take for granted.

In 2006, the United Nations adopted the *Convention on the Rights of Persons with Disabilities* (CRPD) (www.un.org/disabilities/documents/convention/convoptprot-e.pdf), the key aim of which is to:

> *Promote, protect and ensure that full and equal enjoyment of all human rights and fundamental freedoms by all persons with disabilities, and to promote respect for human dignity.* (UN 2006a: Article 1)

Despite these and other mechanisms designed to protect the moral entitlements of people with disabilities, discrimination on the basis of disability still occurs. That is, people with disabilities are still vulnerable to being distinguished by and excluded from social participation *on the basis of their disability*. Once 'marked' on the basis of disability, people with disabilities may experience the impairment, nullification or negation of the enjoyment and exercise of their 'human rights and fundamental freedoms in the political, economic, social, cultural, civil, or any other field' (UN 2006a: Article 2). The flow-on effect of this can also work to undermine the possibility for people with disabilities to 'make friends, express their sexuality, and achieve the family life that non-disabled people take for granted' (WHO 2011b: 147).

The CRPD has identified eight key barriers that are instrumental in restricting participation by people with disabilities; these barriers include (WHO 2011b: 9–10):

- 'inadequate policies and standards' (which do not always take into account the needs of people with disabilities)
- 'negative attitudes' (encompassing negative beliefs about and prejudices against people with disabilities – e.g. school-age children seeking admission to mainstream schools)
- 'lack of provision of services' (people with disabilities are particularly vulnerable to inadequacies in services including health care and rehabilitation)
- 'inadequate service delivery' (e.g. poor coordination of services, inadequate staffing and skill mix and so forth)
- 'inadequate funding' (it has been suggested that, even in high-income countries, between 20% and 40% of people with disabilities do not receive adequate assistance with everyday activities)
- 'lack of accessibility' (this can include difficulties in accessing buildings as well as basic information and communication technologies such as telephones, the internet and television)
- 'lack of consultation and involvement' (people with disabilities are often excluded from decision-making on matters that stand to directly affect their lives)
- 'lack of data and evidence' (owing to a lack of robust comparative data, there is only limited understanding of the enablers and disablers affecting the capacity of people with disabilities to be active participants in social processes).

People's experiences of disability vary across conditions, contexts and cultures. Nonetheless, stereotypical images of being blind, deaf, or confined to a wheelchair prevail, even though in reality disability can be associated with a range of health conditions, and can depend on the personalities of the people affected, the level of support they have and the socio-cultural environments in which they live (WHO 2011b: 8).

As previously noted, not all people who have a disability are equally vulnerable; however, vulnerable populations are disproportionately affected by disability and those with severe disabilities tend to be more disadvantaged than are others. As Cohon (2003: 658) notes:

> *People with disabilities tend to be looked down on, ignored, discriminated against, and otherwise badly treated. Sometimes they are denied education or medical care or excluded from employment. Sometimes they are institutionalized or sterilized against their will. Sometimes they are subjected to violence or other forms of abuse. Often, especially but not only in poor countries, their needs for food and shelter are not met. Many nondisabled individuals are uncomfortable in the presence of the disabled and therefore exclude them from social life. Thus, at times the attitudes of their fellow citizens bar disabled people from carrying out the social roles of students, employees, spouses, and parents.*

As is the case with other vulnerable populations, nurses have a moral responsibility and an important role to play in ensuring that the health and human rights of people with disabilities are upheld. It is also incumbent on nurses to fulfil these responsibilities in their capacity as 'good citizens'. On this point, as Professor Steven Hawking (2011: 3) reminds us,

> we [all] have a moral duty to remove the barriers to participation, and to invest sufficient funding and expertise to unlock the vast potential of people with disabilities. Governments throughout the world can no longer overlook the hundreds of millions of people with disabilities who are denied access to health, rehabilitation, support, education and employment, and never get the chance to shine.

Just as governments can no longer credibly overlook the vulnerabilities and disadvantages experienced by people with disabilities, neither can the nursing profession. Nurses need to collaborate with other community advocates and energise dissent aimed at improving the status quo.

Indigenous peoples

According to the advocacy group *Cultural Survival* (https://www.culturalsurvival.org/issues), there are over 370 million indigenous peoples[6] in the world, living in more than 90 countries and speaking more than 4000 languages. Taken together, these peoples represent a rich diversity of cultures, religions, traditions, languages and histories. Historically, indigenous peoples have suffered unconscionable disenfranchisement and the abrogation of their rights by colonisers who saw fit to construct them as 'savages', 'barbarians', 'backward', and 'inferior and uncivilised' – all dehumanising constructions that were ultimately used by colonisers to justify their subjugation, domination, exploitation, moral exclusion, random killing and genocide of indigenous peoples (International Work Group for Indigenous Affairs (IWGIA) 2013: 452). The legacy of this history continues to affect prejudicially the health and wellbeing of indigenous peoples the world over.

In 2007 the United Nations Declaration on the Rights of Indigenous Peoples (UNDRIP) was adopted by the General Assembly. Although 144 states voted in favour of the declaration, 4 voted against it, notably Australia, Canada, New Zealand and the United States; these four countries later reversed their position, however, and now support the declaration (United Nations (UN) nd). It is acknowledged that since the UNDRIP was adopted, progress has been made in terms of formally recognising indigenous peoples, the devastating history and negative health impact that colonisation has had on their lives and cultures, and the need for reconciliation (see also IWGIA 2017). Despite the progress that has been made, indigenous peoples 'overwhelmingly continue to face discrimination, marginalization and major challenges in enjoying their basic rights' (UN nd) and face ongoing and deep challenges with regard to the lack of domestic remedies to address their concerns.

It remains a confronting reality that indigenous peoples are grossly over-represented 'among the world's vulnerable groups, suffering low incomes, living in poor conditions and lacking adequate access to employment, education, safe water, food and health care services' (ICN 2009: 1). Furthermore, although epidemiological data are 'scanty', the data that do exist show continuing disparities in the morbidity and mortality (including lower life expectancy) rates among indigenous peoples compared with non-indigenous populations.

The health disparities noted in the world's indigenous populations are also reflected in the health status of Australia's indigenous (Aboriginal and Torres Strait Islander) peoples and the New Zealand Māori people (Disney et al 2017; Phillips et al 2017). Moreover, as with other indigenous populations, much of the health disadvantages experienced by Australia's indigenous peoples and Māori 'can be considered historical in origin' (MacRae et al 2013: 13). However, as MacRae and colleagues (2013: 6) correctly point out, this is only part of the story: 'the *perpetuation* of the disadvantages owes much to *contemporary structural and social factors*, embodied in what have been termed the "social determinants" of health' as it does to historical influences [emphasis added].

Health status of Australia's indigenous peoples

Progress is slowly being made in 'closing the gap' in health and disadvantage in Aboriginal and Torres Strait Islander peoples (Australian Indigenous *HealthInfoNet* 2017: 16). Even so, disparities remain, some examples of which are given below. According to the most recent estimates (Australian Indigenous *HealthInfoNet* 2017):

- Life expectancy for Aboriginal males is 69 years – 10 years less than for non-indigenous males; life expectancy for Aboriginal females is 74 years – 10 years less than for non-indigenous females.
- Infant mortality rates (IMRs) in Aboriginal children under 1 year of age is twice that of non-Aboriginal infants.
- Cardiovascular disease (CVD – coronary artery disease, stroke, heart failure and high blood pressure) is a leading cause of death, with Aboriginal and Torres Strait Islander people twice as likely to die from ischaemic heart disease as non-indigenous people; Aboriginal and Torres Strait Islander peoples are also more likely to die from CVD at a younger age (35–44 years), with people in this age group 10 times more likely to die from CVD than non-indigenous people of the same age.
- Other common conditions imposing a significant burden of disease on Aboriginal and Torres Strait Islander peoples are diabetes (the death rate from which is five times higher than for non-indigenous people), kidney disease (the rate of which is seven times more common than for non-indigenous people), chronic obstructive pulmonary disease (COPD) (with admission to hospital three times more likely for influenza and pneumonia and twice as likely for asthma). In the case of communicable diseases, notifications for tuberculosis are 11 times higher for indigenous Australians than non-indigenous Australian-born people.

It is acknowledged that the health of Aboriginal and Torres Strait Islander people is improving. Nonetheless, the morbidity and mortality rates are still unacceptable. In light of the known disparities in indigenous health, in keeping with Morgan and Allen's (1998) call over two decades ago, there is a strong case to be made for indigenous health in and of itself to be treated as 'a special moral imperative' for which all citizens share collective responsibility. To this end, as Morgan and Allen (1998: 732) persuasively argue in relation to the health of Australian Aboriginal peoples, health stands as an 'appropriate site for restitutional action', which accordingly needs to be situated as a primary locus of action encompassing the complex, interwoven and 'enmeshed' processes of *recognition* (of past wrongs), *restorative justice* (to repay some of the 'accrued moral debts' owing to Aboriginal peoples) and ultimately *reconciliation* (see also Johnstone 2007a; Thomas 2004).

Meanwhile, in order to further improve Aboriginal and Torres Strait Islander health, Australian indigenous *HealthInfoNet* (2017: 16) has identified the following changes that need to occur specifically in the health sector:

- more health advancement programs
- better identification of health conditions before they become serious
- more primary health care services that are accessible to Aboriginal and Torres Strait Islander people
- greater cultural competence for service providers.

Health status of New Zealand Māori

Māori health continues to improve although, as is the case in Australia, progress is slow, with Māori continuing to experience significant disparities in health and disadvantage (Disney et al 2017; Houkamau et al 2017; Phillips et al 2017). However, overall the health of Māori children has improved (98% of children were rated by their parents as being in 'good health'). According to New Zealand's Ministry of Health most recent estimates (MOH, 2018):

- Life expectancy for Māori males is 73 years – 7 years less than for non-Māori males; life expectancy for Māori females is 77 years – 6 years less than for non-Māori females (both down from a 9-year gap in the mid-to-late 1990s, representing a 2-year increase in life expectancy from birth).
- Infant mortality rates (IMRs) are 1.5 times higher than of non-Māori infants; with the SIDS rate for Māori infants being approximately 3 times higher than non-Māori infants.
- Cardiovascular disease (coronary artery disease, stroke, heart failure and high blood pressure) is a leading cause of death, with Māori people 1.5–2 times as likely to die from these diseases as non-Māori people.
- Other common conditions imposing a significant burden of disease on Māori are lung cancer, diabetes (with the self-reported prevalence of type 2 diabetes being 50% higher for Māori than non-Māori) and COPD (with the mortality rate among Māori aged 45 years and older being almost 3 times higher than non-Māori in males and 3.5 times higher in females than non-Māori; hospitalisation rates for COPD were also disparate with Māori males 3.5 times more likely to be hospitalised, and Māori female 4.5 times more likely than non-Māori to be hospitalised). In the case of communicable diseases, notifications for meningococcal disease were 1.8 times higher (for infants under 1 year of age) and 3 times higher (for toddlers aged 1–4 years) than the total New Zealand population; Māori had a lower rate of notifications for tuberculosis than the general population.

Inequalities in Māori health are widely acknowledged as posing significant and ongoing challenges to the New Zealand government, which the government itself acknowledges. In 2016 the New Zealand Government refreshed its *New Zealand health strategy* in which the following five principles giving effect to the 'special relationship between Māori and the Crown' were outlined:

- people powered – Māori participation in service delivery
- closer to home – Māori organisations and their unique ability to service their communities
- value and high performance – the importance of achieving health equity and improving outcomes in health status across population groups and Māori health
- one team – acknowledging the role of Māori in the health system, as users of services, as a significant contributor to the health workforce and through Māori institutions
- smart system – ensuring that any technological advances provide an equivalent benefits [sic] to Māori as to the rest of the population (online: http://www.health.govt.nz/our-work/populations/maori-health).

Reduction of health disparities in Māori, however, is going to require more than political rhetoric. As Tobias and colleagues (2009: 1712) contend, it will require sustained political commitment to 'pro-equity health and social policies'. To help foster this commitment, timely monitoring of ethnic health disparities based on high-quality data will be required. In addition, changes in *both* the distribution of the social determinants of health and a responsive health care system will also be required (Tobias et al 2009).

Global call to redress indigenous health disparities

In May 2001, deeply concerned about the disparities in the health conditions of indigenous peoples, the Fifty-Fourth World Health Assembly urged its member states (WHA 2001: 1–2):

1. *to recognise and protect the right of indigenous people to enjoyment of the highest attainable standard of health as set out in the Constitution of the World Health Organization, within overall national development policies;*

2. *to make adequate provisions for indigenous health needs in their national health systems, including through improved collection and reporting of statistics and health data;*
3. *to respect, preserve and maintain traditional healing practices and remedies, consistent with nationally and internationally accepted standards, and to seek to ensure that indigenous people retain this traditional knowledge and its benefits.*

It is almost two decades since this resolution was passed, yet the disparities stubbornly persist. The persistent nature of disparities in the health status of indigenous peoples serves as a potent reminder of the challenges involved in trying to redress past wrongs and the enduring and accumulative negative effects that the processes of dehumanisation, discrimination, moral exclusions and marginalisation can have on the health and wellbeing of a vulnerable population.

Prisoners and detainees

According to the *World prison population list* (11th edition) there are more than 10.35 million people held in penal institutions worldwide, with the world prison rate being an estimated 144 per 100 000 (Institute for Criminal Policy Research 2016). The incarceration of people in penal institutions is one of the main forms of punishment for the commissions of crimes and other offences. Since around the year 2000, the world prison population has grown by almost 20%, with female incarceration rates increasing disproportionately with males (50% for female compared with 18% for males) (Institute for Criminal Policy Research 2016).

In Australia, according to the latest data collected for the period 2013–14, there were 189.3 per 100 000 adults (excluding juvenile offenders) in state and territory prisons; this figure represents an increase in incarcerations – up from 172.4 in 2012–13 (AIHW 2015: 11). As of June 2014, there were 33 170 adults in prison although it is estimated that around 50 000 individuals move through the system in the entire year (AIHW 2015: 11). It has also been estimated that, although indigenous Australians constitute just 2% of the general Australian population, they were significantly over-represented (27%) in the prison population – an incarceration rate 13 times higher than for non-indigenous Australians (AIHW 2015: 11). This over-representation is considered to be due to a complex array of factors, not least the enduring legacy of colonisation and its negative impact on the cultural life-ways (for which read 'cultural dispossession') of Aboriginal peoples.

New Zealand statistics are comparable to those of Australia. As of September 2017, the total prisoner population was 10 470 (Department of Corrections 2018). Like Australia, New Zealand's indigenous population (Māori), while making up only 14.6% of New Zealand's population, were over-represented (51%) in the country's prison population during the data collection period (http://archive.stats.govt.nz/browse_for_stats/snapshots-of-nz/yearbook/society/crime/corrections.aspx). The over-representation of Māori in New Zealand prisons is likewise due to a complex array of factors including the disruption of traditional cultural life-ways of Māori people.

It is often forgotten that 'prisoners are part of society' and that, under various declarations and oaths, while in prison (and upon being released from their custodial sentence) they are entitled to the same quality of health care as is the general population (Gatherer 2013: 1). Although what is variously termed 'custodial nursing', 'prison nursing' and 'correctional nursing' (to be distinguished from 'forensic nursing'[7]) has tended not to have a high profile in the nursing profession, important work has nonetheless been and continues to be done in this 'silent' field (Dhaliwal & Hirst 2016; La Cerra et al 2017; Maruca & Shelton 2016; Schoenly & Knox 2013). The importance and (often overlooked) evolution of this work is reflected in various ways such as via the establishment of correctional nursing as a specialty area, publication of foundational texts in the field – for example, *Essentials of correctional nursing* (by Schoenly & Knox 2013), and the publication of research studies and systematic reviews on the subject (e.g. Dhaliwal & Hirst 2016; La Cerra et al 2017).

The term *prison* refers to an institution that holds people 'who have been sentenced to a period of imprisonment by the courts for offences against the law' (WHO 2007b: xvi). A *prisoner*, in turn, may be defined as 'a person deprived of liberty and kept in prison or some other form of custody as punishment for a crime or other offence against the law' (adapted from *Collins Australian dictionary* 2011: 1310), and whose confinement is the responsibility of a corrective services agency (AIHW 2015: 8).

Many prisoners warrant and even need incarceration for the crimes they have committed, particularly those who are extremely dangerous offenders. And members of the public probably agree that most people who are committed to serve a prison sentence for their offences 'deserve what they get'. They may also have little if any sympathy for prisoners who, upon being incarcerated, face the stress of losing the everyday freedoms that most people take for granted and in some cases even losing their civil liberties – such as the right to vote, the right to the same health care as if one were not a prisoner (e.g. in Australian jurisdictions, upon their entry to prison, prisoners lose access to Medicare – the universal health cover scheme – and the pharmaceutical benefits scheme (PBS); their medical care is determined and provided by the state or territory in which they are imprisoned (AIHW 2015: 3)), the right to privacy, and the right to write letters to family and friends without this being monitored. Some might go even further and contend that prisoners not only deserve to lose their freedoms but, because of violating the rights of their victims, they have also forfeited their rights to these freedoms as well as the right to be treated with respect as a member of society.

Prisons contain some of the most vulnerable, marginalised and disadvantaged people in society. Compared with the general public, prisoners are more likely to have been in social care as a child, unemployed, homeless and to have a low level of educational attainment (AIHW 2015; Ginn & Robinson 2012a; WHO 2014a). Some ethnic minority groups and indigenous groups also tend to be over-represented (as noted earlier, indigenous Australians and New Zealand Māori are significantly over-represented in the respective Australian and New Zealand prison systems). Positioned as 'social outcasts' and already deprived of moral status, prisoners (especially those who have committed heinous crimes) are highly vulnerable to being dehumanised – that is, described and treated as 'animals' or 'monsters' – and thus 'justifiably' excluded from the moral entitlements and protections that would otherwise be afforded them. This may help to explain why, until relatively recently, prison and prisoner health has not attracted the level of attention that is otherwise warranted (see, for example, the ongoing global controversy over what is called 'the health-promoting prison' (Woodall 2016; Woodall & Dixey 2015)).

Over the past few years it has been increasingly recognised that prisoners tend to have poorer health than the average population and that penal institutions are not the best places to address poor prisoner health (Ginn & Robinson 2013; WHO 2014a; Woodall 2016; Woodall & Dixey 2015). Not only this, because of the bullying cultures often found in penal institutions, overcrowding, shared facilities, confined and poorly ventilated spaces, and high staff, prisoner and visitor turnover, prisons are a significant source and 'cause' of poor prisoner health (especially mental illness and infectious disease). Prisoner poor health in this situation is often compounded by a lack of appropriate health care services and inadequate medical attention (Ginn & Robinson 2012b; Jackson 2013). This has led some to argue that, since prisoners come from and are usually returned to the community, taking a proactive stance towards promoting prisoner health is warranted. Taking such a stance stands to benefit not just the prisoners but also the broader community since health promotion in this instance has the capacity to reduce a country's burden of disease (WHO 2014a).

It is now widely recognised that, compared with the general public, prisoners have far greater health needs. Prisoners often enter prison with several pre-existing health problems including mental health problems, certain chronic diseases, communicable diseases, risky drug and alcohol consumption, and tobacco smoking; conversely, others who enter prison healthy are at considerable risk of leaving prison with an acquired health condition such as poor mental health, an illicit drug problem, HIV or tuberculosis

(WHO 2007b, 2014a). In the Australian prison population there is a high prevalence of mental health problems and mental illness (e.g. depression and psychosis), illicit substance use, chronic disease (e.g. asthma, arthritis, cardiovascular disease, diabetes and cancer), communicable diseases (e.g. sexually transmitted infections, hepatitis B, hepatitis C and HIV) and disability (AIHW 2015). Mental health problems and harmful drug use are particularly prevalent (AIHW 2015).

As indicated earlier, there are various declarations and oaths protecting the rights of prisoners to appropriate and equivalent health services to those available in the general community (Coyle 2007). Notable among the measures and instruments advocating this stance are those presented in Box 6.1. Although these and other instruments (including national measures) affirm that health services available in prison should be appropriate and equivalent to that available in the general community, in reality the 'prison environment may make the goal of equivalence and continuity of care between the community and prison difficult to achieve, especially upon entry' (AIHW 2015: 4). In an attempt to redress this situation, the WHO has championed the idea of fostering the 'health-promoting prison' (referred to earlier), a term which is taken as denoting prisons in which:

> the risks to health are reduced to a minimum; essential prison duties such as the maintenance of security are undertaken in a caring atmosphere that recognizes the inherent dignity of every prisoner and their human rights; health services are provided to the level and in a professional manner equivalent to what is provided in the country as a whole; and a whole-prison approach to promoting health and welfare is the norm. (WHO 2007b: xvi)

BOX 6.1 Instruments protecting the rights of prisoners to appropriate health services

- United Nations Universal Declaration of Human Rights 1948 (UN 1949)
  http://www.un.org/en/universal-declaration-human-rights/
- United Nations standard minimum rules for the treatment of prisoners and procedures for the effective implementation of the standard minimum rules (UN 1955)
  https://www.unodc.org/pdf/criminal_justice/UN_Standard_Minimum_Rules_for_the_Treatment_of_Prisoners.pdf
- United Nations International Covenant on Economic, Social and Cultural Rights (UN 1966) Article 12
  http://www.ohchr.org/EN/ProfessionalInterest/Pages/CESCR.aspx
- The Oath of Athens (International Council of Prison Medical Services 1979)
  http://www.medekspert.az/ru/chapter1/resources/The_Oath_of_Athens.pdf
- Principles of medical ethics relevant to the role of health personnel, particularly physicians, in the protection of prisoners and detainees against torture and other cruel, inhuman or degrading treatment or punishment (UN 1982)
  http://www.ohchr.org/EN/ProfessionalInterest/Pages/MedicalEthics.aspx
- United Nations General Assembly basic principles for the treatment of prisoners (UN 1990)
  http://www.un.org/documents/ga/res/45/a45r111.htm
- United Nations Office of the High Commissioner for Human Rights Istanbul protocol: manual on the effective investigation and documentation of torture and other cruel, inhuman or degrading treatment or punishment. (UNOHCHR 2004)
  https://www.ohchr.org/Documents/Publications/training8Rev1en.pdf
- United Nations Office on Drugs and Crime (UNODC) The United Nations standard minimum rules for the treatment of prisoners (the Nelson Mandela rules) (UNODC 2015)
  http://www.unodc.org/documents/justice-and-prison-reform/GA-RESOLUTION/E_ebook.pdf

Nurses are at the forefront of providing prisoner health care in Australia, New Zealand and elsewhere In Australian jurisdictions, for example, registered nurses (RNs) are the most commonly consulted (71%) health professional in prison clinics, followed by general medical practitioners (17%) and mental health nurses (7%); consultation with dentists, psychiatrists and other health professionals constituted just 2%–3% of clinic visits (AIHW 2015: 140).

Nurses working in prisons face significant challenges in their work, not least the challenge of battling the health-injurious effects of the dehumanisation and delegitimisation of their clientele. These challenges do not – and should not – be the domain of prison nurses alone, however, and rightly stand as the province of *all* nurses.

In *The ICN code of ethics for nurses* (ICN 2012a: 2), nurses are reminded that their primary responsibility is to those 'people who require nursing care'. In its position statement on *Nurses' role in the care of detainees and prisoners*, the ICN (2011b: 1) makes clear that 'prisoners are people' and, accordingly, are just as deserving of the professional advocacy of nurses as is the general public. To this end, the ICN (p 1) stipulates that prisoners 'have the right to health care and humane treatment regardless of their legal status' and that, when caring for detainees and prisoners, nurses are expected to adhere to the human rights and ethical principles (such as outlined in the declarations, measures and oaths cited earlier) as well as to the following standards:

- *Nurses who are aware of abuse and maltreatment take appropriate action to safeguard the rights of detainees and prisoners.*
- *Nurses employed in prison health services do not assume functions of prison security personnel, such as restraint or body searches for the purpose of prison security.*
- *Nursing / health research should be based on ethical standards and respect for human subjects and protection of their health and rights. Nurses participate in clinical research on prisoners and detainees only with the prisoner or detainee's informed consent.*
- *Nurses collaborate with other health professionals and prison authorities to reduce the impact of crowded and unhealthy prison environments on transmission of infectious diseases such as HIV, hepatitis and tuberculosis and improve their care and management.*
- *Nurses abstain from using their nursing knowledge and skills or health information specific to individuals in any manner that violates the rights of detainees and prisoners.*
- *Nurses advocate for safe humane treatment of detainees and prisoners including dignity, respect, the provision of clean water, adequate food and other basic necessities of life.* (ICN 2011b: 1)

Several years ago, a forensic psychiatrist, who worked in a large high-security prison housing long-term male prisoners who had committed extremely violent crimes, was asked the question: 'Why do you do this work? How can you work with those "animals"?' To this question, the psychiatrist replied calmly, 'Well someone has to treat those men as human beings, and it might as well be me' (personal communication).

Homeless people

It has been conservatively estimated that approximately 1.6 billion people worldwide live in inadequate housing conditions in urban areas alone (Homeless World Cup Foundation nd). Although reliable data are not available, based on the last global survey conducted by the UN, it is further estimated that more than 100 million people have no housing whatsoever, with almost one quarter of these being children (Homeless World Cup Foundation nd). Although severe housing deprivation can affect *anyone*, those who tend to be disproportionately affected are children and young adults, ethnic minorities and indigenous peoples, women, sole-parent families and people without families. This situation is not confined to individual countries, and is replicated across the globe – even in well-resourced nations like Australia

(Australian Human Rights Commission 2008), Canada (Gaetz et al 2016), New Zealand (Amore 2016), the United Kingdom (Fitzpatrick et al 2018) and the USA (US Department of Housing and Urban Development 2017).

The idea of homelessness often conjures up stereotypical images of 'disheveled vagrants wandering the streets' – people on 'skid row'. The reality of homelessness, however, is far more complex. Moreover, as a team of New Zealand researchers has suggested, since the term *homelessness* is 'burdened by stereotype' a more appropriate term should be used, such as 'severe housing deprivation' (Amore et al 2013: 7). This view has been reiterated by Busch-Geertsema and colleagues (2016) in their attempts to develop a global framework for conceptualising and enabling meaningful comparative measurements of homelessness.[8]

The negative impact of stereotypical views about homeless people should not be underestimated. One reason for this is that homeless people are particularly vulnerable to being treated as 'less than human' (*viz*. dehumanised) and discriminated against (Bower et al 2018; Harris & Fiske 2006). This is because homeless people are often stereotypically perceived as having 'caused their own plight' and hence as moral failures. Once dehumanised, homeless people are at particular risk of being treated prejudicially with disgust and contempt, and denied the moral entitlements and protections that being human would otherwise afford them (Harris & Fiske 2006). This, in turn, leaves them vulnerable to the harms of stigma and discrimination – often without remedy – and even the subjects of unwarranted criminalisation – for example, when arrested for begging or sleeping rough on the streets (see National Law Center on Homelessness and Poverty (NLCHP) 2014; Watts et al 2018).

What is homelessness?

It is perhaps important to state at the outset that there is no *one* definition of homelessness (Australian Bureau of Statistics (ABS) 2012a; Busch-Geertsema et al 2016). Even so, it is generally recognised that homelessness may fall into one of several categories depending on the individual situation and needs of the people concerned. Notable among the categories that have commonly been used are:

- *Primary homelessness* – people who are literally 'roofless' and without shelter (e.g. living on the streets, in parks, in subways or in deserted buildings); this is arguably the most visible form of homelessness.
- *Secondary homelessness* – people with no place of usual residence or 'fixed abode' – i.e. people of 'no fixed address'; they move frequently between various types of accommodation (including transient accommodation with family or friends, or living temporarily in refuges, hostels or boarding houses with shared amenities and without security of tenure) (Chamberlain & MacKenzie 2009).

The European Federation of National Organisations working with the Homeless (nd) (FEANTSA) (a non-governmental organisation established in 1989 to help prevent and alleviate poverty and social exclusion of people threated by homelessness) defines and recognises four categories of homelessness (online: http://www.feantsa.org/en/about-us/faq):

- *rooflessness* (people living rough and people in emergency accommodation);
- *houselessness* (people in accommodation for the homeless, in women's shelters, in accommodation for migrants, due to be released from institutions or receiving long-term support due to homelessness)
- *living in insecure housing* (people living in insecure tenancies, under threat of eviction or violence);
- *living in inadequate housing* (people living in unfit housing, non-conventional dwellings or in situations of extreme overcrowding).

In Australia, homelessness has been defined under Australian federal law as 'inadequate access to safe and secure housing' (*Supported Accommodation Assistance Act 1994*: Preliminary Part 1, Section 4: Definition of *homeless* (p 5)). For the purposes of the Act, 'inadequate access to safe and secure housing' is taken to mean housing to which the person has access:

1. damages, or is likely to damage, the person's health; or
2. threatens the person's safety; or
3. marginalises the person through failing to provide access to:
   (i) adequate personal amenities; or
   (ii) the economic and social supports that a home normally affords; or
4. places the person in circumstances which threaten or adversely affect the adequacy, safety, security and affordability of that housing. (Supported Accommodation Assistance Act 1994 [Cth]: 5)

For research purposes, however, the ABS statistical definition is used, which is informed by an understanding that *homelessness* is literally 'without a home' not mere *rooflessness*; the ABS further understands and recognises that homelessness is 'culturally and historically contingent' (ABS 2012a). Accordingly, the ABS defines homelessness in the following terms:

when a person does not have suitable accommodation alternatives they are considered homeless if their current living arrangement:

- *is in a dwelling that is inadequate; or*
- *has no tenure, or if their initial tenure is short and not extendable; or*
- *does not allow them to have control of, and access to space for social relations.* (ABS 2012a)

In New Zealand, homelessness is officially defined in terms similar to that used in Australia, that is:

living situations where people with no other options to acquire safe and secure housing are: without shelter, in temporary accommodation, sharing accommodation with a household or living in uninhabitable housing. (Statistics New Zealand 2015)

Despite their variations, common to all of the above definitions is the view that a person does not have suitable accommodation when their current living arrangement:

- *is in a dwelling that is inadequate; or*
- *has no tenure, or if their initial tenure is short and not extendable; or*
- *does not allow them to have control of, and access to space for social relations.* (Homelessness Australia nd)

Causes of homelessness

In Australia 1 in 200 people are homeless on any given night. Of the more than 105 000 people who were homeless at the 2016 count, almost 18 000 were children under 10 years of age (Homelessness Australia 2016). In New Zealand, 1 in 120 people were homeless (among the highest in OECD countries). Of the estimated 41 000 who were homeless in the 2013 census, half were under 25 years of age and 25% were children (Amore 2016, https://www.lifewise.org.nz/wp-content/uploads/2016/09/Lifewise-report-final-report-part-1-and-2.pdf).

The causes of homelessness are complex and varied and can range from poverty and financial difficulties (exacerbated by unemployment) to personal and family problems such as domestic violence, family breakdown, family rejection (notably of LGBTIQ youths), poor physical and mental health, substance use and other addictions leading to an inability to cope (Australian Human Rights Commission 2008). These situations are compounded in the case of people who already live on the margins of society (e.g. ex-prisoners, refugees and asylum seekers), have few or no social support networks with either family, friends or the community, and are socially isolated (Australian Human Rights Commission 2008). When these situations are examined in depth, it can be readily seen that when life circumstances beyond a person's control 'strike' then homelessness is a frighteningly real possibility. The lesson here for anyone contemplating making moralising judgments about homeless people is recognising that another's misfortune could so easily be our own – that is, 'there but for the grace of God go I'.

Homelessness and the right to health

Research has shown a strong correlation between homeless and health disadvantage, with homeless people experiencing a disproportionately higher rate of morbidity (disability and chronic illness) and premature mortality compared with the general population (Fazel et al 2014; Jego et al 2018; Rhoades et al 2018; Stafford & Wood 2017). Moreover, as Gerber (2013: 37) notes, the persistently homeless also live in:

> constant chaos, confusion, and fear. Trauma from head injuries, gunshot wounds, stab wounds, lacerations, and/or fractures is a significant cause of death and disability. Hypothermia in the winter and dehydration in the summer are of particular concern.

Homelessness is not just a 'housing' issue; it is also fundamentally a human rights issue (Australian Human Rights Commission 2008).

Given that every person (young and old alike) has a fundamental right to the highest attainable standard of health and health care, homelessness thus stands as a potent threat to the right to health. It is this risk that imposes correlative responsibilities onto others (including nurses) to take action.

Significantly, homelessness can be both a cause and a consequence of ill health. Because of a lack of resources (e.g. the means of transport and the capacity to attend and pay for appointments, the lack of identification and a Medicare card or health insurance card, a lack of facilities to store and administer medications (e.g. refrigeration of insulin, thyroxin)) and a lack of access to appropriate health services generally (Moore et al 2007, 2011), it can also exacerbate existing health problems and complicated care and treatment regimens.

As even a cursory search of the nursing literature will show (too numerous to list here), nurses (particularly those working in community and primary care) have a long history of advocating for and caring about people who are homeless. Their work continues to this day through the efforts of community nurses and nurse-led primary health care clinics operating in liaison with other sectors of the health care system (Roche et al 2017; Savage et al 2006; Su et al 2015).

Like prison nursing, nurse-led care of the homeless has tended not to have a high profile in the nursing profession. Despite the dedicated efforts of nurses working in this 'silent' field, to date the vulnerability and health rights of homeless people have not featured significantly in the nursing ethics literature or nursing policies and position statements. This stands as an area requiring attention and action.

Sexual minorities (LGBTIQ people)

People who identify as lesbian (L), gay (G), bisexual (B), transgender (T), intersex (I) and/or queer/questioning (Q) (commonly referred to by the acronym LGBTIQ or variations thereof) constitute a significant sexual minority of the world's population. The demographics of LGBTIQ people are difficult to accurately quantify owing to a variety of reasons (e.g. flaws in research methodologies and population surveys, reluctance by people to either self-identify or disclose their sexual orientation and gender identities in response to surveys or requests for personal details (e.g. when being admitted to hospital, completing an application for health insurance, etc.), under-reporting and a lack of reliable data generally). Nonetheless, it is conservatively estimated that a significant minority, of around 3% (between 1.5% and 5.5%) of people surveyed, identify as being 'other' than heterosexual (Gates 2011; Wikipedia 2018b, 2018c).

Sexual orientation and gender identities are 'essential elements of identity' and inform how people plan, organise and generally live their lives (Callahan et al 2014: S48). People who are heterosexual often take for granted the 'normalcy' of their sexuality and gender identities and the 'heteronormative' world in which they can openly live. In contrast, people who are not heterosexual and who do not have 'fit' within a heteronormative world (i.e. a world in which heterosexism is regarded as *the norm*) have historically been characterised as 'unnatural' and 'deviant'. This (mis)characterisation of non-heterosexual people has seen LGBTIQ people stigmatised and subjected to unmitigated prejudice, discrimination and hate crimes (many of which have resulted in serious injury and even death). In addition, LGBTIQ people have had their identities ignored, their sexuality pathologised (homosexuality was classified as a mental illness in the *Diagnostic and statistical manual of mental disorders* until 1973) and their sexual behaviour criminalised (noting here that homosexuality remains a criminal offence in some countries, punishable by incarceration and even death) (McGill 2014; Powell & Foglia 2014; Voss 2018). More fundamentally, upon disclosing their sexual orientation and/or gender identities, many LGBTIQ people have been treated as outcasts by their own families and have remained permanently estranged from them even when seriously ill or dying. As noted earlier, estrangement by families is also a major cause of homelessness (with associated risks of mental health issues and suicidality) among LGBTIQ youth (Rhoades et al 2018).

In considering the vulnerability of LGBTIQ people, it is important to place in context the protracted history of stigma, prejudice, discrimination and psychological trauma that many have experienced – especially during their formative years – and the lasting impact that these negative experiences have had on their lives and world views. The US literature identifies at least three distinctive generations of LGBTIQ people and the formative cultural contexts and social periods in which they lived (Foglia & Fredriksen-Goldsen 2014: S40):

- 'Greatest Generation' (born between 1901 and 1924) – affected by deprivations of the Great Depression
- 'Silent Generation' (born between 1925 and 1945) – affected by the laws and medical doctrine that criminalised and pathologised same-sex behaviours and identities
- 'Baby Boom Generation' (born between 1946 and 1964) – influenced by the civil rights era (1960s) and the Stonewall riots (1969).

Although derived from the cultural context of the USA, the generations and social periods identified equally apply to other common-law jurisdictions (e.g. those of Australia, Canada, New Zealand and the UK), which have been similarly affected by the events and socio-cultural norms of the periods in question and who share similar histories regarding the dehumanisation and degradation of LGBTIQ people.

Over the past five decades, progressive liberal democratic countries around the world have enacted many positive social and legal reforms which have resulted in greater social recognition and public acceptance of LGBTIQ people locally and globally. The 'rapid progress' of marriage equality laws (e.g. in Europe, the USA, New Zealand, Australia and elsewhere) is an example. However, as Voss (2018: 1) points out, with rapid progress has come 'harsh backlashes and deterioration of rights'. Despite the many reforms that have been made, LGBTIQ people nonetheless continue to experience prejudice, stigma, discrimination and marginalisation in their everyday lives. Moreover, with the rise of authoritarian (right-wing) populism (whose proponents regard LGBTIQ people as 'eschewing traditional values' and as 'the antithesis of morality'), violence against members of the LGBTIQ community continues despite the enactment of protective laws (Voss 2018: 2). In addition, health inequalities (particularly with regard to mental health issues) remain paramount (Health4LGBTI State-of-the-Art Synthesis Report 2017). As noted by the Australian State of Victoria Better Health Channel, many LGBTIQ people continue to harbour uncertainties about 'whether they will receive acceptance from families, friends, colleagues and services' should they decide to disclose their sexual orientation or gender identities (i.e. 'come out') (Better Health Channel 2018: 1–2). The pressure of these uncertainties, together with both anticipated and actual daily experiences of stigma, prejudice and discrimination, continue to have a significant negative impact on the health and wellbeing of LGBTIQ people, a burden that others who are heterosexual do not have to carry.

It is easy to become complacent about the political gains made by sexual minorities and to assume that equality and justice for this population are 'inevitable' (Powell & Foglia 2014). In light of the growing legitimisation of same-sex marriage, and law reforms permitting LGBTIQ people to adopt children and have access to in vitro fertilisation (IVF) treatments and surrogacy services in order to start a family, it would also be easy think that homophobia in modern societies is 'not an issue any more' and that LGBTIQ people are no longer a vulnerable minority. As a growing body of social and public health research is showing, however, justice is neither 'inevitable' nor 'done' for LGBTIQ people, who continue to experience what Meyer (2003: 3) has classically termed 'minority stress', which he defines as 'the excess stress to which individuals from stigmatized social categories are exposed as a result of their social, often minority, position'. This stress is experienced on account of both anticipated and actual prejudicial and discriminatory behaviours towards them and the related isolation and marginalisation that often follows (see, for example, the study by Synnes & Malterud 2018). In the case of LGBTIQ people who have other stigmatising characteristics (e.g. are of culturally and linguistically diverse backgrounds, live with a disability, are old, suffer from a mental illness, or have been diagnosed with a highly stigmatised disease such as HIV/AIDS or hepatitis C), their vulnerability and risk of minority stress are compounded – i.e. they face a 'double jeopardy'.

Health care contexts have not been immune from the dominant influences of a heteronormative worldview and, historically, have even been overtly hostile to the health needs and interests of LGBTIQ people. This has included 'labeling, judging and forcing wrongful, cruel treatment' upon LGBTIQ people (Powell & Foglia 2014: S2), ignoring their identities, denying them and their partners respect as human beings, and providing inappropriate and less than competent care (Callahan et al 2014). In light of this, it is not surprising that many 'older generations' of LGBTIQ people, who have spent the majority of their lives concealing their sexual orientation and gender identities, are suspicious of 'the system' and may find it difficult to trust health care providers and institutions. Accordingly they may continue to conceal their sexual orientation from their health service providers and may avoid altogether seeking needed medical treatment and health care (including nursing care) even if the health consequences of such avoidance might be dire.

Although many of the 'old prejudices' against LGBTIQ people have shifted, their heritage has lasted such that both conscious and non-conscious biases (the activation of negative stereotypes outside of conscious awareness) persist in modern social contexts (Foglia & Fredriksen-Goldsen 2014). These are particularly problematic in health care settings since, as Foglia and Fredriksen-Goldsen (2014) point out, they can threaten the clinical encounter by undermining patient engagement and shared decision-making, which in turn might (and does) result in patients withholding information that is otherwise essential to correct patient assessment and diagnosis. In either case, the quality and safety of patient care are placed at risk.

It is acknowledged that most LGBTIQ people lead fulfilling and healthy lives. Nonetheless, research is increasingly showing that, as a demographic group, such people have poorer health and wellbeing (particularly in regards to their mental health) compared with the total population (Haas et al 2011; Health4LGBTI State-of-the-Art Synthesis Report 2017; Hughes 2018; King et al 2008; Mayer et al 2008). A key variable contributing to this disparity is the continuing stigma and discrimination that LGBTIQ people can experience in their everyday lives and the minority stress and health-injurious distress that this may engender in them.

Despite the widespread acceptance of patient rights bills and charters in hospital settings and the promulgation of patient engagement and patient-centred care as core principles and standards of the global patient safety movement, biases and prejudices against LGBTIQ people in health care persist (Health4LGBTI State-of-the-Art Synthesis Report 2017). These biases and prejudices can be individual or institutional, subtle or overt, conscious or unconscious, intentional or unintentional. For example, an explicit institutional bias can be found in cases of aged-care facilities that do not allow same-sex partners to room-share when admitted for residential care. Other examples of institutional biases (which may be unintended but discriminate just the same) include the use of 'standard' demographic forms that do not include provisions enabling a patient to indicate that he/she is in a same-sex relationship (e.g. do not contain options for use of terms such as 'life-long partner', or contain options that allow patients only to refer to their life-long partner as a 'friend') and of 'standard' demographic forms that fail to contain provisions enabling patients to indicate that they are transgender or intersex in sexual identity/orientation (e.g. includes options only for indicating whether the patient is male *or* female). Another institutional bias can be found in hospital policies which do not recognise same-sex partners as 'next-of-kin', which in turn enables staff to restrict their visiting rights, to withhold vital information about a partner's health status or medical condition, and to deny partners a legitimate role in surrogate decision-making concerning the care and treatment of their loved one, including at the end of life.

Individual and unconscious biases, in turn, can be expressed ('leaked out') in the following ways:

- declining/refusing to care for LGBTIQ people on grounds of conscientious (religious) beliefs
- averting eye contact
- turning away
- avoiding physical contact – e.g. refusing to shake hands, or declining 'ordinary' acts of comfort, care and kindness
- conveying frank dislike or repugnance either verbally or non-verbally
- ignoring the presence of a partner
- limiting attendance time when caring for or treating LGBTIQ patients
- using derogatory, dehumanising terms when referring to or caring for LGBTIQ patients
- snickering and joking about the patient or his/her partner to others (including staff) (adapted from Foglia & Fredriksen-Goldsen 2014).

It is only in recent years that the human rights of people whose 'sexual orientation and gender identity' (SOGI) differs from the heteronormative population has become the subject of advocacy at the United Nations (UN) Human Rights Council (Daigle & Myrttinen 2018; McGill 2014; Voss 2018). As Voss (2018: 3) contends, however, SOGI is a 'highly contested normative space' and the time being taken to pass resolutions in favour of recognising the human rights of LGBTIQ people is taking an abnormally long time, due largely to the delaying tactics of populist 'counter-SOGI' entities. This delay, he warns, risks not only sending a negative message to LGBTIQ people and SOGI rights advocates, but 'killing momentum' and withering the resources that would otherwise be allocated to progressing the SOGI rights cause (Voss 2018; see also McGill 2014).

Nurses, like others in society, have an ethical responsibility to contribute to the positive project of preventing the dehumanisation, discrimination and degradation of LGBTIQ people in health care contexts. They also have a responsibility to contribute to the positive project of improving the safety and quality of health care for LGBTIQ and redressing their health disparities. This, however, is going to require a multifaceted response encompassing education, research, leadership and ethical practice and making visible the critical (missing) link between *sexuality biases and prejudices* and *patient safety and quality of care*.

Conclusion

It is often said that we can judge a nation or a society 'by the way it treats its most vulnerable citizens' (attributed to Aristotle, 384–22 BC) or, similarly, 'by how it treats its weakest members' (attributed to Mahatma Gandhi, 1869–1948). The same might be said of the health care professions: these too can be judged by the way they treat the most vulnerable and weakest members of society. How well the nursing profession will ultimately be viewed against this measure remains to be seen.

Case scenario 1

In the late 1990s, in what might be regarded as a watershed in the rationalisation of health care debate, Rau Williams, a 63-year-old Māori man with early-stage dementia and suffering a complication of diabetes, was denied kidney dialysis treatment on 'economic grounds' (Field 1997: 10). In keeping with national resource allocation guidelines in operation at the time, clinicians concluded that, since Mr Williams was unable to 'co-operate with active therapy' (he was unable to perform home dialysis independently), was unable to live independently (even though his family were willing to supervise him) and was not expected to derive more than 1 year of life benefit from dialysis, he was 'unsuitable for entry on to the [dialysis] program' (Manning & Paterson 2005: 686–7).

Outraged by the hospital's decision not to treat their father, and in a desperate bid to secure life-saving treatment for him, Rau William's family applied to the New Zealand Court of Appeal to intervene. The patient's evidence was that he did not want to die, and enjoyed some quality of life while on dialysis 'including pleasure from seeing his family' (Manning & Paterson 2005: 687). The court determined, however, that the hospital managers 'did not need to resume kidney dialysis treatment' (Field 1997: 10). In reaching its decision, the court took the stance that it would be 'inappropriate for the Court to attempt to direct a doctor as to what treatment should be given to a patient' (Manning & Paterson 2005: 687). This decision reflected two issues:

> first, a recognition that clinical judgment is beyond the expertise of the courts; and secondly, that a court should not make orders with consequences for the utilization of scarce resources since it lacks knowledge of the competing claims to those resources. (Manning & Paterson 2005: 687)

In response to the case, the then associate Health Minister was reported to have said that 'health rationing was now a fact of life'. It was subsequently observed that:

> Although formal rationing has not previously been acknowledged here [New Zealand], from July every New Zealander referred for surgery in the public health system will be scored for points on clinical and social criteria to determine when they will be treated. (Field 1997: 10)

Case scenario 2

In 2012, the bodies of a woman aged 83 and her carer son aged 51 were found at their Brisbane home 10 days after their deaths. It is believed the mother, who suffered from dementia, was confined to her bedroom and was unable to get out and seek help when her son died, possibly from a cardiac arrest. She died shortly after from natural causes. Described as 'keeping to themselves' and 'living a life of self-imposed solitude', the deaths of these two people stood as a 'sad end to a story of suburban isolation' (Arnold & Sandy 2012: 1). Upon learning of the deaths, a passerby reportedly reflected, 'Your neighbours couldn't care less about you. I could go in my backyard and fall over and no one would know I was there. Years ago everybody knew everybody and you could say hello and have a yarn. That's all gone' (Arnold & Sandy 2012: 1).

CRITICAL QUESTIONS

1 What ethical issues are raised by these cases?
2 If you were to conduct a 'vulnerability assessment' on either Mr Williams or the mother and son featured in these cases, what would your conclusions be? Outline the basis upon which you would make your assessments.
3 If you were involved in providing home care nursing services to either Mr Williams or the elderly mother featured in these cases, what advice would you give the family members caring for them? What, if any, action would you personally take to 'make it better' for the carers involved?
4 How would you judge whether you had 'got it right'?

Endnotes

1 Excerpts taken from Johnstone M-J (2009a) Ethics and human vulnerability. *Australian Nursing Journal* 16(10): 23, reproduced with permission.
2 Excerpts taken from Johnstone M-J (2013c) Ageism and the moral exclusion of older people. *Australian Nursing and Midwifery Journal* 21(3): 27, reproduced with permission.
3 Many different terms are commonly used to describe people's mental health status. Sometimes the terms are used interchangeably, which may be not only incorrect (e.g. a person could have a mental health problem, but not have a mental illness per se) but also confusing. The wrong use of terminology can also be highly stigmatising – particularly if the terms used are perceived as having a negative connotation – for example, 'being disturbed' versus 'being mentally ill' (https://www.mentalhealth.org.uk/a-to-z/t/terminology). In an attempt to dispel some of the myths around mental illness and to improve public perception and understanding of mental health problems, the following key terms have been increasingly defined in the various glossaries included in updated mental health advocacy group and government information and policy documents: 'mental health', 'mental health problem', 'mental illness', 'severe mental illness' and 'severe and complex mental illness' (Australian Government Department Department of Health 2017). The terms 'mental disorder', 'psychiatric disorder' and 'psychiatrically disturbed' have tended to be abandoned and are now more appropriately referred to in information documents and guidelines as 'mental illness' or 'severe mental illness' depending on the symptoms being manifest (Australian Government Department Department of Health 2017). The terms 'mental disorder' incorporating meanings of 'disturbance' and 'defect' continue to be defined and used in mental health legislation, however (see, for example, summaries of Australian State and Territory mental health legislation in Chapter 11 of Staunton & Chiarella 2017). The following is an example of how the key terms have tended to be defined (NB although taken from the Australian Government Department Department of Health (2017) *Fifth National Mental health and Suicide Prevention Plan*, these definitions are consistent with those used in other OECD countries):
   - *Mental health problem* – diminished cognitive, emotional or social abilities but not to the extent that the diagnostic criteria for a mental illness are met.
   - *Mental illness* – a clinically diagnosable disorder that significantly interferes with a person's cognitive emotional or social abilities. Examples include anxiety disorders, depression, bipolar disorders, eating disorders and schizophrenia.
   - *Severe mental illness* – characterised by a severe level of clinical symptoms and often some degree of disruption to social, personal, family and occupational functioning (there are three subcategories: *severe and episodic mental illness*, *severe and persistent mental illness*, and *severe and persistent illness with complex multi-agency needs*).
   - *Severe and complex mental illness* – refers to mental illness that is not directly aligned to any of [the three] subcategories of severe mental illness. Rather it is broader and may include episodic or chronic (persistent) conditions that are not confined to specific diagnostic categories (Australian Government Department of Health 2017: 67, 69).
4 The notion of 'minorities' is essentially political in nature and is used to identify groups distinguished by common ties, for example, of 'descent, race, gender, physical appearance, language, culture or religion, by

virtue of which they feel or are regarded as different from the majority of the population in society' (Bullock & Trombley 1999: 533). As explained by Bullock and Trombley (1999: 533), 'In modern usage the term tends to connote real, threatened or perceived discrimination against minorities, although in exceptional cases (e.g. South Africa under Apartheid) a minority may hold power over a majority.' The notion 'minority group' also connotes a group of people with political claims for 'equality of treatment with that accorded the majority' (Bullock & Trombley 1999: 533).

5   For further information visit (i) https://www.health.govt.nz/our-work/populations/maori-health/he-korowai-oranga/strengthening-he-korowai-oranga/treaty-waitangi-principles; and (ii) https://nzhistory.govt.nz/politics/treaty-of-waitangi

6   Although the term 'indigenous' is used here, its use is by no means universal. In some regions, terms such as 'tribes', 'first peoples / nations', 'Aboriginals' or 'ethnic groups' are preferred (WHO 2007a). The United Nations and WHO, however, understand the term 'indigenous' to include peoples who:
    - *Identify themselves and are recognized and accepted by their community as Indigenous.*
    - *Demonstrate historical continuity with pre-colonial and / or pre-settler societies.*
    - *Have strong links to territories and surrounding natural resources.*
    - *Have distinct social, economic or political systems.*
    - *Maintain distinct languages, cultures and beliefs.*
    - *Form non-dominant groups of society.*
    - *Resolve to maintain and reproduce their ancestral environments and systems as distinctive peoples and communities*
    (WHO 2007a: 1).

7   Forensic nursing has as its focus the application of forensic aspects to nursing practice *viz.* the 'scientific investigation and treatment of trauma, and / or death of victims and perpetrators of violence, criminal activity, and traumatic accidents' (Schoenly nd). Forensic nursing work involves working with the principles and processes of criminal justice; correctional nursing, in contrast, concerns the provision of care to those incarcerated in the justice system. Although distinct specialty areas, the roles of correctional nurses and forensic nurses can overlap – e.g. as reflected in the role of 'correctional forensic nurses' (International Association of Forensic Nurses 2017).

8   With reference to ETHOS (the European Typology of Homelessness and Housing Exclusion), Busch-Geertsema et al (2016: 125) follow the following three domains for assessing whether a standard of housing is adequate: *security domain* (refers primary to security and affordability of tenure), *physical domain* (pertains to the quality and quantity of accommodation and its capacity to meet the needs of inhabitants) and *social domain* (refers to opportunities to enjoy social relations as are culturally appropriate for the community).

CHAPTER 7

Patients' rights to and in health care

KEYWORDS

competency
confidentiality
cultural liberty
dignity
dignity violations
health care
health care economics
human rights
informed consent
informed decisions
nursing care
patients'/clients' rights
privacy
respect
quality care
safe care

LEARNING OBJECTIVES

Upon the completion of this chapter and with further self-directed learning you are expected to be able to:

- Discuss the relationship between patients'/clients' rights and human rights.
- Consider the right to health and health care and:
  - discuss the distinction between the right to *health* and the right to *health care*
  - discuss at least four senses in which a right to *health care* can be claimed
  - outline some controversial arguments raised both for and against the right to health care
  - discuss whether health care economics warrants consideration as an ethical issue in its own right.
- Consider the right to make informed decisions and examine critically:
  - the doctrine of informed consent
  - the right to give an informed consent
  - the five analytical components and seven related elements of informed consent
  - the right of competent patients to refuse consent
  - the right *not to know*
  - the notion of the 'sovereignty of the individual' and its implications for informed consent practices
  - the nature and moral implications of paternalism in nursing and health care.
- Consider the right to confidentiality and:
  - state the International Council of Nurses' position on confidentiality
  - outline the moral basis and requirements of the principle of confidentiality
  - outline the distinction between privacy and confidentiality
  - discuss briefly the conditions under which demands to keep information confidential may be justly overridden.
- Discuss critically the right to dignity.
- Discuss critically the right to be treated with respect.
- Discuss critically the right to cultural liberty.

Introduction

One of the most significant developments in *health care* over the past 40 years has been the *patients'/ clients' rights* movement. With its origins in the US dating back to the late 1960s and early 1970s, the movement was initially spearheaded by an organisation of poor women and their children (the National Welfare Rights Organization [NWRO]), which saw patients' rights as a 'special application of human rights' encompassing the consumer rights of people to universal health insurance (d'Oronzio 2001). Significantly, the focus of the NWRO was not just on the idea of patients' entitlements in a hostile health care environment, but also on 'equality before the law, on economic justice, and on raising the moral standards of the greater society to improve the wellbeing of its most vulnerable and powerless members' (d'Oronzio 2001: 286).

Being characteristic of and, in many ways, an extension of the larger US civil rights movement at the time, the patients' rights movement challenged the status quo: it overturned the idea that being a patient was a 'privilege', made claim to health care as a *positive right*, underscored the health impact of a 'human-rights deprivation', and ultimately saw patients' rights obtain the moral status accorded to other fundamental rights complete with correlative duties, obligations and responsibilities (d'Oronzio 2001: 286).

Today, the idea that the 'end users' of health care should have a voice in how health care is designed and delivered is almost unquestioned. As Tomes (2006: 72) has observed,

> *The concept that the end users of health care – variously conceived of as patients, consumers, or simply 'the public' – should be actively involved in decision making, in both therapeutic and economic domains, has gained widespread acceptance.*

Even so, what might be termed the 'positive project of patient rights' is, as Tomes (2006: 720) puts it, still very much a 'work in progress'. Patient agency and engagement in health care decision-making is continuously vulnerable to being impeded, owing largely to the commonly recognised disablers of: the prevalence of older paternalistic models of medically dominated decision-making, variations in consumer health literacy and desire to co-participate in their care, an increasing lack of appropriate health care resources and service provision (demand exceeding supply), the well-documented fragmentation of health care services, consumerism and the intense politicisation of the health care system by politicians and their bureaucrats (Kaufman 2015; Latimer et al 2017; Mold 2012; Tomes 2006). Thus, upholding patients' rights to and in health care is seen by many to be a daunting project and one that continues to pose many challenges.

In its position statement *Nurses and human rights*, the ICN (2011a) recognises that all individuals have a right to health care and that nurses have an obligation to safeguard and respect this right at all times. This right is taken as including: the right to choose or decline care and to accept or refuse treatment, the right to be treated with respect, the right to informed consent (including to be free of non-consensual medical treatment), the right to confidentiality, the right to dignity (including the right to die with dignity) and the right to be free from pain, torture and other cruel, inhumane or degrading treatment in a health care context. In light of the ICN's (and other related national nursing organisations') statements, it can be seen that the issue of patients' (clients') rights (alias human rights in health care) is of obvious importance to the nursing profession. If nurses are to respond appropriately and effectively to this issue, however, they need to have knowledge and understanding of, first, what patients' rights are and, second, how these rights can best be upheld. It is to advancing an understanding of these matters that this discussion will now turn.

What are patients' rights?

Patients' or clients' rights are generally held to be a subcategory of *human rights*. Statements of patients' or clients' rights serve to highlight particular moral interests that a person might have in health care contexts and that require special protection when a person assumes the role of a 'patient' or 'client'. When the notion *patients' rights* or *clients' rights* is used, a 'signpost' is provided indicating the kind of context and the kind of rights claims that are likely to be encountered by service providers. The notion of patients' rights or clients' rights, in this instance, immediately 'sets the scene' and identifies the domain of concern. In the case of human rights language, the scene that is set is much broader. Some might consider human rights language in health care contexts to be somewhat cumbersome to manage. In many respects, however, using human rights language might be more compelling and more effective in drawing attention to and commanding respect for the deserving moral interests of people in health care domains.

It is perhaps important to clarify that statements concerning patients' rights tend to include a mixture of civil rights, legal rights and moral rights. Popular examples of patients' rights include: a right to health care, a right to participate in decision-making concerning treatment and care, a right to give an informed consent, a right to refuse consent, a right to have access to a qualified health interpreter, a right to know the name, status and practice experience of attending health professionals, a right to a second medical opinion, a right to be treated with respect, a right to confidentiality, a right to bodily integrity, a right to the maintenance of dignity, and others (Box 7.1). Many of these rights statements derive from the broader moral principles of autonomy, non-maleficence, beneficence and justice, already discussed in this book. Unfortunately there is insufficient space here to discuss every type of patients' right that has been formulated at some time or another. For the purposes of this discussion, attention is given to just six broad categories of rights, under which many other narrower rights claims fall. These category claims include the rights: to health and health care, to make self-determining choices (including the right not to have unwanted information imposed), to confidentiality, to be treated with dignity, to be treated with respect, and to cultural liberty.

BOX 7.1 Charters and bills of patient/consumer health rights

- Australian Charter of Healthcare Rights
  http://www.safetyandquality.gov.au/national-priorities/charter-of-healthcare-rights/
- Canadian Patient Bill of Rights (comparative overview)
  http://publications.gc.ca/Collection-R/LoPBdP/BP/prb0131-e.htm
- NZ Health and Disability Commissioner Code of Rights
  http://www.healthpoint.co.nz/useful-information/patient-rights/code-of-rights/
- Scottish Charter of Patient Rights and Responsibilities
  http://www.scotland.gov.uk/Topics/Health/Policy/Patients-Rights/Patients-Rights-Charter
  http://www.scotland.gov.uk/Resource/0040/00407723.pdf
- UK Your Rights in the NHS
  http://www.nhs.uk/using-the-nhs/about-the-nhs/your-choices-in-the-nhs/
- US Patient Bill of Rights
  https://aapsonline.org/patient-bill-rights/

The right to health and health care

In keeping with the *Universal Declaration of Human* Rights (1948) all people have a fundamental right to health – a right that is also recognised in the Constitution of the World Health Organization (adopted by the International Health Conference held in 1946 and which came into force in 1948). It should be clarified that this right does not entail the right to be *healthy* – noting that such a right is unfulfillable given people can develop disease, suffer disabling injuries and remain ill regardless of what and how many resources are spent to prevent or minimise these (Rumbold 2015). Rather, as stated in the Preamble to the WHO Constitution and in general comment 14 of article 12 of the United Nations' *International Covenant on Economic, Social and Cultural Rights* (United Nations CESCR 2000), the right to health entails the right to *the highest attainable standard of health*. The right to the highest attainable standard of health is, in turn, interpreted by WHO as requiring states (governments and public authorities) to:

> *ensure access to timely, acceptable, and affordable health care of appropriate quality as well as to providing for the underlying determinants of health, such as safe and potable water, sanitation, food, housing, health-related information and education, and gender equality.* (WHO 2017c)

The right to health and health care is complex and controversial (Callahan 2009; Daniels 2006; Dyck 2005; Nunes et al 2017; Powers & Faden 2006; Rumbold 2015; Zuniga et al 2013). As well as being a sensitive moral issue, it is also a highly charged political issue, as ongoing media-reported debates on population health and health care resource allocation make plain (see, for example, the debate in the *International Journal of Health Policy and Management* on global developments in priority setting in health, advanced by Baltussen and colleagues (2017), Seixas and colleagues (2017) and Schrecker (2018), and Harris and colleagues' (2017) series of 10 papers reporting the findings of its 'Sustainability in health care by allocating resources effectively' (SHARE) program implemented at Monash Health, the largest health service network in the Australian State of Victoria).

Bioethicists have yet to find a happy medium between the many competing and conflicting views on the subject. Some philosophers have classically argued that health and health care are something all people are equally entitled to, regardless of the cost (Lane et al 2017). Where human life is at stake, they contend, decisions about health and health care should not be constrained by economic considerations (Brody 1986; Powers & Faden 2006). Moreover, in keeping with what is known as the 'rescue principle', which imposes a duty on individuals and communities to 'save and rescue human life' and to 'prevent and avoid illness, injuries, and violations of human rights generally' (Dyck 2005: 280), it is regarded as intolerable when a society 'allows people to die who could have been saved by spending more money on health care' (Beauchamp & Childress 2001: 246). If more money is required, the solution is relatively simple: redirect society's resources – for example, away from gross expenditures on arsenals of arms and other life-threatening instruments of war, and towards improving health promotion and illness–injury prevention programs and redressing existing inefficiencies in the system (Dyck 2005: 317 pe) and the growing 'inappropriate allocation' of finite health care resources (Kaufman 2015) (see also Porter's (2010) highly cited commentary on the question of 'What is value in health care?'; Welch and colleagues' (2011) *Over-diagnosis*, in which consideration is given to the ramifications of unnecessary testing, drugs and surgeries, and the recent burgeoning literature on 'over-diagnosis' and 'medical overuse' (see, for example, systematic reviews by Morgan and colleagues (2018) and Jenniskens and colleagues (2017), and commentaries by Armstrong (2018) and Hofmann (2017)); and Callahan's (2009) *Taming the beloved beast*, followed by the equally provocative works of Kaufman's (2015) *Ordinary medicine: extraordinary treatments, longer lives, and where to draw the line* and Fourie and Rid's (2016) *What is enough?: Sufficiency, justice and health*; in these works robust calls are made for a radical re-thinking about health care, how to ensure the sufficient and just distribution of health care in the face of ever-dwindling resources and the need to achieve economically sustainable reform).

Others argue that it is implausible and impossible to ensure 'good health' and to provide a high standard of health care to all persons equally. In the case of health care, at best, all that people can reasonably claim is a 'decent minimum' of health care, as measured in terms of the amount necessary to secure a minimally decent or 'tolerable' life (Buchanan 1984; see also Engelhardt 1986; Fried 1982; Nunes et al 2017; Rumbold 2015; Sreenivasan 2007). Some theorists further argue that having access to only a 'decent minimum' of health care is a more plausible idea, particularly when it is considered that social determinants are a more reliable precursor of health and that having universal access to health care as such does not necessarily ensure *health* (Engster 2014; Rumbold 2015; Sreenivasan 2007). Not all agree, however. Some counter that even a 'decent minimum' of health care can still not be 'decent' since even this level can leave people who are less well off with poorer health outcomes relative to those who are more affluent (Ter Meulen 2011). Others, meanwhile, have argued that there is no such thing as a right to health care. One philosopher has even claimed that it is *immoral* to speak of health care as a 'right' (Sade 1983), and another that the expression 'a right to health care' is nothing but a 'dangerous slogan' (Fried 1982: 395).

Charles Fried (1982: 400) claims that the 'impossible dilemma posed by the promise of a right to health care' is really nothing more than a product of 'our culture's inability to face and cope with the persistent facts of illness, old age, and death'. He goes on to assert provocatively that:

> *Because we are little able to come to terms with the hazards which illness proposes, because the old are a burden and an embarrassment, because we pretend that death does not exist, we employ elaborate ruses to put these things out of the ambit of our ordinary lives.* (Fried 1982: 400)

Whether the right to health and health care is a bogus claim, a dangerous slogan or a cultural quirk will, however, depend very much on how the notions of 'health' and 'health care' are interpreted (see, for example, Nunes et al 2017; Rumbold 2015). For instance, there is room to suggest that criticism of the right to health care derives from the erroneous equation of 'health care' with 'medical care' (Schneiderman 2011). Since medical care makes up only a small proportion of overall health care, it is obviously not synonymous with health care. Moreover, as the vast body of literature on the social determinants of health makes plain, even if medical care were the major form of health care, it would not necessarily guarantee 'good health' (Sreenivasan 2007; Wilkinson & Marmot 2003). Once the notions of 'health' and 'health care' are understood in more holistic terms, the right to these things may not seem so outrageous, fraudulent or even culturally odd as a claim.

Every culture has its way of promoting health and preventing ill-health, of dealing with sickness, illness, pain and suffering, and of caring for the ill and injured, and the dying. However, not every culture embraces Western scientific medicine as the most effective way of dealing with health, sickness and related illness and/or end-of-life experiences. Thus not every culture is posed with the dilemma of economic restrictions on resource allocation. Once health and health care, in their more holistic and socially determined sense, are seen as an important means of promoting a person's *total* (and not merely physical) wellbeing, it becomes increasingly difficult to deny that claims to it are valid and morally justified. What makes a claim to health and health care compelling is that, once it is accepted, it has the moral power to prescribe actions to relieve the distressing symptoms caused by illness and injuries, to promote human wellbeing (a moral end) and, indeed, promote human life itself (also a moral end) (Nunes et al 2017; Rumbold 2015). If the entitlements to health and health care are denied, then people's entitlements to a range of other interests must also be denied, including those of life, happiness and even the exercise of self-determining choices.

It is beyond the scope of this text to deal with the many arguments and counter-arguments raised in response to the question of whether people have a right to health and health care. What is of concern here is to clarify the *nature* of the claim to a right to health and health care, and what might be meant by such a claim.

People's entitlement to receive health and health care first received global recognition with the signing of the United Nations *Universal Declaration of Human Rights* on 10 December 1948. Article 25 states:

> Everyone has the right to a standard of living adequate for the health and wellbeing of himself [sic] and his [sic] family, including food, clothing, housing and medical care and necessary social services, and the right to security in the event of unemployment, sickness, disability, widowhood, old age or other lack of livelihood in circumstances beyond his [sic] control. (United Nations 1978: 8)

Since the signing of this declaration, the question of the right to health and health care has taken on a new meaning, and has emerged largely as a result of what people perceive to be an 'unjust or unfair state of affairs' involving present structures of health and social care, which are seen as diminishing and even eliminating possibilities for the enhancement of the quality of human life and for human life itself (Powers & Faden 2006).

In speaking of the more specific right to health care, it is important to distinguish at least four different senses in which it can be claimed – that is, the right to equal access to health care, the right to have access to appropriate care, the right to quality care, and the right to safe care.

The right to equal access to health care

Access to health care refers to 'whether people who are – or should be – entitled to health care services receive them' (Emanuel 2000: 8; see also Lane et al 2017; Nunes et al 2017; Rumbold 2015). The right to equal access to health care raises questions of distributive justice and of how the benefits and burdens associated with health care service delivery ought to be distributed. It also raises questions of whether people or institutions can be found morally negligent for failing to provide equal access to health care for the people requiring it. Responses refuting this sense of a right to health care typically centre on such arguments as: 'there is not a "bottomless pit" of health care resources, and somebody has to do without'.

Specifically, the 'scarce resources, but unlimited wants' argument tends to be constructed as follows:

1. the demand for health care has outstripped supply
2. this is fundamentally because health care resources are limited
3. different people have different health needs, and different views on how existing resources should be used to meet these needs
4. it is true that existing health care resources can be used in alternative ways
5. nevertheless, health care resources are limited, so it is not possible to satisfy everybody's needs and wants (Beauchamp & Childress 2013; Dyck 2005).

The ultimate conclusion drawn from these premises is that, inevitably, choices will have to be made. In particular, borrowing from Sheehan and Wells (1985: 59), choices will have to be made about:

1. the conditions for which scarce resources should be made available
2. the priority with which given conditions should be treated.

It remains an open question, however, whether the premises of the 'scarce resources, but unlimited wants' argument are to be accepted and, further, whether its apparent 'inevitable' conclusions must also be accepted. Given the politicisation of the health care resources debate, it is far from clear that the 'scarce resources' argument must be accepted – at least not in its conventional form. Further, it is also open to question whether we are obliged to accept that economic principles ought to supplant morality as the ultimate test of conduct, as an economic rationalisation approach to health care seems to demand. Human life is not something that can be reduced, like an object, to mere economic worth. Attempts to do so risk seeing 'worthless' human beings (increasingly characterised as 'unproductive burdens on society') denied the health care entitlements they would otherwise be entitled morally to receive. This is not to say that there is no place for the economics of health care to be regarded as an important ethical issue requiring attention. For example, Baily (2011), a US health economist, has persuasively argued that *health care economics* is – and should be seen as – *an ethical issue in its own right* and it is time that it was placed firmly back on the public agenda.

It is important to recognise meanwhile that the issue of resource allocation in health care goes far beyond the simple question of merely *how to allocate dollars and cents*. It involves much broader questions of how 'equity in health care' should itself be defined (Lane et al 2017), how to measure quality of life, quality of care, the value and efficacy of health care and medical treatment (defined as 'outcomes relative to costs' (Porter 2010: 2477)), and how to calculate cost-effectiveness as well as complex socio-cultural questions pertaining to power, politics and profit (Callahan 2009; Engster 2014; Fourie & Rid 2016; Kaufman 2015; Porter 2010; Schneiderman 2011; Scott 2014; Ter Meulen 2011; Welch et al 2011). Fundamentally, it also involves questions of how best to promote *health*, not merely how to *access* health care services in 'bricks and mortar' hospitals and specialist clinics.

The right to have access to appropriate care

The right to have access to appropriate care is a second sense in which a right to health care can be claimed. This sense raises important questions concerning the conventional models of health care delivery (their value and effectiveness), the ability generally of health care services to accommodate people's personal preferences, health beliefs, health values and health practices, and, of relevance to multicultural societies, the capacity of health care services to uphold agreed standards of cultural *competency* and cultural safety when caring for people of diverse cultural and language backgrounds. As examples given in Chapter 4 have already shown, failure to provide health care in a culturally appropriate, responsive and informed manner can have harmful consequences (clinically, legally and morally). Other examples given throughout this book will lend further weight to claims that failure to provide people with access to appropriate care can result in otherwise preventable adverse outcomes for patients and health service providers alike.

Many other examples can be given here. The complementary therapy movement, for instance, has posed all sorts of ethical issues for health service providers, particularly in instances where patients prefer to use untested vitamin or herbal remedies, and other 'alternative' therapeutic agents for serious diseases, rather than risk the known and unpleasant side effects of more orthodox medical treatments. To some extent this type of problem has been overcome on account of alternative therapies becoming better researched and more widely accepted by health professionals. Thus, today, it is not uncommon for patients to receive a combination of orthodox and unorthodox treatments.

Another aspect of 'appropriate care' entails patients having access to people (lay folk and professional) of their own choosing. It also includes patients' entitlements to seek a second medical opinion, to refuse a recommended medical therapy, to choose an alternative health therapy, to be surrounded by family and friends and for them to have unrestricted visiting rights, and to decline to be 'ordered' to do anything they do not wish to do. As the Australian Consumers' Association (1988: 16) stated three decades ago, patients do not need a doctor's or nurse's 'permission' (to be distinguished here from *advice*) for anything.

The right to quality care

A right to appropriate *quality care* is the third sense in which the right to health care can be claimed (Nunes et al 2017).

Quality in health care (to be distinguished from *safety in health care*) has been defined as 'the degree to which health services for individuals and populations increase the likelihood of desired health outcomes consistent with current professional knowledge' (Runciman et al 2009: 22). In keeping with the

Australian Commission on Safety and Quality in Health Care framework (ACSQHC 2010), high-quality care is always:

1. *consumer centred – which means: providing care that is easy for patients to get when they need it; making sure that health care staff respect and respond to patient choices, needs and values; forming partnerships between patients, their family, carers and health care providers*
2. *driven by information – which means: using up-to-date knowledge and evidence to guide decisions about care; collecting and analysing data on quality and safety and feeding back information for improvement; taking action to improve patients' experiences.* (ACSQHC 2010: 2)

In light of the above provisions, it can be seen that the 'quality care' sense of the right to health care imposes a range of obligations and responsibilities on health care providers including having the 'right attitude' as well as the 'right knowledge' and 'right skills' – in short being *competent* in their practice.

The right to safe care

Safety, which is often included as a component of quality, is different from quality in that it has a different emphasis, notably 'the reduction of risk of unnecessary harm associated with healthcare to an acceptable minimum' (Runciman et al 2009: 21). In keeping with the *Australian safety and quality framework for health care* (ACSQHC 2010: 2), *safe care* is also *consumer centred* and *driven by information* (as outlined above). In addition, safe health care is *organised* for safety, by which is meant that safety is made a '*central feature* of how healthcare facilities run, how staff work and how funding is organised' [emphasis added] (ACSQHC 2010: 2).

It is generally accepted that all people receiving health care have the *right to be safe* (Kohn et al 2000; Sharpe 2004). This right has been interpreted to mean 'the right to be kept free of danger or risk of injury while in health care domains', which in turn has been further interpreted as entailing 'a correlative duty on the part of health service providers to ensure that people who are receiving care are kept free of danger or risk of injury while receiving that care' (Johnstone & Kanitsaki 2007c: 186). These moral requirements are unremarkable in that they 'reflect the well-established principle in health care of "do no harm" and the associated moral duty on the part of health care providers to avoid commissions and omissions that could otherwise result in preventable harm to patients' (Johnstone 2007b: 82). Underpinning this stance is the universal recognition that 'people generally have a special interest in their significant moral interests (e.g. to life, quality of life, dignity, respect) in not being harmed and that this special interest ought to be protected – provided this can be done without sacrificing other significant moral interests' (Johnstone 2007b: 82).

The International Council of Nurses regards patient safety as being 'fundamental to quality health and nursing care' and asserts that all nurses have a fundamental responsibility to 'address patient safety in all aspects of care', including (but not limited to) 'informing patients and others about risk and risk reduction', 'advocating for patient safety' and 'reporting adverse events' (ICN 2012b: 1). In keeping with the principles of a 'system approach' to human error management, the ICN explains:

> Early identification of risk is key to preventing patient injuries, and depends on maintaining a culture of trust, honesty, integrity, and open communication among patients and providers in the health care system. ICN strongly supports a system-wide approach, based on a philosophy of transparency and reporting – not on blaming and shaming the individual care provider – and incorporating measures that address human and system factors in adverse events. (ICN 2012b: 1)

(The issues of reporting patient safety concerns will be discussed in Chapters 11 and 12.)

Challenges posed by the right to health and health care

Nurses, individually and collectively, have a moral responsibility to act in ways that promote and protect people's rights to health and health care. How well they can and will succeed in fulfilling this responsibility, however, will depend on how they view justice and the demands it places on them. As Dyck (2005: 322) reminds us, 'In the end, health care is one of the areas that test whether members of the community in question are aware of, and willing to meet, the moral demands of the moral requisites of community.' Moreover, in the context of claims to a 'decent minimum of health care':

> *To ask what justice demands of us, to ask what we owe one another, is to ask what kind of community we aspire to be in our relations to one another, particularly when some among us are ill and otherwise in need. What we do about health care reflects what kind of community we are, and what we think ought to be done about health care reflects what kind of community we think we ought to be.* (Dyck 2005: 307–8)

The question of health care justice, and in particular the problem of health inequities, will be considered in more detail in the final chapter of this book.

The right to make informed decisions

Obtaining informed consent to care and treatment from patients or their surrogates (i.e. if lacking the capacity to give consent) is a fundamental ethical and legal obligation of attending health professionals, including nurses. Inherent in nursing practice is recognition of the right of people to make *informed decisions* and to formally consent (or refuse to consent) to care and treatment related to their health needs. To this end *The ICN code of ethics for nurses* (ICN 2012a: 2) prescribes: 'The nurse ensures that the individual receives sufficient information on which to base consent for care and related treatment'. This responsibility is reiterated in national codes of conduct for nurses; some examples include: the NMBA (2018a) *Code of conduct for nurses* (Principle 2.3), the NCNZ (2012a) *Code of conduct for nurses* (Principle 3), the NMC (2015) *The code: professional standards of practice and behaviour for nurses and midwives* (Principle 4), the CNA (2017) *Code of ethics for registered nurses* (Part 1c), the ANA (2015) *Code of ethics for nurses with interpretive statements* (Provision 1.4) and the SNB (2018) *Code of conduct for nurses and midwives* (Standard 2).

In recent years the adoption of 'consumer engagement', 'patient participation' and 'patient-centred care' as fundamental standards of safety and quality in health care has seen significant improvements in consent processes, including the provision of essential information to enable engaged decision-making by patients. Nonetheless, problems remain. Of concern to nurses are the daily challenges they face when, due to contextual factors that are often beyond their control, they are hindered in their attempts to enable patients and their loved ones to obtain the information they need and which is required to enable them to make an informed consent to care and treatment. Individuals who are vulnerable (e.g. the frail elderly, children, people with cognitive impairment, patients who do not speak or understand English, people with mental health problems/mental illness) are particularly at risk of having their entitlements to make informed decisions overlooked and even violated – especially when being cared for in time-pressured and rapidly changing environments such as the emergency department, a busy surgical ward or the operating room.

As noted in the opening paragraph of this subsection, people have a fundamental right to make informed decisions and to formally consent (or refuse to consent) to care and treatment in health care contexts. This right has both a legal and ethical basis and is widely recognised in a range of policy documents and health care standards, as well as in the codes of conduct and ethics of the health care professions. The issue of informed consent has obvious implications for nurses, not least on account of their being at the forefront of receiving requests from patients and relatives for information. Also, nurses are at the forefront of being expected to take appropriate action when patients' information needs are not being met and/or when their (the patients') entitlements in regard to consent practices are unjustly violated. It is therefore important that nurses have a thorough understanding of the nature and function of informed consent, as well as their responsibilities as nurses in relation to facilitating patients making informed decisions about recommended care and treatment options, as specified in their respective codes of ethics and conduct. It is to exploring these two issues that this discussion will now turn.

What is informed consent?

Informed consent is defined by the Australian Commission on Safety and Quality in Health Care (ACSQHC) as a 'process of communication between a patient and a clinician about options for treatment, care processes or potential outcomes' (ACSQHC 2017: 289). This communication process is aimed at (and is expected to result in) obtaining 'the patient's authorisation or agreement to undergo a specific intervention or participate in planned care' (ACQSHC 2017: 289). The key purpose of the communication is to ensure that the patient 'has an understanding of the care they will receive, all the available options and the expected outcomes, including success rates and side effects for each option' (ACSQHC 2017: 289).

Positioned as a national safety and quality health service accreditation standard, all public health services are expected: to implement processes to enable partnership with patients in decisions about planning and delivering their care including informed consent to treatment, to have in place mechanisms to monitor and improve documentation of informed consent, and to have in place mechanisms to align the information provided to patients with their capacity to understand.

It should perhaps be clarified that the doctrine of informed consent, although having a profound ethical dimension, is essentially a legal doctrine developed partially out of recognition of the patient's right to self-determination and partially out of the doctor's duty to give the patient 'information about proposed treatment so as to provide him or her with the opportunity of making an "informed" or "rational" choice as to whether to undergo the treatment' (Robertson 1981: 102; see also Beauchamp & Childress 2013; Staunton & Chiarella 2017). In distinguishing the differences between a legal and a moral approach to informed consent, Faden and Beauchamp (1986: 4) explain that, from the perspective of legal law, the approach taken to informed consent 'springs from pragmatic theory', which focuses more on a doctor's duty *to disclose information to patients* and not to injure them. By contrast, from the perspective of moral philosophy, the approach taken to informed consent 'springs from a principle of respect for autonomy that focuses on the patient or subject, who has a right to make an autonomous choice' (Faden & Beauchamp 1986: 4). The overall purpose of informed consent is, however, a moral one in that it seeks to protect patients and their loved ones from preventable harm and to improve the safety and quality of health service provision.

Whether such a clear-cut distinction can be drawn between a legal and a moral approach to informed consent is a matter of some controversy. The moral demand to respect autonomy is clearly the prime motivator of the doctor's duty to disclose information, and the moral principle of non-maleficence is the prime motivator of the doctor's duty not to injure or harm patients. It seems that, although the moral and legal approaches to informed consent can be loosely distinguished, they are nevertheless inextricably linked. It is this linkage which highlights the other important functions, besides the promotion of patient autonomy, that the application of the doctrine of informed consent also serves, namely those of protecting patients, avoiding fraud and duress (i.e. as occurs when information is not disclosed, or is disclosed in a manner that seeks to manipulate choice), of encouraging self-scrutiny by health professionals, of promoting 'rational' and systematic moral decision-making, and of involving the public 'in promoting autonomy as a general social value and in controlling biomedical research' (Beauchamp & Childress 1983: 67; see also Capron 1974; Gert et al 1997).

There is no question that consent practices have improved considerably over the past four decades (Wolf et al 2018). Health professionals have increasingly recognised the benefits of ensuring that patients (and their proxies) are informed appropriately about their care and treatment options, and patients (and their proxies) are more willing to question the information that they have been provided in order to inform their choices and consent to treatment (Kerridge et al 2013). Even so, some unresolved issues remain. For example, when seeking consent to treatment, health professionals must also inform patients of their entitlement to refuse a recommended medical or nursing procedure, and the opportunity to refuse must always be presented without prejudice to them. This entitlement holds even when health care providers do not agree with refusal or when refusal may cause them to experience distress.

A lack of qualified health interpreters in health care contexts can also compromise informed consent processes. For example, a 2005 Australian study (Johnstone & Kanitsaki 2007a) has suggested that, in some situations, because of not having ready access to qualified health interpreters, doctors sometimes rely on diagnostic testing (often subjecting patients to an unnecessary barrage of expensive diagnostic investigations) rather than direct diagnostic questioning of patients to find out what might be wrong with them. Consent practices in these situations were, at best, 'dubious'. The study revealed that a *testing* rather than a *therapeutic communication* (questioning) approach to medical care was most likely to occur in situations where attending health professionals took the stance of treating patients 'as if' they were unconscious – sometimes referred to colloquially as 'veterinary medicine' (Johnstone & Kanitsaki 2007a: 101). In a US case, a patient who was 'continuously crying' was deemed to be 'non-verbal' on account of going all day without an interpreter enabling her to voice what was wrong (she was in pain) (Taira 2018). Progressive commentary and a growing body of published research (too numerous to list here) has underscored ongoing issues concerning the need to improve communication and consent procedures with patients with limited English proficiency (see, for example, Basu G et al 2017; Lee et al 2017; Taira 2018).

The analytic components and elements of an informed consent

The concept of informed consent is comprised of five analytic components: *disclosure, comprehension (understanding), voluntariness, competence* and *consent* itself (Faden & Beauchamp 1986). In their classic work on the subject, Faden and Beauchamp (1986: 54) argue that, for consent to be regarded as *informed*, it must satisfy a number of criteria, notably:

> *(1) a patient or subject must agree to an intervention based on an understanding of (usually disclosed) relevant information, (2) consent must not be controlled by influences that would engineer the outcome, and (3) the consent must involve the intentional giving of permission for an intervention.*

More recently, Beauchamp and Childress (2013) have argued that, for consent to be informed, the following seven elements must be evident:

1. *Threshold elements (preconditions)*
    (i) *Competence (to understand and decide)*
    (ii) *Voluntariness (in deciding)*
2. *Information elements*
    (iii) *Disclosure (of material information)*
    (iv) *Recommendation (of a plan)*
    (v) *Understanding (of 3 and 4)*
3. *Consent elements*
    (vi) *Decision (in favour of plan)*
    (vii) *Authorization (of the chosen plan).* (Beauchamp & Childress 2013: 124)

The plausibility of the analytic components and elements of informed consent as outlined above will be considered further in Chapter 8.

Informed consent and ethical principlism

As stated above, informed consent is in essence a legal doctrine. Even so, it also rests heavily on ethical principlism (discussed in Chapter 3), for both its content and its justification as an action guide. The principles of particular importance here include those of:

- *autonomy* – which demands respect for patients as self-determining choosers, and justifies allowing them the option of accepting risks
- *non-maleficence* – which demands the protection of patients from battery, assault, trespass, exploitation and other harms that may result from inadequate or inappropriate consent processes (including inadequate, inappropriate or manipulative disclosures of information)
- *beneficence* – which demands the maximisation of patient wellbeing via consent processes
- *justice* – which demands fairness and that patients not be unduly or intolerably burdened by consent processes.

It should be noted that, although autonomy is *a* value underlying the doctrine of informed consent, it is not *the* value, nor an *absolute* value. As Faden and Beauchamp (1986: 18) point out, at best autonomy is only a prima-facie value, and to regard it as having overriding value would be both historically and culturally 'odd'. This is not to say that autonomy does not have a significant place in a moral approach to informed consent. It merely means that it does not have a *sole* place, and may be justly overridden or restricted by other moral considerations and principles, such as those already mentioned.

The right not to know

Developments in the field of genomics over the past two decades have rekindled debate on the so-called 'right to genetic ignorance' and the right of people not to be burdened with 'unwanted knowledge' about their genetic constitution (Chadwick et al 2014). Central to this debate is the question of whether, counterbalancing the right *to know*, people also have the right *not to know* – that is, to remain consciously ignorant of their genetic constitutions or other information about themselves or others.

Some argue, unequivocally, that there can be no right to genetic ignorance; quite the reverse: people in fact have *a duty to know* their genetic constitutions (Bortolotti & Widdows 2011; May & Spellecy 2006; Räikkä 1998; Rhodes 1998; Takala 1999, 2001; Turner 2009; Wilson 2005). Key reasons for this include: to prevent harm to others (i.e. passing on harmful genetic diseases to offspring), to prevent harm to self (i.e. the early diagnosis of genetic diseases, or predispositions to them, will enable people to obtain timely medical management and treatment), and to protect autonomy (having access to relevant information is essential to self-determination and the exercise of autonomous choice) (May & Spellecy 2006; Räikkä 1998; Takala 1999, 2001). Accordingly, informing people of their genetic constitution – even if they do not want to know about it – is justified (*reasonable paternalism* argument) (Wilson 2005). Second, there are no grounds for plausibly claiming a right to 'self-regarding foolishness', of which a claim to genetic ignorance is seen to be an example (Takala 1999).

Others, however, are more circumspect. Although acknowledging that the right *not to know* is controversial, they hold that it can nonetheless be justified. First, respect is due to people's preferences (*self-determination and autonomy* argument); by this view there is no duty to know (Häyry & Takala 2001). Second, people have a right to genetic *privacy* and to be free of trespass (individuals are sovereign and are entitled to protect their private sphere, notwithstanding that this private sphere also includes genetic information about their forebears, which they may have preferred were kept private). Once known it can be difficult to maintain the confidentiality of personal information; as Turner (2009: 300) notes, 'it is sometimes impossible to learn something without permitting others to learn that information as well' and to prevent them from making harmful disclosures of that information. Third, imposing unwanted information on people violates their sovereignty and risks 'smuggling' medical paternalism back into practice (*anti-paternalism argument*) (Häyry & Takala 2001; Takala 2001). Finally, the predictive power of genetic profiling is overstated; people could be harmed by information about their genetic constitution – particularly if, on the basis of the information received, they take drastic action aimed at preventing a disease that, on the balance of probabilities, may never develop (e.g. undergoing a bilateral mastectomy to avoid the risk of breast cancer, or committing suicide out of a fear of developing Alzheimer's disease).

Questions concerning *the right to know versus the right not to know* have relevance to other areas in health care, not just in the domain of genetic profiling. For instance, there are some circumstances in which patients do not always want to receive information that might otherwise be necessary to meet the criteria of providing an informed consent to treatment (e.g. for the treatment for a cancer-related illness) (Stahl & Tomlinson 2017). Moreover, as discussed in Chapter 4, there are situations (e.g. having a cancer diagnosis disclosed) where a patient might, on the basis of strongly held cultural health beliefs and practices, unequivocally decline the opportunity to receive the 'unwanted' information. In these kinds of situations, when patients make an authentic choice not to receive certain information and, on reflection, are not open to changing their minds about receiving the information in question, then to impose this information upon the patients would count as a paternalistic act – which might not be justified (the subject of 'paternalism' will be considered below).

In weighing up the right to know and the right not to know, it is important to be mindful that knowledge is not a neutral force: while knowledge can empower people, it can also constrain and restrict them. As Turner (2009: 308) explains,

> *Knowing enlarges our set of possibilities but also narrows it. It can reinforce our beliefs or overturn them. It is, in short, a chaotic force, one often beyond our control, that sculpts our very persons as it (a) reduces the world of unlimited options to a restricted set of rational objectives, dividing conduct into the rational and the impermissibility irrational, and (b) changes the way we see ourselves and the world around us. Even when knowledge is not toxic […] it might be a dangerous weapon capable of being turned against us by others.*

In light of this, it is understandable that, in some situations, people would rather remain ignorant than be burdened with a knowledge that stands to disrupt their meaning and place in the world at large (recall the example of 'Mr G' given in Chapter 4, and the harmful consequences of the attending doctor imposing information about his cancer-related diagnosis and prognosis in a manner that was against his and his family's wishes). Where deciding the right *not to know* stands as a conscious decision and poses no risks to the significant moral interests of others, health professionals ought to respect this preference – although noting that ascertaining this preference may, in reality, be difficult. As Turner (2009: 351–2) goes on to point out:

> *Without asking directly, it is impossible to be absolutely certain whether an individual wants, at a given moment, to learn some piece of information. But, asking that question itself conveys information, diminishing to at least some degree the ignorance that individual might have wanted to maintain.* [emphasis added]

For example, although well intended, the common practice in Australian hospitals of independently seeking the wishes of non-English speaking patients through the use of an interpreter risks violating their right 'not to know'. This practice generally entails a doctor or another member of the health care team getting patients aside from their family members and independently questioning them through the use of an interpreter about whether they want to be told the results of diagnostic tests directly (e.g. for ascertaining a cancer diagnosis), or whether they prefer this information be relayed to their family instead. This approach is problematic since it risks 'letting the cat out of the bag': by asking the patient the question, the very thing the patient does not want to know is revealed – that is, that he is facing a cancer-related illness.

Informed consent and the sovereignty of the individual

Foundational to the doctrine of informed consent is the view that the individual is sovereign: alias the *sovereignty of the individual*. This highly individualistic and idealistic notion characterises the person (patient) as a solitary competent individual who possesses 'a sphere of protected activity or privacy free from unwanted interference'; by this view, although 'influence is acceptable', coercion in any form is not (Kuczewski 1996: 30). Kuczewski explains that:

> Within this zone of privacy, one is able to exercise his or her liberty and discretion. Within this protected sphere take place disclosure, comprehension, and choice, which express the patient's right of self-determination ... The person is opaque to others and therefore the best judge and guardian of his or her own interests. Although the physician may be the expert on the medical 'facts', the patient is the only individual with genuine insight into his [sic] private sphere of 'values'. Because treatment plans should reflect personal values as well as medical realities, the patient must be the ultimate decision-maker. (Kuczewski 1996: 30)

A significant implication of this view is that the patient's family, friends and/or chosen carers are conceived 'as comprising competing interests'; they are also seen as having no entitlements whatsoever in regard to any consent to medical treatment processes in which the 'sovereign individual' might otherwise engage (Kuczewski 1996). This may help to explain some of the tensions examined previously in Chapter 4 in regard to family members seeking active participation in consent to medical treatment processes for their loved ones and the reluctance by some doctors and nurses to involve these family members in such processes.

Negative attitudes towards family involvement in patient decision-making and consent to treatment are, however, shifting. It is being increasingly recognised that family members and chosen carers have a vital role to play in advocating the safe and high-quality care of their loved ones. By being intimately acquainted with ('knowing well') the patient, family members and chosen carers are able to provide appropriate and meaningful feedback to their loved ones, and to generally assist in 'reality checking' their loved one's decisions and the values, beliefs (new and old) and deliberations influencing these decisions. The role of family members and loved ones in consent processes is particularly important given that, in stressful and unfamiliar situations, patients are vulnerable both to information overload and to short-term memory loss. The stress of being admitted to hospital; of coping with feelings of pain, fear and anxiety; of being separated from the familiarity of one's home, family and friends; the general disruption of one's life, not to mention the effort required to adapt to a new (hospital) environment characterised by strange smells, sights, noises, tastes, routines, faces, procedures and sensations – all these may contribute to lessening an individual's capacity to pay attention to and to recall information that has been disclosed.

To complicate matters, health professionals seeking consent or giving information do not always manage their encounters with patients very well. Some use a hurried, uninterested and sometimes intimidating approach when seeking a patient's consent. When seeking consent from a patient, health professionals may fail to give due attention to such things as: controlling their tone of voice, choosing a suitable time and place to approach the patient, ensuring privacy, using the appropriate body language and facial expressions, choosing the right words, avoiding complicated jargon, sitting physically at the same level as the patient, being generally respectful, and so on. It such situations, a patient's family or loved ones can be especially supportive and can play a vital role in restoring the otherwise-diminished autonomy that their sick loved ones might be experiencing.

Paternalism and informed consent

The word *paternalism* comes from the Latin *pater* meaning 'father', and literally means 'in the manner of a father, especially in usurping individual responsibility and the liberty of choice' (*Collins Australian dictionary* 2011: 1210). In the bioethics literature, paternalism has been defined in a variety of ways. Literature published in the early 1970s, for example, defined paternalism (construed as a principle *viz* the *paternalistic principle* (Beauchamp 1980: 98)) as:

> *the interference with a person's liberty of action justified by reasons referring exclusively to the welfare, good, happiness, needs, interests or value of the person being coerced.* (Dworkin 1972: 65)

Subsequently, paternalism was defined more specifically as:

> *interference with a person's freedom of action or freedom of information, or the deliberate dissemination of misinformation, where the alleged justification of interfering or misinforming is that it is for the good of the person who is interfered with or misinformed.* (Buchanan 1978: 372)

A further modification in definition resulted in the suggestion that for an act to be paternalistic:

> *There must be a violation of a person's autonomy … There must be a [sic] usurpation of decision-making, either by preventing people from doing what they have decided or by interfering with the way in which they arrive at their decision.* (Dworkin 1988: 123)

A more recent definition of paternalism holds it to be:

> *the intentional overriding of one person's preferences or actions by another person, where the person who overrides justifies this action by appeal to the goal of benefiting or of preventing or mitigating harm to the person whose preferences or actions are overridden.* (Beauchamp & Childress 2013: 215)

Early literature on the subject distinguished between two types of paternalism: (1) harm paternalism, and (2) benefit paternalism (Beauchamp 1978; Beauchamp & Childress 1994). *Harm paternalism* (underpinned by the principle of non-maleficence) was thought to be justified where it had as its objective protecting individuals from self-inflicted harm. In contrast, *benefit paternalism* (underpinned by the principle of beneficence) was thought to be justified where it had as its objective securing a good or a beneficence that an individual would not otherwise get — for example, because their liberty is limited. These two forms of paternalism were, in turn, categorised still further, with the following distinctions being made: (1) strong (or hard) paternalism and (2) weak (or soft) paternalism, considered below.

In the case of *strong paternalism*, it was thought to be 'proper to protect or benefit a person by liberty-limiting measures' *even when his [or her] contrary choices are informed and voluntary* (Beauchamp 1978: 1197). An example of 'strong paternalism' would be where a consultant physician refuses to release a competent although seriously ill patient from hospital even though the patient has requested discharge and knows the potentially fatal consequences of his/her request.

Strong paternalism is in contradistinction to *weak paternalism*, where interference with an individual's conduct is justified only in cases where that person's conduct is 'substantially nonvoluntary or when temporary intervention is necessary to establish whether it is voluntary or not' (Feinberg 1971: 113, 116). In short, where a person's autonomy has been compromised in some way (e.g. as a result of pain, drug ingestion, psychogenic distress, physical trauma to the head that interferes with memory, and the like), it is acceptable to paternalistically override a person's choices or restrain their liberty of conduct. This form of paternalism has been widely accepted in law, medicine and moral philosophy. An example of 'weak paternalism' would be where an attending health care professional attends the scene of a motor vehicle accident and picks up an injured, partially coherent victim and takes him/her to hospital even though the victim has refused an ambulance (Beauchamp 2004: 1985).

As a point of clarification, it should be noted that harm paternalism is thought to be easier to justify and uphold than benefit paternalism. One reason for this is that it was (and is) generally thought, controversially, that we have a greater duty to avoid harm than to promote good — which may not always be within our capacity in given contexts and thus not something for which we could be held morally responsible for not doing. If it was our duty to do or promote good — even where we lacked the resources to do so — this would risk us being condemned as 'unethical' for not doing something that we could not do anyway, which would be untenable.

However defined or conceptualised, it should be noted that paternalism remains morally controversial since it always entails the choices or actions of one person being overridden by another without consent. Even if a person's stated preferences do not originate from a substantially autonomous and authentic choice, overriding his or her preference can still be paternalistic (Beauchamp & Childress 2013). This is because, even in the case of 'diminished autonomy', persons (e.g. young children, the intellectually disabled and the mentally ill) can still be capable of exercising self-interested choices. It is against this backdrop then that a key question arises, namely: 'Is paternalism ever justified and, if so, under what conditions?'

Is paternalism justified?

The literature reveals at least three possible answers to the question of whether paternalism is justified:

1 pro-paternalism (always justified)
2 anti-paternalism (never justified)
3 prima-facie paternalism (sometimes justified).

These three possible answers are discussed below.

Pro-paternalism (always justified)

Proponents of the pro-paternalism position hold that paternalism is *always justified* to 'protect individuals against themselves' (Hart 1963: 31). This position is supported by an appeal to the principles of human welfare, beneficence (e.g. as in the case of overriding the harmful choices of children) and/or 'rational consent' (meaning consent that 'would otherwise have been given'); in this instance, paternalism is thought to be justified as a kind of 'social insurance policy' for our own protection (Beauchamp 2004: 1986). Further, it is held that sometimes an immediate act of paternalism may, paradoxically, protect a person's 'deeper autonomy' – for example, in the case of someone who is depressed and suicidal (Beauchamp 1980). Justificatory considerations for strong (hard) paternalism, include the following conditions:

1. *A patient is at risk of a significant, preventable harm.*
2. *The paternalistic action will probably prevent the harm.*
3. *The prevention of harm to the patient outweighs risks to the patient of the action taken.*
4. *There is no morally better alternative to the limitations of autonomy that occurs.*
5. *The least autonomy-restrictive alternative that will secure the benefits is adopted.* (Beauchamp & Childress 2013: 222)

Anti-paternalism (never justified)

Proponents of the anti-paternalism position hold that paternalism is *never justified*. This is because paternalism always involves a violation of moral rules – for example, that we ought to respect people's choices even if we do not agree with them, provided they do not harm others; the individual is sovereign and any coercion or interference with his/her self-determining choices is morally unacceptable. Acts of paternalism also violate people's privacy and fail to treat them as the moral equals of others (Childress 1982, cited in Beauchamp 2004: 1986).

Prima-facie paternalism (sometimes justified)

Proponents of prima-facie paternalism (also known as ambivalent paternalism) hold the view that paternalism is *sometimes justified*, though severely limited. Any action of coercion against or interference with another's conduct carries a heavy burden of justification. Paternalism is justified only where:

1. *the evils prevented from occurring to the person are greater than the wrongs [if any] caused by the violation of the moral rule*

FIGURE 7.1
Three positions on paternalism

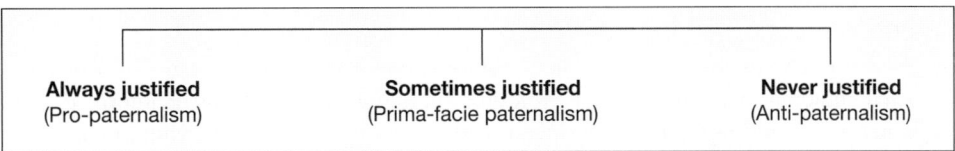

  2. *it can be universally justified under relevantly similar circumstances always to treat persons in this way.*
     (Silber 1989: 453)

These three positions may be expressed diagrammatically, as shown in Fig. 7.1.

Despite the apparent differences between these three positions, there is some agreement between the positions of 'weak paternalism' and 'anti-paternalism'. These are:

  1. *it is justifiable to interfere in order to protect persons against harm from their own substantially non-autonomous decisions; and*
  2. *it is unjustifiable to interfere in order to protect persons against harm from their own substantially autonomous decisions.* (Beauchamp 2004: 1986)

One reason for this closeness in position is that, as some contend, 'weak paternalism' is not really paternalism at all since it cannot be substantively distinguished from anti-paternalism. In the ultimate analysis, both rest on the principles of beneficence and non-maleficence, and both reject strong paternalism (which justifies overriding strongly autonomous choices). However, when it is considered that even strong paternalism rests on the principles of beneficence and non-maleficence, the differences between all three positions may, in the end, be overstated.

Applying the 'paternalistic principle' in health care

Application of the 'paternalistic principle' in health care contexts is not clear-cut and indeed raises a number of important questions, such as: 'How are we to justify overriding another's choices?', 'What constitutes beneficial and harmful outcomes for the patient?', 'What constitutes a patient's "best interests"?', 'How are we to measure the quality of another's autonomy and autonomous choices?', 'Do people have the right to refuse life-saving/enhancing treatment?' and 'What if treatments are "harmful"?'

The abuses of paternalistic decision-making and the rise of individualism and patients' rights in the 1970s and 1980s saw a backlash against paternalism in health care. The past four decades have, however, seen a tempering of this rejection (Beauchamp & Childress 2013). As Beauchamp has prophetically noted (2004: 1989):

  Paternalism seems likely to continue to be a viewpoint that will gain or lose adherents as the issues and larger social context shift. We may never again see the concentrated flurry of scholarly interest in this subject that was exhibited from the mid 1970s to the mid 1980s, but paternalism is not likely to be an issue that will soon disappear.

One author has argued controversially that medical paternalism in health care contexts (which he states is often practised 'covertly') is not only here to stay, but is also 'essential' to ethical practice and the promotion of patient autonomy; he writes:

  Although patient autonomy is dominant in current ethical discussions, medical paternalism is not extinct. Indeed it cannot become so, for the exercise of paternalism is essential to the practice of medicine. After all, we are the medical experts, and we are required to recommend what is medically best for the patient. It is therefore arguable that some measure of paternalism is involved in most treatment decisions. This covert paternalism is not necessarily bad, provided it is recognised for what it is, and is used appropriately to guide and support patient autonomy rather than to override it. (Tweeddale 2002: 236)

Informed consent and nursing care

The issues of informed consent and the right to refuse consent or receive unwanted information are all issues of moral importance to the nursing profession. Although the doctrine of informed consent has traditionally been discussed primarily in regard to medical treatment, the underlying moral values, moral principles and moral requirements of this doctrine apply equally to other kinds of health care practices and procedures, including *nursing care* and procedures (Aveyard 2004; Cole 2012). A rare example of the application of the doctrine of informed consent in nursing care domains can be found in Dudzinski and Shannon's (2006a, 2006b) case study of a competent patient's refusal of nursing care, including turning and incontinence management (see also the commentary on this case by Tong (2006)). In light of this, nurses are no less exempt than are any other health care professionals from the moral standards governing consent procedures, including the moral requirements to:

- disclose all relevant information necessary for making an informed decision about proposed nursing cares and procedures
- ensure that the patient understands the information received and the implications of giving consent
- ensure that the consent is given voluntarily (that is, that nurses do not coerce or manipulate the patient into giving consent)
- ensure that the patient has the capacity to make an informed decision, and, if not, that any surrogate decision-making on the patient's behalf is in accordance with rigorous moral standards.

Likewise the issue of paternalism: although paternalism has primarily been discussed in regard to the profession of medicine (medical paternalism), the issues raised apply just as well to nursing (nursing paternalism). These issues both stand as fertile ground for further debate, research and scholarship.

The right to confidentiality

The principle of *confidentiality* has long been recognised as an important and fundamental guide to action in – and even the cornerstone of – effective health professional–client relationships (McMahon 2006). This principle is maintained in law via statutory provisions, common law and principles of equity (Forrester & Griffiths 2015) and reflected in professional ethics via position statements, codes of conduct and codes of ethics. There are, however, notable exceptions to this duty, for instance, when:

- the patient / client (or his / her lawful representative) has given express consent to the proposed disclosure of information (including health records)
- disclosures are mandated or permitted by law (e.g. notification of known or suspected cases of child abuse / elder abuse, suspicious injuries, commission of serious offences, manifestation of 'notifiable diseases' – for example, infectious diseases such as hepatitis, typhoid fever; sexually transmitted diseases such as syphilis, gonorrhoea, acquired immunodeficiency syndrome (AIDS); and non-infectious diseases such as cancer)
- disclosures are 'in the public interest' – that is, the obligation to maintain the confidentiality of patient information may be overridden in circumstances where the public interest is at risk (e.g. where the patient has been identified as posing a threat either to a third party or to themselves) (Forrester & Griffiths 2015; Staunton & Chiarella 2017).

There are widely divergent views among health professionals and patients / clients about the nature and 'bindingness' of confidentiality, and the degree to which it is – and ought to be – upheld in practice (Bozzo 2018; Bute et al 2015; Jansen & Friedman Ross 2000; McMahon 2006; Mendelson & Wolf 2017; Piel & Opara 2018; Spooner 2015; Winslade 2004). Furthermore, whereas the professional duty to maintain patient confidentiality was once regarded as being absolute, growing dissatisfaction with this stance has seen a significant shift in both policy and practice over the past four decades, with most health professional codes and guidelines now recognising the duty to maintain confidentiality as being at best prima facie (discretionary), not absolute in nature (McMahon 2006; Spooner 2015). For example, whereas the 1983 version of the World Medical Association (WMA) *International code of medical ethics* took an absolutist position on confidentiality, stating: 'A physician shall preserve *absolute confidentiality on all he [sic] knows about his [sic] patient* even after the patient has died' [emphasis added] (p 6), the current revised 2006 version of the code takes a much more circumspect position; it states (p 2):

> *A physician shall respect a patient's right to confidentiality. It is ethical to disclose confidential information when the patient consents to it or when there is a real and imminent threat of harm to the patient or to others and this threat can be only removed by a breach of confidentiality.*

The revised Australian Medical Association's (2016) *AMA code of ethics* also recognises that, although doctors have an obligation to maintain confidentiality, exceptions may arise; Section 2.2.2 of the revised Code states:

> *Maintain the confidentiality of the patient's personal information including their medical records, disclosing their information to others only with the patient's express up-to-date consent or as required or authorised by law. This applies to both identified and de-identified patient data.*

Nursing codes and guidelines take a similar stance. *The ICN code of ethics for nurses*, for example, states: 'The nurse holds in confidence personal information and uses judgment in sharing this information' (ICN 2012a: 2). The NMBA (2018a) *Code of conduct for nurses* (Principle 3.5), in turn, states:

> *Nurses have ethical and legal obligations to protect the privacy of people. People have a right to expect that nurses will hold information about them in confidence, unless the release of information is needed by law, legally justifiable under public interest considerations or is required to facilitate emergency care.*

Likewise, the NZNC (2012a) *Code of conduct for nurses*; Principle 5 of the Code states simply: 'Respect health consumers' privacy and confidentiality', under which eight standards are described.

Confidentiality as an absolute principle

As briefly mentioned in the opening paragraphs of this section, there has been a significant shift in the way in which the duty of confidentiality is regarded and practised in health care contexts. Historically, the principle of confidentiality was interpreted as an *absolute* principle. In application it was (and still is in some contexts, e.g. the priest confessional) taken as demanding that information gained in a professional–client relationship must be kept secret, even when its disclosure might serve a greater public good. An example of the extent to which confidentiality was once regarded by professionals (especially doctors) as being absolute can be found in a 1904 case in which a physician refused to warn a prospective victim that her fiancé had syphilis, thereby risking both her and her offspring being exposed to the disease (Bok 1980). Commenting on the case, the physician wrote:

> *A single word […] would save her from this terrible fate, yet the physician is fettered hand and foot by his cast-iron code, his tongue is silenced, he cannot lift a finger or utter a word to prevent this catastrophe.*
> (Bok 1980: 147)

In another case, reported in the *British Medical Journal* (*BMJ*) in 1906, the duty of the doctor to maintain absolute confidentiality was again emphasised. The case involved a man who suffered from asthma and who sometimes became distressed and had even collapsed with his condition – although never while at work. Employed as the sole operator of a railway signal box, and fearing he would lose his job if his employer knew of his medical condition, the man refused to disclose his condition to his employer. Of this case, the editor of the *BMJ* commented:

> *The circumstances, extreme though they be, cannot be held to justify a breach of the law of professional secrecy [...] the doctor ought not to write direct to the railway company without the patient's consent, and unless he fully understands the nature of the communications to be made.* (BMJ 1906, cited in McMahon 2006: 567)

It is now widely recognised that, in cases where innocent victims stand to be significantly harmed by a failure to disclose, the demand to breach confidentiality becomes morally compelling. This was the view taken in the highly cited US legal case *Tarasoff v Regents of the University of California* (1974), credited with marking the turning point in contemporary attitudes towards the duty to maintain confidentiality in the professional–client relationship. The case involved a university student, Prosenjit Poddar, who had met and became infatuated with a young woman, Tatiana Tarasoff. Unfortunately, Tarasoff did not share Poddar's feelings, and told him so. Consequently, Poddar became very depressed and sought psychiatric help on a voluntary outpatient basis at the Cowell Memorial Hospital at the university. During a consultation with his psychologist, Dr Lawrence Moore, Poddar revealed that he seriously intended to kill Tarasoff. After receiving this information the psychologist wrote to the campus police and informed them that Poddar was 'at this point a danger to the welfare of other people and himself', also pointing out that Poddar had been threatening to kill an unnamed girl who he felt had 'betrayed him' and had 'violated his honour' (Daley 1983: 243). The psychologist then went on to ask the police for assistance in detaining Poddar for psychiatric assessment. Daley writes that the campus police detained Poddar 'but released him when he appeared rational and promised to stay away from Tarasoff' (p 235).

Following this, Poddar's psychologist was directed by a superior to take no further action and to destroy his client's records (a practice which is sometimes followed by psychologists, psychotherapists and psychiatrists in order to ensure confidentiality). Two months later, as he had threatened to his psychologist, Poddar carried out his intention and killed Tarasoff with a butcher's knife.

Daley (1983) notes that neither the girl nor her parents were warned of Poddar's threat. It seems that none of the psychotherapists involved considered it part of their professional morality to warn the victim. Even the California Supreme Court acknowledged recognition of the general rule that 'there is ordinarily no duty to control the conduct of another or to warn those endangered by such conduct' (p 235). However, the Supreme Court also recognised certain exceptions to the general rule, and its final decision in the Tarasoff case imposed a new duty to warn upon doctors and psychiatrists under its jurisdiction. Although the psychiatric profession 'reacted with alarm' to the California Supreme Court's ruling at the time (it claimed that it would 'cripple the use of psychotherapy by destroying the confidentiality vital to the psychiatrist–patient relationship' (p 234)), the 'duty to warn intended victims' is now accepted. The ethical and legal issues raised by the landmark Tarasoff case (specifically the requirement to disclose patient confidences in the interests of protecting third parties) were revisited in 2016, when another case *Volk v DeMeerieer* (in Washington State), again involving the duty to warn third parties, became the subject of public scrutiny and debate (Piel & Opara 2018). In Australia, the duty to warn an intended victim at risk of harm by another became the subject of media commentary and controversy after a Sydney woman who had contracted HIV from her husband 'successfully sued the medical practice where the couple had received premarriage testing for sexually transmitted diseases' (Lamont 2003: 1). The woman (who was in her late twenties) sued the practice for failing to tell her of her husband's HIV-positive status. Damages of $727 000 were awarded to the woman on the grounds that 'the doctors had not adequately counselled either partner about their results' (*The Age* 2003: 14). The woman learned about her husband's HIV-positive status only 15 months after they had both been tested when she found a laboratory report showing that her husband was HIV-positive; previously, the husband had shown her a falsified report declaring him to be HIV-negative. Although the court upheld the principle of doctor–patient confidentiality and affirmed that 'doctors cannot be sued for damages by maintaining the confidential relationship', it also affirmed that doctors 'must safeguard patients through proper counselling protocols and, if necessary, notify the Director of General Health, who has the power to breach confidentiality and directly warn someone they are at risk of infection' (Lamont 2003: 1). An editorial appearing in *The Age* concluded (2003: 14):

> *Doctor–patient confidentiality is an important principle and policy-makers are right to do their utmost to uphold it. But human life is even more precious and doctors have a duty to do all they can to protect those whom they believe are at risk.*

The Tarasoff case and others like it (such as the Sydney case, cited above) have served to raise interesting and thought-provoking questions about the nature and force of the principle of confidentiality and the extent to which health professionals are obliged morally to uphold it.

In general, the demand to keep secret information disclosed in a professional–client relationship is thought to derive from the broader moral principles of autonomy, non-maleficence, justice and the obligation to keep one's promises. In the case of autonomy, it is held that individuals are entitled to choose who should have access to information about themselves, as well as what information should be disclosed, if any. Non-maleficence, on the other hand, demands that people are entitled to be protected from the harms that might flow from disclosure (which can be considerable). Justice demands that a person about whom 'private' information is known deserves to be treated fairly. Promise-keeping, simply put, demands that 'added respect is due for that which one has promised to keep secret' (Bok 1980: 149), although it is generally recognised that a promise to do morally evil things is either not binding at all or 'deficient in its binding power' (Freedman 1978: 12).

In health care contexts, the supremacy of the principle of confidentiality is thought to be particularly justified on grounds that it is crucial to preserving the fiduciary (trust) nature of the health professional–patient relationship (Beauchamp & Childress 2013; Mendelson & Wolf 2017). If patients/clients can trust their attending health professionals to keep secret certain information disclosed in the professional relationship, it is thought that patients/clients will be more likely to reveal information crucial for making a correct assessment/diagnosis, and thus a correct prescription of care and treatment.

Understandably, if it were common practice to breach confidentiality, patients/clients would probably lose their trust and confidence in their attending health care professionals, and would probably refrain from divulging critical information to them. Worse, they might not seek professional help at all – something which might have the undesirable consequence of individuals, groups and indeed the community at large suffering a health status inferior to that which might otherwise be enjoyed.

The question remains, however, of whether the principle of confidentiality really is as binding as professionals seem to think it is. Where does it come from? Also, as Bok (1980: 154) correctly asks: 'Was it ever meant to stretch so far as to require lying?' and 'Why is it so binding that it can protect those who have no right to impose their incompetence, their disease, their malevolence on ignorant and innocent victims?'

In answering these questions, it is important to understand the nature of the principle of confidentiality and why, up until recently, it has been problematic in health professional practice.

Confidentiality as a prima-facie principle

On close analysis it can be seen that, at best, the principle of confidentiality is, and can only ever be, a prima-facie principle. Confidentiality has a special link to a person's *right to privacy*, which may be loosely defined as the right to 'have control over information about ourselves' or 'control over who can sense us' (McCloskey 1980; Parker 1974; Thomson 1975). This in turn is connected with the principle of autonomy, which demands that people should be respected as autonomous choosers, and have the right to act on their choices provided these do not seriously impinge on the moral interests of others. Given this, it seems reasonable to hold that, where the maintenance of confidentiality results in the moral interests of others being violated, the principle can and must be overridden. This conclusion is also partially supported by the principles of non-maleficence and justice. Thus, in instances where keeping a confidence or a secret has the unhappy consequence of causing or failing to prevent an otherwise-avoidable harm, and/or indeed results in an unequal distribution of harms over benefits, there is a very strong case supporting disclosure of the information being kept secret.

When subjected to the scrutiny of broader moral principles, it can be seen, first, that there are serious limits to the duty of secrecy and of maintaining confidentiality. Second, it is clear that, although in some instances the norm of confidentiality might justifiably extend to include lying, this does not hold unconditionally in all cases. (Given a consequentialist analysis, lying can only ever be justified on the grounds that it is necessary to prevent an otherwise-avoidable harm from occurring, and where there is no other alternative action which can be taken to prevent the foreseen harm in question.) Third, it can be seen, given the competing demands of the moral principles of non-maleficence and justice, that the principle of confidentiality can never be used morally to protect those who would impose their incompetence, their diseases and their malevolence on innocent and uninformed victims.

Unfortunately, the moral principle of confidentiality has sometimes been abused to prevent the disclosure of unscrupulous practices. For example, in the 1987 National Commission of Inquiry into the 'unfortunate experiment' at the National Women's Hospital in New Zealand, it was alleged that nurses were warned not to give evidence to the Inquiry on grounds that 'it was an offence [under the Hospital Act concerning confidentiality of patient information] to disclose information concerning the condition or medical history of any patient' (cited in Johnstone 1999a: 26–7). In the early 2000s, respective inquiries into nurse whistleblowing events concerning alleged breaches of patient safety and substandard practices at the MacArthur Health Service (MHS) in the Australian State of New South Wales (ICAC 2005a, 2005b) and the Bundaberg Base Hospital (BBH) in the Australian State of Queensland (Queensland State Archives 2005), evidence was submitted suggesting that demands to uphold confidentiality were similarly used as a mechanism to prevent nurses from disclosing their concerns to appropriate authorities when seeking to have the situations they had observed remedied (Cleary 2014).

This misuse of the principle of confidentiality stands as an example of how conventional ethical principles of conduct can be (ab)used to maintain and reinforce the status quo rather than to challenge it. Further, when more parochial interpretations and applications of the principle of confidentiality are considered, what emerges is not a respect for ethical conduct, but rather what Bok (1980: 149) describes as 'primeval tribal emotions: the loyalty to self, kin, clansmen, guild members as against … the unrelated, the outsiders, the barbarians'. Bok (p 149) concludes by warning that the principle of confidentiality can sometimes serve little more than the drive for 'self-preservation' and 'collective survival in a hostile environment'.

It is not being suggested here that the principle of confidentiality ought not to be respected. On the contrary: confidentiality is an important moral requirement of any health care professional–patient/client relationship, and one that is crucial to ensuring the protection of a patient's/client's wellbeing and moral interests. Arbitrary, indiscriminate and capricious breaches of confidentiality can have morally undesirable and even devasting consequences for patients/clients, including difficulties in obtaining employment or housing, and forming/maintaining social relationships.

As noted earlier, the principle of confidentiality is at best prima facie in nature, meaning there are situations in which it can be justly overridden. The grounds upon which a decision to disclose information about a patient must, however, be carefully evaluated against and be compliant with formally recognised legal and ethical requirements – noting that upholding the principle of confidentiality is not always straightforward, particularly in cases requiring mandatory reporting (e.g. child abuse and elder abuse). Ethical quandaries posed by mandatory reporting requirements will be considered further in Chapter 12 of this book.

The right to be treated with dignity[1]

According to Article 1 of the *Universal Declaration of Human Rights* (1948) 'All human beings are born free and equal in *dignity* and rights.' The right to dignity as implied in this statement (and which encompasses the rights of people to uphold their own dignity as well as to be treated with dignity by others) and its implications for the health and wellbeing of people have, however, been poorly addressed in the health professional literature. Although the right to *die with dignity* has been widely considered in the bioethics and nursing literature (too voluminous to list here), and has gained popular usage in contemporary debates on the provision and limits of invasive medical treatment at the end stages of life, it is important to clarify that the right to dignity involves considerably more than merely the right to *die* with dignity. Furthermore, although the terms 'dignity' and 'dying with dignity' have been and are being freely used in discussions and debates on end-of-life care, there is room to question whether those who use them have a clear understanding of what precisely they mean.

Another concern is that these terms have come to be used in a rather clichéd sense, and thus could have the undesirable consequence of a blanket definition of dignity being applied uncritically in all situations, regardless of their ethically significant differences, and in a way which could result in a serious distraction from (rather than a focus on) the moral issues at stake. For example, some speak of the removal of a life-support system, or the withdrawal of some other orthodox medical therapies, as tantamount to 'letting a person die with dignity'. What such views presume, however, is that the terms 'dignity' and 'dying with dignity' in these contexts have a clear-cut, commonsense meaning and use and, furthermore, implicitly justify the acts or omissions in relation to which they have been expressed. This usage also seems to treat the *right to dignity* as being synonymous with the *right to die with dignity*, which is wrong and misleading since the right to die with dignity is just one of several kinds of dignity rights claims that a person might exercise.

Two key questions arise here: 'What is dignity and what is meant by the right to be treated with dignity?' and 'What might be the implications of, given definitions of dignity, the right to be treated with dignity for members of the nursing profession?'

What is dignity?

The notion of dignity, what it is and what entities have it (e.g. whether non-human animals can also be characterised as having dignity) are all highly contested issues (Düwell 2011). In an attempt to unravel the rival meanings in play, it is useful first to consider the etymological origins and dictionary definitions of the term.

The word dignity comes from the Latin *dignitas*, meaning 'merit', and *dignus*, meaning 'worthy'. Today, there are as many definitions of 'dignity' as there are dictionaries. *Collins Australian dictionary* (2011: 470), for example, defines dignity as:

> [1] … *a formal, stately, or grave bearing* … [2] *the state or quality of being worthy of honour* … [3] *relative importance; rank* … [4] *sense of self importance* …

According to the *Oxford English dictionary* (2014 online), dignity is:

> 1. a. *The quality of being worthy or honourable; worthiness, worth, nobleness, excellence* … 2. a. *Honourable or high estate, position, or estimation* … 4. a. *Nobility or befitting elevation of aspect, manner, or style*

The question of dignity has also been a topic of significant philosophical debate, with little consensus being reached. For example, in 1651 the English philosopher Thomas Hobbes defined it as (1968: 52):

> (T)he publique worth of a man [sic], which is the Value set on him [sic] by the Common-Wealth … And this Value of him [sic] by the commonwealth, is understood, by offices of Command, Judicature, public Employment; or by Names and Titles, introduced for distinction of such Value.

Later philosophers, however, rejected this 'social worth' view and sought to define dignity in more sophisticated moral terms. The German philosopher Immanuel Kant, for instance, defines dignity in quite different terms as 'an intrinsic, unconditioned, incomparable worth or worthiness' (1972: 35). Rejecting the 'market value' or 'social worth' interpretations of dignity, he goes on to assert that:

> Morality or virtue – and humanity so far as it is capable of morality – alone has dignity. In this respect it cannot be compared with things that have economic value (a market price) or even with things that have an aesthetic value (a fancy price). The incomparable worth of a good man [sic] springs from his [sic] being a [moral] law making member in a kingdom of ends. (Kant 1972: 35)

More recent definitions and interpretations have tended to capture the essence of Kant's views. One philosopher, for example, argues that dignity is akin to 'justified happiness' (a happiness which is 'interpenetrated with a sense of meaning, reason, and worth') and the attainment of 'just goals' – that is, morally valuable ends (Swenson 1981: 23). The behaviourist B F Skinner (1973: 48–62) sees dignity and what he calls the 'struggle for dignity' as having many features in common with freedom and the 'struggle for freedom'.

Others meanwhile have suggested that a more fruitful approach to defining dignity is by taking into account what dignity is *not* and the various forms in which '*dignity violations*' can manifest, such as humiliation, degradation and dehumanisation (Kaufmann et al 2011a, 2011b).

Some of the most revealing and instructive definitions of dignity, however, come from a group of undergraduate nursing students completing the first year of their university nursing program. Comments were sought from the students after their clinical placement at a residential care home for the elderly. The results are summarised as follows.

- 'Dignity is concerned with self-respect, and how this is related to society – your social worth.'
- 'Dignity is a feeling of pride … of feeling good about yourself.'
- 'Dignity is having pride without shame.'
- 'Dignity is being accepting of one's self, and of what's to come … the problem is, however, that a lot of people base their self-worth on what other people think of them.'

Dying with dignity, in turn, was described by the students in the following terms:

- 'Dignity and dying with dignity is being happy with oneself, and what one has achieved in life.'
- 'Dying with dignity is dying the way you want to die.'
- 'Dignity and dying with dignity is maintaining self-value, self-respect and self-image …'
- 'Dying with dignity is having no pain, no fear. Feeling valued, and having your opinions valued. Yes. That's it! It involves having control and being valued.'
- 'Dying with dignity is putting yourself above whatever is going on around you.'

In considering all these definitions, it soon becomes apparent that there may be as many definitions of 'dignity' and 'dying with dignity' as there are people trying to define it. The lesson to be learned from this is that nurses – and indeed health care professionals generally – must never take the notion of dignity (and its usage) for granted. They must also be cautious in treating these terms as if they had clear-cut, commonsense interpretations. What one person might consider 'dignity', another person might equally reject – and this has important implications for nursing care delivery in particular, and health care management generally.

How, then, should dignity be defined? Further, what is meant by the 'right to dignity'?

Dignity and the right to dignity

Despite the variety of definitions and interpretations of the notion 'dignity', it may be broadly understood as belonging to a cluster of interrelated concepts, namely: respect, status, privacy, self-esteem and (freedom from) shame (McGee 2011: ix). Some suggest that a modern account of human dignity should minimally encapsulate the following elements, notably that the ascription of the status of human dignity:

- applies equally to all human beings
- is other regarding (i.e. it aims to regulate the relationships between humans and between humans and political institutions)
- affirms the inherent moral worth of the individual
- has overriding moral authority in the context of human rights (i.e. as a normative consideration it 'trumps' other considerations) (Düwell 2011).

Taking these concepts and attributes into account, dignity and the right to dignity in health care (encompassing the rights to uphold one's own dignity and to be treated with dignity by others) may thus be taken to mean: *a special interest that persons have in being treated as entities with intrinsic moral worth, whose autonomy and capacity for exercising self-determining choices ought to be respected by others, and who ought to be supported and facilitated in their attempts to maintain their humanity, self-respect and a sense of their own moral worth and self-esteem when in a health care context.*

Dignity violations

Before concluding this discussion on the right to dignity, some further comment on the notion of 'dignity violations' and its possible implications for the health and social wellbeing of people is warranted.

According to the late Jonathan Mann, Professor of Health and Human Rights at the Harvard School of Public Health, there exists a critical relationship between dignity – or rather 'dignity violations' – and the health and social wellbeing of people (Mann 1997: 11). Although conceding that a satisfactory definition of dignity is both complex and elusive, Mann is adamant that we can nonetheless know when our 'dignity is violated or impugned'. Moreover, by undertaking an exploration of dignity (what it means and what forms violations of it might take) we may uncover new and important understandings of human suffering and progress the human effort that is needed to redress this suffering as a health and human rights issue (Mann 1997: 11). Mann's thoughts on this are worth quoting in full; he states:

> it seems we all know when our dignity is violated or impugned. Perform the following experiment: recall, in detail, an incident from your own life in which your dignity was violated, for whatever reason. If you will immerse yourself in the memory, powerful feelings will likely arise – of anger, shame, powerlessness, despair. When you connect with the power of these feelings, it seems intuitively obvious that such feelings, particularly if evoked repetitively, could have deleterious impacts on health. Yet most of us are relatively privileged, we live in a generally dignity-affirming environment, and suffer only the occasional lapse of dignity. However, many people live constantly in a dignity-impugning environment, in which affirmations of dignity may be the exceptional occurrence. An exploration of the meanings of dignity and the forms of its violation – and the impact on physical, mental, and social well-being – may help uncover a new universe of human suffering, for which the biomedical language may be inapt and even inept. (Mann 1997: 11–12)

For Mann, dignity is a fundamental precursor of the realisation of human rights that, in turn, is a linchpin to the realisation of the goals of health (Mann 1997; Mann et al 1994, 1999). Realisation of this connection, meanwhile, serves to reveal also 'the rights-related responsibilities of physicians and other health care workers' to make allies of public health and human rights and to push for a 'new' ethics of the public's health (Mann 1997; Mann et al 1994, 1999).

The right to be treated with respect

Related to the right to be treated with dignity is the right to be treated with *respect*. People (whatever their age, cultural backgrounds, cognitive and physical abilities, sexuality, social position, and so forth) have a special interest in being treated with respect. Furthermore, there are significant moral reasons why this interest ought to be protected. Thus, the claim that people have a right to be treated with respect is a meaningful one.

Underpinning most moral claims is the principle that people ought to be treated with respect. Otherwise referred to in moral philosophy as 'respect for persons', this principle is generally regarded as being of paramount importance to the establishment, development and maintenance of moral relationships between people, and to moral practice generally (Tadd 1998: 1–3).

The notion of 'respect for persons' is widely used, often without qualification, in the bioethics literature (its meaning more or less taken for granted) and, of significance to this discussion, it is widely used in codes of professional ethics. For instance, common to most nursing codes of ethics is a prescribed demand to 'respect patients' in the provision of nursing care. This demand tends to be interpreted in varying ways as including an obligation to treat with respect a patient's needs, values, beliefs and culture. Also, nursing codes of ethics prescribe respect for patients' rights. Consider the following examples.

The Preamble to *The ICN code of ethics for nurses* states:

> Inherent in nursing is respect for human rights, including cultural rights, the right to life and choice, to dignity and to be treated with respect. Nursing care is respectful of and unrestricted by considerations of age, colour, creed, culture, disability or illness, gender, sexual orientation, nationality, politics, race or social status.
> (ICN 2012a: 1)

The NMBA (2018a) *Code of conduct for nurses* prescribes 'Nurses engage with people as individuals in a culturally safe and respectful way' (Principle 3).

The Nursing Council of New Zealand (NCNZ 2012a) *Code of conduct for nurses* places a particular emphasis on the importance of respect – both generally and in terms of patients' rights. In the preamble to the code, it states:

> Treating health consumers, families and colleagues with respect enables nursing relationships that support health consumers' health and well-being. Treating someone with respect means behaving towards that person in a way that values their worth, dignity and uniqueness. It is a fundamental requirement of professional nursing relationships and ethical conduct. (NCNZ 2012a: 4)

Despite the term's common use in the ethics literature and in codes of ethics, however, just what constitutes 'respect' and 'respect for persons' has received surprisingly little attention by authors. In the remainder of this chapter an attempt will be made to remedy this oversight. Specifically, brief attention will be given to exploring the nature and moral implications of 'respect' and 'respect for persons' – particularly as these pertain to the ethical practice of nursing and the promotion of patients' rights generally.

Every culture has its own conception of *respect* and 'its own norms of behaviour and ways of being that are considered respectful' (Sugirtharjah 1994: 739). Asian cultures, for example, tend to treat respect as a moral duty expressed through such concepts (tautologically) as: *duty, respect* and *honour* (Sugirtharjah

1994). Western cultures, however, tend to give greater primacy to respect as an individual moral *right* (Sugirtharjah 1994: 740).

Western conceptions of *respect* and, specifically, *the principle of respect for persons* have borrowed heavily from the work of the 18th century German philosopher, Immanuel Kant. In his celebrated work *Fundamental principles of the metaphysics of ethics*, Kant (1959: 56) prescribes the (now famous) practical imperative: 'So act as to treat humanity, whether in thine own person or in that of any other, in every case as an end withal, never as means only.' This practical imperative has been variously translated to mean that *people should always be treated as ends in themselves, and never as mere means (for instance, as objects) to the ends of others*. Although commonly accepted, this conception of 'respect for persons' is, however, inadequate and requires expansion to enhance its usefulness as a guiding principle in health care domains. There is, for instance, considerable scope to suggest that respecting persons entails something far more than fulfilling the negative duty of not treating individuals as 'mere means' to the ends of others. It also involves the positive duty of treating people in a manner that is affirming of their *personal identity* and *worth* as human beings – that is, affirming of who and what they are.

In clarifying the nature and moral implications of rights claims involving respect in health care contexts, it is important first to draw a distinction between respecting *persons* per se, and respecting the *rights* of persons. Although the latter is obviously a critical ingredient of the former, the two are nevertheless distinct. In regard to the latter, respecting the *rights* of persons means honouring a range of special interests (moral entitlements) that people might have, say, upon entering a health care domain – for example, the right to health care, to make informed choices, to decline the receipt of unwanted information, to have information about themselves treated as confidential, to be treated with dignity, to cultural liberty and to be treated with respect itself. Moral demands to treat *persons* with respect, in contrast, is fundamentally tied to enhancing the self-identity of persons and involves, in complex ways, acknowledging persons for who they are as human beings and responding to them in a manner that prima facie preserves the integrity of their self-identity and the promotion of moral goods that this preservation will facilitate. Let us explore this claim further.

Respect (from the Latin *respicere*, meaning 'to look back, pay attention to', from *specere*, meaning 'to look') is essentially a moral attitude that when translated into action is manifest as the showing of admiration, regard, esteem and/or kindly consideration for another. In short, respect manifests as the 'good' treatment of people, and invariably results in their being 'humanised' (i.e. enabled to experience their 'beingness' both as human persons and as moral entities, and/or characterised as having moral worth). Disrespect, in contrast, manifests as the 'bad' (or ill) treatment of people, and invariably results in them being 'dehumanised' (deprived of qualities that otherwise enables them – and others – to feel they are 'human beings' of moral worth). Or, to borrow from Asian thought, disrespecting another is to 'take away' that other's 'face'; to 'lose face', in turn, is to diminish that person's very identity and dignity, and consequently to 'pollute the web of relationship' (Rivers 1996: 54–5). Respect, in contrast, keeps 'the door of relationship' open (Rivers 1996: 55).

What then are the ingredients of respectful health-professional (nurse–patient) interactions? In conclusion to this discussion on the right to be treated with respect, there is scope to suggest that minimally a nurse's respectful interactions with patients, chosen carers and significant others must contain the following:

- acknowledgment of the moral worth and dignity of human beings
- a positive regard for and valuing of persons for who they are as human beings
- focused attention on persons (i.e. being 'fully present' and being fully alert to another's presence, *viz* not treating persons in a dismissive, dehumanising, belittling or marginalising manner)
- empathically attuned listening (taking seriously what another says and knows)

- supportive actions aimed at promoting another's moral interests and wellbeing
- strategies aimed at 'saving face' and preserving the web of relationship.

The right to cultural liberty

When in health care contexts, people have the right to *cultural liberty* – that is, the right to maintain their 'ethnic, linguistic, and religious identities' – otherwise referred to as 'cultural rights' (Fukuda-Parr 2004). Cultural rights claims entail a corresponding duty on the part of health professionals to respect cultural difference as an active component of human rights and development (Marks 2002). Central to the notion of cultural rights is the recognition that culture is not a static process encompassing a frozen set of values, beliefs and practices. Rather it is a process that is 'constantly recreated as people question, adapt and redefine their values and practices to changing realities and exchanges of idea' (Fukuda-Parr 2004: 4). Thus, claims to cultural liberty are not about 'preserving values and practices as an end in itself with blind allegiance to tradition'; they are fundamentally concerned with expanding individual choice and the 'capability of people to live and be what they choose, with adequate opportunity to consider other options' (Fukuda-Parr 2004: 4).

The right to cultural liberty is inherently linked to dignity and the right to be treated with respect. Although policy texts overtly champion recognition of cultural rights in health care contexts (see Johnstone & Kanitsaki 2008b), the degree to which cultural liberty and cultural rights are actually respected in such contexts remains a moot point. As with the other patients' rights discussed in this chapter, the right to cultural liberty is also a right that the nursing profession has a responsibility to protect and uphold. This responsibility is perhaps best articulated in the cultural competency and cultural safety literature (briefly referred to in Chapter 4), which has burgeoned in recent years due to the increasingly diverse and complex ethno-cultural and language profiles of patient populations in multicultural societies the world over.

Conclusion

The issue of patients' rights to and in health care is an important one for members of the nursing profession. Although a patients' rights approach to ethics in health care is not free of difficulties, it nevertheless serves a number of important functions. Among other things, discourse on patients' rights helps to remind both health professionals and the laity alike: first, that upon entering health care domains for care and treatment, people have special interests and entitlements which ought to be recognised and protected; second, and related to this first claim, people (patients) are not – and never have been – obliged to be the passive recipients of unnegotiated care. Third, patients' rights discourse helps to remind health professionals (nurses included) that their relationships with patients and their chosen carers are constrained by morally relevant considerations. Fourth, patients' rights discourse highlights the vulnerability of people in health care contexts and the 'special' actions that are required by others (including nurses) to help reduce this vulnerability and to promote generally the significant moral interests of patients and their chosen carers. Finally, patients' rights discourse helps to remind us that moral decision-making in health care is not just a matter of 'working through normative hierarchies of values', but is also 'a matter of personal extension into the lives and values of other human beings' which deserve respect (Thomasma 1990: 250).

Despite the enormous progress that has been made over the past four decades in regard to the whole issue of patients' rights to and in health care, patients' rights violations continue to occur across the continuum of care. In light of this, it is morally imperative that the nursing profession takes a proactive stance on the matter of patients' rights and continues to support and promote them, as and when the need arises.

Case scenario 1

A 20-year-old Jehovah's Witness woman has given birth to her first child. Unfortunately, following the delivery of her child, she starts to bleed badly. Her attending doctors offer the woman and her husband a stark choice: 'One hour to decide between a blood transfusion and a hysterectomy', or else death (Magazanik 1998: 1). If the woman has a hysterectomy, this means that her first child will be her last. The blood transfusion, however, is not an option since it is against her religion. Her refusal to have a blood transfusion is expressed clearly and frequently (both verbally and in writing), has been formally documented, and is widely known by hospital staff. The woman is observed by her husband to be very 'strong, confident and calm about the whole matter' (p 2).

A hysterectomy is performed, but the woman continues to bleed and she is transferred to the intensive care unit of a major hospital for further care. She starts to drift in and out of consciousness, and her condition becomes poor. Worried that the woman could die, her attending doctors seek legal advice. The advice received is recorded as follows: 'Continue supportive measures. Not for blood unless at direction of court.' (Magazanik 1998: 2).

The woman's condition continues to deteriorate and it is probable that, within an hour, she will suffer irreversible brain damage. Distraught at the prospect of his wife dying, the husband changes his mind about a blood transfusion and, upon seeking advice from hospital authorities, successfully obtains a court order giving him legal guardianship over his wife and hence the lawful authority to consent to a blood transfusion being given. The husband provides his consent to hospital authorities immediately and his wife is given a blood transfusion. The woman recovers quickly and is well enough to leave hospital 1 week later.

According to media reports, however, the husband feels 'guilty' about the transfusion and the woman is 'furious' that the blood was given to her against her wishes. According to a Supreme Court document, the woman stated:

> *I view the blood transfusion that was forced upon me at the [name of hospital deleted] as equivalent to rape. To me, it feels as if someone has forced an abortion on me while I was under sedation. I am angry about what has happened and I have cried about it a number of times.* (quoted in Magazanik 1998: 2)

The woman is also reported as stating that she 'would have "screamed" and "fought" against the transfusion had she not been sedated' and that she is 'considering suing the hospital, doctors, nurses and lawyers involved in giving her blood' (Magazanik 1998: 2). The Jehovah's Witness organisation is reported to be deeply involved in the legal action that is being pursued, stressing its position that 'We want to be certain that if people say "I do not want blood", then that is respected' (p 2).

Case scenario 2

A 42-year-old woman, suffering from severe abdominal pain, is brought by ambulance to the Emergency Department (ED) of a major metropolitan hospital. Upon admission to the ED she is immediately recognised by an attending nurse, who remarks in a terse tone of voice 'You used to be one of my lecturers. I obviously didn't do what you wanted me to as you failed me on one of my assignments'. The woman had been a senior lecturer at a local university, but neither recognised the ED nurse nor remembered ever failing an assignment written by her. Later, she heard the nurse making disparaging comments about her to other staff in the ED. During the remainder of her stay in the ED, the woman was largely ignored by nursing staff (even her vital signs were not checked) until she was admitted to the ward.

CRITICAL QUESTIONS

1. What patients' rights have been violated in these two cases?
2. What were the moral duties of the nurses in these scenarios in regard to upholding and protecting the rights of the patients concerned?
3. How might the violations that occurred in these cases have been prevented?
4. What might be done to assist the patients in the cases whose rights have been violated to come to terms with the aftermath of their experiences?

Endnote

1. Section 4, 'The right to dignity and dying with dignity', is revised from Johnstone M-J (1989a) 'Dying with dignity', *New Zealand Nursing Journal* 81(12): 34, 37.

CHAPTER 8

Ethical issues in mental health care

KEYWORDS

competency to decide
cybersuicide
ethics
human rights
mental health
mental health ethics
mental illness
parasuicide
psychiatric advance directives
self-harm
suicide
suicidal behaviour
suicide intervention
suicide postvention
suicide prevention
'Ulysses contracts'

LEARNING OBJECTIVES

Upon the completion of this chapter and with further self-directed learning you are expected to be able to:

- Discuss critically why a charter of rights and responsibilities specific to mental health care is required.
- Identify eight domains deemed relevant to the rights and responsibilities of both users and providers of mental health care services.
- Examine the notions of competency and its implications for persons with impaired decision-making capacity.
- Discuss critically the notions of 'surrogate/substitute decision-making' and 'supported decision-making' in the case of people deemed to be rationally incompetent.
- With reference to the idea of psychiatric advance directives in mental health:
  – define what a psychiatric advance directive is
  – discuss critically the different theoretical frameworks and forms that psychiatric advance directives can take
  – discuss critically the different functions that psychiatric advance directives might serve
  – examine the purpose of 'Ulysses contracts'
  – discuss critically the possible risks and benefits of psychiatric advance directives.
- With reference to the ethics of suicide prevention, intervention and postvention:
  – discuss the distinction between suicide, suicidal behaviour and parasuicide and why making this distinction is important
  – examine critically at least five criteria that must be met in order for an act to count as suicide rather than some other form of death (e.g. euthanasia)
  – consider arguments both for and against the proposition that people have a 'right to suicide'
  – examine critically the conditions under which a person's decision to suicide may warrant respect
  – discuss critically the ethics of suicide prevention, intervention and postvention.
- Explore ways in which the nursing profession might improve its advocacy of people with mental health problems and severe mental illnesses.

Introduction

The issue of patients' rights to and in health care, discussed in the previous chapter, has obvious relevance and application for people with mental illness admitted to hospital for the care and treatment of non-psychiatric conditions (e.g. injuries sustained as a result of a road traffic accident, an acute appendicitis, complications of diabetes, renal failure, etc.). It also has obvious relevance for people admitted to mental health care facilities for psychiatric care and treatment. There is, however, one notable caveat to this stance: because the rights of people with mental illness are disproportionately vulnerable to being infringed in health care contexts (both psychiatric and non-psychiatric), a more nuanced approached to the issue is required. Specifically, an approach is required that places strong emphasis on consolidating the *mental health* interests of those who have or who are at risk of developing mental illnesses and which also emphasises the 'special' responsibilities that health care providers have towards this vulnerable group. Underpinning this caveat is the reality that in most jurisdictions around the world there are legislative provisions that enable people with severe mental health illness to be detained, restrained, coerced and/or treated *without their consent*. This is so even in jurisdictions which have progressive legislative provisions enabling patients to determine in advance their 'will and preferences' apropos care, treatment and supported decision-making options (Callaghan & Ryan 2016; Hem et al 2018; Molodynski et al 2014; Tingleff et al 2017).

Coercive measures commonly used in mental health care contexts have been classified as basically involving four types: 'seclusion, mechanical constraint, physical restraint/holding, and forced medication' (Krieger et al 2018; Tingleff et al 2017); these can be imposed in either institutional or community health care settings (e.g. community treatment order (CTO) contexts) (Corring et al 2017; Nagra et al 2016; Molodynski et al 2014). In Australian, New Zealand and other common-law jurisdictions, legislative provisions also enable psychiatrists to override a person's will and preferences and admit ('commit') them involuntarily to hospital for treatment, which, in effect, grants psychiatrists the authority to 'act as substitute decision-makers, rather than as advisers and service providers' (McSherry 2012: 1).

The need of a highly nuanced approach to upholding the rights of persons with mental illness and related problems in health care rests on at least three considerations. First, as discussed previously in Chapter 6, people with mental illness are among the most stigmatised, discriminated against, marginalised, disadvantaged and hence vulnerable individuals in the world. Moreover, despite the efforts of mental health consumer groups and other mental health advocates, people with mental health problems and psychosocial disabilities continue to experience the infringement of many of their basic human rights (including the right to mental health and to mental health care). This is so despite what Callaghan and Ryan (2016: 601) describe as a 'revolutionary paradigm shift' that is occurring as a result of Article 12 of the UN Convention of the Rights of Persons with Disabilities (CRPD)[1] 'objecting to the automatic use of substituted decision-making whenever a person fails to meet a functional test of decision-making capacity'.

A second consideration is that many people with mental illness have experienced high rates of trauma during their lifetime. Thus, there is an ever-present risk that, when admitted to a psychiatric facility as an involuntary or non-voluntary patient, their institutional experiences may trigger previous trauma, provoke feelings of fear, anxiety and anger and thereby aggravate their psychiatric symptoms (a burden which others who do not have a history of trauma or mental illness do not carry) (Cusack et al 2018; Goulet et al 2017; McKenna et al 2017). This can sometimes mean that, rather than providing a 'psychiatric sanctuary', an involuntary admission to a psychiatric facility may sometimes be experienced as a 'psychiatric sentencing' – akin to a penal incarceration. This is especially likely in cases where involuntary or non-voluntary hospitalisation involves unconsented, coercive institutional procedures such as seclusion, restraints, forced medication and forced feeding (Borckardt et al 2007; Cusack et al 2018).

Third, even when persons with mental illness later acknowledge the need for their earlier involuntary or non-voluntary admission to hospital, they are sometimes left feeling very dissatisfied with the situation – not least because they feel that their humanity and dignity have been violated in the process. This, in turn, may be counter-therapeutic because of the harmful emotional effects of the dehumanisation and dignity violation that are sometimes experienced as well as the undermining of trust in the professional–client relationship (Belcher et al 2017; Borckardt et al 2007; Cusack et al 2018; Gustafsson et al 2014).

In seeking to redress the implications of these considerations, mental health advocates have increasingly sought to emphasise and champion a suite of rights and responsibilities that are specific to the context of mental health care. In this chapter an attempt will be made to contribute to this positive project by providing an overview of stated rights and responsibilities in mental health care. Because one of the most ethically confronting issues in mental health care is the coercive treatment[2] of persons admitted as involuntary or non-voluntary patients to a psychiatric facility or program, particular attention will also be given to the issues of informed consent and competency to decide, and ongoing proposals to develop and operationalise 'psychiatric advance directives' (PADs) in jurisdictions around the world. Attention will also be given to the vexed issue of the ethics of suicide prevention, suicide intervention and suicide postvention. While drawing primarily on the Australian experience, this discussion nonetheless has relevance for nurses working in other countries.

Vulnerability, human rights and the mentally ill

It has long been recognised at a social, cultural and political level that people suffering from mental illnesses and other mental health-related problems need to have their moral interests as human beings protected from abuse and neglect, which, for a variety of reasons, are especially vulnerable to being violated. This need of protection has also been recognised at an international level as evident from the United Nations General Assembly's adoption in 1991 of the *Principles for the protection of persons with mental illness and for the improvement of mental health care* and, a decade later, by the World Health Organization's release of *The world health report 2001: mental health: new understanding, new hope* (WHO 2001a). A little over a decade later, in the cultural context of Australia, the need to assure the rights of people with mental illness and the 'provision of recovery-orientated practice in mental health services' was positioned as a core principle in the Australian Commonwealth Government's *National framework for recovery-oriented mental health services* (Australian Health Ministers Advisory Council (AHMAC) 2013) and the Council of Australian Governments' (2012) *Roadmap for national mental health reform 2012–2022*. A similar stance was taken in New Zealand with the Ministry of Health releasing its *Rising to the challenge: the mental health and addiction service development plan 2012–2017* (New Zealand Ministry of Health 2012).

In attempting to secure protection of the rights of the mentally ill from abuse and neglect, a human rights model of mental health care ethics has been adopted. Underpinning the selection of this model is the view that 'all people have fundamental human rights' and that people with mental health problems or mental illness should not be precluded from having or exercising these rights just because of their mental health difficulties. As the Mental Health Consumer Outcomes Task Force argued almost three decades ago (1991: ix):

> The diagnosis of mental health problems or mental disorder is not an excuse for inappropriately limiting their [people with mental health problems or disorders] rights.

In March 1991, the Australian Health Ministers acknowledged and accepted the above viewpoint and adopted, as part of Australia's national mental health strategy, the final report of the Mental Health Consumer Outcomes Task Force, titled *Mental health statement of rights and responsibilities*. First published in 1991, with a 2012 revised edition of the statement launched in early 2013, this document stands as an influential guide for other public policy initiatives and statements such as the *National mental health policy* (released in 2008 and committed to by all Australian governments), and successive national mental health plans (including the most recent *Fifth national mental health and suicide prevention plan* released in 2017, the *National standards for mental health services 2010* and the *National carer strategy* in 2011 (Australian Government Department of Health 2010, 2011, 2017) and other documents (e.g. *Mental health statement of rights and responsibilities* (Australian Government Department of Health 2012: 3)).

The primary objective of the 2012 revised version of the *Mental health statement of rights and responsibilities* document is to inform stakeholders of the rights of people experiencing a mental illness to have access 'to timely assessment, individualised care planning, treatment and support' and the related rights and responsibilities that consumers, carers, support persons, service providers and the community all have in relation to these rights (Australian Government Department of Health 2012: 3). To this end, the document addresses the following eight domains:

1. *Inherent dignity and equal protection* – encompassing the right of all people to respect the human worth and dignity of people with mental illnesses, and to support people who are mentally ill or intellectually disabled to exercise their rights when their own capacity to do so is impaired.
2. *Non-discrimination and social inclusion* – encompassing the rights to: privacy and confidentiality; health, safety and welfare; equal opportunities to access and maintain health and mental health care, and other social goods; contribute to and participate in the development of social, health and mental health policy and services.
3. *The promotion of mental health and the prevention of mental illness* – encompassing the responsibilities of governments and health service providers to: promote mental health; support, develop, implement and evaluate programs for preventing mental health problems and illnesses; support the ongoing development of comprehensive, flexible, integrated, and accessible community, primary health and hospital-based social support, health and mental health services.
4. *The rights and responsibilities of people who seek assessment, support, care, treatment, rehabilitation and recovery* – encompassing the right of people (including children) to 'participate in all decisions that affect them, to receive high-quality services, to receive appropriate treatment, including appropriate treatment for physical or general health needs, and to benefit from special safeguards if involuntary assessment, treatment or rehabilitation is imposed' (p 12).
5. *Rights and responsibilities of carers and support persons* – encompassing the rights and responsibilities of carers and support persons in relation to the rights to: respect the human worth and dignity of people; privacy and confidentiality; seek and receive appropriate training and support; participate in and contribute to the development of social, health and mental health policy.
6. *Rights and responsibilities of people who provide services* – encompassing rights and responsibilities in regards to upholding the highest possible standards of mental health care, including the development and implementation of social, health and mental health policy and service delivery policies and guidelines.
7. *Rights and responsibilities of the community* – encompassing the responsibility of communities to be adequately informed and educated about mental health issues, and to uphold the rights of mental health consumers and their carers.
8. *Governance* – encompassing the responsibility of governments and other stakeholders to ensure that mental health initiatives (including service provision, mental health legislative reform, and other forensic

matters) are appropriately resourced and supported. (adapted from *Mental health statement of rights and responsibilities* (Australian Government Department of Health 2012)).

At first glance, the content and intent of the *Mental health statement of rights and responsibilities* (2012) seem to provide an important basis for the protection of the human rights of people made vulnerable by mental health problems. On closer examination, however, the practical guidance that this statement can offer is also limited – like other codes and statements, they cannot tell people *what to do in particular cases*.

As previously explained, a moral right can be defined as a special interest or entitlement which a person has and which ought to be protected for moral reasons. The claim of a moral right usually entails that another person has a corresponding duty to respect that right. Fulfilling a corresponding duty can involve either doing something 'positive' to benefit a person claiming a particular right or, alternatively, refraining from doing something 'negative' which could harm a person claiming a particular right. For example, if a patient claims the right to make an informed consent concerning prescribed psychotropic medication or electroconvulsive therapy (ECT), this imposes on an attending health care professional a corresponding duty to ensure that the patient is fully informed about the therapeutic effects and the adverse side effects of the treatments in question as well as to respect the patient's decision to either accept or refuse the treatment, even where the health professional may not agree with the ultimate decision made. The moral force of the right's claim in this instance is such that if an attending health care professional does not uphold or violates the patient's decision in regard to the treatment options considered, that patient would probably feel wronged or that an injustice had been done. The health care professional in turn could be judged, criticised and possibly even censured on grounds of having infringed the patient's rights.

An important question to arise here is: 'If statements on mental health rights and responsibilities fall short of providing clear-cut guidance in cases of this nature, is there any point in having them?' The short answer to this question is, yes. Whatever the faults, weaknesses and difficulties of such statements, they nevertheless achieve a number of important things; like bills and charters of patient rights generally,

- they help to remind mental health patients/consumers, service providers, caregivers and the general community that people with mental health problems (including mental illnesses and mental health problems) have special moral interests and entitlements that ought to be respected and protected
- they help to inform stakeholders (patients/consumers, service providers, caregivers and the community) of what these special entitlements are and thereby provide a basis upon which respect for and protection of these can be required
- they help to delineate the special responsibilities that stakeholders (patients/consumers, service providers, caregivers and the community) all have in ensuring the promotion and protection of people's moral interests and entitlements in mental health care and in promoting mental health generally
- they help to remind all stakeholders (patients/consumers, service providers, caregivers and the community at large) that their relationships with each other are ethically constrained and are bound by certain correlative duties.

Competency to decide

As discussed in the previous chapter under the subject heading 'The analytic components and elements of an informed consent', an essential criterion to satisfying the requirements of an informed consent is *competency to decide*. Determining whether a person has the competency to make an informed decision about whether to accept or reject a recommended treatment is not a straightforward matter, however. This is because there is no substantial agreement on the characteristics of a 'competent person' or on how 'competency' should be measured. To complicate this matter further, there is also no substantial agreement on what constitutes *rationality*, which, as has been argued elsewhere, is very much a matter of subjective interpretation. As Gibson (1976) pointed out in an early article on the subject, rationality cannot escape the influences of the social patterns and institutions around it and, for this reason, any value-neutral account of rationality is quite inadequate. She further suggested that, at most, rationality should be regarded as a *value*, rather than a property that all 'normal' people have (Gibson 1976: 193). In summary, the notion of 'rational competency' is problematic because there is no precise definition of, or agreement on, what it is.

Philosophical disputes about what constitutes 'rationality' and 'competency to decide' have particular ramifications for people who have what has been termed 'fringe decision competence' (Hartvigsson et al 2018), who are cognitively impaired and/or who, because of the manifestations of severe mental illness, are involuntarily admitted to psychiatric facilities for treatment. The lack of conceptual clarity in this instance risks 'pushing ethics to their limits' – especially in cases 'where patients have not reached out for help' yet treatments are imposed without their informed consent (Gustafsson et al 2014: 176).

Even if there were agreement on what constitutes rational competency, there remains the problem of 'whereby the definition of competence changes in different clinical situations' (Gert et al 1997: 135). For example, an elderly demented resident may be deemed competent to eat his/her evening meal alone, but deemed not competent to refuse treatment – for example, surgery for a fractured hip. As Gert and colleagues (p 132) go on to explain, we need to appreciate that persons as such are 'not globally "competent" but rather "competent to do X", where X is some specific physical or mental task'. In other words, competence is always 'task specific' and determining or measuring competence is thus always 'context dependent'.

Significantly the issue of competency rarely arises in contexts where the patient agrees with and consents to a doctor's recommended or prescribed treatment. Rather, it tends to be only in cases of 'treatment refusals, especially those that appear to be irrational, that the question of a patient's competence most frequently and appropriately arises' (Gert et al 1997: 142; see also Light et al 2016). An instructive example of this can be found in the much-publicised Australian case of John McEwan that occurred in the mid 1980s and which sparked an unprecedented public inquiry into the so-called 'right to die with dignity' (Social Development Committee 1987).

John McEwan, a former Australian water-skiing champion, was left a ventilator-dependent quadriplegic after a diving accident at Echuca, Victoria. Throughout his hospitalisation, he repeatedly asked to be allowed to die. At one point, desperate to achieve his wish, he went on a hunger strike and instructed his solicitor to draw up a 'living will', which stated 'that he did not wish to be revived if and when he fell into a coma' (*Bioethics News* 1985: 2). According to media reports, this act led to a psychiatrist certifying him as rationally incompetent, thereby enabling John McEwan to be treated (fed) against his will. The psychiatrist's judgment was revoked a few days later, however, when John McEwan 'agreed to end his hunger strike and accept a course of antidepressants' (p 2).

A little over a year after his accident, and despite still being ventilator dependent, John McEwan was discharged home. The round-the-clock day care he required was given by family members and friends who had received special training in how to care for him. In the weeks following his discharge from hospital, John McEwan continued to express his wish to be allowed to die (Social Development Committee 1987: 310–11). This prompted the general practitioner who was medically responsible for him to inform the senior nursing assistant that:

> *John McEwan at his own request could come off the ventilator from time to time but had to be reconnected if he became distressed* even if it was against his own wishes. [emphasis added] (Social Development Committee 1987: 312)

During one incident, while at home, John McEwan was observed to be angry at having been reconnected to the ventilator against his wishes. Also, in another incident shortly before his death, he talked openly with his general practitioner about 'hiring someone to blow his [John McEwan's] brains out or kill him as he felt his wish to die was being frustrated' (Social Development Committee 1987: 316). There was no reason to suspect that John McEwan's wishes were irrational. Before his accident he had been a committed sportsman and for him the life of a helpless quadriplegic was intolerable.

At four o'clock in the morning on 3 April 1986, John McEwan was found dead by his nursing attendant. At the time of discovery he was disconnected from his ventilator.

It is perhaps easy to think of competency in cases such as this in purely medical or psychiatric terms. In an early work on the subject, Roth and colleagues (1977) argue, however, that the concept of competency is not merely a psychiatric or medical concept, as some might assume, but is also fundamentally social and legal in nature. They go on to warn that there is no magical definition of competency, and that the problems posed by so-called 'incompetent' persons are very often problems of personal prejudices and social biases, or of other difficulties associated with trying to find the 'right' words. In a more recent work on competency, Light and colleagues (2016: 34) argue that 'all definitions of capacity [for decision-making] involve intrinsically normative judgments and inevitably reflect the influence of context and values'. These views have been underscored in an insightful essay by Stier (2013) who explores the fundamentally normative nature generally of assessing, diagnosing and treating mental illness – including determining whether something is a *mental illness* (which relies on normative judgments about 'normal' versus 'deviant' behaviour), *irrational* (which includes judgments about 'impaired reality testing'), or *harmful and distressing* (which relies on value-laden judgments about whether something is 'bad and dysfunctional').

Historically the critical issue in developing tests of competency is how to strike a contented balance between *serving a rationally incompetent person's autonomy* and also *serving that person's health care, nursing care and medical treatment needs*. Also of critical concern is finding a competency test which is comprehensive enough to deal with diverse situations, which can be applied reliably and which is mutually acceptable to health care professionals, lawyers, judges and the community at large.

Roth and colleagues (1977) suggest that competency tests proposed in the literature basically fall into five categories:

1. evidencing a choice
2. 'reasonable' outcome of choice
3. choice based on 'rational' reasons
4. ability to understand
5. actual understanding.

The test of *evidencing a choice* is as it sounds, and is concerned only with whether a patient's choice is 'evident'; that is, whether it is *present* or *absent*. For example, a fully comatose patient would be unable to evidence a choice, unlike a semi-comatose patient or a brain-injured person, who could evidence a choice by opening and shutting their eyes or by squeezing someone's hand to indicate 'yes' or 'no'. The *quality* of the patient's choice in this instance is irrelevant. One problem with this test, however, is whether, say, the blinking of a patient's eyelids can be relied upon as evidencing a choice; in a life-and-death situation one would need to be very sure that a patient's so-called 'evidencing a choice' is more than just a reflex.

The test of *reasonable outcome of choice* is again as it sounds, and focuses on the outcome of a given choice, as opposed to the mere presence or absence of a choice. The objective test here is similar to that employed in law, and involves asking the question: 'What would a reasonable person in like circumstances consider to be a reasonable outcome?' The reliability of this measure is, of course, open to serious question — as might be objected, what one person might accept as reasonable another might equally reject.

The test of *choice based on 'rational' reasons* is a little more difficult to apply. Basically, it asks whether a given choice is the product of 'mental illness' or whether it is the product of prudent and critically reflective deliberation. A number of objections can be raised here. For example, contrary to popular medical opinion, there is nothing to suggest that a person's decision to suicide is always the product of mental disease or depression. A patient could without contradiction 'rationally' choose suicide as a means of escaping an intolerable life characterised by suffering intractable and intolerable pain. Alternatively, a depressed and so-called 'irrational' person might refuse a particular psychiatric treatment, such as psychotropic drugs, electroconvulsive therapy or psychosurgery, out of a very 'rational' and well-founded fear of what undesirable effects these treatments might ultimately have.

The test of *ability to understand*, on the other hand, asks whether the patient is able to comprehend the risks, benefits and alternatives to a proposed medical procedure, as well as the implications of giving consent. Here objections can be raised concerning just how sophisticated a patient's understanding needs to be. The problem also may arise of patients perceiving a risk as a benefit. Roth and colleagues (1977: 282), for example, cite the case of a 49-year-old psychiatric patient who was informed that there was a one-in-three-thousand chance of dying from ECT. When told of this risk she replied, happily: 'I hope I am the one!'

The fifth and final competency test is that of *actual understanding*. This test asks how well the patient has actually understood information which has been disclosed. This can be established by asking patients probing questions and inviting them to reiterate the information they have received. On the basis of educated skill and past experience, the health professional is usually able to ascertain the level at which the patient has understood the information received and what data gaps or misunderstandings remain.

A variation of this test was further developed and advanced by Grisso and Appelbaum (1998: 31), and includes assessing patients for their abilities to:

1. express *a choice*
2. understand *information relevant to treatment decision-making*
3. appreciate *the significance of that information for [their] own situation, especially concerning [their own] illness and the probable consequences of [their] treatment options*
4. reason *with relevant information so as to engage in a logical process of weighing treatment options.* [emphasis original]

In a later appraisal and application of this test, Appelbaum (2007: 1835) reiterates that legal standards for assessing the decision-making capacity of patients still generally embody 'the abilities to communicate a choice, to understand the relevant information, to appreciate the medical consequences of the situation, and to reason about treatment choices'. In relation to these criteria, he goes on to clarify that the *patient's* task in consent situations is to:

- *clearly indicate their preferred treatment options;*
- *grasp the fundamental meaning of the information being communicated by their attending doctor (apropos the nature of patient's condition, nature and purpose of proposed treatment, possible benefits and risks of that treatment, and alternative approaches (including no treatment) and their benefits and risks);*
- *acknowledge (have insight into) their medical condition and likely consequences of the treatment option available (noting that 'delusions or pathologic levels of distortion or denial are the most common causes of impairment');*
- *engage in a rational process of manipulating [sic] the relevant information (this criterion focuses on the process by which a decision is reached, not the outcome of the patient's choice, since patients have the right to make 'unreasonable' choices).* (Appelbaum 2007: 1836)

He further clarifies that the *doctor's* commensurate task in consent situations is to:

- *ask the patient to indicate a treatment choice;*
- *encourage the patient to paraphrase disclosed information regarding their medical condition and treatment options;*
- *ask the patient to describe their views of medical conditions, proposed treatment and likely outcomes;*
- *ask the patient to compare treatment options and consequences and to offer reasons for selection of the option chosen.* (Appelbaum 2007: 1836)

Since the publication of the foundational works by Grisso and Appelbaum (1998) and Appelbaum (2007), a number of competency assessment tools have been developed[3] (Wang S-B et al 2017). Of these, the MacArthur Competence Assessment Tools (MacCATs) developed and trialled by Appelbaum and Grisso (Appelbaum & Grisso 1995; Grisso & Appelbaum 1995; Grisso et al 1995, 1997) are generally regarded 'as having the most reliability and validity for assessing competence related to functional abilities, and have been widely used in psychiatry' (Wang S-B et al 2017: 56). Criteria stipulated in other jurisdictions are reflective of these original proposals. For example, in Australian jurisdictions, ascertaining whether a patient has the capacity to make informed decisions requires that the following processes be examined and shown:

- the comprehension and retention of information about the treatment
- the capacity to formulate a reasonable belief about the information that has been given
- the capacity to weigh up that information in the balance so as to arrive at a prudent choice
- the capacity to communicate the decision made (after Kerridge et al 2013: 384–6).

Similarly in the United Kingdom – for example, Section 3(1) of the UK *Mental Capacity Act (2005)* stipulates that, in order to be deemed rationally incompetent, a patient must be suffering from a condition that makes him or her unable to:

(i) understand information relevant to the decision

(ii) retain that information

(iii) use or weigh that information as part of the process of making the decision, or

(iv) communicate his decision. (cited in Banner 2012: 1079)

These and like criteria remain problematic, however. Because of unresolved uncertainties concerning how the concept of competency is to be interpreted and applied by clinicians, and the tendency to overlook what Banner describes as the 'inherent normativity of judgments made about whether a person is using or weighing information in the decision-making process', there remains the ever-present risk of patients failing on the criteria 'to the extent that they do not appear to be handling the information given in an appropriate way, on account of a mental impairment disrupting the way the decision process ought to proceed' (Banner 2012: 3078; see also Stier 2013 and Light et al 2016 – both referred to earlier).

It should be noted that competency is a key issue not just in psychiatric care, but in any health care context where judgments of competency are critical to deciding: (1) whether a patient can or should decide and/or be permitted to decide for herself or himself, and (2) the point at which another or others will need to or should decide for the patient – that is, become what Buchanan and Brock (1989) term *surrogate decision-makers* and what is variously referred to in Australian jurisdictions as involving 'substitute decision-making' and 'supported decision-making', with the latter placing the person who is being supported 'at the front of the decision-making process' (Australian Law Reform Commission (ALRC) 2014: 51). The question remains, however, of how these things can be decided in a morally sound and just way. This question becomes even more problematic when it is considered that persons deemed 'rationally incompetent' (or, at least, cognitively impaired) can still be quite capable of making 'reasonable' self-interested choices, and, further, that the choices they make − even if 'irrational' − are not always harmful (Williams 2002; see also Light et al 2016; Stier 2013).

Commenting on the moral standards which should be met when deciding whether to respect or override the expressed preferences of a patient deemed 'incompetent', Buchanan and Brock (1989) have classically argued in their foundational text that it is important to be clear about *what* statements of competence refer to. Like Gert and colleagues (1997), cited earlier, they argue that statements of competence (i.e. in clinical contexts) usually refer to a person's competence to *do something*, in this instance, to *choose and make decisions*; according to this view, competence is, therefore, 'choice and decision-relative'. Given this, determining competence in health care contexts fundamentally involves determining a person's ability *to make particular choices and decisions under particular conditions* (Buchanan & Brock 1989: 311–65; see also Light et al 2016)).

An important problem here, particularly in psychiatric contexts, is that severe mental illness can significantly affect the capacities needed for competent decision-making (for instance, understanding, reasoning and applying values), and hence the ability generally of severely mentally ill persons to make sound decisions about their own wellbeing − including the need for care and treatment. For example, as Buchanan and Brock (1989: 318) comment:

> a person may persist in a fixed delusional belief that proffered medications are poison or are being used to control his or her mind. Such delusions or fixed false beliefs obviously may also impair a person's capacity to reason about whether hospitalisation and treatment will on balance serve his or her wellbeing. Severe mental illness can also affect and seriously distort a person's underlying and enduring aims and values, his or her conception of his or her own good, that one must use in evaluating hospitalisation and treatment for an illness.

It is precisely in situations such as these that attending health care professionals need a reliable framework within which to decide how best to act − notably: (1) whether to respect a patient's preferences even though the patient is deemed 'incompetent', or (2) whether to override patients' preferences in the interests of protecting or upholding what has been deemed by *others* to be in the patient's overall 'best interests'. Just what such a framework would − or indeed should − look like is, however, a matter of some controversy. Nevertheless, as Buchanan and Brock's highly cited work *Deciding for others: the ethics of surrogate decision-making* (1989) has shown, it is possible to devise at least a prima-facie working framework to guide professional ethical decision-making in this sensitive, complex and problematic area. Specifically, Buchanan and Brock (1989: 84–6) suggest that the whole issue hinges on:

1. setting and applying accurately standards of competency to choose and decide; and
2. achieving a balance between (i) protecting and promoting the patients' wellbeing (human welfare), (ii) protecting and promoting the patients' entitlement to and interest in exercising self-determining choices, and (iii) protecting others who could be harmed by patients exercising harm-causing choices.

With regard to setting and applying accurately standards of competency to choose and decide, Buchanan and Brock suggest that, among other things, ethical professional decision-making in this problematic area should be guided by the following considerations (1989: 85):

> No single standard of competence is adequate for all decisions. The standard depends in large part on the risk involved, and varies along a range from low / minimal to high / maximal. The more serious the expected harm to the patient from acting on a choice, the higher should be the standard of decision-making capacity, and the greater should be the certainty that the standard is satisfied.

In other words, the extent to which an attending health care professional is bound morally to respect the choices of a person deemed 'rationally incompetent' depends primarily on the severity of the risks involved to the patient if her or his choices are permitted. The higher and more severe the risks involved, the higher and more rigorous should be the standards for determining the patient's decision-making capacity, and the more certain attending health care professionals should be that the patient has met these standards. Appelbaum likewise asserts that when a patient's decisions are of a life-and-death nature a 'relative high level performance with respect to the relevant criteria should be required' (Appelbaum 2007: 1838). This framework is expressed diagrammatically in Fig. 8.1.

For example, if a patient with severe mental illness decides to refuse hospitalisation, the extent to which an attending health professional is obliged morally to respect this decision will depend on how severe the risks to the patient are of not being hospitalised — for instance, whether a failure to hospitalise the patient will result in her or him suiciding, or will result only in her or him being left in a state of moderate, although not life-threatening, depression. In the case of suicide risk, the grounds for not honouring a patient's decision do seem at least prima facie stronger than possible grounds for overriding the decision of a patient who is only moderately depressed. (Whether or not the risk of suicide does provide strong grounds for overriding a patient's decision to refuse hospitalisation and treatment is another question, and one which is considered shortly in this chapter.)

While Buchanan and Brock's (1989) 'sliding scale' framework is useful, it is not free of difficulties. For instance, there remains the problem of how to determine what is a harm, what is a low/minimal and high/maximal risk of harm, and who properly should decide these things — the answers to which involve complex value judgments. Consider, for example, the following case (personal communication).

An involuntary psychiatric patient refuses to take the psychotropic medication he has been prescribed. In defence of his refusal, the patient argues 'reasonably' that the adverse side effects of the drugs he is being expected to take are intolerable, and that he would prefer the pain of his mental illness to the intolerable side effects of the drugs that have been prescribed to treat his mental illness. Staff on the ward in which he is an involuntary patient are divided about what they should do. The more experienced

FIGURE 8.1

Assessing risk and permitting choices of patients deemed 'rationally incompetent'

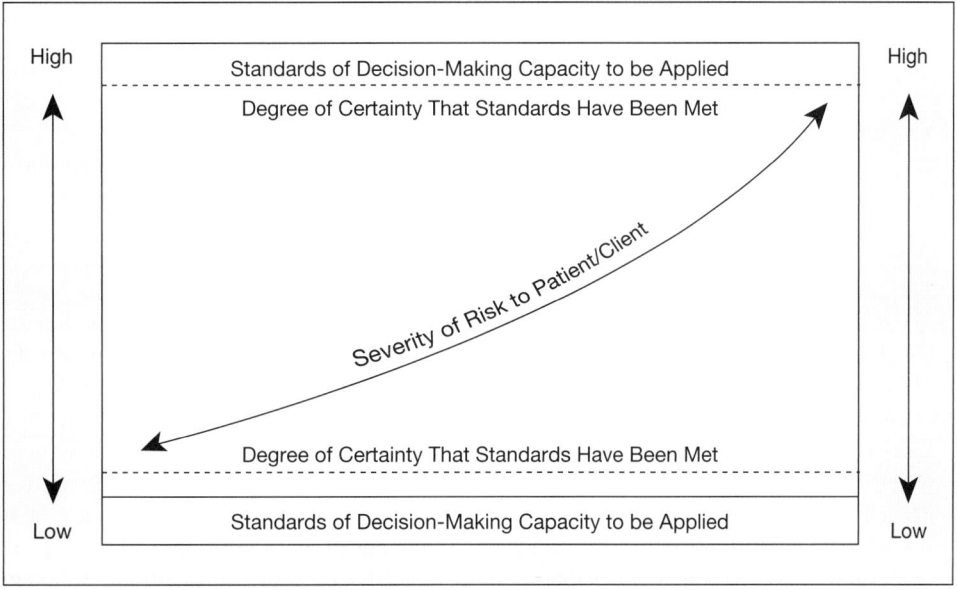

staff members in this case insist that the patient should be given his medication forcibly by intramuscular injection. They argue in defence of this decision that the patient's condition is deteriorating rapidly, and that if he does not receive the medication prescribed he will 'spiral down into a psychiatric crisis' (in other words a total exacerbation of his condition), which would be even more intolerable and harmful than the unpleasant side effects he has been experiencing as a result of taking the psychotropic drugs in question. They make the additional value judgment that it would be 'better' for the patient if his psychiatric condition were prevented from deteriorating, and that their decision to administer his prescribed medication forcibly against his will is justified on these grounds.

The less experienced staff members on the ward disagree with this reasoning, however, and argue that, even though the patient's psychiatric condition is deteriorating, and this is a preventable harm, the patient is nevertheless able to make an informed decision about this and therefore his wishes should be respected. In defence of their position, they argue that the patient's complaints are justified – the adverse side effects of his psychotropic drugs have indeed been 'awful', and are commonly experienced by other patients as well; and that he has experienced a decline in his psychiatric condition before, and hence knows what to expect. Further, they argue, if he is given the medication against his will, an even greater harm will follow: specifically, he will trust the nursing staff even less than he does already, and will be even less willing to comply with his oral medication prescription than he is now.

In this case, the more experienced staff outnumbered the less experienced staff, and the patient was held down and forcibly given an intramuscular injection of the medication he had refused. Later, after recovering from this incident, the patient was, as predicted by the less experienced nursing staff, grossly mistrustful of the nursing staff on the ward, and even less willing to comply with his oral medication prescription. His requests for different and less drugs, and more counselling, went unheeded.

This case scenario demonstrates the difficulties that can be encountered when accepting/rejecting a patient's ability to choose and decide care and treatment options, and deciding when and how to override a patient's preferences. Not only is there the problem of how to determine accurately what a harm is and how a given harm should be weighted morally when evaluating whether a patient's choices should be respected or overridden; there is the additional problem that attending health care professionals may disagree radically among themselves about how these things should be determined – to a point that may even cause rather than prevent harm to the patient, as happened in this case. What else then should health care professionals do?

One response is to insist on the development of reliable (research-based) criteria for deciding these sorts of problematic issues. The need to do this becomes even more acute when the problem of determining and weighing harms is considered in relation to the broader demand to achieve a balance between protecting and promoting the patient's wellbeing, protecting and promoting the patient's autonomy, and protecting others who could be harmed if a mentally ill person is left free to exercise harm-causing choices (as happened in the *Tarasoff* case, considered in Chapter 7).

Just what these criteria should be, however, and how they should be applied, is an extremely complex matter, and one that requires much greater attention than it is possible to give here. Nevertheless, Buchanan and Brock (1989) provide an important basis for identifying the following three factors which need to be taken into consideration when deciding whether to override a mentally ill person's decisions, namely: (1) whether the person is a danger to herself or himself, (2) whether the person is in need of care and treatment, and (3) whether the person is a danger to others. In regard to the consideration of being a danger to self, Buchanan and Brock (1989: 317–31) correctly argue that what is needed are stringent criteria of what constitutes a *danger to self*; in the case of the need for care and treatment, that what is needed are stringent criteria for *ascertaining deterioration and distress*; and in the case of harm to others, that what is needed are stringent criteria of what constitutes *a danger to others*. Also, although applying the criteria developed may inevitably result in a health care professional assuming the essentially paternalistic role of being a surrogate decision-maker for a given patient, this need not be problematic provided the model of surrogate decision-making used is *patient centred* – that is, committed to upholding the patient's interests and concerns insofar as these can be ascertained.

A patient-centred model of surrogate decision-making, in this instance, would have as its rationale *preventing harm to patients*, and would embrace an ethical framework which is structured 'for deciding *for* patients for *their benefit*' (Buchanan & Brock 1989: 327, 331). This is in contrast with a non-patient or 'other'-centred decision-making model, which would have as its rationale *preventing harm to others*, and which embraces an ethical framework 'for deciding *about* others for *others' benefits*' (Buchanan & Brock 1989: 327, 331). It should be noted, however, that these two models are not necessarily mutually exclusive and indeed could, in some instances, be mutually supporting (a man contemplating a violent suicide involving others is a danger not only to himself but also to the innocent others he plans to 'take with him'). Just which model or models are appropriate, and under what circumstances they should be used, will, however, depend ultimately on the people involved (and the relationships between them), the moral interests at stake, the context in which these moral interests are at stake, the resources available (human and otherwise) to protect and promote the moral interests that are at risk of being harmed, and, finally, the accurate prediction of possibilities and probabilities in regard to the achievement of desirable and acceptable moral outcomes. This, in turn, will depend on the competence, experience, wisdom and moral integrity of the decision-makers, and the degree of commitment they have to: (1) ensuring the realisation of morally just outcomes and (2) protecting and promoting the wellbeing and moral interests of those made vulnerable not just by their mental illnesses, but also by the inability of their caregivers to respond to the manifestation of their illnesses in an informed, morally sensitive, humane, therapeutically effective and culturally appropriate way.

Psychiatric advance directives

As previously indicated in this section, an integral and controversial component of psychiatric practice is involuntary care and treatment. Although practised under the rubric of benevolent paternalism, the tenets of involuntary treatment have nonetheless seriously challenged and, in many instances, infringed the rights of mentally ill persons – particularly those whose decision-making capacity has been seriously compromised by their illness – to make informed and self-determining decisions about their care and treatment. Thus, the right to make informed and self-determining decisions has the distinction of provoking controversy in the field – a controversy that has been classically described as:

> *the apparent clash between two highly revered values: the 'right to be let alone' and the patient's interest in the full and effective exercise of medical [sic] professionals' healing skills.* (Dresser 1982: 777)

On account of the tension between patient autonomy and therapeutic paternalism in psychiatric contexts – and the extraordinarily difficult and sometimes tragic situation in which this has often placed people (consumers and caregivers alike) – advocates and commentators have searched for ways to reconcile or at least accommodate the opposing values at issue (Dresser 1982). Underpinning this search has been the commensurate pressing need to find a balance between promoting autonomy and preventing harm and, equally important, finding a way to advance a genuine ' "supported decision-making" model in which a person makes treatment decisions for themselves, with support where required' (Ouliaris & Kealy-Bateman 2017: 574).

Striking a balance between promoting autonomy, supporting decision-making and preventing harm

People with serious mental illnesses can often experience periods of profound distress during which their capacity to make prudent and self-interested decisions about their care and treatment options can be seriously compromised. During such periods, the mentally ill can also be at risk of harming themselves and/or others. In either case, timely and effective psychiatric treatment and care are imperative.

In many instances, people with serious mental illnesses might not comply with, and might even refuse altogether to accept, recommended psychiatric treatment (e.g. oral or intramuscular psychotropic medication, or electroconvulsive therapy). In such instances, because of the psychiatric imperatives to treat their conditions (particularly if extremely distressed and 'out of control'), the mentally ill are vulnerable to having medical treatments paternalistically imposed on them against their will. Enforced treatments in such cases may, however, compound their distress and make future treatment difficult, especially if the patient later feels (i.e. during a moment of restored competency to decide) that the fiduciary nature of the professional–client relationship has been violated.

Situations involving the enforced medical treatment of the mentally ill can cause significant distress to caregivers as well who, while wanting to respect the preferences of their patients, may nevertheless recognise that, without treatment, patients in distress (and their families or supporters) will not be able to be consoled and, worse, may remain unnecessarily in a state of 'psychiatric crisis'. Here very practical questions arise of what, if anything, can be done to strike a balance between respecting the patient's autonomous wishes and constraining their freedom where its exercise could be harmful to themselves and/or to others?

For many, the answer lies in the systematic development and formal adoption of psychiatric advance directives (PADs). Widdershoven and Berghmans (2001: 92) explain that:

> By using psychiatric advance directives, it would be possible for mentally ill persons who are competent and with their disease in remission, and who want timely intervention in case of future mental crisis, to give prior authorisation to treatment at a later time when they are incompetent, non-compliant, and refusing treatment.

Later works have consistently reaffirmed this view (Ouliaris & Kealy-Bateman 2017; Sellars et al 2017; Zelle et al 2015a). Although 'gold standard' evidence is lacking, the authors of a 2009 Cochrane Database Systematic Review on 'Advance treatment directives for people with severe mental illness' nonetheless concluded that advance directives were 'well suited to the mental health setting for the purpose of conveying patients' treatment preferences should they become unable to articulate them in the future' (Campbell & Kisely 2009: 10).

But what are PADs, and are they capable of achieving the outcomes that their proponents anticipate and expect? It is to providing a brief overview of PADs – their origin, their rationale, their basic function, the perceived risks and benefits of adopting them, and the possible enablers and disablers to their uptake – that this discussion now turns.

Origin, rationale and purpose of psychiatric advance directives

Psychiatric advance directives have been defined as 'documents that allow users with severe and chronic mental illnesses to notify their treatment preferences for future crisis relapses and to appoint a surrogate decision-maker for a period of incompetence' (Nicaise et al 2013: 1). A review of the literature has found that the information and options most frequently cited by users when preparing a PAD are:

1. contact details of the user, the consultant, the general practitioner, the psychiatric nurse and the nominee (trusted person nominated by the user)
2. mental health problem or diagnosis
3. current medication and dosage
4. early signs of crisis
5. instructions to follow at the beginning of a crisis (Nicaise et al 2013: 10).

The main purpose of providing this information and alerting service providers to their preferred options is to ensure the continuity of their care, although research demonstrating this purpose remains inconclusive.

Variously named 'psychiatric wills', 'self-binding directives' (SBDs), 'advance directives', 'advance statements', 'advance agreements', 'advance instructions', 'crisis cards' and 'Ulysses contracts', the idea of notifying treatment preferences in advance, or making a 'psychiatric will' (a term that is analogous to 'living wills'), is credited with originating in the work of the eminent American psychiatrist, Thomas Szasz (1982), and the identified need for psychiatric patients to have an instrument that enabled them to refuse unwanted treatment. It was (and continues to be) believed that, when completing PADs during periods of 'competency', persons with severe mental illnesses will be enabled to feel 'empowered' and to have a sense of 'self-determination' (Nicaise et al 2013: 8; see also Berghmans & van der Zanden 2012).

In a 2013 systematic review of the literature on the subject, Nicaise and colleagues (2013) identified three main theoretical frameworks or rationales for PADs:

- enhancement of the user's autonomy
- improvement in the therapeutic alliance between the users and clinicians
- integrations of care through health providers working in partnership with clients and families.

Subsequent literature published on the subject (too numerous to cite here) has reaffirmed these findings (to be discussed further under the following sections on anticipated risks and benefits of PADs).

Forms and function of psychiatric advance directives

Since first being proposed in the early 1980s, PADs have evolved and tend to take one or both of the following two forms, notably:

- *an instructional directive* 'that provides specific information about a patient's treatment preferences'
- *a proxy directive*, in which a patient 'appoints a surrogate decision-maker who has legal authority to make treatment decisions on behalf of the patient when incapacitated' (Srebnik 2005: S42).

Depending on the legal regulations governing a given PAD, a directive can contain provisions for either 'opting-out' (refusing) treatment (both general and specific – e.g. ECT), or 'opting-in' (consenting to services as well as to specific treatments) (Atkinson et al 2003; Swartz et al 2006). To put this more simply, PADs stand to serve the basic functions of:

- *prescription* (advance consent to treatment options)
- *proscription* (advance refusal or rejection of treatment options)
- *surrogate decision-maker designation*[4] (identification and advance nomination of substitute decision-makers)
- *irrevocability during a crisis* (also known as a 'Ulysses contract' – see below)
(Swartz et al 2006: 67).

Of these four functions, the *Ulysses contract* is arguably the most reflective of the moral justification of PADs. The origin of the term 'Ulysses contract' is not clear although it probably originated in a commentary by Ennis (1982: 854) in which reference is made to 'Odysseus at the mast', published in response to Szasz's (1982) original article on 'The psychiatric will' (see also Hastings Center Report 1982a).

The idea of a Ulysses contract derives from Homer's story of the mythological character Ulysses (known as Odysseus in Greek mythology) who escaped being seduced to his death by the 'sweet songs' of the Sirens, the magical women of Cyrene, who cast spells on the sailors of ships so that their vessels would be wrecked and subsequently could be scavenged. Being previously warned of the evil intentions of the Sirens, Ulysses took the precaution of commanding his sailors to bind him to the mast of his ship (effectively restraining him), and to plug their ears with wax so that they could not hear and hence be seduced to their deaths by the Sirens. Ulysses further ordered his sailors not to release him from the mast until they were safely past the Sirens. By taking these steps, Ulysses was able to investigate the power of the Sirens without being seduced to his death by them as well as ensure the safety of his ship and his crew as they sailed past them. This story is used controversially in philosophy to demonstrate the difference between freedom and autonomy: in this case, although Ulysses had his freedom constrained (i.e. by having his body tied to the mast of his ship), his autonomy (rational preference) was essentially left intact – including during the momentary period of his incompetence while under the bewitching spell of the magical Sirens. This myth has been taken by PAD proponents as analogously justifying psychiatric patients abdicating their 'freedom' to substitute decision-makers during periods of incapacitation: although restrained during these periods, like Ulysses, their autonomy nonetheless remains intact.

Anticipated benefits of psychiatric advance directives

Despite the expectations reflected in the stated purposes and theoretical frameworks of PADs, their overall acceptance and uptake remain patchy. Moreover, there is little evidence showing that PADs have, in fact, achieved their intended purpose (Campbell & Kisely 2009). Nonetheless PADs have been touted as having the capacity to realise a number of benefits including: 'decrease hospitalizations, reduce coercion in treatment, and improve relationships between consumers, families and clinicians' (Peto et al 2004; Sellars et al 2017; Zelle et al 2015a), and destigmatising patients with mental illness on account of giving them the same rights to refuse psychiatric treatment as patients who wish to refuse general medical treatment (Atkinson et al 2004). To date, however, the anticipated benefits of PADs have yet to be realised. One reason for this is the systemic barriers to their use including a 'lack of resources deployed to assist patients in preparing PADs (unless assistance is provided, completion rates for PADs tend to be low), and a lack of "buy-in" and acceptance of PADs by clinicians' (Swanson et al 2007: 78). Lack of awareness and education about PADs (on the part of consumers and clinicians alike) has also been identified as a contributing factor (Peto et al 2004). This, in turn, has contributed to a lack of competence on the part of both health service providers and service users to honour and implement PADs (Nicaise et al 2013: 2). Other barriers that have been identified include:

- concerns about the 'legal and ethical issues relating to the liability for implementing or overriding (PAD) statements'
- the lack of capacity of 'the system' to organise therapeutic alliances and care around service user preferences (Nicaise et al 2013: 2).

Some studies have suggested that, overall, clinicians are broadly supportive of the 'advance-consent' function of PADs (termed 'prescriptive function'); however, clinicians are more reticent about their 'advanced-refusal' function (termed 'proscriptive function') – especially if used to refuse all future treatment (Swartz et al 2006).

Although barriers to the implementation of PADs persist, research has found that consumers continue to have a high interest in and demand for PADs. This is in contrast to clinicians, who have consistently been found to be somewhat ambivalent about and even afraid of them (Amering et al 1999; Appelbaum 2004, 2006; Atkinson 2004; Atkinson et al 2004; Elbogen et al 2006; Hobbs 2007; Kaustubh 2003; Kim et al 2007; Puran 2005; Srebnik & Brodoff 2003; Swanson et al 2006a, 2006b, 2006c, 2007; Swartz et al 2006; Varekamp 2004). In one US study, for example, although 66%–77% of consumer respondents stated they would like to complete a PAD if given the opportunity and assistance to do so, only 4%–13% had actually done so (Swanson et al 2006b). In a UK study, whereas 89% of voluntary organisations and more than two-thirds of stakeholder groups surveyed thought that PADs were needed, only 28% of psychiatrists surveyed thought they were (Atkinson et al 2004).

Comparable studies conducted in Australia and New Zealand have had similar findings. For example, in what is believed to be the first published national study of its kind, an Australian survey of 143 psychiatrists found that less than 30% supported PADs which involved treatment refusals (e.g. cessation of medication, remaining out of hospital and not being the subject of an involuntary admission to a psychiatric facility) (Sellars et al 2017). Of those who reported they did not support PADs, the key rationale was concern for the 'clinical profile of the patient and the professional imperative regarding the psychiatrist's duty of care' (Sellars et al 2017: 70). In short, those who did not support PADs placed more importance on clinical outcomes than on upholding patient autonomy.

A New Zealand survey of 110 mental health service users and 175 clinicians had similar findings (Thom et al 2015). The researchers reported that, although most (93%) of both clinicians and users supported the idea of PADs, they differed significantly on the preferred content of such directives – particularly with regard to the use of seclusion as a method of de-escalation. Whereas most clinicians believed that New Zealand's mental health legislation should be able to *override* a user's preferences outlined in a PAD, in contrast most mental health service users disagreed that legislation should enable their preference to be overridden (Thom et al 2015).

Also, although some studies have suggested that clinicians are broadly supportive of the 'advance-consent' function of PADs (termed 'prescriptive function'), clinicians are more reticent about their 'advance-refusal' function (termed 'proscriptive function') – especially if used to refuse all future treatment (Swartz et al 2006).

Despite this reticence, the PAD is increasingly being regarded as an important instrument that enables respect of not only the patient's wishes, but also their values (i.e. in regard to what is important in life). Further, although PAD instruments should not 'replace deliberation about possible future changes in the patients' condition' (Widdershoven & Berghmans 2001: 93), they are nonetheless seen as having an important role to play in eliciting and guiding communication about such matters (see also Spellecy 2003).

Anticipated risks of psychiatric advance directives

It is important to acknowledge that, despite their envisaged benefits, PADs are not without risk. Some commentators are especially worried about their moral authority (particularly if patients change their minds at some point) and their vulnerability to being abused and misused (Spellecy 2003). As Dresser (1982: 842) cautioned over three decades ago, if insufficiently informed persons enter into commitment contracts 'only to please their psychiatrists, the contracts would become an avenue for the abuse of psychiatric paternalism, thus decreasing individual liberty'. Dresser further cautions that, in the absence of an opportunity for patients to withdraw consent to treatment, PADs in reality could well stand as a 'coercive treatment mode that would take us a step backward – or at least sideways – from a more sensitive and realistic solution to a very difficult situation' (Dresser 1982: 854). The inability to get 'quick determinations' of illness and competency – and hence healing treatment – has also been identified as a risk that could serve ultimately to undermine the effectiveness of PADs (Cuca 1993: 1178; see also Nicaise et al 2013). These risks may be accentuated in cases where the PADs are 'competence-insensitive' and service providers wrongly judge the point at which a PAD applies and apply it prematurely (Bielby 2014).

Earlier in this chapter, under the discussion of competency to decide, the case was given of an involuntary psychiatric patient who was held down and given an intramuscular injection of psychotropic medication against his will (see pp 213–14). It will be recalled that this incident resulted in the patient being left highly mistrustful of nursing staff and even less willing to comply with his prescribed oral medication. There is room to speculate that, had a PAD been in force at the time for this patient, a very different outcome might have resulted in this case.

Current trends in the legal regulation of psychiatric advance directives

The enactment of formal legislation regulating PADs has a protracted history dating back to the USA, which has the longest history of their use, with Minnesota in 1991 becoming the first American state to enact legislation giving recognition to the 'advance psychiatric directive' allowing its citizens to 'draft directives for intrusive mental health treatments' (Cuca 1993: 1165). Currently almost two-thirds of the states in the USA have legal processes in place for allowing and managing PADs (Zelle et al 2015b).

Early proponents of PADs in the US expected that their use would spread (Appelbaum 1991). Progress has been slow, however. Only a few countries (e.g. Australia, Austria, Germany, Canada, Switzerland, the Netherlands and the United Kingdom) have introduced or are working to introduce and uphold PADs or 'psychiatric wills' (Amering et al 1999; Atkinson et al 2003; Varekamp 2004). In the UK, for example, the passage through parliament of the *Mental Capacity Bill 2004* (which was given Royal Assent in 2005, and came into force in 2007) authorises a limited form of PADs (i.e. instruments provided for by this legislation can only be used to *refuse* rather than to *give consent to* treatment) (Meredith 2005: 9; Swartz et al 2006).

Arguably the most profound change (described as an 'evolving revolution' by Callaghan and Ryan 2016) has occurred in Australian jurisdictions. Prior to 2014 there seemed to be little optimism that PADs will be formally adopted in Australian jurisdictions as a legal mechanism for promoting and protecting the rights of mentally ill people to participate effectively in decision-making concerning their psychiatric care and treatment. Since then a substantive paradigm shift has occurred, which has seen PADs incorporated into mental health legislation in the Australian Capital Territory (2015), Queensland (2016), Victoria (2014) and Western Australia (2014), with the Australian Capital Territory legislation regarded by commentators as the most progressive (see comparative table in Ouliaris & Kealy-Bateman 2017: 576). There is, however, still work to be done, noting that provisions for PADs have not yet been incorporated in the mental health legislation of all Australian jurisdictions and that, even where it has been (e.g. Victoria), patient preferences can still be overridden under defined circumstances (Callaghan & Ryan 2016; Maylea & Ryan 2017). However, in compliance with the provisions contained in the CRPD, there is now recognition that 'persons with disabilities enjoy legal status on an equal basis with others in all aspects' and that this requires recognition that competent persons, at least, have the right to refuse psychiatric treatment (Maylea & Ryan 2017: 88).

The changes that are occurring are not merely cosmetic and reflect a substantive move away from models of clinical decision-making based on determinations of 'best interests' and 'harm minimisation' (and which have tended to be over-reliant on assessment of capacity and rational competency) towards a model of 'supported decision-making' (SDM). As noted earlier, SDM places the person who is being supported at the front of the decision-making process (ALRC 2014). This paradigm shift in mental health is challenging traditional evaluation criteria and conventional justifications for involuntary treatment. On this point, with reference to the provisions contained on the CRPD, Callaghan and Ryan (2016: 610) explain:

> *Capacity assessment must not be used as a tool to deprive people of the right to participate in decision-making. Capacity must be presumed, and people with mental illness must be offered the support to exercise capacity.*

Several years ago, a consumer advocate pleaded:

> *Psychiatric Advance Directives can fulfil a real need – almost everyone I talk with about them immediately recognises that [...] I'd like to see Psychiatric Advance Directives legally enforceable throughout Australia [...] At the very least, I'd like to see changes to mental health legislation, removing any impediments to*

the use of Advance Directives in mental health settings. That said — I think Advance Directives can be used effectively, even in states where they have no formal legal status. (Strong, nd)

It has taken a very long time but, it would seem, this advocate's plea is at last being heard.

Ethical issues in suicide and parasuicide

Suicide fundamentally involves a person intentionally taking their own life (WHO 2001a, 2007c). For a death to be classified as a suicide in Australia, New Zealand and other jurisdictions, it must be:

established by coronial enquiry that the death resulted from a deliberate act of the deceased with the intention of ending his or her own life (intentional self-harm). (Simon-Davies 2011: 2)

Parasuicide, in turn, has been defined as 'any non-fatal act in which an individual deliberately causes self-injury or ingests a substance in excess of any prescribed or generally recognised dosage' (O'Connor & Armitage 2003 – citing Kreitman, 1977).

The precursor to suicide and parasuicide is *suicidal behaviour*, which has been conceptualised as 'a complex process that can range from suicidal ideation, which can be communicated through verbal or non-verbal means, to planning of suicide, attempting suicide, and in the worst case, suicide' (WHO 2012a: 4).

Scope of the problem

Suicide is recognised internationally as being a major public health issue and its prevention a global priority (WHO 2014b). WHO estimates that approximately 800 000 people die from suicide each year (being around 1 death every 40 seconds somewhere in the world) and that for every adult suicide they may be more than 20 others attempting suicide. Put another way: attempted suicide occurs up to 20 times more frequently than completed suicides (WHO 2014b: 13).

Worldwide, suicide is the second leading cause of death in 15–29 year olds. Although a serious problem in high-income countries, it is the low- and middle-income countries that bear the larger burden of the global suicide problem where an estimated 75% of all suicides occur (WHO 2014b: 15).

Australian suicide statistics mirror global trends. For the period 2012–16 the average number of suicide deaths was 2795 per year, equating to around 7.85 suicide deaths by suicide in Australia each day (Mindframe 2017). During this period, suicide was identified as being one of the leading causes of death for people aged 15–44 years and the second leading cause of death for people aged 45–54; it is also the leading cause of death in children aged between 5 and 17 years (ABS 2016).

Suicide and suicidal behaviour is also a significant health and social issue in New Zealand. Although relatively stable, the New Zealand statistics mirror global and regional trends, with the highest rate of suicide among youths aged 15–24 years (Ministry of Health 2017).

Cybersuicide

A relatively unusual dimension of the suicide problem to emerge in recent years has been the increasing incidence of *cybersuicide* (also called 'net suicide') and cyberspace suicide pacts. Cybersuicide refers to the phenomena of suicidal behaviour (ideation) and completed or attempted suicide influenced by the internet (Birbal et al 2009; Kingsley 2017). Cyberspace suicide pacts, in turn, entail two or more people 'meeting' on the internet and entering into an agreement 'to commit suicide together at a given time and place' (Rajagopal 2004: 1298). Research has suggested that the most 'preferred' platforms for forming suicide pacts are *Twitter* (Lee & Kwon 2018) and *Instagram* – the latter due to its inclusion of visuals as part of its messaging, noting that visuals work to increase online engagement (Carlyle et al 2018).

As the internet has grown (it has been estimated that there are now almost 3 billion users of the internet), so too has cybersuicide and 'webcam suicide', which is spreading across countries, cultures and generations. Among the reasons why the internet is so alluring to those contemplating and completing suicide relates to its unique features of being accessible, convenient, anonymous, private and even invisible (Bell et al 2018; Carlyle et al 2018); its interactivity (especially when forming pacts) is another alluring feature (Kingsley 2017).

It has been estimated that there are well over 100 000 websites that contain graphic information on how to suicide, with suicide notes, death certificates as well as colour photographs depicting actual suicidal acts (Alao et al 2006: 490); some sites also actively *encourage* suicidal acts (Westerlund 2011). This information is found not just on 'the dark net' (parts of the net that are not visible on search engines – that is, they are 'hidden' and uncensured and can be accessed only via special software) but is also freely available via popular search engines such as Google, Bing and Yahoo and via popular reference sites such as Wikipedia (2018d) (Kingsley 2017). Suicide information is also available via various chat rooms, as even a cursory search on the internet quickly reveals (Biddle et al 2008). Cybersuicide is also enabled by opportunities to purchase potentially lethal drugs from online pharmacies, which do not require a valid prescription from a qualified medical practitioner (Alao et al 2006).

Adolescents have been identified as a population that is particularly vulnerable to the allure of internet influences cultivating suicidal behaviour (Alao et al 2006; Bell et al 2018; Biddle et al 2008; Birbal et al 2009). They are also vulnerable to pact suicides. Although suicide pacts are not a new phenomenon, the composition of pacts has changed. Whereas most suicide pacts are generally between people who are well known to each other (e.g. spouses, siblings, friends), what has been particularly unusual about the phenomenon of cybersuicide pacts is that they have been between complete strangers who, as stated by Rajagopal (2004: 1298), 'have met over the internet and planned the tragedy via special suicide websites'. In South Korea, which has the highest suicide rate in the world, it has been reported that suicide pacts account for almost one-third of all suicides (Lee & Kwon 2018: 22).

Commentators are worried that the cyberspace suicide networks will become 'breeding grounds for real-life tragedies' (Dubecki 2007a: 1, 2007b) and will spark an epidemic of internet death pacts as despondent young people in particular – especially those immersed in a youth sub-culture of online networking – will 'log out of life' (Cameron 2005: 6; 2006).

The moral challenge of suicide

It is almost five decades since Thomas Szasz published his landmark article on 'The ethics of suicide' and its ramifications in the context of psychiatric care (Szasz 1971). Since then *mental health ethics* has generally been marginalised by the mainstream bioethics movement (Johnstone 1995; Williams 2016). To date there has been relatively little published on the subject in the bioethics literature, which has largely been overshadowed by works on the subject of euthanasia and physician-assisted suicide. With the notable exception of two early articles published in the international journal *Nursing Ethics* (Farrow & O'Brien 2003; Long et al 1998) and Cutcliffe and Links' (2008a, 2008b) two-part article on contemporary ethical issues pertaining to the nursing care of suicidal patients, even less has been published in the nursing ethics literature on the subject, which, like the mainstream bioethics literature, has been overshadowed by works on the subject of euthanasia and physician-assisted suicide and, more recently, 'moral distress' in relation to these issues.[5]

Suicide and its counterpart parasuicide (attempted suicide) warrant special attention since they pose a range of particularly challenging ethical issues for health service providers and for society as a whole. There are at least two underpinning reasons for this. The first of these relates to the fact that suicide and parasuicide (and the moral harms they stand to cause) are *relatively preventable*. The second relates to the stubbornly enduring *stigmatisation of suicide* itself and the barriers this poses to the successful prevention of suicide and the treatment of those who have unsuccessfully attempted suicide.

It is no small measure of the enduring legacy of stigmatisation that, despite improved understanding of the causes and consequences of suicide, efforts to prevent it in many countries remain stymied (WHO 2012a, 2014b). As WHO (p 11) has observed:

> Those who have lost someone to suicide, as well as those who have a history of suicide attempts, often face considerable stigma within their communities. Stigma may prevent people from seeking help and can become a barrier to accessing suicide prevention services including counselling and postvention support; this is of particular concern in countries where suicidal acts are illegal. Also, high levels of stigma may negatively affect proper reporting and recording of suicidal behaviours with its public health consequences.

WHO goes on to explain that 'while efforts to reduce the stigma of suicidal behaviours can benefit from being incorporated into the more general process of destigmatising mental illness, typically, *additional efforts* to reduce stigma attached to suicidal behaviours are required' [emphasis added] (p 11). This stance is reiterated by the WHO in its *Comprehensive mental health action plan 2013–2020* (WHO 2013b), *Preventing suicide: a global imperative* (WHO 2014b) and by the respective Australian and New Zealand Governments (i.e. in the Australian Government Department of Health's (2017) *Fifth national mental health and suicide prevention plan*, and the New Zealand Ministry of Health's (2012) *Rising to the challenge: the mental health and addiction service development plan 2012–2017*).

The problem of stigmatisation of suicide in Australia was revealed in a 2014 media report published in the Greek newspaper, *Neos Kosmos*, in which an account was given of how members of the Greek-born immigrant community still feel the need to 'tip-toe' around the issue of mental illness generally and suicide in particular (Velissaris 2014). Because family members tend to take responsibility for each other's wellbeing, they will automatically 'blame and shame' themselves if a loved one suicides (Velissaris 2014). This tendency has been fuelled by miscommunications by some priests who have not kept pace with contemporary understanding of mental illness and reportedly have denied Greek-orthodox burial services to persons who have suicided. Fearful of their loved ones being denied an orthodox burial, some families have requested the coroner not to write 'suicide' on their loved one's death certificate (Velissaris 2014).

Suicide, by its very nature, is an extremely difficult and complex issue to address. At a personal level, the suicide of a loved one, a friend or an associate can be a devastating experience. Those 'left behind' may find themselves struggling 'to make sense of the suicidal act and the causes of suicidal behaviour' (Davis 1992: 90). They may also find themselves overwhelmed by feelings of grief, shame, remorse, anger, despair and possibly even guilt at the thought that 'perhaps they could have done more' or that 'if only I had been there … it might never have happened'. It has been estimated that, for every suicide, six people (including family, friends, co-workers) are 'deeply affected' and 30 more are 'affected' (e.g. members of the community, first-response personnel such as police, ambulance and fire brigade staff) (Connetica 2016: 2)). Current research is also confirming that people bereaved by suicide are at a significantly higher risk of attempting suicide compared with bereavement caused by sudden natural causes – regardless of whether they are a blood relative (Pitman et al 2016; Spillane et al 2017). There is also growing evidence that people bereaved by suicide may be at risk of developing adverse physical health outcomes, although evidence of this is patchy and inconsistent (Spillane et al 2017).

Suicide is also difficult to address at a professional / therapeutic level. Even the very best of psychotherapies may still fail to prevent a person from completing a suicide, and even the very best of medical and nursing care may still fail to restore someone who has attempted suicide to a life that person regards as being 'worthwhile' and worth living. Equally if not more problematic are the difficulties of addressing the suicide issue at a moral level. Included among these difficulties is the challenge that suicide and attempted suicide pose to fundamental moral notions about the value, sanctity and meaning of life. An important question here is not 'how to achieve a better more fruitful [good] life' – a central question in Western moral philosophy – but, as Heyd and Bloch (1981: 185) point out, 'whether to live at all'.

More seriously, suicide challenges the very basis of ethics itself, and not least the values, standards and principles comprising it which might otherwise be appealed to for guiding deliberation on such issues as the entitlements and responsibilities of people contemplating suicide, the moral permissibility and impermissibility of suicide prevention, the entitlements and responsibilities of others towards those contemplating or attempting suicide, and other similar issues. Compounding the moral complexity of these issues is the additional consideration that, unlike other causes of death, suicide (or, more specifically, death from suicide) is, as has already been stated, relatively preventable.

Nurses who have either cared for a person who has attempted suicide, or who have been involved in the care of family members and friends of someone who has attempted suicide or succeeded in committing suicide, will be only too familiar with the deep emotional agony that inevitably comes with this kind of situation. They will also be very aware of the complex moral problems that are commonly associated with implementing interventions aimed at preventing suicide, with caring for those who have attempted unsuccessfully to suicide and with the difficulties of addressing these problems in a satisfying and helpful way.

It is not the purpose of this discussion to examine or present a treatise on the clinical aspects of suicide (its underlying causes and means of prevention) or, indeed, on the philosophy or sociology or anthropology of suicide. Such a task would require major works in their own right – as have already been undertaken (see, for example, foundational works by Battin 1982, 1996; Battin & Mayo 1980; Clemons 1990; Colt 1991; Durkheim 1952; Farberow 1975a, 1975b; Firestone 1997; Hendin 1998; Kaplan & Schwartz 1993; Miller 1992; Stengel 1970). Rather, the task here is to acquaint nurses with the ethical dimensions of suicide and suicide prevention, and the nature of nurses' moral obligations when caring for people who are contemplating or who have attempted suicide. In undertaking this task, attention will be given to examining briefly:

- linguistic challenges in defining suicide, and possible criteria that must be met in order for an act to count as suicide
- the nature and implications of the ethics of suicide prevention, intervention and postvention
- fundamental questions of whether people can meaningfully claim a 'right' to suicide and, if so, what corresponding duties such a rights claim might impose on others.

Defining suicide

Notwithstanding the definition of suicide given in the opening paragraph to this section, a further examination is warranted of given definitions of suicide – a term which, incidentally, entered the English language only in 1651 (Battin 1982: 22–58; Wennberg 1989: 17).

Suicide is a very distinctive kind of death and one which is generally distinguished from other kinds of deaths (e.g. from natural causes, homicidal acts, accidental deaths and other undetermined causes). The word suicide comes from the Latin *sui,* 'of oneself' and *cidium,* 'a slaying' (from *caedere,* 'to kill'). Like many other terms used in moral discourse, suicide is, however, a contested notion. Moreover there are no universally agreed criteria that should be met in order for an act to count as an instance of suicide or attempted suicide per se. The practical implications of this will be considered shortly, particularly in regard to the continual stigmatisation of suicide and parasuicide, and the sometimes-pejorative characterisations of suicide attempts as 'not being genuine'.

According to Stengel (1970: 77), a commonsense notion of suicide can be expressed in the following terms:

> *A person, having decided to end his [or her] life, or acting on a sudden impulse to do so, kills himself [or herself], having chosen the most effective methods available and having made sure that nobody interferes. When he [or she] survives he [or she] is said to have failed and the act is called an unsuccessful suicide*

> *attempt. Death is the only purpose of this act and therefore the only criterion of success. Failure may be due to any of the following causes: the sense of purpose may not have been strong enough, or the act may have been undertaken half-heartedly because it was not quite genuine; the subject was ignorant of the limitations of the method; or he [or she] was lacking in judgment and determination through mental illness.*

This definition is not, of course, without controversy — for example: 'What constitutes a "genuine" suicide attempt?' and 'When is a suicide attempt to be regarded as "half-hearted" as opposed to "whole-hearted"?' Further, as Stengel himself points out, the definition may not do justice to what has become 'a very common and varied behaviour pattern' (1970: 77). Nevertheless, it provides an important insight into the kinds of criteria that should be met in order for an act to count as suicide. One such criterion is that of *intention* — specifically, the intention to end one's life (Margolis 1975, reprinted in Beauchamp & Perlin 1978: 95).

As Beauchamp points out (1980: 70), central to what is called the 'prevailing definition' of suicide is the following premise: 'Suicide occurs if and only if there is an intentional termination of one's own life.'

Beauchamp suggests that other criteria should be met in order for an act to count as suicide, including the following:

1. *death is chosen voluntarily (that is, is free of coercive or manipulative influences)*
2. *an active means of death is chosen*
3. *death is caused by the person desiring death (one dies by 'one's own hand')*
4. *death is self-regarding (rather than altruistic or other-regarding)*
5. *the person seeking death does not have a fatal or terminal illness.* (Beauchamp 1980: 73–9)

Windt suggests similar criteria of suicide (all of which have been mentioned in the suicide literature). These are:

1. *death [must be] caused by the actions or behaviour of the deceased*
2. *the deceased wanted, desired, or wished death*
3. *the deceased intended, chose, decided or willed to die*
4. *the deceased knew that death would result from his [or her] behaviour; and that*
5. *the deceased was responsible for his [or her] own death.* (Windt 1980: 41, tabulations added)

At first glance, these and similar criteria of suicide appear helpful. On closer analysis, however, a number of problems quickly become apparent — not least the problem of so-called 'exceptional cases', and whether the criteria listed are relevant to or can be applied appropriately and meaningfully to these cases. Consider, for example, the cases of people engaging in dangerous and potentially life-threatening ('suicidal') sports (e.g. bungee jumping, mountain climbing, racing car driving, hang gliding), dangerous work activities (being a member of a bomb disposal squad or a combat soldier), or other life-threatening activities such as cigarette smoking, eating and drinking excessively, illicit drug taking and so on. In all these cases, it is probably true that the people concerned: chose the activities in question; were aware of the potential threats the activities posed to their lives and wellbeing; voluntarily engaged in the activities chosen; and, were they to die as a result of engaging in these activities, were 'responsible for their own deaths' insofar as they were willing accomplices to the activities and their associated risks. Further, while the people concerned might not have intended their own (accidental) deaths, they nevertheless foresaw their deaths as a possibility associated with the risky activities they had engaged in, and thereby, ipso facto, can be said to have intended their own demise. Given the criteria for suicide outlined above, it seems we are committed to accepting that people who die as a result of their deliberately engaging in dangerous sporting activities, work activities or lifestyles have, in essence, suicided.

Yet, this does not seem to accord with our intuitions on the matter – nor does it sit comfortably with what we would perhaps ordinarily regard as suicide. Let us examine another example to see if this will clarify the matter.

In 1982, Barney Clark, aged 62, became the first human being to receive an artificial (mechanical) heart. Recognising that this medical experiment had the potential to make Mr Clark's life burdensome, his doctor, Willem Kolff, gave him a key that could be used to turn off the compressor sustaining the artificial heart's action. Defending his decision to supply this key, Dr Kolff argued that if Mr Clark:

> *suffers and feels it isn't worth it any more, he has a key that he can apply … I think it is entirely legitimate that this man whose life has been extended should have the right to cut it off if he doesn't want it, if life ceases to be enjoyable.* (cited in Beauchamp & Childress 2001: 188)

The conceptual dilemma which arises here is this: if Mr Clark had chosen to use the key he had been given, and had turned off the compressor driving his artificial heart, which of the following statements would have been the most accurate description of his action and the cause of his death:

1 forgoing extraordinary means of life-sustaining treatment
2 withdrawing from an experiment
3 letting nature take its course
4 natural death
5 euthanasia
6 suicide?

To complicate the issue, as Beauchamp and Childress point out (2001: 188):

> *If [Clark] had refused to accept the artificial heart in the first place, few would have labelled his act a suicide. His overall condition was extremely poor, the artificial heart was experimental, and no suicidal intention was evident. If, on the other hand, Clark had intentionally shot himself with a gun while on the artificial heart, the act would have been characterised as suicide.*

To complicate the issue still further, what if Mr Clark had consented to receiving the heart in the belief that the risks associated with the experiment were so great that a hastened death would be assured? Could this be classified as a kind of suicide?

Part of the difficulty in sorting out the conceptual confusion surrounding the development of an adequate definition of and criteria for suicide can be linked to the lingering legacy of varying socio-cultural historical and religious taboos against suicide. Beauchamp and Childress (1989: 223) suggest, for example, that we often shield acts of which we approve (or at least acts of which we do not disapprove) from the stigmatising label of 'suicide' – preferring instead to use terms that are more socially acceptable, such as 'euthanasia' or 'withdrawing extraordinary life-saving treatment' and similar notions.

In light of these considerations, perhaps an important first step in developing a workable definition of and criteria for suicide is to demystify it, and to strip it of the taboos and stigmatisation which still linger around it – and which may encourage people to be less than intellectually honest when speaking of its incidence and cause. A second and related step is to modify the negatively connoted language that tends to be used in referring to and discussing suicide. In this instance, the problem of language is highly significant, and should not be underestimated. As Wennberg explains (1989: 17):

> *'suicide' is not a neutrally descriptive term like 'cat', 'car', or 'flower'. Rather, it carries with it a strong negative connotation, especially when it is part of the phrase 'commit suicide'. For one typically does not commit X where X is either something approved or something of neutral standing (cf. 'commit murder', 'commit a felony', 'commit a crime', 'commit adultery', 'commit a sin', 'commit treason', 'commit a faux pas', etc.).*

The lesson here is important: the use of the phrase 'committed suicide' (as opposed to the phrase 'completed suicide' or the term 'suicided') is misleading and unhelpful – not least because it seems to imply the commission of a crime, or even a sin, when clearly there has been none.

A third and final step towards developing a working definition of and criteria for suicide is to reinstate the authority of our own ordinary commonsense experience of the world, and our collective experience-based knowledge of what is and what is not an act of suicide or attempted suicide. One reason for this is that, in the ultimate analysis, the distinction between suicide and other types of death (e.g. euthanasia) may rest not on sophisticated philosophical criteria, but on our fine intuitions informed by life experience. Thus, ultimately, this matter may well be decided by appealing to:

1. the known intentions and motivations of the person who has died (for instance, whether the death was pursued as 'an alleged solution for the ills of dying' [euthanasia], or as an 'alleged' cure for the ills of living [suicide] (Donnelly 1990: 9))
2. the context in which the person died
3. whether the person who died genuinely believed there was no alternative besides death in order to alleviate his or her suffering, or to transcend the life circumstances which for him or her had become unbearable.

The problem remains, however, that ascertaining these things may be just as difficult as establishing reliable criteria for suicide. Nevertheless, it is important that suicide be defined. One reason for this is that without an adequate definition of suicide it will remain extremely difficult to assess accurately the incidence, cause and appropriate means of preventing suicide. It will also be difficult to eradicate the spurious distinction which is sometimes drawn between 'genuine' and 'non-genuine' suicide attempts, with the tragic consequence that some who are suffering and needing help will be dismissed as malingerers and, worse, as not suffering or needing help at all.

Finally, the lack of an adequate definition of suicide will make it difficult to engage in substantive moral debate on the ethical aspects of suicide, and to respond effectively and appropriately to the many moral problems raised by the suicide question, some of which are considered below.

Before continuing, however, a brief clarification is required on the working definitions of the terms 'suicide' and 'parasuicide' to be used in the remainder of this chapter, and on the distinction which might otherwise be drawn between 'suicide' (as presently being considered in this chapter) and 'euthanasia' (to be considered in Chapter 10).

Although there is no universally agreed criteria of suicide, suicide is generally recognised as being one of the five medical–legal classifications of modes of death, which are taken to include (in addition to suicidal death): accidental, natural, homicidal and undetermined death (Colt 1991: 263–4). Furthermore, while acknowledging the many difficulties associated with formulating a precise and universally agreed definition of suicide, there is a strong sense in which suicide (at least in the Western world) can be meaningfully understood as:

> *a conscious act of self-induced annihilation, best understood as a multidimensional malaise in a needful individual who defines an issue for which the suicide is perceived as the best solution.* (Shneidman 1985: 203)

A more elaborate explication of this view is as follows:

> *suicide has two branches. The first is that suicide is a multifaceted event and that biological, cultural, sociological, interpersonal, intrapsychic, logical, conscious and unconscious, and philosophical elements are present, in various degrees, in each suicide event.*
>
> *The second [...] is that, in the distillation of each suicide event, its essential element is a psychological one; that is to say, each suicidal drama occurs in the mind of a unique individual. Suicide is purposive. Its purpose is to respond to or redress certain psychological needs. There are many pointless deaths but there are*

no needless suicides. Suicide is a concatenated, complicated, multidimensional, conscious and unconscious 'choice' of the best possible practical solution to a perceived problem, dilemma, impasse, crisis or desperation. (Shneidman 1993: 3)

Parasuicide (a term which came into usage in the late 1960s in an attempt to overcome the confusion associated with using the term 'attempted suicide') can, in turn, be defined as:

An act with non-fatal outcome, in which an individual deliberately initiates a non-habitual behaviour that, without intervention from others, will cause self-harm, or deliberately ingests a substance in excess of the prescribed or generally recognised therapeutic dosage, and which is aimed at realising changes which the subject desired via the actual or expected physical consequences. (Williams 1997: 69)

Both suicide and parasuicide are the 'unequivocal expression of raw suffering' or the 'psychache' (Shneidman 1993) of individuals – a suffering from which, for a variety of reasons (not always known or understood by others), these individuals have not been able to secure relief (Heckler 1994: xxiv). Suicide ideation (suicidal thoughts) and suicidal behaviour are also taken here as being 'the result of extreme and unusual human predicaments' which require people's deepest and most empathic understanding (Heckler 1994: xxv).

Distinguishing suicide from euthanasia

Suicide, as discussed in this section, is taken here as referring to a different kind of death that might otherwise be brought about by voluntary active euthanasia or physician-assisted suicide. While euthanasia, physician-assisted suicide and 'unassisted' suicide (as being considered here) share several features in common, there are also some significant differences between them. One such difference was captured by the following insightful comments of a former university student:

As I see it, in the case of euthanasia / assisted suicide, the person wants to live, but cannot (and it is too hard to die); whereas in the case of 'suicide proper', the person can live, yet does not want to (it is too hard to live). (Su Chia Hsian, personal communication)

Another key difference that warrants mention here is that, whereas euthanasia and physician-assisted suicide tend to be conducted in the context of a breakdown in physical health and wellbeing, suicide (as being considered here) tends to occur in the context of a breakdown in mental health and wellbeing – that is, it is linked in important ways to a lethal combination of the psychogenic distress states of depression, hopelessness, despair and apathy.

Ethical dimensions of suicide

Orthodox religious traditions have, for the most part, tended to regard suicide as the gravest sin imaginable, and as constituting the most serious violation of one's duties to oneself, to others and to God (Gearing & Lizardi 2009). These views have been extremely influential and continue to be the subject of philosophical debate today. However, as Knight (1992: 262) points out, 'religiously speaking, the notion of suicide as an unforgivable sin has few, if any, defenders in contemporary moral philosophy'. Further, unlike the days when religious prohibition saw suicide condemned as a grossly immoral act, it is difficult today to find tenable moral arguments against the suicide of people who are able to choose autonomously to end their own lives (Knight 1992: 262). Nevertheless, a number of troubling questions remain about the ethics of suicide, such as: 'Is there a right to suicide?', 'If so, what conditions must be satisfied before this right can be claimed?', 'What are the obligations of others in regard to those contemplating or attempting suicide?', 'Is there a duty to prevent suicide?' and 'If so, under what conditions should a suicide be prevented?' It is to briefly answering these questions that the remainder of this discussion now turns.

Autonomy and the right to suicide

Fundamental to Western moral thinking is the principle of autonomy. As discussed in Chapter 3, the moral principle of autonomy prescribes that a person's considered preferences should be respected – even if others disagree with them or regard them as foolish – provided they do not interfere with or harm the significant moral interests of others. If this principle is accepted, then the entitlement of people to choose autonomously to suicide must be respected; it must also be accepted that it would be morally indefensible to prevent these people from exercising their choice. By this view, as Beauchamp explains (1980: 100):

> If people are autonomous, then they have the right to be left alone and to do with their lives as they wish, so long as they are sufficiently free of responsibilities to others. From this perspective, the intervention in the life of a suicide is simply an unjust deprivation of liberty.

Jonathan Glover argues along similar lines (1977: 171), explaining that once it is admitted that suicide need not always be regarded as an 'irrational symptom of mental disturbance', then:

> [it] is a matter for each person's free choice: other people should have nothing to say about it, and the question for someone contemplating it is simply one of whether his [or her] future life will be worth living.

It is far from certain, however, that people contemplating or attempting suicide are, in fact, entitled to be 'left alone and to do with their lives as they wish' (Beauchamp 1980: 100), or that 'other people should have nothing to say about it' (Glover 1977: 171). There are a number of reasons for this. First, an act of suicide is never without moral consequences: not only does it have an impact on the significant moral interests of the person suiciding, but also it can significantly affect the important moral interests of others (as stated earlier, between 6 and 30 people can be affected by the suicide of another). As experience tells us, suicide can shatter, injure and destroy the lives of other people; it can also cause substantial loss to society. Where suicides do affect the significant moral interests of others, there are at least prima-facie grounds for justifying paternalistic intervention to prevent those suicides occurring. As well as this, where other people's significant moral interests are at stake, there may even be an obligation on the part of people contemplating suicide not to proceed with planned actions aimed at ending their own lives (Brandt 1978) – although it is an open question just how realistic this demand is in the case of people suffering severe psychological distress.

In the light of these circumstances, it is evident that claims to autonomy *alone* are not sufficient to justify an unequivocal acceptance of a person's decision to suicide, or to justify non-intervention or 'non-postvention' (counselling and therapy after a suicide attempt (Battin 1982: 16)) in the case of contemplated or attempted suicide. There is always the possibility, however, that the concerns or interests of others may not be strong enough to override a person's autonomous wish to suicide. Even so, this is something which must be determined by careful evaluation and a 'balancing of considerations' of all the moral interests involved (Beauchamp & Perlin 1978: 91), not just by an uncritical deontological acceptance of the moral principle of autonomy. Such a calculation might ultimately show that a contemplated suicide, once carried out, should indeed be permitted in the interests of others.

A second reason why it is not clear that people contemplating or attempting suicide should not have their wishes interfered with is that the *quality* of the autonomy behind the choice may not be optimal. As was discussed in Chapter 3, as a *concept* (to be distinguished here from a *principle*), autonomy refers to a person's independent and self-contained ability to decide. At issue in the case of suicide is the question of whether a person contemplating suicide is really capable of making the evaluative, deliberative and reflective choices that are fundamental to an authentic, prudent and autonomous decision to suicide. Although it is true that even so-called 'incompetent' people are still capable of making self-interested choices (see, for example, the discussion on competency earlier in this chapter), the extent to which the choices of these people should be respected is not something that can be decided solely on the basis of the demands prescribed by the moral principle of autonomy; there are other moral considerations that need to be taken into account – including the moral demand to prevent otherwise-avoidable harm to people, which a suicide death stands to cause.

The issue of the quality of a suicidal person's autonomous choice to kill himself or herself is an important one and, even when considered from a clinical as opposed to a philosophical perspective, has an important bearing on deciding the ethical acceptability of paternalistic interventions aimed at preventing people from completing suicide.

It is known, for example, that depression is a major contributing factor in suicide and that the improved detection and treatment of depression is generally regarded as a major component of effective suicide prevention strategies (Ribeiro et al 2018). Although depression alone may not result in suicide, when it is coupled with abiding and intolerable feelings of hopelessness about the future, despair and apathy the risk of suicide is extremely high. Of importance to the discussion at this point is the consideration that feelings of depression, hopelessness, apathy and despair can have a significant and far-reaching impact on a person's ability to make 'truly' autonomous choices. As has long been recognised in the bioethics literature, these feelings can:

- restrict people's abilities to evaluate and calculate correctly the range of possibilities and probabilities available when planning and making judgments about their lives and future prospects (Beauchamp 1980; Brandt 1978, 1980)
- skew calculations of the probable harms and benefits that may flow from suicide (as Beauchamp (1980: 101) points out, 'without depression, persons might make quite different calculations even when their situation is dire')
- result in suicidal people overestimating the magnitude and insolubility of their problems (Knight 1992)
- result in impulsive and imprudent choices that might otherwise not have been made (Heyd & Bloch 1981).

In short, feelings of depression, hopelessness, apathy and despair can undermine in significant ways a person's ability to make sound autonomous choices. The question remains, however, of whether these feelings and a possible associated diminution in the ability to make sound autonomous choices are of a nature that justifies paternalistic intervention to prevent a person completing suicide – including using invasive procedures to resuscitate someone who has attempted suicide. Or would such intervention – no matter how benevolent – still constitute an unacceptable violation of the moral principle of autonomy?

The short answer to these questions is that intervention may not only be justified, but may even be required, in the interests of both promoting a person's autonomy and saving a worthwhile life. On this point, Jonathan Glover explains (1977: 176–7):

> Where we think someone bent on suicide has a life worth living, it is always legitimate to reason with him [or her] and to try and persuade him [or her] to stand back and think again. There is no case against reasoning, as it in no way encroaches on the person's autonomy. There is a strong case in its favour, as where it succeeds it will prevent the loss of a worthwhile life. (If the person's life turns out not to be worthwhile, he [or she] can always change his [or her] mind again.) And if persuasion fails, the outcome is no worse than it would otherwise have been.

Glover goes on to contend that where suicidal tendencies are the product of temporary depressive mood-swings – for instance, where the person 'alternates between very much wanting to go on living and moods of suicidal depression' – then intervention aimed at overriding a decision to suicide 'is less disrespectful of autonomy than overriding a preference that plays a stable role in a person's outlook' (Glover 1977: 178). If, for example, a person repeatedly and persistently attempts suicide, and the underlying preference (i.e. to die) informing these attempts remains constant, then the onus is on would-be 'rescuers' or interveners to reconsider their own judgments about whether the life of the person attempting suicide is, in fact, worthwhile and worth living, or whether they have been mistaken in their views. Confronting as it may be, the demand in the latter instance may be an overriding one in favour of not intervening to save the person's life (Glover 1977). Before this position is accepted, however, there are at least prima-facie grounds for asserting that the following five conditions must be met:

1. that the decision to suicide is based on a realistic assessment of the life-circumstances or situation at hand (Knight 1992: 254; Motto 1983: 443–6)
2. that the person contemplating suicide has made an 'exhaustive examination' of all available options and has taken into account the 'various possible "errors" and [made] appropriate rectifications of his [or her] initial evaluation' (Brandt 1978: 132; Brandt 1980)
3. that the thought processes used in reaching the decision to suicide have not been impaired by severe emotional distress, feelings of hopelessness and despair, mental illness or the adverse side effects of drugs (Knight 1992: 254)
4. that the degree of ambivalence between wanting to live and wanting to die is minimal (Donnelly 1990: 8; Glover 1977: 178; Motto 1983: 443–6)
5. that the desire and motivation to suicide is of a nature that 'uninvolved observers from their community or social group [would find] understandable' (Knight 1992: 254).

Although the satisfaction of these criteria may not always result in the prevention of morally undesirable consequences in situations involving people wanting to suicide, it may nevertheless result in more appropriate assessments of when it is right and when it is not right to paternalistically override a person's autonomous decision to suicide.

One problem which emerges here, however, is that, even if these criteria are not satisfied, does that necessarily justify paternalistic intervention to prevent a person from completing a suicide? What if the suicidal person in question is in a state of intolerable suffering, as suggested in the Chabot case (discussed in Chapter 10)? Here the additional questions arise: 'Can those who are suffering intolerably and intractably (whether on account of physical or mental illness or some other state of physical or psychogenic distress) be expected decently to go on living?', 'Or should people in these situations be released from the "obligation to live" – if, indeed, it is an obligation – irrespective of their ability to decide autonomously what is in their own best interests?' and 'Are others entitled morally to force a person to go on living a life characterised by excruciating feelings of depression, hopelessness, apathy, despair and a sense that life has lost all meaning and purpose?' It is not unreasonable to hold that a person in this state would prefer death to life. As Glover points out (1977: 174):

> Most of us prefer to be anaesthetised for a painful operation. If most of my life were to be on that level, I might opt for a permanent anaesthesia, or death.

Margolis (1975, reprinted in Beauchamp & Perlin 1978: 96) argues, however, that although prolonged anaesthesia may indeed be 'prudentially preferable to enduring pain' the desire to reduce pain in itself 'cannot justify suicide to end pain as a decision of a prudential sort'. One reason for this is that enduring even intolerable pain may, in the ultimate analysis, still be preferable to no life at all (Margolis 1975, reprinted in Beauchamp & Perlin 1978: 96; see also Glover 1977). Another reason is that to allow suicide as a means of alleviating suffering is to compound the hopelessness underpinning the suffering of suicide; it is also to abandon as hopeless those who have abandoned themselves as hopeless, and thereby to violate a fundamental professional ethic of care and responsibility to aid the distressed.

If suicide is viewed as a 'violent statement about human connections, broken and maintained' (Lifton 1979: 239), and not simply as a matter of exercising an autonomous choice (as Hauerwas (1986: 107) reminds us, 'life has a purpose beyond simply being autonomous'), perhaps our moral obligations towards those contemplating or attempting suicide will become clearer. In particular, as Knight's (1992) discussion on the suffering of suicide clarifies, there needs to be a much greater understanding of the excruciating sense of hopelessness and despair that underlies and motivates many a decision to suicide. Drawing on the landmark work by Heckler (1994), there also needs to be a much greater appreciation by others that behind every suicide and parasuicide is a life story of 'overwhelming circumstances'. As Stubbs (1994: xii) reminds readers, in the foreword to Heckler's insightful study *Waking up alive: the descent to suicide and return to life*:

> *Suicide is caused by feelings not by facts – a similar event may be borne by one person and may lead another to suicide or attempted suicide. Events, feelings and experiences add strands to a net that can drag you under. The final straw can be the weight of gossamer but the combined effect can be devastating. Or the final straw can weigh like an iron girder ... Unless we have stood on the edge of the precipice of our own life, we can only begin to grasp how it feels.*

Once these and related considerations are understood, it may become clearer that the way to remedy the suffering underlying a decision to suicide is not to do away with the sufferer, but rather to do away with the sense of hopelessness and despair fuelling the suffering. This, however, requires great compassion, empathy and commitment on the part of those intervening and preventing people from suiciding. As Knight puts it (1992: 266):

> *Intervention in suicide involves walking down that 'dark road' and immersing oneself into that world in which the suicidal person is living. One soon discovers that most suicidal persons have a predisposition to overestimate the magnitude and insolubility of their problems. Coupled with this, as has been emphasised by those 'who have been there', is an exaggerated negative view of the outside world, of themselves, and of the future. An awareness of what and how a suicidal person is thinking and feeling may lead those intervening to see quickly that the suicidal person's plight has a way out, and soon hope begins to dawn.*

The ethics of suicide prevention: some further considerations

It is probably true that most health care professionals feel obliged to:

- try and persuade people contemplating suicide to change their minds
- counsel those who have lost their sense of hope, purpose and meaning in life, in order to modify their perceptions so that they regain a more optimistic outlook on the future
- resuscitate people who have attempted suicide and who are on the brink of death
- treat the injuries of people whose suicide attempts have failed.

Whether health care professionals do, in fact, have these obligations may, in the end, be a matter to be decided not by moral theory, or even by law, but by empathy, compassion, kindness and wisdom, informed by a profound understanding of human vulnerability and suffering, together with a commitment to take each case on its own unique and individual merit. Either way, it is important not to forget that our obligation to render aid to a person contemplating or attempting suicide is as strong as it would be to aid any person in distress, and that this may require more than merely protecting a person's autonomy; it may require the more substantive task of protecting a person's genuine human welfare, and restoring in them a sense of hope that, often due to circumstances beyond their control, has abandoned them.

Some may find it amenable to view suicide as the manifestation of a mental illness, and hence something that is 'irrational' and 'irresponsible' and ipso facto quite beyond the realms of moral inquiry.

This discussion has shown, however, that even if suicide is the product of mental illness or extreme emotional distress, depression or other psychogenic pain states it still has a profound moral dimension, and still requires those involved in suicide prevention and intervention to justify their views and actions, and not to merely assume that these are in themselves morally correct just because they have as their end the preservation of life or the maximisation of autonomy.

Suicide and parasuicide are issues of importance and concern to all nurses, not just to those working in the area of mental health. How well nurses and others respond to the moral issues raised depends, however, on a variety of factors – including the success with which suicide is stripped of the taboos which still surround it, and the degree to which suicide is demystified as a desperate act aimed at transcending a situation which a distressed person has come to perceive as hopeless.

Many years ago I was involved in the care of a woman who had attempted suicide by pouring a can of petrol over herself and setting fire to it. She arrived in casualty with 100% burns to her body. Incredibly, despite the horrendous injuries her body had sustained, her eyes were unharmed. The extent of her burns made it impossible to insert an intravenous line in the usual way, and a cut-down (which involves a surgical incision to expose a deeply situated vein) had to be performed. I remember the doctor looking at me while he was performing the cut-down, and gasping in horror as the woman's burnt flesh parted in his hands. Nevertheless, this compassionate man succeeded in inserting the intravenous line, and consoled the woman as he did so. As we all worked diligently to retrieve this injured life, the woman looked on smiling, and reassuring us all with the words, 'Don't worry dears, I will be all right'. I remember looking up at this woman and, on observing her terrible injuries, thinking how desperate she must have been to have engaged in such an act. She, however, looked back at me with eyes that were clear and shining, and, bizarre as this whole scene was, I could see that she had found incredible peace within herself. The image of her burnt and tortured body did not sit well with the peace expressed in her eyes, but I knew that she had achieved her goal, and that it would be only a matter of time before she would be released from the suffering that had motivated her to undertake such a desperate act. Her death a day or two later was no surprise. Yet I still cannot help thinking that this woman paid a terrible price for the peace she eventually found in death, and could not find in life.

During the same year, I was involved in the care of a man who had also attempted suicide, in this instance by placing the muzzle of a gun in his mouth and shooting himself. He failed in his attempt to kill himself, however, and succeeded only in destroying one side of his face. After receiving plastic surgery to repair the serious gunshot wound sustained, he was admitted to intensive care. Unlike the woman who had set fire to herself, however, he was not at peace within himself. As he lay corpse-like on his bed, I remember noting that his eyes were like the eyes of a dead man – dilated, dull, and unresponsive to light. It was as though his soul had died, and nothing mattered any more. Once, when his plastic surgeon visited to check his wounds, the man handed the doctor a note. Written on the note were the words: 'Dear Dr X – did you do this [the surgical repair] for your sake or mine?' Understandably, the surgeon, who was a compassionate and gentle man, was devastated. Shortly after being transferred out of the intensive care unit to a general ward, the man climbed out through a toilet window and plunged to his death several storeys below. Many of the staff were left feeling that they had failed this man. The circumstances motivating his initial suicidal attempt had not seemed insurmountable to them, and they sincerely believed he was 'better' – but he was not better, and eventually he too achieved his goal of death. As I recall the case of this desperate and hopeless man, I cannot forget the costly suffering and distress of those he left behind – especially his wife and young children. How different things would have been if he, like the people caring for and about him, could have perceived that his problems were not as overwhelming as he thought, and that it was not necessary to take the desperate action that he ultimately took. To this day, I am reminded by this case of the importance of never underestimating the capacity of human beings to feel deeply and to suffer profoundly on account of things which seem (though they may not necessarily be) insurmountable, and of how feelings of desperation and hopelessness associated with problems perceived as insurmountable can so easily override the desire to go on living.[6]

Conclusion

Addressing ethical issues in mental health care is a strongly warranted project. This project must, however, take into account that people with mental illnesses tend not so much to be affected by the so-called 'big' ethical issues so often deemed 'paramount' in the mainstream bioethics literature (e.g. informed consent, confidentiality and so forth). Rather, they tend to be affected by much more 'basic' day-to-day relationship and existential issues which, while perhaps lacking the intrigue of other 'exotic' bioethical issues, nevertheless have a profound moral dimension and warrant just as much attention as do the 'big' ethical issues. Such issues include:

- *the desperate need for understanding*
- *the need to be able to speak openly and to be heard*
- *the longing for acceptance by others of the mystery and the unpredictability of their illness, without constantly having to defend and explain to those who have little interest in understanding*
- *the desire to be equal with others and to have basic human rights respected*. (adapted from Burdekin et al 1993: 439–40).

Other fundamental issues requiring ongoing attention and critical evaluation concern the delivery of effective *recovery-focused* (Çam & Yalçıner 2018), *trauma-informed* (Muskett 2014; Moloney et al 2018; Wilson et al 2017) and genuinely *person-centred* (Waters & Buchanan 2017) mental health care in community and institutional settings.

Nurses have a fundamental role to play in promoting access, equity, compassion and social justice in mental health care domains. The main responsibility, however, may not be so much to promote the autonomy of people with mental illnesses, which may be misdirected. Rather the higher priority is to recognise the vulnerability of people when at risk of or already in the grip of a psychiatric crisis, to ensure that those who are mentally ill are as safe as they can possibly be and that they get the care they need, and which ultimately may enable them to obtain a state of health and the peace of mind and ease of being that most others take for granted.

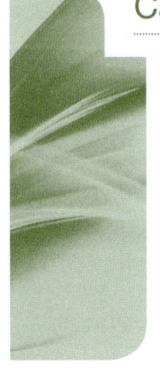

Case scenario

A 16-year-old girl, who had a history of being ruthlessly bullied via social media, was feeling overwhelmingly suicidal and went to the emergency department (ED) of the local hospital seeking help. This was not the first time she had attended the ED over the past year when feeling suicidal. Although the ED did not appear busy, she nonetheless had to wait 4 hours before being seen. When she was seen, she was told 'we couldn't help you before and there is little we can do for you now' and so 'go home'. A few days later, the girl suicided by hanging herself. An inquest into her death concluded that her death could have been prevented. Contributing factors included: failure to keep adequate medical records of her attendances at the facility, dismissive attitudes of the staff towards the seriousness of her suicide ideation, lack of regard for the insights of family members who had accompanied her previously to the hospital, and a lack of responsiveness and compassion by the staff.

CRITICAL QUESTIONS

1. What are your responsibilities as a professional caregiver in regard to caring for people who present with suicide ideation?
2. How might you have maximised the moral interests, welfare and wellbeing of the 16-year-old girl who presented to the ED for help?
3. What action, if any, would you take if you encountered a co-worker treating a suicidal person seeking help in a dismissive and uncompassionate manner?

Endnotes

1. Article 12 can be accessed at: https://www.un.org/development/desa/disabilities/convention-on-the-rights-of-persons-with-disabilities/article-12-equal-recognition-before-the-law.html.
2. According to Belcher and colleagues (2017) medication refusal and non-adherence is regarded by mental health care professionals as one of the most critical ethical and as well as clinical issues they have to deal with in both short-term and long-term patient care.
3. See the *Hopkins Competency Assessment Test (HCAT)*, the *Competency Interview Schedule (CIS)*, and the *Structured Interview for Competency/Incompetency Assessment Testing and Ranking Inventory (SICIATRI)* as cited in Wang S-B and colleagues (2017).
4. As noted earlier, there is, however, a growing shift away from the notions of 'surrogate' or 'substitute' decision-maker to that of 'supported decision-making' (ALRC 2014; Callaghan & Ryan 2016).
5. Mental health ethics has largely been estranged in the nursing ethics literature. For example, a cursory search of the international journal *Nursing Ethics*, the pre-eminent journal in the field of nursing ethics, found only a handful of substantive articles on ethical issues specifically related to mental health or psychiatric care (in the period 1994–2018), notably: Ohnishi and colleagues' (2008) discussion on whistleblowing in a Japanese psychiatric hospital; Edwards and Hewitt's (2011) critical examination of the ethics of nurses overseeing 'supervised self-harm' regimes; Moe and colleagues' (2012) exploration of the ethics of mental health nurses 'working behind the scenes' when caring for patients experiencing first-episode psychosis; Eren's (2013) exploration of nurses' ethical beliefs and ethical problems encountered in Turkish psychiatric settings; Norvoll and Pedersen's (2018) study of patients' moral views on coercion in mental healthcare; and Warrender's (2017) essay on the ethics of risk management in patients with borderline personality disorder.
6. Names and details of times and places have been suppressed, but these are true stories that reflect the experience of all nurses everywhere.

CHAPTER 9

Ethical issues in end-of-life care

KEYWORDS

advance care planning
advance directive
Do Not Resuscitate (DNR) directives
end-of-life decision-making
living wills
medical futility
Not For Resuscitation (NFR) directives
Not For Treatment (NFT) directives
quality of life
respecting patient choices (RPC) programs
withdrawal of treatment

LEARNING OBJECTIVES

Upon the completion of this chapter and with further self-directed learning you are expected to be able to:

- Discuss critically 'Not For Treatment (NFT)' directives and 'Not For Resuscitation (NFR)' directives.
- Discuss critically the moral criteria that might be used to justify an NFT or NFR directive.
- Examine critically the ethical dimensions of NFT and NFR directives.
- Discuss critically ways in which NFT and NFR policies and procedures could be improved.
- Discuss the notion of 'medical futility' and its implications for the profession and practice of nursing.
- Explain why medical futility has been controversially abandoned as an explicit decisional criterion in end-of-life decision-making.
- Examine critically the criterion 'quality of life' and its relevance to end-of-life decision-making.
- Discuss critically three senses in which the notion of quality of life might be used.
- Explore the possible risks to patients of making faulty quality-of-life judgments.
- Define 'advance directives' and 'advance care planning'.
- Discuss critically how advance directives work.
- Differentiate between advance directives, advance care planning and respecting patient choices (RPC).
- Examine critically the risks and benefits of advance directives and advance care planning.
- Explore how nurses can make a significant contribution to care and treatment decisions at the end stage of life.

Introduction

At the end stages of life there invariably comes a point at which decisions have to be made about whether to start, stop or withdraw life-sustaining treatment. The life-sustaining treatment in this instance can include the use of invasive ('aggressive') treatments (such as mechanical ventilation/life-support machines, surgery, emergency cardiopulmonary resuscitation, haemodialysis and chemotherapy), or the use of less-invasive ('less-aggressive') treatments (such as the administration of antibiotics, cardiac arrhythmic drugs, blood transfusions, and intravenous and/or nasogastric hydration). Whether involving invasive or non-invasive treatments, decisions have to be made either way (i.e. to treat or not to treat) *even* when it is 'obvious' (or at least highly probable) that their administration will not result in improved clinical outcomes for the patient – for example, the patient will continue to experience 'grievous bodily deterioration' and/or will ultimately die, regardless of the treatment given (Cantor 2004: 1400). The question remains, however, of who should decide these things, and on what basis?

The questions of who ultimately should decide whether to provide, withhold or withdraw life-sustaining treatments at the end stage of life, as well as when, where and how best to decide, are all matters of moral controversy. In clinical contexts, controversies surrounding these issues can also give rise to serious conflict and moral quandary among those involved – that is, health care providers, patients, their families, and/or persons legally authorised to make decisions on behalf of the patient. Conflict, in this instance, can take the form of health care providers being asked to 'do everything' when they believe that a *withdrawal of treatment* is more appropriate, or their being asked to 'do nothing' (or, at least, to withdraw treatment) when they believe that it should be continued. When unable to agree to either request, this situation can pose a morally challenging and at times emotionally burdensome situation for decision-makers – and one that is not easily resolved. The dilemmas and associated discomfort among decision-makers in these instances can be compounded when there is also disagreement among clinicians about: the nature and stage of a patient's illness, how responsive a patient's illness might be to treatment, and whether proposed therapeutic measures are worth it if 'the gain in weeks or months that might reasonably be expected' by a given therapeutic intervention is significantly outweighed by the loss of quality of life due to the toxic side effects of the treatment.(Ashby & Stoffell 1991: 1322).

Protracted disputes about end-of-life care are rare, with most being resolved through the use of effective conflict resolution strategies (Willmott et al 2014). Intractable disputes, however, are more challenging and may require tribunal or judicial intervention (MacCormick et al 2018; Willmott et al 2014). Commentators contend that tribunals and courts (especially the Supreme Court) have an important role to play in resolving end-of-life care disputes, not least because they provide definitive guidance to clinicians in their decision-making (Close et al 2018; MacCormick et al 2018; Willmott et al 2014).

At the forefront of the moral controversies and dilemmas about *end-of-life decision-making* are the issues of *Not For Treatment (NFT) directives*, *Not For Resuscitation (NFR) directives* (also sometimes called Do Not Resuscitate (DNR) directives), withholding or withdrawing the administration of artificial nutrition and hydration (ANH) (to be discussed in Chapter 10) and the criteria or bases used for justifying these directives (e.g. 'medical futility', quality-of-life considerations, and advance directives/advance care planning/respecting patient choices programs). The practical and moral significance of these issues for attending health care providers (particularly those caring for an ageing population) has been underscored by an international study (a world first) comparing the percentage of deaths occurring in hospital and residential aged care facilities in 45 populations (Broad et al 2013). The study found that, with the notable exception of China, Taiwan, Chile and three Eastern European countries (Albania, Lithuania and Serbia), the majority of the deaths reported occurred in hospitals and residential care facilities (Broad et al 2013: 261). As these settings are places where high levels of end-of-life care are provided, there is room to speculate that the vast majority of deaths probably occurred after a decision was made to forgo life-sustaining therapy (e.g.

cardiopulmonary resuscitation). One team of researchers has suggested that a significant majority, >75% of people, who die in hospital do so with a NFR/DNR order in place (Mockford et al 2015).

These issues are of demonstrable significance for the nursing profession. Nurses are often at the forefront of requests either for life support to be withheld or withdrawn or, alternatively, 'for everything possible to be done'. The 'rightness' or 'wrongness' of such requests, however, are not always clear-cut and, in contexts where different values, attitudes and beliefs prevail, deciding these things can be extremely challenging. Since these issues have significant moral implications for the profession and practice of nursing, some discussion of them here is warranted.

Not For Treatment (NFT) directives

Sometimes, during the course of end-of-life care, an explicit medical directive might be given to the effect that a patient is Not For Treatment (NFT). Sometimes the patient or his or her proxy will agree with (and may even have requested) the NFT decision that has been made; sometimes they will not. It is when there is disagreement about a treatment choice – that is, where a decision is 'contested' – that the matter becomes problematic. Here an important question arises, namely: 'When is it acceptable, if ever, to provide, withdraw or withhold life-sustaining medical treatment of a patient during their illness trajectory?'

The problem of treatment in 'medically hopeless' cases

In the past, decisions about what treatments to provide – when, where and by whom – were made autonomously (some would say paternalistically) by attending doctors. This sometimes led to a situation in which people were being 'aggressively' treated even when their cases were deemed 'medically hopeless'. In other words, people were treated 'aggressively' even where it was evident to experienced bystanders that such treatment would not make a significant difference to their health outcomes or life expectancy. Sometimes treatment of this nature was imposed without the patient's knowledge or consent (e.g. those in a so-called 'persistent vegetative state'), and gave rise to varying degrees of suffering by both patients and their families/friends.

This situation began to change, however, as the public started to become wary of and started to question the wisdom of people being 'hopelessly resuscitated'. This public questioning saw a number of key cases reaching the public's attention. Rosemary Tong (1995: 166) explains:

> As a result of various factors, the withholding and withdrawing cases that captured the imagination of the public in the 1960s and 1970s were ones in which patients or their surrogates resisted the imposition of unwanted medical treatment. The media portrayed dying patients as routinely falling prey to physicians who, out of fear of subsequent litigation … or out of obedience to some sort of 'technological imperative' … insisted on keeping them 'alive' irrespective of the quality of their existence.

Tong (1995) suggests that during the 1960s and 1970s, economic resources permitted everything possible to be done. During the 1980s and 1990s, however, it became increasingly evident that neither individuals nor society as a whole could sustain the 'technological imperative' to treat regardless of the outcomes. Thus communities in the Western world entered into a new era that was characteristically 'burdened with new obligations of social justice' in health care (Tong 1995: 167). Whereas end-of-life issues in the 1960s and 1970s were more concerned with *patient autonomy versus medical paternalism*, in the 1980s and 1990s they had become chiefly concerned with *patient autonomy versus distributive justice* (Tong 1995: 166–7), a concern that persists to the present time. Over the intervening decades, however, two key questions have come to dominate bioethical thought, namely: 'Are people faced with severe illnesses and approaching the ends of their lives (or their proxies) morally entitled to request "medically inappropriate", "non-beneficial" and "expensive" (futile) medical treatment?' and 'Is it right to refuse such requests?', or, as Quill et al (2009) ask, 'when patients or their proxies ask for "everything possible to be done", should clinicians ignore the face value of such requests and instead use the request merely as a basis for a "broader discussion" on what the patient "really wants" and what "doing everything" really means to the patient?' At stake in answering these questions are not just the entitlements of dying individuals but also, as Tong (1995: 167) concludes:

> the future wellbeing of the health care professional–patient–society relationship – a relationship best understood not in terms of competing rights (though that is an aspect of it), but in terms of intersecting responsibilities.

Disputes about futile or useful treatments at the end stages of life invariably represent 'disputes about professional, patient and surrogate autonomy, as well as concerns about good communication, informed consent, resource allocation, under-treatment, over-treatment, and paternalism' (Kopelman 1995: 109). They also represent dispute about 'how to understand or rank such important values as sustaining a life, providing appropriate treatments, relieving suffering, or being compassionate' and the bearing these values may have on deciding questions of resource allocation (Kopelman 1995: 111).

Who decides?

The question of who and how to decide end-of-life treatment options is a difficult one to answer. Choices include:

- the medical practitioner (unilateral approach)
- the health care team (consensus approach)
- the patient or his/her surrogate (unilateral approach)
- the health care provider and patient/nominated support person (consensus approach)
- society (consensus approach).

While all plausible, none of the above approaches is without difficulties (even in the case of a consensus being reached, this alone is not enough to confer moral authority on the decisions made). For example, although all may entail respect for the autonomy of individuals, they nevertheless risk decisions being made that are arbitrary, biased, capricious, self-interested and based on personal preferences. This is unacceptable (especially in contested cases) since, as Kopelman points out (1995: 117–19):

> If one ought to do the morally defensible action in the contested case, then the final appeal cannot be solely preferences of someone or some group. Preference or agreements may be unworthy because they result from prejudice, self-interest or ignorance. In contrast, moral justification requires giving and defending reasons for preferences, and by doing so relying on methodological ideals of clarity, impartiality, consistency and consideration of all relevant information. Other important, albeit fallible, considerations in making moral decisions include legal, social, and religious traditions, stable views about how to understand and rank important values, and a willingness to be sensitive to the feelings, preferences, perceptions and rights of others. The evolution of contested cases often illustrates the pitfalls of failing to take the time and clarify people's concerns, problems, feelings, beliefs or deeply felt needs or even to consider if people are treating others as they would wish to be treated … Over-treatments may be burdensome to patient and costly to society, yet under-treatments can compromise the rights or dignity of the people seeking help.

In the case of requests being made for 'everything possible to be done' some have suggested that there is no obligation (legally or morally) to comply with such requests in so-called medically hopeless ('futile') cases. In Australian and UK jurisdictions this stance has also been upheld by the courts, which, unlike US courts, have usually deferred to medical opinion on whether a contested treatment is 'inappropriate' or 'futile' (Close et al 2018; Paris et al 2017; Willmott et al 2014). Jecker and Schneiderman (1995: 160) clarify, however, that 'saying "no" to futile treatment should not mean saying "no" to caring for the patient'. They conclude:

> [saying 'no'] should be an occasion for transferring aggressive efforts away from life prolongation toward life enhancement. Ideally, 'doing everything' means optimising the potential for a good life, and providing that most important coda to a good life — a 'good death'. (Jecker & Schneiderman 1995: 160)

Decisions about whether or not to initiate or to withhold and/or remove medical treatment on patients deemed 'medically hopeless' will rarely be without controversy (sometimes referred to in the bioethics literature as the 'not starting versus stopping' debate (see, for example, Gert et al 1997: 282–3)). Nurses are not immune from the controversies surrounding these decisions, and may even find themselves unwitting participants in them. It is essential, therefore, that nurses are well appraised of the relevant views for and against decisions aimed at limiting or withdrawing the medical treatment of patients deemed (rightly or wrongly) to be 'medically hopeless'.

Not For Resuscitation (NFR)/Do Not Resuscitate (DNR) directives

Cardiopulmonary resuscitation (CPR) was developed in the 1960s and evolved to become standard practice in hospitals around the world (MacCormack et al 2017; Mills et al 2017). When a patient suffers a cardiac or respiratory arrest, CPR is the default option, which may be applied as an emergency treatment without consent (Levinson et al 2018; Sritharan et al 2016). CPR is generally taken to include:

> external cardiac massage, assisted ventilation via face-mask, cardiac defibrillation, and also the advance life-support measures of medications, intubation and ventilation. (Hayes 2010: 112)

The CPR process starts by a call being made to an emergency response team (called 'medical emergency team' (MET), or 'rapid response team' (RRT) in Australia), compromised of senior medical and nursing clinicians. This process will usually commence unless there are specific and clearly documented instructions to the contrary — for example, where a patient has been validly deemed 'Not For Resuscitation' (NFR) or 'not for RRT' (Brown et al 2014; Coventry et al 2013; Sidhu et al 2007).

At some stage during their clinical practice, nurses will be confronted with the difficult moral choice of whether to initiate, participate in decision-making about, follow or refuse to follow a NFR directive (also called a Do Not Resuscitate (DNR) directive, and 'Do Not Attempt Resuscitation' (DNAR) directive) (Bjorklund & Lund 2017; De Gendt et al 2007; Ganz et al 2012; Giles & Moule 2004)). NFR/DNR/DNAR orders are described by the Australian Commission on Safety and Quality in Health Care (ACSQHC 2015: 34) as relating 'solely and specifically to decisions to not perform cardiopulmonary resuscitation if the patient has a cardiac or respiratory arrest.' The ACSQHC further explains that 'In some organisations, decisions about other specific limitations of medical treatment may also be listed as part of a resuscitation plan (e.g. decisions to call a medical emergency team or transfer a patient to intensive care if they deteriorate)'.

The NFR/DNR directive ('order') is given by a doctor. Typically, a NFR/DNR directive directs that, in the event of a cardiac or pulmonary arrest, neither emergency nor advance life-support measures will be initiated by physicians, nurses or other hospital staff (Martin et al 2007). The stated aim of NFR/DNR directives is unequivocal: to limit the administration of CPR where it is considered (usually by the patient's treating doctor) that such efforts would be futile, burdensome or contrary to the patient's wishes (Mills et al 2017). NFR/DNR is thus a form of NFT, and is probably the most common NFT directive operationalised in health care contexts today.

A decision not to resuscitate a person generally derives from a medical judgment concerning the irreversible nature of that person's disease, their probable poor or hopeless prognosis, and the related futility or 'inappropriateness' of performing CPR (Willmott et al 2014). This is a controversial position, however. As an NFR / DNR decision is based on normative judgments about what constitutes a patient's 'best interests', 'quality of life', 'dignity' and whether a patient's preferences and autonomous wishes ought to be respected, deciding whether to make a patient the subject of an NFR / DNR directive is as much a *moral decision* as it is a medical decision. Others, however, contend that although the decision to perform or not perform CPR has a *moral dimension* (and one that deserves respect) it nonetheless still primarily involves a *medical* not an *ethical* judgment. Hayes (2012: 80), for example, contends that CPR decision-making comprises three steps:

> *(i) technical analysis and judgment about the patient's illness, disease trajectory and expected response to CPR; (ii) moral analysis about the application of that technical judgment and (iii) a discussion with the patient and / or family that seeks to understand the patient, their values and the moral implications of providing or withholding CPR for that patient.*

Up until the late 1990s, few health care organisations had operational NFR policies and guidelines – and those that did had poor compliance rates – a situation that placed patients, staff and hospitals at risk (Collier 1999; De Gendt et al 2007; Giles & Moule 2004; Honan et al 1991; Kerridge et al 1994; Sidhu et al 2007). As a consequence, NFR practices tended to be 'secret', characterised by ad hoc, ambiguous and disparate decision-making and communication, with directives often being given without the patient's or family's knowledge or consent (see discussion on DNR / NFR in the first edition of this book – Johnstone 1989b).

Today, a different situation exists in Australian jurisdictions. This is due largely to the problems associated with DNR / NFR directives being made public,[1] which eventually resulted in change. Following recommendations made by various government authorities for hospitals to have NFR / DNR policies, standardised forms for authorising and communicating NFR / DNR directives, and patient information leaflets, as well as the provision of a framework for policy content, health care institutions in Australia, as elsewhere (e.g. New Zealand, South Asia, the United Kingdom (UK), Europe and the United States (US)) now have transparent, operational and appropriately supported NFR / DNR policies, guidelines and practices in place. Even so, problems remain. Although there have been notable improvements in the prevalence and content of NFR / DNR policies and practices in Australian and New Zealand public hospitals and health care institutions over the past three decades, research over the past decade has found that wide variations in NFR / DNR practices and processes continue to exist (Brown et al 2014; Hardy et al 2007; Hayes 2012; Sidhu et al 2007). Notable among the issues identified are: a low rate of documentation (as low as 12% in one case) (Mills et al 2017), 'social loafing' (the expectation that someone else will assume responsibility for giving an NFR directive) (Levinson et al 2018: 56), readiness by doctors to shift responsibility for making NFR orders onto others (Sritharan et al 2016), and the association of NFR / DNR directives with substandard care (Sritharan et al 2016). UK researchers have made similar findings identifying, as additional problems, erroneously conflating 'do not resuscitate' with 'do not provide active treatment' as having unintended consequences, and relatives experiencing distressing ambiguous discussions about the issue (MacCormick et al 2018; Perkins et al 2016). Issues identified by researchers in other jurisdictions include inconsistencies across five areas: in understanding and implementing the concept of NFR, in decision-making, in communication, and in the management of NFR processes (Arabi et al 2018, Fox & Muir 2016).

One of the more controversial problems, however, concerns the lawful authority of doctors to impose an NFR / DNR directives *without* the consent of the patient or those authorised to act of the patient's behalf – an issue first raised 30 years ago in Australia by Johnstone (1988; see also Endnote 1 in this chapter). Sritharan and colleagues (2016) correctly explain that laws concerning NFR directives differ across different jurisdictions. In some jurisdictions (e.g. Canada, UK, USA), policies and legislative changes have been operationalised requiring doctors to obtain consent to withhold CPR. For example, in the UK, two important legal challenges in the courts (in 2014 and 2015 respectively) have created legal precedent and have clarified the unequivocal duty of health care professionals to consult patients or their surrogates when making resuscitation decisions (MacCormick et al 2018). The position in other jurisdictions is less clear, however. For example, according to Sritharan and colleagues (2016), in the Australian State of Victoria, consent is required only:

> where a procedure or medical treatment is on offer. Withholding of a futile or overly burdensome treatment, in the case of CPR, does not require consent from anyone other than the treating doctor [emphasis added] (Sritharan et al 2016: 685).

This view seems to rest on the assumption that because NFR does not entail the *active provision* of medical treatment (technically no medical treatment is on offer – that is, the order is *not* to provide treatment), then consent is not required. (This presumably is because the order essentially entails that 'not a finger will touch the body'.) They go one to contend that, although good communication is essential when discussing the imposition of an NFR order with families, doctors must nevertheless 'exercise caution in ensuring discussion around NFR orders is *not misconstrued as the seeking of consent*' ostensibly because 'this may unfairly place a burden of responsibility for the decision on the family' [emphasis added] (Sritharan et al 2016: 685).

An analysis of Australian judicial deliberations has found that the Supreme Court tends to defer to medical opinion when assessing 'best interests' of patients (a standard decision criterion used for adjudicating end-of-life care cases) and to accept the conclusions drawn by medical practitioners on the matter of futile medical treatment (Willmott et al 2016). Adding to the authority of doctors to determine medical futility, the ACSQHC (2015) *National consensus statement: essential elements for safe and high-quality end-of-life care* likewise upholds the view that doctors are not obliged to provide treatment they deem medically futile. Guiding principle 14 of the *Statement* reads: 'Unless required by law, doctors are not obliged to initiate or continue treatments that will not offer a reasonable hope of benefit or improve the patient's quality of life' (ACQSHC 2015: 5).

In light of these findings, there is room to suggest, as Youngner (1987) prophetically contended over three decades ago, that DNR directives may be 'no longer secret, but they are still a problem'. Thus, although the policy situation may have improved, there are still risks (moral, legal and clinical) associated with current NFR/DNR practices (see also Ehlenbach & Curtis 2011; Sanders et al 2011).

Issues raised

Issues raised by current (and past) NFR/DNR practices can be broadly categorised under three general headings:

1. NFR/DNR decision-making criteria, guidelines and procedures
2. documentation and communication of NFR/DNR directives
3. implementation of NFR/DNR directives.

These issues are of obvious importance, as is the need to ensure that attending clinicians comply with carefully formulated and clearly documented policies and guidelines governing NFR/DNR practices. Without such guidelines and associated compliance by attending health care staff:

- patients' rights and interests will be at risk of being infringed (e.g. patients could be resuscitated when they do not wish to be, or not resuscitated when they do wish to be)

- nurses and other allied health workers will be at risk of having to carry a disproportionate burden of responsibility in regard to actually carrying out NFR/DNR directives (although an NFR/DNR directive might be given in 'good faith' medically speaking, it may nevertheless be 'wrong' – not just on moral grounds, but on legal grounds as well, especially if it contravenes a patient's or lawful proxy's expressed wishes) (see, for example, *Northridge v Central Sydney Area Health Service* (2000)).[2]

Problems concerning NFR/DNR decision-making criteria, guidelines and procedures

Criteria and guidelines used

Despite the existence of NFR/DNR policies and guidelines, different doctors and nurses may nevertheless appeal to different *criteria* (to be distinguished here from *procedures*) for making NFR/DNR decisions. For example, some doctors and nurses might appeal to *quality-of-life* criteria (the issue of quality of life is discussed under a separate subheading in this chapter), while others might appeal to *sanctity-of-life* criteria when making NFR/DNR decisions (discussed in Chapter 10). Although NFR/DNR decisions based on either of these criteria might well be in accordance with a patient's preferences, they might equally be in contravention of them. There have been some notable instances of this. For example, in one case in which end-of-life criteria were applied, a previously fit 90-year-old man who required admission to hospital for multiple medical problems was not resuscitated following a cardiac arrest. The decision not to resuscitate him was made by attending medical staff even though both the patient and his wife had clearly indicated that they wished 'everything possible' to be done to try and preserve his life – including CPR in the event of a cardiac arrest (Hastings Center Report 1982b: 27–8).

In contradistinction to this case, in another case this time involving an appeal to sanctity-of-life criteria, a 70-year-old woman 'was resuscitated over 70 times within a few days' (Annas, cited in Bandman & Bandman 1985: 236). In another similar case, a patient was resuscitated 52 times before 'family members literally threw themselves across the crash cart to prevent the team from reaching the patient' for the 53rd time (Dolan 1988: 47). Although these cases occurred some time ago, they nonetheless serve to provide important reminders of the moral risks involved when different people use different criteria to inform their NFR/DNR decisions and practice.

Another troubling practice is that of hospital staff deeming patients to be NFR/DNR on the basis of a DNR decision made during a previous hospital admission. For example, if a patient is made DNR during an admission to hospital in March, is discharged, but comes back into hospital in April, the patient is made DNR again on the basis of the March hospital admission decision. Although the degree to which this practice occurs is not known, the study by Sidhu and colleagues of NFR policies and practices in Australian public hospitals (cited earlier) found that, in the case of patients who had an NFR order from a previous admission, only 34% of policies of the hospitals surveyed indicated that 'a new order was required' (Sidhu et al 2007: 73). In other words, 66% of respondent hospitals left open the possibility of patients being deemed NFR/DNR on the basis of a previous hospital admission. In the case of patients being admitted from another institution with a standing NFR order, only 3% of the policies surveyed contained provisions for dealing with this situation. The rationale behind this is not entirely clear. What is clear, however, is that such a practice is in contravention of acceptable standards of safe and quality care and should be abandoned (Sanders et al 2011).

Equally concerning is the over-reliance on age as a decisional criterion when making NFR/DNR decisions. Many residential care homes for the aged, for example, have a default policy of not resuscitating their residents in the event of either a cardiac or a respiratory arrest. Likewise palliative care units/hospices, where NFR/DNR directives are taken as 'implicit' and are assumed – without discussion or consent – to come into effect upon admission. Finally, also not addressed in guidelines are how to resolve disagreements about what criteria should be used to inform NFR/DNR decisions – and how to resolve disagreement generally about whether to prescribe NFR/DNR or reverse a NFR/DNR directive once made. The 2007 study by Sidhu and colleagues, for example, found that 58% of policies neither anticipated nor outlined procedures for reversing NFR/DNR orders that had been given.

The exclusion of patients from decision-making

Despite the widespread acceptance of the principle of patient autonomy and informed consent, patient preferences concerning resuscitation are not documented, inconsistently documented, ambiguously documented, or if documented (such as via an advance care plan) are not taken into consideration – that is, they are ignored (Levinson et al 2018; Mills et al 2017).

Excluding patients or their proxies from participating in NFR/DNR decisions is contrary to the accepted ethical standards of contemporary health care practice and indeed of the health care professions (ACSQHC 2015). It also risks unnecessary suffering for the patient (if he/she survives) and their loved ones. For example, when informed that no attempt had been made to resuscitate her husband, the wife of the 90-year-old man (referred to above) reportedly stated that the decision was 'against her wishes' and that:

> *Doing everything [...] is the difference between life and death. The doctor was playing God when he decided he should not try to save my husband. You're not playing God when you've tried everything and exhausted all methods. All I wanted was for them to try. My husband knew how to love and be loved. That was his quality of life. That suited him and it suited me.* (Hastings Center Report 1982b: 28)

In the past, health care professionals have strongly believed that patients should not be 'burdened' with having to decide whether they should be resuscitated in the event of a cardiac arrest – particularly if the patient's condition is 'medically hopeless' and any further treatment – including CPR – would be 'futile' (Loewy 1991; Scofield 1991; Tomlinson & Brody 1990). Some have gone even further to suggest that, in some instances, health care professionals have no obligation to engage the patient in decision-making – pointing out that, 'under certain circumstances, arousing a dying patient to inform them of their imminent demise runs counter to the principle of beneficence in health care' (Tonelli 2005: 637). This stance has resulted – and continues to result – in patients (or their proxies) sometimes not being consulted about an NFR/DNR directive even though institutional policy has required that their consent be obtained and even though research has consistently shown that a majority of patients and their proxies want to be involved in decision-making concerning NFR/DNR directives (see Willmott et al 2016). An important lesson here, as Sidhu and colleagues (2007: 75) warn, is that 'the presence of a policy does not guarantee that it will be followed'.

Misinterpretation of directives

Another difficulty associated with current NFR/DNR policies and guidelines is that they are vulnerable to being misinterpreted, which, in turn, can result in the under-treatment and substandard care of patients (Brown et al 2014). An example of the way in which a NFR/DNR directive can be misinterpreted can be found in the case of a dying patient who had pulmonary congestion and pneumonia, and, associated with these two conditions, copious mucus production. In this case, the nurses (mis)interpreted the DNR directive to include withholding oropharyngeal/nasopharyngeal suctioning. As a result, the patient was left, quite literally, to drown in his own secretions – until another nurse detected the error and took immediate action to correct the other nurses' misinterpretation of the directive. The lesson to be learned from this case – and others like it – is that *'no code' does not mean 'no care'* (Heyland et al 2006).

Problems concerning the documentation and communication of NFR/DNR directives

A second issue of concern in the NFR/DNR debate involves the use of disparate means by which DNR directives are documented and communicated to members of the health care team. In the past, NFR/DNR directives were communicated using the following questionable processes:

- Directives being given verbally only (i.e. they were not formally documented in the patient's medical or nursing notes). This practice came about largely because doctors were 'loathe to indicate in written notes in patient records that a patient [was] not for resuscitation' (Social Development Committee 1987: 108).
- Directives being 'confirmed' by sticking coloured dots (usually black ones) or scribbling an asterisk either on the patient's medical history chart and/or by the patient's name on the ward's bed allocation board. As a point of interest, in 1988 the Association of Medical Directors of Victorian Hospitals recommended to the Victorian Hospital Association that 'a round white sticker with "sky" blue border and an oblique "sky" blue stripe be adopted by hospitals to denote Not For Resuscitation'. They advised that the sticker should be 'placed on the front of the patient record, on the bed card and on the patient's wristband' (*Victorian Hospital Association Report* 1988: 3).
- Directives being 'confirmed' by pencilling the initials 'NFR' or 'DNR' or some other equivalent in an inconspicuous place on the patient's medical history or nursing care plan, or both.
- Directives being written euphemistically as 'routine nursing care only', or 'comfort care only'.

Although once commonly accepted throughout institutional health care settings, these modes of communicating NFR/DNR directives are unacceptable. Not only do they fall far short of accepted standards of documentation, but they risk miscommunication and misinterpretation of care plans, which, in turn, creates the potential for 'inadequate and poor quality' medical and nursing care (Brown et al 2014: 99; see also Chen et al 2009; Sidhu et al 2007). Even so, acronyms and ambiguous terminology continue to be used. For example, Brown and colleagues (2014) found that the variations of the following ambiguous terms were frequently used in patient charts: 'ward measures', 'ward measures only', 'active ward measures', 'active ward management', 'medical ward care'. Because the meaning of these terms was unclear, the capacity for good communication was impaired. Even the acronyms 'NFR' and 'DNR' themselves have been called into question on account of their also being vulnerable to misinterpretation. In its background paper on *End-of-life care in acute hospitals*, for example, the Australian Commission on Safety and Quality in Health Care (ACSQHC) (2013: 36) noted that, during its consultation process, it found that:

> *different participants could mean quite different things when using the terms NFR and DNR. Some participants used NFR very specifically to mean not for chest compressions in the event of a cardiopulmonary arrest, while others used them interchangeably with terms such as 'for palliation' or 'for comfort care'. It appears that confusion about what such terms actually mean in practice is common.*

Problems concerning the implementation of NFR/DNR directives

Even when all proper processes have been followed, a nurse might still be left in a quandary about whether to uphold a given NFR/DNR directive and may, in practice, experience difficulties implementing a directive even though 'medically indicated' and lawfully prescribed. Compounding this problem is that 'nurses are often excluded from the resuscitation decision-making process despite their desire to participate' (Ganz et al 2012: 848). This, in turn, may delay the initiation and/or avoidance of resuscitation being actively practised by some nurses (Ganz et al 2012).

Most nurses probably feel comfortable carrying out NFR/DNR directives and may even be at the forefront of encouraging doctors to prescribe them. Some nurses, however, may experience significant difficulties because of poor or ambiguous organisational practices.

For instance, there have been a small number of cases in which nurses have been dismissed from their places of employment because of deciding not to initiate resuscitation on a patient even though no NFR/DNR directive was in place. In a little-known Australian case, for example, a registered nurse was dismissed from her job and also faced disciplinary action for allegedly 'disobeying a written directive to continue medical treatment' on a seriously ill elderly woman and, on her own volition, deciding that the patient should be 'classified as not for resuscitation' (Collier 1999: 2). Although the patient's physician is reported to have later agreed that a 'not for resuscitation order' would have been given, hospital authorities apparently took the position that the dismissal was justified on the grounds that the nurse had contravened hospital policies (Collier 1999).

The issue of implementing NFR/DNR directives is of particular concern to nurses since they are the ones often left with the ultimate decision of whether or not to initiate CPR in an arrest situation. They are thus also invariably left with the burden of having to accept the responsibility for the consequences of both their actions and their omissions in cardiac and respiratory arrest situations.

Improving NFR/DNR practices

Most in the field agree that the status quo is not acceptable and that clear guidance in the form of standards, policies and protocols is needed to remove the ambiguities that continue to undermine safe NFR/DNR practice and ensure the safety and quality of care of patients whose severe illnesses may render CPR in the event of a cardiopulmonary arrest unviable (Arabi et al 2018; Coventry et al 2013; Perkins et al 2016). Others suggest that, due to the problems that continue to be associated with NFR/DNR/DNAR directives and their demonstrable shortcomings, they should quite simply be replaced with a more effective clinical process (Fritz et al 2017; Thomas et al 2014). One proposal (trialled and implemented in some Australian jurisdictions) is a clinical framework called 'goals of care' (GOC) (Thomas et al 2014). Widely used in the US, the framework has been designed specifically to replace NFR/DNR orders, containing instead provision for three treatment categories: curative/restorative, palliative and terminal. The GOC are devised in consultation with the patient or proxy and revised as appropriate (i.e. depending on the patient's medical condition, the patient can move between categories; when GOC are changed, they are documented on a new form) (Thomas et al 2014).

A second proposal has been developed in the UK and is known by the acronym ReSPECT – 'recommended summary plan for emergency care and treatment' (Fritz et al 2017). This framework, like the GOC framework, has been developed to replace NFR/DNA forms, 'to provide additional support for conversations about goals of care and to provide guidance to clinicians about which treatment would or would not be wanted in an emergency event of a patient having to make a decision themselves' (Fritz et al 2017: 3).

In institutions where NFR/DNR practices are likely to continue, the following recommendations are made in the interests of redressing the framework's shortcomings:

- There needs to be a recognition that NFR/DNR decisions are not just 'technical decisions' based on 'medical facts' about a patient's probable poor prognosis or illness trajectory; they are also fundamentally moral decisions involving normative judgments about the 'best interests', value, meaning and quality of patients' lives – something that clinicians may not always be well placed to judge.
- Any NFR/DNR decision made ought to reflect the *patient's [or the proxy's] informed decision*.
- NFR/DNR decisions/directives should be *clearly written* on patients' medical and nursing charts, and should include all the relevant information upon which the decisions have been

based (including descriptions of the patients' statements relevant to their request that life-saving measures be withheld, who has been involved in the decision-making, and whether the family has been informed); a standardised 'NFR/DNR authorisation' or a 'Limitation of Medical Treatment' form should also be signed.

- Mechanisms must be established to ensure the *correct interpretations* are made of non-treatment directives.
- Once a NFR/DNR decision has been made, it should be *reviewed* and *reaffirmed* in writing at intervals which are appropriate to the patient's changing condition.
- A NFR/DNR directive should be *able to be revoked* at any time at the request of the competent patient or, in the case of the incompetent patient, by the cited next-of-kin or legal representative, or as is morally appropriate (Sidhu et al 2007).
- A NFR/DNR decision should be carried out only by those who have freely, and possessing the necessary information, agreed to carry out such directives. Where nurses or doctors have a genuine conscientious objection to following a NFR/DNR directive, morally they ought to be *permitted to abstain* conscientiously from being actively involved in caring for the patient in question.

By incorporating these and other similar considerations in NFR/DNR policies and guidelines, nurses and doctors can rest assured that they truly have done all that is possible to ensure that patients' rights and interests have been properly respected in life-threatening situations, and that they have not overstepped their authority as health care providers. Members of the community at large can also rest assured that their assumptions about being well cared for upon coming into hospital or other related health care agencies are not misplaced, and that they can most assuredly trust and rely on those people who will most probably care for them during those delicate, life-threatening moments which are all too often characterised by intense personal need and human vulnerability.

Medical futility

One criterion that is commonly used to justify non-treatment (e.g. NFT/NFR/DNR) decisions is that of '*medical futility*'. The notion of 'medical futility' first appeared in the 1980s and is generally used to refer to medical treatment that fails to achieve the goals of medicine insofar as it offers no discernible medical benefit to the patient (i.e. it fails to overcome the patient's medical problem, or results in the patient surviving, but only to lead a 'useless life') (Fine 2017; Moratti 2009; Youngner 2004). This idea (medical futility) was advanced largely in an attempt to convince the public of the need to establish a public policy that would enable treating doctors to 'use their clinical judgment or epidemiological skills to determine whether a particular treatment would be futile in a particular clinical situation' (Helft et al 2000: 293; Moratti 2009; Taylor & Lantos 1995). Underpinning this movement was the idea that:

> once such a determination had been made [that a particular treatment was futile], the physician should be allowed to withhold or withdraw the treatment, even over the objections of a competent patient. (Helft et al 2000: 293)

Medical futility proved to be an extremely controversial idea, however, and sparked a debate of unprecedented vehemence in the medical literature – particularly during the early 1990s (Fine 2017; Helft et al 2000; Moratti 2009; Nelson 2003). Around the mid-to-late 1990s, interest in the topic waned and debate languished primarily because a consensus could not be achieved on either the clinical or the ethical reliability of using medical futility as an end-of-life decision-making frame: for every thoughtful definition of 'medical futility' that was put forward, critics successfully raised counter-objections, pointing out exceptions that made broad acceptance of the notion and its operationalisation impossible (Helft et al 2000; Nelson 2003).

Around the late-1990s to the early 2000s, despite the relative lack of published research on the topic, interest in the notion of medical futility was revitalised. In Western liberal democratic nations, changes to the health care system, the emergence of the evidence-based practice movement, the adoption of clinical risk management strategies aimed at improving patient safety, ongoing advances in medical technologies capable of prolonging life in the incurably ill, and an increasing emphasis on the need to rationalise health care services to ensure their viability, all placed renewed emphasis on the need to re-visit the medical futility debate.

Among the leaders of this debate were intensive care physicians who had become increasingly perplexed about the public expectations being placed on them to 'mechanically prolong life beyond reasonable limits' and the personal dissatisfaction they experienced when expected to practise what they regarded as 'unrewarding' and even 'bad' medicine (i.e. medicine that failed to achieve the goals of medicine). In response to what was perceived by many as a futile use of intensive care services, a growing consensus emerged on the need to: (i) improve understanding of the ethical dimensions and implications of treating (or not treating) incurably ill and life-supported patients admitted to adult intensive care units; and (ii) develop mechanisms by which 'futility' could be operationalised.

The global medical futility debate that ensued during the 1980s and 1990s was driven by at least three processes:

1. The contemporary nature of medicine and its ability, through the use of technology (particularly that used in intensive care units), to not only extend the lives of critically ill patients but to change the way people die making it necessary 'to make choices about when to use and when to forgo these powerful but imperfect interventions'
2. The current re-examination of the dominance of the principle of patient autonomy and its conflict with the benevolent paternalism and integrity of clinicians (medical and nursing)
3. The emergence of managed care, escalating health care costs, and socio-political demands to 'reduce health care expenditures by eliminating nonbeneficial interventions' (Capron 1997: x–xi).

Observers had long acknowledged that, 'many, if not most, patients who die in our hospitals today die not because life at that particular point in time could not have been prolonged but because a conscious decision to discontinue or refrain from starting treatment was deliberately made' (Loewy & Carlson 1993: 429; see also Asch et al 1995; Ayres 1991). Further, there was general agreement in the literature that there is a point at which providing life-prolonging treatment to incurably ill persons is 'medically futile' and hence ethically problematic and, in such circumstances, intensive care practitioners should not be obliged to provide life-sustaining or life-prolonging treatment (Atkinson et al 1994; Faber-Langendoen & Lanken 2000; Lo 2000; Loewy & Carlson 1993; Schneiderman & Jecker 2011; SUPPORT Principal Investigators 1995; Taylor & Lantos 1995; Zucker & Zucker 1997). There was, however, no consensus on what that point was, or on the moral grounds that might otherwise be appealed to in order to justify claims that the point in question has been reached (see, for example, Asch et al 1995: Carnevale 1998; Cogliano 1999; Fisher & Raper 1990a, 1990b, 1990c; Kopelman 1995; Levin & Sprung 1999; Moratti 2009; Schneiderman et al 2017; Veatch 2017).

Compounding these difficulties, there was also no consensus on what constituted *medical futility* per se and there was no agreement about what the sufficient and necessary conditions were for a medical intervention to be deemed 'futile'. Adding to this uncertainty, there was a paucity of published research on the experiences of patients, families/chosen carers, medical and nursing staff, and others in regard to the administration and monitoring of medically futile treatment in adult intensive care or the values and meanings such people may have attributed to their experiences. In sum, there was a paucity of research on the lived experiences of patients, families and chosen carers, and medical and nursing staff from which grounded remedies and strategies could be devised to help resolve moral controversies and disputes in this area. About the only point on which there was consensus was that the issue of medical futility was perplexing, complex, complicated and largely unresolved.

As debate on the subject waxed and waned, the explicit use of 'medical futility' as an end-of-life decision-making frame was largely abandoned, primarily because its advocates were unable to overcome the objections raised against it. In recent years, however, there has been another resurgence of interest in the notion of medical futility, spearheaded in part by the publication of a revised second edition of Schneiderman and Jecker's (2011) influential work *Wrong medicine: doctors, patients and futile treatment* (first published in 1995) and by the 2017 Charlie Gard case in the UK (Montello 2017). The Charlie Gard case involved an infant boy from London who was born with a rare genetic disorder. As his condition deteriorated, hospital staff determined that further medical treatment (including experimental treatment) would be futile and would also prolong his suffering. The infant's parents disagreed with this determination, however, and challenged it in the British courts and ultimately the European Court of Human Rights. All courts unanimously rejected the parents' appeal (Paris et al 2017).

Also underpinning resurgence in the medical futility debate are increasing concerns about the costs of end-of-life care and the 'hard rationing choices' that need to be made in cases where treatment will provide 'no net benefit for all' (Baily 2011: 176, 180). As one intensive care physician reflected on what he perceived as unrealistic demands to 'provide more and more expensive ways of maintaining life in the face of futility', the intensive care unit has more often than not served as 'a surrogate end-of-life service at enormous and unsustainable cost to society' (Hillman 2009: 169, 8). Contending that intensive care units were originally intended only to 'temporarily sustain life until recovery', the physician goes on to argue that the time has come to seriously question 'just how many resources should be used to manage the seriously ill at the end of life, and who should make decisions about resource allocation' (Hillman 2009: 9, 12).

It is not clear whether the notion of medical futility per se will ever achieve mainstream parlance as an overt policy frame. Conceptual and definitional issues remain problematic and advocates still seem unable to overcome the objections that have historically been raised against it (Coonan 2016; Lantos 2017; Moratti 2009; Pope 2012). These objections continue to be serious and are not without foundation. For example, a 2010 systematic review of the literature on the empirical basis for determinations of medical futility concluded that determinations of futility are 'based on insufficient data to provide statistical confidence for clinical decision-making' (Gabbay et al 2010: 1083). Moreover, problems with the determinations extended beyond statistical confidence to include 'bias, lack of uniform criteria, and the risk of ignoring potential for improved outcomes with technological advances and the accumulation of clinical experience' (Gabbay et al 2010: 1088).

To date, those on either side of the debate continue to be unable (or unwilling) to reach a consensus on the subject. This has been unequivocally demonstrated by the collection of articles published in a 2017 special issue of *Perspectives in Biology and Medicine* (https://muse.jhu.edu/issue/37924). In this special issue, veteran scholars (some of whom have been writing on the subject for 40 years) advance a range of contested views on the subject. Taken together, these essays serve to highlight not just the complexity of the issue, but the profound intractability of the disagreements between proponents and opponents of medical futility as a reliable and ethical clinical decision framework. Whereas proponents ('medical futilitarians') view the medical futility frame as enabling medical decision-making that will optimise the rights and dignity of people at the end-stage of their lives, opponents see it as disturbingly ambiguous and as involving judgments more of value than of fact (Lantos 2017: 392). Due to its normative orientation and vulnerability to subjective interpretations, critics worry that the frame as it stands exposes clinicians to the risk of making harmful errors of judgment and wrong decisions about life-prolonging medical treatment. Proposed alternatives – notably the terms 'potentially inappropriate' and 'inappropriate' medical treatment (as proposed by Bosslet et al (2015, 2017)) fare no better and reap similar criticisms to those directed at the concept of medical futility.

Despite the seriousness of the conceptual, empirical and moral problems associated with the notion of medical futility, this had not been sufficient to stop the notion from being operationalised informally in clinical settings. This is most evidenced by the widespread use of policies and guidelines that have as their basis the notion of medical futility, even if not explicitly stated (Joseph 2011; Pope 2009). The primary process by which the notion has been operationalised is via the 'regulation of the allocation of decision-making powers among the various actors involved in the decision-making process' (Moratti 2009: 372). The key mechanisms by which decision-making authority has been regulated include advance care directives, advance care planning, and respecting patient choices programs, each of which works by 'nudging' people towards making a particular decision when at the end of life, usually to forgo life-prolonging treatment (Blumenthal-Barby & Burroughs 2012). In this instance, 'nudging' (also called 'choice architecture') is achieved through the often-stated aims of these instruments, notably to improve education, to improve communication and documentation concerning end-of-life care and, via these processes, to minimise the risk of intractable conflict between stakeholders (patients, families, and attending health care providers) and improve care. (Advance care directives, advance care planning, and respecting patient choices programs will be briefly considered under separate sub-headings later in this chapter.)

Quality of life

A key decisional criterion commonly appealed to when making decisions about care and treatment for patients at the end stages of life is that of *quality of life*. Quality-of-life considerations are deemed to be particularly important in situations where a patient's life 'might be saved only to be lived out in severely impaired conditions' (Walter 2004: 1388). In such situations, quality-of-life considerations might be used, albeit controversially, to justify withholding or withdrawing life-sustaining medical treatment from a particular patient. Here questions arise of: 'What is quality of life?', 'Who decides this?' and 'Is quality of life a reliable criterion upon which to decide whether to start, stop or withhold life-sustaining treatment?'

Origin of the phrase

The idea of and accompanying phrase 'quality of life' is believed to have come into use shortly after World War II (Meeberg 1993). It was later popularised in the 1970s as a global taxonomy 'used in the context of healthcare where it has been linked with sociology, medicine, psychology, economics, geography, social history, philosophy and nursing' (Milton 2013: 121). It was not until the 1990s, however, that literature on the subject began to proliferate and the subject assumed the importance that it has today. It is telling, for example, that, whereas in the 1960s and 1970s there was hardly any literature on the subject, a review of PubMed databases ending in 2005 revealed a dramatic increase to over 550 000 works (Moons et al 2006). At the time of writing this book, using the medical subject heading (MeSH) term 'quality of life', a cursory search using the internet search engine http://scholar.google.com.au/ yielded a result of over 4.6 million 'hits' on the subject.

Despite its conventional usage, the quality-of-life criterion is not without controversy. One reason for this is that the notion is difficult to define and can be used to refer to different though equally valid (subjective) realities. In short, as Welch-McCaffrey (1985: 151) points out: 'Quality of life is not a term that has unequivocal meaning nor is it unambiguously determinable in any given case.'

Defining quality of life

Defining quality of life can be a lesson in linguistic humility. As both past and recent literature reviews and conceptual analyses have shown: there is no consensus on how quality of life should be defined, measured or used as a decisional criterion in health and end-of-life care (Condon 2013; Ferrans 1990; Leplège & Hunt 1997; Martinez-Martin 2017; Meeberg 1993; Moons et al 2006, 2010; Zaal-Schuller et al 2018). Significantly, although popularly used in nursing discourse, the concept itself has also been poorly addressed from a nursing perspective (Condon 2013; Plummer & Molzahn 2009). About the only thing on which there does appear to be a consensus is that:

- quality of life is a highly subjective notion that can be meaningful only if it has input from the person 'living the life' (Parse 2007: 217)
- as a 'life status' it is not static and is subject to variances depending on the individual circumstances of the person whose 'quality of life' is in question (Moons et al 2006; Plummer & Molzahn 2009)
- what definitions and models are in use are generally weak because they rely too heavily on a medical model of deliberation and fail to give due attention to cross-cultural and existential concerns (Leininger 1994; Leplège & Hunt 1997).

In regard to cross-cultural concerns – as Leplège and Hunt (1997) point out – as a definition of quality of life is inevitably bound up with the issues of translation, meaning and conceptual equivalence in different cultures and, given the ethnocentric biases of past research, a universal definition of quality of life is simply not feasible.

The ongoing quandary about how best to define quality of life has led some scholars to suggest that, at best, quality of life (at least in a nursing care context) can be defined only in terms of being 'an intangible, subjective perception of one's lived experience' (Plummer & Molzhan 2009:140).

Why defining quality of life is difficult

One reason why defining quality of life is difficult is that what is at issue here is not just defining '*quality* of life' per se, but '*life*' itself. In the case of the term 'life', this can be used to refer to two different realities, namely the:

> *(1) vital or metabolic processes that could be called human biological life; or (2) human personal life that includes biological life but goes beyond it to include other distinctively human capacities, for example, the capacity to choose and to think.* (Walter 2004: 1389)

Likewise with the term 'quality', which can refer to several different realities including: a formal state of excellence, the attributes or properties of either a personal or biological life, the minimum attributes necessary for a personal life (e.g. the capacity or potential capacity to have human relationships, to pursue human purposes, to live life independently), the value (worth) of life itself, and so on (Kuhse 1987; Walter 2004). Each of these realities, in turn, can be variously interpreted, and their interpretations variously interpreted, and so on ad infinitum – further demonstrating the complexities involved in trying to devise an agreed operational definition of the criterion.

As already stated, to date, no consensus has been reached on how 'quality of life' should be defined or interpreted. Nevertheless, as Downie and Calman (1987: 190) argue:

> *Most ... would agree that quality of life relates to the individual person, that it is best perceived by that person, that conceptions of it change with time, and that it must be related to all aspects of life.*

Different conceptions of quality of life

When appealing to end-of-life considerations in health care contexts it is important for health care professionals (including nurses) to recognise that 'quality of life' can mean very different things to different people. For example, in a foundational article on the subject, Ferrans (1990: 249–50) proposed that definitions of quality of life as used in health care contexts tend to fall into five broad categories:

- *normal life* – defined as 'the ability to function at a level similar to healthy persons or typical of persons of the same age' (noting, however, that what constitutes 'normal' can be a matter of dispute) (p 248)

- *happiness / satisfaction* — taken as encompassing short-term positive feelings and long-term 'cognitive experience resulting from a judgment of life's conditions' — in other words 'general life satisfaction' (it is noted, however, that 'happiness' and 'satisfaction' are not synonymous, are subjective states that rely on patient perceptions, and are difficult to measure) (p 250)
- *achievement of personal goals* — related to the above and taken as referring to the satisfaction that the achievement of life goals brings, and the dissatisfaction that failure brings (noting, however, this can be highly variable depending on what goals and their achievement individuals regard as important) (p 250)
- *social utility* — generally taken to mean 'the ability to lead a socially useful life', for example being valued as a spouse, grandparent, teacher, citizen or 'making contribution to the national economy through gainful employment' (this notion is problematic, however, as it leaves unanswered whose criteria of 'social utility' is to be used)
- *natural capacity* — which focuses 'on a person's physical and/or mental capabilities (actual or potential)', for example to decide medical treatment options (this view is problematic, however, since it ignores the fact that quality of life depends on much more than 'physical and intellectual endowment').

These categorisations are variously reflected in other published accounts (see, for example, Zaal-Schuller and colleagues' (2018) study on quality-of-life decisions concerning severely disabled children, and Martinez-Martin's (2017) critical essay on quality-of-life considerations for people with Parkinson's disease and movement disorders), as well as personal accounts of what individuals believe to be 'quality of life'. For example, since the late 1980s I have had the opportunity to ask successive classes of nursing students (both undergraduate and postgraduate) for their views on what they regard as constituting a 'quality of life'. In response to this question, the following (differing) characteristics have been commonly identified:

- enjoyment and being happy, further defined as:
  - feeling contented
  - having no worries
  - being stress-free
  - feeling fulfilled
- being healthy (and not having to suffer in any way)
- being valued and respected
- having freedom and independence (being self-determining)
- being able to function effectively
- actual achievement and/or being able to achieve important goals
- having the love of family and friends.

The fact that these students held differing views about what constitutes quality of life is not, in itself, problematic. However, were these students to impose their personal views on their patients and/or to use their personal views to influence care and treatment decisions involving patients with life-threatening illnesses, this would be a different matter. Of particular concern would be the risks that such an imposition of views could pose to patients, especially if they were to influence treatment decisions that could be shown later not to have accorded with the patients' end-of-life views.

Health care providers (nurses among them) sometimes assume that people who suffer devastating injuries (or illnesses) have — or will have — a poor quality of life. Further, this belief is sometimes translated into the judgment that 'those who cannot lead normal lives would be better off dead'. Not infrequently, these kinds of judgments influence decisions about whether or not to treat patients deemed 'medically hopeless' and who, if treated, could at best live only an 'impaired life'. It is important to note, however, those who provide health care and those who receive it may not always share the same view about the conditions under which a quality of life is possible (Hammell 2007).

End-of-life judgments can have a significant bearing on *quality* (and *quantity*) of *care / treatment* decisions. The views and attitudes of health care providers may not only significantly affect the care they provide, but may also 'influence patients and families struggling with critical treatment decisions' (Gerhart et al 1994: 807). It is therefore vital that health care providers exercise great care when making end-of-life judgments, and act in a morally responsible way when using these judgments to inform clinical decisions.

Using quality-of-life considerations to inform treatment choices

As the discussion thus far has shown, quality of life as a decisional criterion can be interpreted only subjectively and can mean quite different things to different people. This finding is important as, among other things, it warns that using quality of life as a decisional criterion when making end-of-life treatment choices is not without risks (e.g. what might be an appropriate non-treatment decision for one person might be quite inappropriate and even wrong for another). It also warns that members of the health care team involved in making end-of-life treatment decisions need to take great care to ensure that what *they* consider to be 'quality of life' is congruent with what their *patients* consider to be 'quality of life' and, further, that such considerations are in fact relevant to deciding the care and treatment options in the situation at hand. Some have gone even further and contended that, unless patients have the capacity to judge and communicate what constitutes quality of life for themselves, it is inappropriate and wrong for it to be used as a decisional criterion at all – either by health care teams or by patients' proxies (Walter 2004). There is also the risk that if used as a decisional criterion without the patient's input this could ipso facto emerge as being exclusory – that is, result in that patient being excluded from treatment options on grounds of what others have (inappropriately) decided is in 'the patient's best interests' (Walter 2004: 1391).

Three senses of quality of life

Accepting that the notion of quality of life defies precise definition, there are nevertheless three different senses in which it can be used when deciding care and treatment options; these are: (i) a *descriptive sense*, (ii) an *evaluative sense* and / or (iii) a *prescriptive sense* (i.e. morally required or prohibited) (Morreim 2004; Reich 1978b; Walter 2004).

Descriptive sense of quality of life

Reich (1978b: 830) explains that, where the term 'quality of life' is used as a descriptive statement, an observation is being made merely about the *properties or characteristics* of a human individual. In other words, quality of life in this sense simply refers to an *observable* and *'objective' description* about certain features or traits a person might have, and thus is morally neutral. An example of a descriptive end-of-life statement would be: 'this person has pain', 'this person has lost her or his functional ability', or 'this person is totally dependent on others for care'. By this view, to say someone has lost quality of life would be to say nothing more than that she or he has lost a particular property or characteristic (or set of characteristics) of life, not the value of life itself.

Evaluative sense of quality of life

Quality of life in the evaluative sense has a different focus and purpose. In this instance a quality-of-life statement would make explicit that 'some *value or worth* is attached to the characteristic of a given individual or to a kind of human life' (Reich 1978b: 831; see also Walter 2004). For example, an evaluative quality-of-life statement might assert that 'the pain suffered by this person is bad' and 'the absence of pain in this person is good', or that 'the loss of functional ability experienced by that person is bad' and 'the regaining of function by this person is good', or that 'this person's dependency on others for care is bad' and the 'regaining of independence by this person is good', and so on. To say a person has lost quality of life in this sense would be to assert merely that *some property or aspect of her or his life has lost value*, not that life itself has lost value – although the attachment of value to certain qualities or characteristics, in this instance, often becomes the very basis upon which an individual human life might be judged worth living or not worth living, and clinical decisions made accordingly (Walter 2004).

Prescriptive sense of quality of life

Quality of life in the prescriptive or morally normative sense, in contrast, has a different focus again. Here, a quality-of-life statement would entail a *moral judgment* on a given (already evaluated) quality or set of qualities of an individual human life. Quality of life expressed as a moral judgment in this instance would seek to prescribe what would be a good or bad, right or wrong way of regarding a given individual human life or, more specifically, on the basis of its qualities, what ought and ought not to be done 'to support and protect' it. An example of a morally prescriptive end-of-life statement would be:

- a life marked by intense pain is a life which is not in an individual's best interests to go on living; ending such a life would thus be a morally just thing to do, or
- a life free of pain is a minimally decent life, and thus one worth living; to take such a life would be morally objectionable, or
- a life which cannot be lived independently is a life not worth living; therefore, ending such a life would be a morally decent thing to do, or
- a life which can be lived independently of others is a minimally decent life and therefore a life worth living; taking such a life would be morally objectionable.

In this instance, a statement concerning the loss of quality of life could be interpreted as indicating that the life in question no longer has worth and thus could be justly terminated. Alternatively, a statement concerning an increase in quality of life could be interpreted as indicating that the life in question has improved worth and thus justly warrants preservation and protection.

In light of these three different senses of quality of life, it can be seen that there is considerable potential for making mistakes when deciding end-of-life treatment options based on quality-of-life considerations. This observation raises a number of important points for nurses. First, it wisely instructs the need for nurses to distinguish carefully the senses in which they might be using, or rather misusing, quality-of-life statements. This is particularly important in situations where decisions need to be made about which interventions should be implemented in order to enhance or promote the objective *qualities* of a person's life, and, further, about which quality or qualities ought to be enhanced or restored over others. For example, once it is identified that a person is in a state of pain, which can be observed and described 'objectively', and that the pain in question is evaluated negatively by that person, an attending nurse will be in a relatively strong position to assert that interventions aimed at alleviating pain ought to take priority in that situation. If, however, it is determined that the person in question does not regard the pain as a disvalue, or at least regards its relief as being less valuable than, say, maintaining mental alertness, an attending nurse might be in quite a different position. Chosen interventions aimed at alleviating pain might assume quite a different priority, and indeed might take on a different form.

A second important point is that, by distinguishing the different senses in which the term quality of life can be used, the nurse may become more aware of the logical leap between making a *descriptive* judgment on the quality or qualities of a person's life and then making a *prescriptive* judgment (on the basis of that descriptive judgment) concerning what ought or ought not to be done in relation to that person's life. For example, if we distinguish between these different senses of 'quality of life', it soon becomes apparent that it is one thing to say a given person has lost one or two objective (descriptive) *qualities* or *properties* of their life, but it is quite another to say that, on the basis of those lost properties or qualities, the *life* itself of the person in question has less moral value or ought to be treated in one particular way rather than another.

Lastly, when examining the fragile connection between the descriptive, evaluative and morally prescriptive senses of quality of life, fundamental questions emerge of *who should decide* which values ought to be given to certain qualities or properties of life, and, further, on the basis of these ascribed values, of whether an individual human life in a particular context ought to be regarded as having one type or degree of moral value rather than another.

It can be seen that, in using the notion of quality of life, nurses must exercise care to distinguish the exact sense in which they are using it. They must also be aware of how easy it is to leap from a *descriptive statement* concerning a person's quality of life to a *prescriptive statement* on what should be done for that life — morally, medically or otherwise. Furthermore, they must take steps to guard against making this leap in judgment, particularly in instances where doing so might result in another person not only losing a minimally decent *level* of life, but losing *life* itself.

Advance directives

In common law and in most civil jurisdictions, all competent adults have the right to refuse medical treatment, including life-sustaining / saving treatment, whether or not it is documented (Australian Law Reform Commission 2014, DP81, 10. 47). Underpinning this common-law right is the presumption that every adult has the mental capacity to consent or refuse to consent to any medical intervention 'unless and until that presumption is rebutted' (Ashby & Mendelson 2003: 261 supra note 11). At an international level, this right is expressed under the UN *Convention on the rights of persons with disabilities* (UN, 2006a), which states that a person has a 'right to respect for his or her physical and mental integrity on an equal basis with others'. Sometimes, however, people who are suffering from serious illnesses and / or who are dying will not be able to exercise their right to decide on account of having lost their capacity to make prudent and responsible life choices (i.e. they have become incompetent). In such situations, treatment decisions invariably fall to someone else — for example, the patient's proxy (partner or next-of-kin) or the health care team. Proxies and health care professionals who find themselves in this surrogate decision-making role may not, however, know what to decide. This is especially so in cases where the patient's wishes are not known or, if known, are open to a variety of interpretations and hence dispute. Problems can also arise where proxies 'express certainty' regarding the preferences of the patient when, in fact, there is no clear basis for their opinions and / or where preferences collide with the values and beliefs of caregivers (Johns 1996). A critical question to arise here is: 'How is it best to deal with this situation and the dilemmas it poses?' It was in response to this question that the idea of *advance directives* was formed.

What is an advance directive?

In Australian jurisdictions an *advance directive* (to be distinguished from an advance care plan) encompasses the 'formal *recording* of an advance care plan' [emphasis added] (Australian Health Ministers Advisory Council 2011: 10). Specifically, as clarified by the ACSQHC (2015) in its *National consensus statement*, an advance directive is a:

> *type of* written *advance care plan recognised by common law or specific legislation that is completed and signed by a competent adult. It can record the person's preferences for future care, and appoint a substitute decision-maker to make decisions about health care and personal life management* [emphasis added] (p 32).

In New Zealand, an advance directive is defined in the country's *Code of health and disability services consumers' rights* (2012) (https://www.hdc.org.nz/your-rights/the-code-and-your-rights/) as:

A written or oral directive –

(a) By which a consumer makes a choice about a possible future health care procedure; and

(b) That is intended to be effective only when he or she is not competent:

"Choice" means a decision –

(a) To receive services:

(b) To refuse services:

(c) To withdraw consent to services (Definitions, p 2).

The *advance directive* (also called a 'living will') is a relatively modern phenomenon dating back to the late 1960s in the cultural context of the US. Based on the principles underpinning the doctrine of informed consent and respect for the sovereignty of the individual to decide what is to count as being in his or her own best interests (see discussion on informed consent in Chapter 7), advance directives take as their starting point the right of the individual to be self-determining in the matter of medical treatment when incapacitated – especially at the end of life.

In recognition of this assumed right, most common-law countries now have 'living wills' legislation of some kind upholding the entitlement of individuals to make known in advance their wishes about, and to provide instructions regarding, what medical care and treatment they would or would not want should they become incompetent.

In Australia, the right to make an advance directive (i.e. to make anticipatory or pre-emptive decisions to refuse medical treatment) is recognised as a fundamental right of self-determination and has statutory recognition in most Australian states and territories, although the content of this statutory recognition varies across the different jurisdictions (Carter et al 2016). As previously stated, it is also recognised as a right in New Zealand. Interestingly, despite the rhetoric surrounding a patient's right in the case of advance directives, the rights of patients to *request* medical treatment is less clear and, for reasons to be considered shortly, rarely features in advance directives discourse. It is similar in New Zealand, where the issue has gained momentum only in recent years (Ministry of Health 2011; New Zealand Medical Association nd).

How do advance directives work?

An advance directive works by 'directing' one or all of the following things:

- *designate another person to make decisions (a proxy directive)*
- *provide instructions about a person's values and goals or treatment preferences (an instructional directive)*
- *both of the above (a combined directive).* (Fischer et al 2004: 75)

In either case, the directives can be expressed formally or informally. Whereas formal advance directives take the form of *a signed and legally authorised written document* (such as a living will, an enduring power of attorney), informal advance directives take the form of *unwritten oral communications* between the patient and his/her family, friends and/or attending health care professionals (Fischer et al 2004). Although both can be used to inform treatment choices at the end stage of life, the formal (written) advance directive is thought to be preferable since it can:

- provide documentary evidence of the patient's values, goals of treatment and preferences
- reduce opportunities for conflict among family members/substitute decision-makers and the health care team
- reduce opportunities for fraud and duress
- reduce ambiguity about what has been authorised

- authorise the termination of treatment that 'commits all future decision-makers to a course of action and offers legal enforcement for the patient's preferences' (Buchanan & Brock 1989: 118; Fischer et al 2004: 75).

Risks and benefits of advance directives

Although morally warranted, advance directives (both formal and informal) are not free of difficulties. As Buchanan and Brock (1989) have argued in their foundational work on the subject, advance directives are vulnerable to a number of 'weighty objections' on account of the following considerations (adapted from Buchanan & Brock 1989: 152–3; see also Denniss 2016; Dresser & Robertson 1989; Sass 1998):

- *a person's previously expressed preferences (no matter how well informed) can change as therapeutic options and hence prognosis change;*
- *people may not always be the best judges of their interests (interests anticipated to be at stake when an advance directive was made initially might change radically under future unforeseen conditions);*
- *'important safeguards that tend to restrain imprudent or unreasonable contemporaneous choices are not likely to be present, or, if present, to be effective' in contexts involving advance directives (e.g. if a competent patient refuses life-sustaining treatment his or her caregivers can urge the patient to reconsider this choice – which, in some cases, can 'prevent a precipitous and disastrous decision'; in the case of advance directives being activated, however, the same protective response is less likely);*
- *the expected condition of a patient when a treatment decision is required may be substantially different to that envisaged when an advance directive was originally made; in instances where the patient's actual condition is substantially different to what was expected, the authority of the advance directive is called into question.*

Advance directives can also be problematic on account of imprecise language being used (leaving them vulnerable to a variety of contentious interpretations), and/or designated proxies (who may, at best, have only 'bystander recollections' of a patient's wishes (Perkins 2007: 53)) disagreeing among themselves about what was in fact meant by statements contained in a directive. Underscoring this difficulty is the additional problem that advance directives of similar content can be the subject of disparate degrees of discretion in regard to whether they are binding upon surrogates. In contexts requiring expedited decision-making about medical treatment and care, a patient's anticipatory statements – and what they meant – can be difficult to validate (Stewart 2006). Taking into account all of the above, it can be seen that, rather than promoting 'good' end-of-life decision-making, an advance directive could inadvertently lead to disastrous (non-)treatment choices being made.

Another, although largely overlooked, problem is the failure by proponents and practitioners to take into account cross-cultural considerations when seeking advance directives from ethnic minority patients and the moral risks that are inherent in taking an assimilationist 'one size fits all' approach to the practice. As Johnstone and Kanitsaki (2009a) have shown, many ethnic minority groups find the idea of advance directives not only inappropriate and rude, but also offensive on account of their being perceived as tantamount to wishing death ('willing ill') on a person. For such groups, autonomy and sovereignty of the individual is not a priority. Rather what matters are: family relationships, interdependency, family advocacy and protection, 'burden sharing', love and being well cared for (Johnstone & Kanitsaki 2009a). In the cultural context of Australia, despite the multicultural and multi-religious nature of its population, the importance of culture and religion on advance care planning (ACP) remains poorly understood (Pereira-Salgado et al 2018). Contributing to this situation is a lack of online resources which health care professionals can access to obtain reliable information to help guide their practice (Pereira-Salgado et al 2018). Also problematic is that, despite being characterised as 'absolute', advance directives are ironically a 'right without remedy' (Stewart 2006: 47). This is because they are difficult to enforce and lack legal remedy in cases where they are not honoured. Advance directives are especially difficult to enforce in cases where patients have directed that treatment should be provided and not withheld or withdrawn, since there are generally no positive or affirmative rights to health care (Freckelton 2006; Manning & Paterson 2005). As noted earlier, doctors may decide that a requested treatment (e.g. CPR) is 'potentially inappropriate', 'inappropriate' or 'futile' and not agree to provide it. In such instances the courts usually defer to medical opinion on whether a contested treatment is 'inappropriate' or 'futile' (Close et al 2018; Paris et al 2017; Willmott et al 2014). Although patients have a 'nuanced' right to treatment (Flood et al 2005), legal challenges to the rationing of health care (sometimes referred to as the 'micro allocation of health care resources') have been rare (Manning & Paterson 2005: 686). When legal challenges have been mounted, the courts and policy-makers have been 'extremely reticent in legislating guarantees of access to health services' (Manning & Paterson 2005: 691). This situation seems unchanged. As Yamin and Lander (2015) note, in general, the judiciaries have tended to display an aversion to adjudicating upon matters concerning the right to health care and the allocation of resources.

Despite these and other difficulties, advance directives are nevertheless regarded as having significant moral importance and authority in clinical contexts, not least on account of serving the following important values:

- preserving patient wellbeing by protecting patients from intrusive and 'futile' medical treatments
- promoting patient autonomy and self-determination
- serving altruism by 'authorising the termination of treatment that would impose financial or emotional costs on others' (Buchanan & Brock 1989: 152).

Other values that can be served include:

- enabling patients to plan for death and dying
- strengthening relationships by facilitating communication among loved ones and the settling of 'unfinished business' (Martin et al 2000; Singer et al 1998).

The moral authority of advance directives is thought to be particularly strong in cases where it can be shown that:

> *The patient clearly understood the clinical situation that was likely to occur, the directive itself is readily understood, the treatment possibilities have not changed substantially since the patient's directive was written (e.g., by an advance in medical therapy possibilities), the discretion allowed to contemporaneous decision makers is clear, and the choices articulated are congruent with what is otherwise known about the patient.*
> (Lynn & Teno 1995: 573)

Initially there were high expectations that advance directives would become prevalent and would 'effectively guide end-of-life decisions' (Hammes & Rooney 1998). These expectations have not, however, been realised. Research and practical experience to date strongly suggest that uptake has tended to be poor and that, for the most part, advance directives are under-utilised in clinical contexts, appear not to play a major role in guiding treatment decisions to withhold or withdraw life-sustaining treatment, and have even failed to protect a patient's wishes at the end of life (Denniss 2016; Johnson S et al 2017; MacKenzie et al 2018). In response to this situation some commentators concluded that advance directives and 'living wills' increasingly looked like 'failed social policy' (Jordens et al 2005: 566). Moreover, were health care professionals, patients and bioethicists to persist with their allegiance to advance directives, they would 'persist in error' and allow 'the triumph of dogma over inquiry and hope over experience' (Fagerlin & Schneider 2004: 30).

Warning against programs 'intended to cajole everyone into signing living wills' (Fagerlin & Schneider 2004: 39), proponents of the idea called for a new approach – notably one that places less emphasis on 'signing documents', and more emphasis on improving processes of communication and 'preparing patients and families for the uncertainties and difficult decisions of medical crises' (Perkins 2007: 51). This call prompted a change in thinking about processes for planning end-of-life care, and a shift away from the notion and nomenclature of *advance directives* to that of advance care planning (ACP) and respecting patient choices (RPC). The rationale for and outcome of this change is briefly considered below.

Advance care planning

In an attempt to redress the failings of the advance directives initiative, proponents of pre-emptive and anticipatory decision-making in health care contexts strongly argued that advance directives were never meant to entail the mere signing of documents confirming one's 'living will', but rather 'the *planning* for care and treatment in the event of future incapacity' (Jordens et al 2005: 565). In light of this, proponents further argued that processes for facilitating ACP 'must evolve' past merely completing an advance directive to something more substantive (Perkins 2007: 51). To this end, the issue of advance directives was reframed as a matter of *planning* future care and treatment (as opposed to merely *consenting* to it and *recording* that consent) and, related to this, 'respecting patient choices' notably to refuse future care and treatment that would otherwise be 'medically futile' (Department of Health 2014; Jordens et al 2005; Perkins 2007; Seal 2007; Shanley & Wall 2004). As noted earlier, despite the rhetoric surrounding a patient's right in the case of advance care planning, the rights of patients to *request* medical treatment continues to be less clear and rarely features in advance care planning or respecting patient choices discourse.

Until recently, despite widespread interest in ACP, there has been no consensus on how to define it. Believing this made the process vulnerable to being challenged and its consistent implementation difficult, a multidisciplinary panel of 52 ACP experts from four countries used a formal Delphi consensus process to help develop a formal definition for use in both research and clinical domains (Sudore et al 2017). The panel achieved a final consensus one-sentence definition and accompanying goals statement, as follows:

> *(1) Advance care planning is a process that supports adults at any age or stage of health in understanding and sharing their personal values, life goals, and preferences regarding future medical care.*
>
> *(2) The goal of advance care planning is to help ensure that people receive medical care that is consistent with their values, goals and preferences during serious and chronic illness.* (Sudore et al 2017: 826)

The panel clarified that 'For many people, this process may include choosing and preparing another trusted person or persons to make medical decisions in the event the person can no longer make his or her own decisions' (Sudore 2017: 826).

The European Association of Palliative Care likewise used a formal Delphi method (involving 109 experts from Europe, North America and Australia) to develop a definition of ACP for its purposes (Rietjens et al 2017). This panel achieved both a brief and extended definition of ACP. The brief definition is as follows:

> *Advance care planning enables individuals to define goals and preferences for future medical treatment and care, to discuss these goals and preferences with family and health-care providers, and to record and review these preferences if appropriate.* (Rietjens et al 2017: e546)

In the cultural context of Australia, ACP has been formally defined in similar terms, notably as:

> *A process of planning for future health and personal care, whereby the person's values and preferences are made known so that they can guide decision-making at a future time when the person cannot make or communicate their decisions.* (ACSQHC 2015: 32)

In the cultural context of New Zealand, in turn, ACP has been formally defined in the following terms:

> *Advance care planning is a process of discussion and shared planning for future health care. It is focused on the individual and involves both the person and the health care professionals responsible for their care. It may also involve the person's family/whānau and/or carers if that is the person's wish. The planning process assists the individual to identify their personal beliefs and values and incorporate them into plans for their future health care. ACP provides individuals with the opportunity to develop and express their preferences for care informed not only by their personal beliefs and values but also by an understanding of their current and anticipated future health status and the treatment and care options available.* (Ministry of Health 2011: 1)

These definitions are in contradistinction to *advance directives*, which, as stated above, constitute one form of formally *recording* a person's advance care plan. Other forms that an advance directive can take include 'statutory advance care directives', including an Enduring Power of Attorney for health or personal decisions, an Advance Health Directive, a Medical Power of Attorney, a Refusal of Treatment Certificate, and other documents recognised in state legislation (AHMAC 2011: 10).

ACP and its counterpart *respecting patient choices* (RPC), discussed below, have increasingly been devised as 'programs' with the aim of increasing the uptake of provisions for pre-emptive decision-making in health care contexts. The primary purpose of such programs, however, is still strongly linked to an advance directive framework, in that their key aim is to improve advance directive *utilisation* 'through providing a supportive framework for ACP-ing (Advance Care Planning) and primarily equipping nurse(s) as RPC (Respecting Patient Choices) consultants' (Seal 2007: 29). Just what the outcome of these programs will be, however, and whether they will be more successful than their predecessor advance directive initiative, remains to be seen.

Whatever the risks and benefits of advance directives, ACP and RPC programs, it is likely that they will gain increasing authority in health care domains to guide end-of-life decision-making. To ensure that they achieve their intended purpose, it is vital that those completing advance directives and advance care plans ensure that they are carefully written and clearly understood by those who may be left to implement them.

The limitations of ACP, however, also need to be acknowledged. According to Johnson and colleagues (Johnson B et al 2017: 392) there are at least two reasons for this: first, the assumption that ACP is an 'unequivocal good' risks nudging policy-makers and decision-makers in a direction that may not result in the needs of dying people being met (also noting here that not all people trust or even want to engage in the ACP process); second, assumptions about the efficacy and positive cost–benefits of ACP may undermine critical questions that warrant being raised about whether the costs (in both economic and human terms) are acceptable given the 'modest and variable impact' that ACP has on end-of-life care.

Respecting patient choices

Respecting patient choices (RPC) programs (a form of advance care planning) have their origins in a 1991 'collaborative, systematic, community wide advance directive education program' called *Respecting Your Choices*, which was implemented in major health systems in the La Crosse area of Wisconsin in the United States of America (Hammes & Rooney 1998). Defined by the La Crosse-based Gundersen Lutheran Medical Foundation (2007: 2) as a 'comprehensive, community-based advance care planning program with a key message: "Advance care planning is a process of communication rather than a signature on a document"', this initiative has been widely operationalised under the Gundersen Lutheran Medical Foundation's official trade mark for the program *Respecting Choices* in other American states, and other countries (e.g. Canada, Spain) (Hammes 2003).

A modified version of the Gundersen Lutheran Medical Foundation's *Respecting Choices* program has also been operationalised in Australia. The Australian program commenced as a pilot program in 2002 under the auspices of Austin Health, a metropolitan health service in Melbourne, Victoria. It was subsequently expanded to other health services and aged care facilities in Victoria and other Australian states and territories. The stated aims of this program, which is strongly reminiscent of its precursor 'medical futility' as a decision-making frame, is to assist individuals and families to become informed about *the realities and possibilities of modern medicine* and, together with their attending health care providers, make decisions about and plan future medical treatment. Defined in the Australian socio-cultural context as a 'process of communication between a person and the person's family members, health care providers and important others about the kind of care the person would consider appropriate if the person cannot make their own wishes known in the future' (Shanley & Wall 2004: 32), the respecting patient choices program was positioned as a process designed to enable end-of-life decision-making to become a part of routine and expected care (Lee et al 2003).

A key, although rarely acknowledged, driver of the Australian respecting patient choices model is the economic imperative to reduce the admission rates and length of stay in emergency and critical care services of older people. By enabling older people to 'opt out' of life-prolonging medical regimens that are otherwise available to them, respecting patient choices programs were heralded as helping to reduce significantly the costs that would otherwise be associated with their care (in the case of Austin Health, the metropolitan health service that initiated the respecting patient choices program, the cost savings of the program were estimated to be around $250 million per annum) (Austin Health 2006a, 2006b, 2011). In keeping with a general reluctance by Australian courts and policy makers to affirm a positive right to health care (Flood et al 2005), 'opting in' for life-prolonging treatment is less well supported by the respecting patient choices program. A review published by MacKenzie and colleagues (2018), however, has found that RPC initiatives may not be as successful as its advocates would have hoped, with research suggesting it has had only a limited (if any) impact on the quality or cost of end-of-life decision-making and care.

Rethinking 'end-of-life care'[3]

In light of the growing fiscal pressures on health care services, it has been suggested that health care as a whole stands in urgent need of reform. Some have suggested that one domain in which reform is especially needed and where health expenditure could be adjusted to get 'better value for money' is end-of-life care. The 'unnecessary' admission and re-admission to hospital and intensive care units of older patients who are at the end of their lives and who would be better served by other services (e.g. palliative care) have been highlighted as particular issues in need of attention. As quoted earlier, one intensive care physician has contended controversially that the intensive care unit to where the health care system frequently brings older persons 'often acts as a surrogate end-of-life service at enormous and unsustainable cost to society' (Hillman 2009: 8).

Health care reform aimed at improving end-of-life care is not – and has never been – a simple matter. In the absence of a robust body of evidence on patients' experiences and outcomes of end-of-life care and considered debate on the ethical issues raised, there remains the question: 'What would a reformed health care system that could deliver high-quality care at the end of life look like?' (Palliative Care Australia 2010). Other factors complicating the matter include: unrealistic expectations of what modern medicine can offer, 'reinforced by everyday stories of the latest medical miracle' (Hillman 2009); inadequate funding and insufficient alternatives for managing end-of-life care; and the difficulties associated with progressing discussion on this topic in a society characterised by diverse cultural values, beliefs and attitudes concerning life and death issues. These considerations are significant and underscore the need for nurses intending to participate in public debate on the topic to be well informed about the issues at stake and to resist oversimplifying them as being 'just a matter of respecting patient choices'.

Not all agree that health reform per se is the principal solution to ensuring the sustainability of future health care services. As noted in Chapter 7, medical technologies pose a much greater risk to future sustainable health care than do demographic and health trends. As noted by Callahan (2009) although medical technology may 'cure disease', it does not (and cannot) cure death; instead 'it just moves it [disease] to some other lethal condition, and the cost thereby moves with it' (p 23).

Health care reform is not just a matter of making the system 'work better'. As Callahan (2009) concluded a decade ago, if the common good is to be achieved, we need to rethink some of our fundamental values about health and health care. This, he suggests, is going to require a 'cultural revolution' in our thinking about medical technology, progress, death and ageing, because the brutal reality is that 'there are no reliable or seriously envisioned practical and politically accepted means of managing costs anywhere near the extent that is necessary' (Callahan 2009: 6).

Palliative Care Australia (2010: 1) makes the important point that the proposed national health care reform in Australia 'presents an opportunity to review how systems of care might better enable a more dignified, peaceful and respectful death' for people at the end of life. Pointing out that challenges to achieving better end-of-life care for people exist from the 'individual patient level to communities, health professionals and care systems', Palliative Care Australia (2010: 1) goes on to underscore the need for improved community and health professional awareness of end-of-life issues, including: dying at home, understanding a shared and common language about end-of-life care, the societal reluctance to talk about death and the inevitability of death, the lack of understanding of the 'indistinct boundaries between chronic and complex health problems, ageing and dying', cross-cultural considerations in end-of-life care, and the unnecessary confusion that surrounds planning palliative care and end-of-life services – all issues that apply to cultural contexts outside of Australian jurisdictions.

These and related issues – and possible responses to them – do not, however, occur in a moral vacuum, nor are they free of moral risk. Thus, in addition to being well informed about the practical issues at stake, people need also to be well informed about the ethical values and standards that are at risk of being compromised as new and emerging values and belief systems – including economic values and related considerations – alter the ways in which people think about and respond to end-of-life care and what it is that, ultimately, they will or will not be willing to sacrifice.

Conclusion

There is an emerging consensus on the practical and moral importance of communication at the end stages of life and the use of a 'fair process' for dealing with end-of-life decision-making. Fundamental to the 'fair process' being advocated are the following six steps:

1. *prior deliberation on the values of the doctors, patient and family / nominated carers*
2. *joint decision-making at the bed-side with reference to outcome data and the intention or goals of treatment*
3. *facilitated discussion and conflict resolution within the accepted limits of all parties*
4. *the use of institutional ethics or patient care committees in the event of unresolved disputes*
5. *transfer to another treating institution in the event that patients' wishes cannot be upheld*
6. *court intervention in the case that another treating institution cannot be found and the patient's or the proxy's request is offensive to the agreed and accepted ethical standards of a majority of health care professionals.* (adaptation with tabulations, Council on Ethical and Judicial Affairs, American Medical Association 1999)

In addition to the above, due consideration must also be given to cultural imperatives in end-of-life decision-making and care, and ensuring that health care providers who are at the forefront of deciding treatment options and refusals are not only *morally competent*, but also *culturally competent* to care for patients whose cultural and language backgrounds – and cultural knowledge, values and beliefs – they do not share (previously discussed in Chapter 4).

It is acknowledged that nurses do not make the final decisions in relation to overall medical care planning and that they do not have legitimated authority to make life-and-death decisions in clinical contexts. Nevertheless, on account of the time they spend communicating with patients and their families / nominated carers, nurses have an important role to play in initiating discussion about future treatment options, particularly in regard to end-of-life treatment. Nurses also have an important role to play in ensuring that planned end-of-life care and treatment accords with the patient's values, beliefs and preferences – where these are known and are not in contravention of the law. Although not always preventing the dilemmas commonly associated with end-of-life decision-making, the involvement of nurses – and the communication processes that they can facilitate – may nevertheless provide an important safety and quality check that could help to prevent disastrous end-of-life care and treatment decisions from being made.

Case scenario 1[4]

At a seminar on ethical issues in clinical nursing practice, an experienced intensive care nurse asked for advice on 'what more she could have done' in the situation, which she then related as follows.

She had been involved in the care of a middle-aged woman who, after suffering a massive myocardial infarction, had been admitted (deeply unconscious) into the local intensive care unit. The woman had been intubated before admission to the unit, and was placed immediately on a respirator. A few days later the medical hopelessness of the patient's condition was confirmed, and a medical decision was made to remove the artificial life-support system that was sustaining her life.

The woman's husband, who had been present most of the time since his wife's admission, objected strongly to this decision, however, and became very aggressive towards the medical and nursing staff. He also threatened to sue the hospital. Recognising the husband's reaction as a manifestation of extreme grief, the intensive care nurse approached the woman's adult children, who were also present, and, in a private setting, discussed with them what they thought should or could be done to help their father deal with the situation better. The children were unanimous that what was required was 'extra time' – specifically requesting that the removal of the life-support system be delayed so that they could console their father and help him to see that the situation really was 'hopeless', and that, tragic as it was, nothing further could be done.

Upon learning of the family's wishes, the nurse offered to act as a mediator between them and the medical staff, to herself remove the life-support from their mother at the appropriate time, and to seek support for their wishes from the attending medical staff. This the family accepted. Over the next hour, the nurse was able to fulfil her role as 'mediator', and succeeded in obtaining full support from the medical staff involved in the case. This support included the medical staff agreeing to the nurse deciding when and how to remove the life-support system from the patient. As a result of this mediation, extra time was 'bought', and the woman's husband and children were able to come to terms with the tragic decision that had been made. The family members were all able to sit with the woman as the nurse progressively turned off the artificial life-support system. Later, the husband returned to the intensive care unit and thanked the nurse for her intervention.

Case scenario 2[5]

A 72-year-old Greek-born male, with only limited capacity to understand and speak English, was admitted to hospital for care and treatment following the progression of a prostate cancer-related illness. The man had a history of repeated admissions to hospital for the treatment of kidney failure, urinary retention and infection, to which he had responded well. That is, on each occasion of his admission, following treatment, his temperature dropped to normal and his kidney function and urine output improved, and he was discharged home into the care of his family.

During the current admission, a family conference was called to discuss 'choices' with attending medical staff and nurses – including NFR, which was already in place without the patient's or family's consent. When the family rejected the NFR 'option', they were presented with the following 'choices':

- the patient cannot stay in the ward because it is for acute care patients only
- the patient can be admitted to palliative care, but if he arrests there will be no CPR initiated (i.e. an NFR directive will be in place)
- the patient cannot be admitted to a rehabilitation unit, as rehabilitation is not an appropriate option for him at this stage of his illness
- the patient can go home, but if he arrests CPR will not be initiated as family members don't know how to perform CPR (even if his wife did know how to perform CPR she is herself too ill to be able to perform the procedure)
- the patient can go home and if he arrests the family can call an ambulance; however, if they call an ambulance and the patient is intubated and taken to hospital, he will not be admitted to ICU (the family is told: 'the tubes will be taken out' and the patient 'allowed to die' upon arrival at the hospital).

When challenged by a family member about the ethics of these 'choices', medical and nursing staff defended their stance on the following grounds:

- 'to save the family from being distressed'
- 'the patient's body cannot be repaired' (the family was told 'We cannot replace his lungs, liver and kidneys').

The outcome of the meeting was that members of the family were left feeling extremely distressed. They felt very strongly that their views had not been *respected* (they later revealed to a family friend that 'we were not asking for a kidney, liver or lung transplant', but simply for *care* – specifically for *palliative care*, with the option of at least one CPR attempt in the event of a cardiac arrest, so that 'we could know that "at least the doctors and nurses tried everything" and that truly nothing more could be done – that it was in God's hands'). Meanwhile, the patient also 'caught wind' of his family's distress and, upon learning of the full extent of the situation, started to cry, declaring, 'I'm obviously worthless in their eyes. If they won't care for me then obviously they think I am worthless. I'm worthless. I might as well die. They might as well kill me now.' The patient's wife (also suffering from multiple medical problems) expressed great fear and distress at the prospect of her husband of over 40 years dying at home, telling her sister and daughters 'I can't cope'.

Although the patient was discharged home with the support of domiciliary nursing services, the patient and his family remained adamant that they were given no 'real choice' other than the 'choice to die'. Regrettably, even after the patient had died, the family remained angry, distressed, bitter and mistrustful of the hospital, which they felt had abandoned them in their moment of greatest need.

CRITICAL QUESTIONS

1. What are your responsibilities as a professional caregiver in regard to caring for people at the end stages of life?
2. How would you have handled the above situations?
3. In regard to the first case scenario, what advice would you have given the intensive care nurse in response to her request for advice on 'what more she could have done'?
4. In regard to the second case scenario, what advice would you have given the family in response to their request for 'palliative care with the option of at least one CPR attempt in the event of a cardiac arrest'?

Endnotes

1. Australian NFR/DNR practices were first exposed in 1988 by Megan-Jane Johnstone in a conference paper titled 'The nature and moral implications of "Not For Resuscitation" orders', presented at the 'First Victorian State Nursing Law and Ethics Conference: Matters of life and death' (30 September 1988, Melbourne) and subsequently published in the Proceedings of the conference (School of Nursing, Phillip Institute of Technology, Melbourne)(Johnstone 1988a), *Bioethics News* (formal publication of the Centre for Human Bioethics, Monash University, Melbourne) (Johnstone 1989c), and Australian Nursing Federation monograph (Johnstone 1989d) and the first edition of this book (Johnstone 1989b). Discussion of the NFR issue has been updated in all subsequent revised editions of the book (1994, 1999, 2004, 2009, 2016). The original paper attracted mainstream media attention, which, at the time, was unprecedented for a nursing conference paper (see Craig 1989; Miller 1988, 1989; Schumpeter 1988; *The Standard* (Warrnambool) 1989).
2. The case of *Northridge v Central Sydney Area Health Service* (2000) NSWSC 1241 involved a 37-year-old man who had been admitted to the Royal Prince Alfred Hospital in Sydney in an unconscious state, following a cardiac arrest as a result of a heroin overdose. Four days later, the hospital decided to withdraw treatment without seeking the family's consent. The family became suspicious when the patient was transferred to a renal transplant ward and made an application to the Supreme Court for an order that treatment continue. The Court upheld the family's application. In making his determination, Justice O'Keefe criticised the hospital's 'premature diagnosis, a lack of communication with the family and a failure to adhere to relevant hospital policies' (Bowen 2005: 13).
3. This section is an expanded version of Johnstone M-J (2010) Equitable health care reform and end-of-life care. *Australian Nursing Journal* 18(2): 22, reproduced with permission.
4. Details of this case have been altered to disguise the identity of the patient, the staff and the hospital concerned. Any resemblance the case might have to an actual case is therefore purely coincidental.
5. Details presented with the permission of the family (personal communication, confidential source).

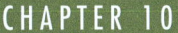

The moral politics of abortion and euthanasia

KEYWORDS

abortion
assisted suicide
clinically assisted nutrition and hydration
doctrine of double effect
euthanasia
fetal/maternal rights
fetus
human being
involuntary euthanasia
mercy killing
moral politics
morality policy
non-voluntary euthanasia
paediatric euthanasia
palliative sedation
paternal rights
personhood
pre-emptive euthanasia
psychiatric euthanasia
reproductive autonomy

LEARNING OBJECTIVES

Upon the completion of this chapter and with further self-directed learning you are expected to be able to:

- Discuss critically the nature of morality policy and what it involves.
- Examine critically the distinction between morality policy and other commonplace policies.
- Examine critically the primary concern of morality politics.
- Compare and contrast the moral politics of abortion and euthanasia.
- Examine critically the definitions of abortion used respectively by pro-abortionists and anti-abortionists.
- Identify two key issues upon which the abortion issue has traditionally turned.
- Discuss critically the following three positions on abortion:
  1. the conservative position
  2. the moderate position
  3. the liberal position.
- Outline at least six contemporary developments informing the 'new ethics of abortion' and its possible implications for the abortion debate generally.
- Discuss briefly the common arguments advanced both for and against the view that the fetus is not a person.
- Discuss at least three instances in which the rights of a fetus (once granted) might come into conflict with the rights of others.
- Define and differentiate between the terms 'euthanasia', 'assisted suicide' and 'mercy killing'.
- Differentiate between six types of euthanasia commonly discussed in the bioethics literature.
- Discuss critically arguments commonly raised for and against euthanasia.
- Discuss critically the nature and moral implications of 'psychiatric euthanasia'.
- Discuss critically the issue of palliative sedation.
- Examine critically the distinction between palliative sedation and euthanasia.
- Examine critically the ethical implications of withholding or withdrawing clinically assisted nutrition and hydration at the end stage of life.

- reproductive rights
- sanctity of life
- slippery slope
- voluntary euthanasia

- Examine critically the issue of patients with serious advanced illness voluntarily stopping eating and drinking.
- Construct critical arguments for and against the proposition that the nursing profession should adopt a definitive position (e.g. for, against, or a neutral position) on these issues.
- Discuss critically the emerging role of nurse practitioners in providing assisted deaths.

Introduction

Abortion and euthanasia are arguably among the most controversial bioethical issues to have captured the public's attention in Western liberal democracies. Because people have deeply held personal values and beliefs about these issues, when they are raised in public forums they tend to elicit highly emotive responses and a deep polarisation between those who are 'for' and those who are 'against' their public acceptance and legitimisation.

It is widely recognised that both these issues are extremely divisive and, as such, are unlikely to be resolved to the satisfaction of all concerned. This, in turn, has given rise to an extremely sophisticated 'moral politics' aimed at securing partisan support for the respective positions at stake. This situation is largely driven by one of the confounding factors in the abortion and euthanasia debates – notably, that both these issues constitute 'morality policy' issues.

In this chapter, attention will be given, first, to providing a brief overview of the nature of 'morality policy' and 'moral politics' and the core objectives of stakeholders who seek to use these processes to advance their respective stances on controversial moral issues such as abortion and euthanasia. Following this, an in-depth examination will be made of the respective issues of abortion and euthanasia, and the philosophical arguments that are commonly raised for and against their legalisation. Finally, brief attention will be given to the vexed question of whether the nursing profession ought to adopt a formal and definitive stand on these issues and the emerging role of nurse practitioners in directly providing 'medically' assisted deaths.

Morality policy[1]

'*Morality policy*' is a relatively new field of scientific inquiry, with focused scholarship on the subject emerging around 2012 (Hurka et al 2018; Studlar & Cagossi 2018). Although a consensus has yet to be reached on the nature of morality policies, it is generally agreed that 'there is a core of political issues that contain more potential for moral contestation than others' (Hurka et al 2018: 430). In western democracies such 'core political issues' have been identified as primarily involving birth, sex and death – namely abortion, same-sex marriage, euthanasia, stem cells / assisted reproduction technology and capital punishment (Studlar & Cogossi 2018).

In practice, morality policy basically involves an interest group, first, framing an issue as a 'public policy' issue and then, once positioned as a public policy issue, further framing it as a *morality issue* to engender public and ultimately political support for the position desired by its advocates. In other words, morality policy involves taking a highly strategic approach to framing a public policy whereby emphasis is placed on 'adherence to principle above instrumental rationality as a way of advocating for or against policies' (Mucciaroni 2011: 201). Morality policy is generally distinguished from other commonplace policies (such as economic policies) on grounds that they concern conflicts and disagreements about a polity's basic moral values, are not amenable to compromise, are widely salient and generally easy to understand, and tend to be determined more by values and moral argument than by expertise (Mooney 1999; Mooney & Schuldt 2008; Mucciaroni 2011; Norrander & Wilcox 1999). It is theorised that the reason the core political issues identified above generate intense (even violent) moral contestation is because they fundamentally involve a clash between public and private values, as opposed to a conflict over 'tangle resources' (Budde et al 2018a: 427). To put it another way: these issues centre on 'conflicts over principles rather than material interests' (Budde et al 2018b: 45). Of relevance to this discussion is that morality policies – for example, abortion, euthanasia – tend to be adopted in greater congruence with public opinion than are other more ideological (e.g. economic) policies.

Linchpin to the success of morality policy is favourable public opinion (see discussion on public opinion in Chapter 2). The influence of public opinion may not always succeed in securing a policy change, however. This is because public opinion on morality policy issues might be mitigated, for example, when 'policy makers themselves hold highly salient personal positions, influenced by religion, interest groups distort aggregate public opinion significantly, and parties position themselves to attract the energies of interest group activists rather than the median voter' (Norrander & Wilcox 1999: 709). In such instances, politicians who are otherwise the gatekeepers to public policy reform are able to (and mostly prefer to) sidestep taking action (see also Studlar & Cagossi 2018).

Like other morality policy issues (e.g. gay marriage, stem cell research), abortion and euthanasia involve a conflict in the polity's basic moral values (in this case about autonomy, life and death), are controversial and 'newsworthy' (have the capacity to generate media hype), are not amenable to compromise (tend to involve polarised views and intractable disagreements), are widely salient with nearly everyone having an opinion (the issues quickly elicit intense personal points of view), and rely on the mass media rather than on professional literature in moving the issue onto the public (moral) policy agenda (after Glick & Hutchinson 1999). Further, and like other morality policy issues, whether or not abortion and euthanasia will ultimately be adopted and legitimated as a public policy will depend largely on its level of congruency with public opinion.

In the case of abortion, it has always been the ultimate objective of abortion politics to achieve a high level of congruency between a pro-abortion stance and public opinion on its permissibility as a public policy. Likewise euthanasia politics (Johnstone 2013a); it too aims to achieve a high level of congruency between a pro-euthanasia stance and public opinion on its permissibility as a public policy. Just where health professional groups (including nursing) ought to 'sit' in relation to these politics, however, is open to question and also a matter of some controversy. It is an important aim of this chapter to assist nurses to navigate these politics and decide whether, how and where to position themselves in the debates that these issues continue to engender.

Moral politics[2]

Politics is fundamentally concerned with 'who gets what; how resources and people are organised; and who is licensed to take these decisions' (Louw 2010: 8–9). It is also about the disagreements and struggles that occur in relation to these things. According to Dupré (2011), disagreement constitutes the very essence of politics. He goes on to contend that without disagreement there would be no incentive to 'cooperatively establish the laws and build the institutions on which social order and justice depend' (Dupré 2011: 3).

Like 'basic' politics, abortion and euthanasia politics are fundamentally concerned with *who gets what* (e.g. abortion as a medical regimen in preference to other options such as adoption, ectogenesis; euthanasia as a medical regimen in preference to other medical regimens such as palliative care, terminal sedation and the like), *how resources and people are organised* (e.g. providing abortion/euthanasia services, which could include public and private hospital resources; in the case of euthanasia this could also involve 'mobile' and domiciliary services providing assisted deaths in a patient's own home), and *who is licensed to take these decisions* (e.g. the patient in consultation with his or her attending physician). The primary objective of both abortion and euthanasia politics is *political* in that it also seeks to cooperatively establish pro-abortion / pro-euthanasia laws and the institutions needed to enable the safe enactment of those laws.

Abortion

Unsafe abortion has been identified as one of the most easily preventable causes of maternal ill-health and death, yet it continues to threaten the health and lives of women and girls globally. For instance, in countries that have restrictive abortion laws, maternal mortality rates are estimated to be three times higher than in countries where women and girls have access to safe abortion services (Johnson B et al 2017). The well-documented and longstanding risks of unsafe abortion to women and girls has led some commentators to declare that 'ending the silent pandemic of unsafe abortion is an urgent public-health and human-rights imperative' (Grimes et al 2006: 1908). In response to the issues and challenges raised by this situation, in 2012 the WHO deemed preventing unsafe abortion a strategic priority underpinned by the following two goals:

- in circumstances where abortion is not against the law, to ensure that abortion is safe and accessible
- in all cases, women should have access to quality services for the management of complications arising from abortion (WHO 2012d).

In 2017, this stance was underscored by a collaborative of international organisations which included, among others, the United Nations Development Program (UNDP), World Health Organization (WHO), Development and Research Training in Human Reproduction (HRP) and the United Nations Department of Economic and Social Affairs (UN DESA) launching a new database designed to 'strengthen global efforts to eliminate unsafe abortion by producing an interactive open-access database and repository of current abortion laws, policies, and national standards and guidelines' (available: http://www.srhr.org/abortion-policies/). It is hoped that, despite its acknowledged limits, this new database will provide comprehensive information on the laws, health standards, policies and practices of different countries and thereby improve transparency and enabling initiatives aimed at improving the status quo to be better informed (Johnson B R et al 2017).

Even though the WHO has identified safe abortion as a strategic global priority, abortion as such remains a deeply contentious and divisive issue. Of all the bioethical issues that command public attention today, next to the ethics of euthanasia (to be considered later in this chapter) the ethics of abortion is among the most controversial. Although abortion has been legal in many countries for several decades, its moral permissibility and legal status continue to be the subject of heated public and academic debate. Some notable examples include debates surrounding:

- The restrictive abortion laws in the Republic of Ireland, which, up until the success of the historic 25 May 2018 referendum to repeal that country's constitutional ban on abortion, were regarded as being amongst the most restrictive in the world. However, the landmark success of the referendum, which saw a resounding majority (almost 67%) of people vote in favour of repealing the ban, created a major political problem for the minority Conservative UK government of Theresa May (Koubaridis 2018). Following the success of the referendum, May faced increasing pressure to 'allow a free vote on the abortion issue in Northern Ireland' where strict laws ban abortion even in cases of rape and severe fetal genetic abnormalities. The problem she faced (and faces) is that her minority Conservative government is in power only because of the support of Northern Ireland's Democratic Unionist Party, 'which is staunchly in favour of keeping the strict laws in place' (Koubaridis 2018). It is reported that the issue created a rift in the Conservative party, with a number of May's colleagues pushing for reform. Meanwhile, in June (just a few weeks after the Republic of Ireland referendum) an appeal brought by the Northern Ireland Human Rights Commission (NIHRC) against Northern Ireland's anti-abortion laws was dismissed by the Supreme Court, despite a majority of the judges indicating that the laws needed to be reformed. At the time of writing, the Northern Ireland government is reportedly 'not obliged to change the law' (BBC News 2018).

- Three controversial judgments by the European Court of Human Rights addressing the issue of access to abortion, declining in one case to affirm abortion as a human right per se (Westeson 2013).
- The legal case of *Right to Life New Zealand Inc. v Abortion Supervisory Committee* [2008] challenging the lawfulness of the way in which the mental health exception in New Zealand abortion law was being applied (Leslie 2010).

Significantly, over the years, the polarity of values and views underpinning the abortion controversy has threatened to divide nations, has seen abortion clinics firebombed and abortion workers fatally shot by pro-life fanatics, and has even brought down governments (Hadley 1996).

Despite the legislative and moral reforms of the past six decades, women's so-called '*reproductive rights*' (including the right to safe abortion) are still constantly being challenged. Also, despite being 'sensationally and bewilderingly public', abortion for many women remains a deeply private, personal and even taboo subject (Hadley 1996: xi). Even in so-called 'liberal' democratic countries where individualism and a person's right to make important life choices (including the right to choose death) is highly respected and enshrined in law, women are often forced to justify their need of an abortion in a way 'that many find to be degrading and intrusive' (Greenwood 2001: ii3). Further, although there is much rhetoric about women having 'reproductive autonomy', it is governments, members of the medical profession and the courts legitimating their authority that ultimately have the power to decide if, when, how and under what circumstances a woman's reproductive rights will be exercised (Greasley 2017; Sifris & Belton 2017; see also essays by Goodwin (2017) and Andaya & Mishtal (2017) on the erosion of women's rights to abortion care in the US following the election of Donald Trump). Women can also face other significant barriers when seeking access to safe reproductive health services – for example, availability of services (particularly for women in rural and remote areas), waiting times for an appointment, travelling distance to a clinic (which can include having to travel from rural to metropolitan areas as well as interstate), abortion stigma (i.e. perceived stigma of attending a clinic and having the procedure; staff can also experience being stigmatised for their work), financial barriers, and conscientious objection by doctors (Cockrill & Hessini 2014; Harris et al 2018; Kumar et al 2009; Lowe & Hayes 2018; Martin L A et al 2017, 2018; Regan & Glasier 2017; Sifris & Belton 2017).

Over the past two decades, a 'new ethics of abortion' has emerged (Gillon 2001; Greenwood 2001; Wyatt 2001). This 'new ethic' has rekindled the fires of old controversies surrounding the moral status of the *fetus* and has posed new challenges to contemporary moral thought about the permissibility and impermissibility of abortion (see, for example, Martin T 2001). Processes informing the 'new ethics of abortion' include the following five developments, which Wyatt (2001: ii15–ii18) believes 'have irreversibly altered the ethical debate about abortion in Western societies':

1 *advances in fetal physiology* (these have made it possible to confirm that fetuses have 'a range of sophisticated abilities with well-developed sensory perception in all systems: vision, hearing, touch, taste and smell'; it is now known that even very young fetuses have the capacity to imitate facial expressions, breathe and initiate hand–face contact, startle, sucking and swallowing movements)

2 *development of fetal medicine as a specialty* (making it possible to discern major abnormalities and to 'provide seamless medical care for the fetus through the intrauterine period and on into the critical first hours and days of birth'; it is now possible to provide such intrauterine treatment as blood transfusions and curative surgery for congenital defects)
3 *development of neonatal intensive care and improved survival of extremely preterm infants* (with developments in specialised neonatal intensive care techniques, it is now commonplace for preterm babies of just 23–4 weeks of gestation to survive; the survival of preterm babies of just 22 weeks weighing less than 500 g at birth has also been described)
4 *changed perspective on the rights of the disabled* (many in the disabled rights movement regard the abortion of fetuses with genetic disorders or other disabling conditions to be discriminatory and as being prejudicial against disabled people)
5 *changes in professional counselling* (research has shown that the way information is given to parents can significantly influence the choices they make; this, in turn, has given rise to a new imperative for so-called 'non-directive counselling').

Other developments prompting new debate and bioethical controversies on the abortion issue are the global growth of 'wrongful conception', 'wrongful life' or 'wrongful birth' lawsuits as well as 'wrongful abortion' suits driven largely by advances in preimplantation and prenatal diagnostics (Fox 2017; Frati et al 2017; Yakren 2017). In the case of wrongful conception, action is taken by a parent or parents to recover damages for the birth of an unplanned child, such as an unsuccessful sterilisation procedure (Forrester & Griffiths 2015: 216).

Wrongful birth/life suits, in turn, are based broadly on the argument that a pregnancy should never have been enabled to go full term and ipso facto the resulting infant should never have been born. For example, a baby may have been born with severe and irremediable disabilities in circumstances where, if appropriate medical advice and care had been provided, a decision not to continue the pregnancy would have been made (Forrester & Griffiths 2015; Frati et al 2017). In such cases, an infant's mother generally seeks compensation on grounds that she was deprived of the opportunity to have an abortion within a relevant time because of a health worker's (e.g. a doctor's or a counsellor's) negligence (e.g. failed abortion, misdiagnosis of fetal abnormality after screening, misdiagnosis of maternal illness which could have resulted in fetal abnormality) (Frati et al 2017). 'Wrongful abortion' lawsuits, in contrast, concern situations in which a pregnant woman is 'induced to undergo an abortion by a negligent conduct (usually a medical misrepresentation)' (Perry & Adar 2005: 507). For example, a woman might decide to have an abortion based on advice received from her attending medical practitioner that her fetus is at risk of being born with severe birth defects because of a drug she has taken. After the abortion is performed, however, she learns that the medical advice she was given about the risks to her fetus 'was a negligent misrepresentation, and that the termination of the pregnancy was unnecessary' (Perry & Adar 2005: 507). In such cases, the woman might sue for compensation for the catastrophic loss she has suffered, notably, the 'nonbirth of a wanted child' (Fox 2017: 167).

The above issues help to demonstrate the complexities of the abortion issue and the tensions involved. Just what the outcome of the 'new ethics of abortion' will be remains an open question. What is clear, however, is that there is 'no Olympian perspective from which these issues can be viewed in benign and omniscient neutrality' (Wyatt 2001: ii19).

The abortion issue is not 'new' to the nursing profession. As shown by the examples given in the previous editions of this book, nurses historically have had to face a range of personal, political and professional difficulties on account of moral disagreements in the workplace concerning the abortion issue. Research has also revealed that nurses (including those who choose to work in abortion services) may face a range of other complexities, tensions and dilemmas inherent in abortion work on account of trying to 'accommodate the requirements of society, the women patients, and their own beliefs' (Huntington 2002: 276; see also Chiappetta-Swanson 2005; Martin et al 2017). To help gain a better understanding of the complexities of the issues involved, a critical examination of the ethics and politics of abortion is warranted. It is to providing such an examination that this chapter will now turn.

What is abortion?

Before advancing this discussion, it is important first to clarify the meaning of the term *'abortion'*. In keeping with lay dictionary definitions, abortion may be defined simply as the 'premature termination of a pregnancy by either spontaneous or induced expulsion of a nonviable fetus from a uterus' (*Collins Australian dictionary* 2011: 4), and usually entails the death of the fetus (Warren 2014). Greasley (2017: 2) offers the following more definitive definition of abortion, notably: 'as the deliberate ending of a pregnancy with the known or desired result that the embryo or fetus will die'. Not all participating in the abortion debate subscribe to such 'simple' or 'definitive' definitions, however. Instead, most lean towards definitions of abortion that, although appearing to be value-neutral (objective), are in essence ethically loaded and hence at risk of misleading moral debate on the issue. For instance, those who are opposed to abortion tend to use the following terms in their discourse: 'unborn child'/'unborn human life' (versus fetus) and 'mothers' (instead of pregnant women) (Greasley 2017). Accordingly, they typically define it in such terms as 'artificially causing the miscarriage of an unborn child', or 'killing an innocent human being'. Definitions of abortion using these or similar terms are not just defining the 'act' of abortion, however. They also seem to be conveying the conclusion that abortion is morally wrong (at the very least, the terms used — 'unborn child'/'innocent human being' — seem to appeal to our moral intuition that killing another person who is a non-aggressor is a morally terrible action). In contrast, those who support abortion tend to use the terms 'pregnancy' and 'fetus' (versus 'child'/'unborn human being') in their discourse. Accordingly, they tend to define abortion in such terms as 'terminating pregnancy' or 'ridding the products of unwanted/unviable conception'. Definitions of abortion using these and similar terms seem to imply that abortion is not only not morally wrong but may even be morally neutral (the term used 'ridding the products of unwanted conception' seems to invite the 'reasonable' question: 'What is so morally terrible about getting rid of something that is 'unwanted' and/or incapable of normal growth and development?').

It is unlikely that a consensus will be reached among contesting parties on a working definition of abortion and that various ethically loaded definitions will continue to be used. This is so despite research suggesting that both the terms 'abortion' and 'termination of pregnancy' are distressing even to those providing abortion services, although use of the term 'termination of pregnancy' is less so (Kavanagh et al 2018). Either way, it is important to remember that the issues at hand need to be decided by careful deliberation, not by definitions; they also need to be examined in a manner that will question rather than reinforce the status quo.

Arguments for and against the moral permissibility of abortion

Arguments for and against abortion have tended to be advanced from three distinctive positions: a conservative position, a moderate position and a liberal position. These three positions are considered briefly below, noting that little has changed since they were first debated in the early 1970s and 1980s, with foundational works on the subject still being widely cited and/or reprinted in contemporary anthologies today.

The conservative position

According to the conservative position (see, for example, Brody 1982; Noonan 1983), abortion is an absolute moral wrong, and thus something which should never be permitted under any circumstances

– not even in self-defence, such as cases where a continued pregnancy would almost certainly result in the mother's death. A common concern among conservative anti-abortionists is that, if abortion is permitted, then respect for the sanctity of human life will be diminished, making it easier for human life to be taken in other circumstances. Arguments typically raised against abortion here are almost always based on the sanctity-of-life doctrine. One example of the kind of reasoning which might be employed to argue against abortion is as follows:

> *It is wrong to kill innocent human beings; fetuses are innocent human beings; therefore it is wrong to kill fetuses.* (Warren 1973: 53)

Or, to use another example:

> *Human beings have a natural right to life; fetuses are human beings; therefore fetuses have a natural right to life and killing them is wrong.* (Pojman & Beckwith 1994)

Whether human beings do in fact have a natural right to life, and whether fetuses are in fact human beings, are matters of ongoing philosophical controversy.

The moderate position

According to the moderate position (see, for example, Bolton 1983; Werner 1979) abortion is only a prima-facie moral wrong, and thus prohibitions against it may be overridden by stronger moral considerations. Werner (1979), for example, argues that abortion is permissible provided that it is procured during pre-sentience (i.e. before the fetus has the capacity to feel). Since a pre-sentient fetus cannot feel, it cannot be meaningfully harmed or benefited. Thus, as with other non-sentient or pre-sentient entities, it makes no sense to say a fetus has rights, much less a right to life. In the case of post-sentience, Werner argues that abortion may still be justified on carefully defined grounds, namely: *self-defence* (e.g. where the life or health of the mother would be at risk if the pregnancy were allowed to continue); or *unavoidability* (e.g. where abortion cannot be avoided, such as in the case of ectopic pregnancy or accidental injury). Abortions performed on lesser grounds are, according to Werner, unjustified. A more recent articulation of this position similarly holds that abortion is 'seriously wrong', except in rare instances – for example, after rape, during the first 14 days after conception when the fetus 'is definitely not an individual', where the woman's life is threatened by the continuation of the pregnancy and where the fetus has anencephaly or, if born, is highly likely to have a life of prolonged unrelievable suffering (Marquis 2014: 141; Nuccetelli 2017).

Bolton (1983) takes a slightly different line of reasoning. She argues that, as fetuses are not undisputed persons, they do not have the same rights not to be killed as do actual undisputed persons. Thus, in the case of life-threatening pregnancy, at least, a woman's right to life overrides that of the fetus. Bolton also argues, controversially, that if women are not permitted to have abortions, the community might find itself deprived of the beneficial contributions that a woman freed of the burdens of child rearing would otherwise be free to make (p 335). She concedes, however, that there are also cases 'in which others stand to benefit from the pregnant woman's bearing a child' (p 337), and that this too might contribute to the community's benefit. The bottom line of Bolton's position is that abortion is morally permitted in some situations, and might even be 'morally required' in others, but it is not morally permitted in some other types of situations. Either way, the facts of the matter need to be carefully assessed and analysed before an abortion decision is deemed justified.

Another moderate argument raised in defence of abortion is that a woman is under no moral obligation to bring a pregnancy to term, particularly in instances where the pregnancy has been forced upon her (as in the case of rape), or where the pregnancy has not resulted from a voluntary and informed choice (as in cases involving contraceptive failure or ignorance). In her classic and still widely cited article 'A defence of abortion' (reproduced in LaFollette 2014: 124–31), Judith Jarvis Thomson (1971) contends, for example, that even if it is conceded, for the sake of argument, that a fetus is a person, this still does not place an obligation on a woman to carry it to full term. This is because morality does not generally require individuals to make large sacrifices to keep another alive. Thus, if pregnancy requires a woman to make a large sacrifice – and one which she is not willing to make – it is morally permissible for her to terminate the pregnancy.

A more recent moderate argument in defence of the permissibility of abortion takes an entirely different stance. Some philosophers, for example, have rejected the 'competing rights' view of the permissibility of abortion, and its basis in, what one scholar describes as, a 'profoundly misleading view of gestation and a deontological crude picture of morality' (Little 2014: 151). What is primarily at issue in the abortion debate, they contend, is not a 'fetus's rights' or a 'woman's rights' as has been conventionally argued, but having the 'right attitude' to parenthood and family relationships (Hursthouse 2014b; Little 2014). This includes recognising that, although pregnancy is one of many physical conditions a woman can experience, it does not mean it is without vice (e.g. women can be in very poor health and/or have to deal with extremely demanding circumstances that make continuing a pregnancy intolerable). In such instances, women who decide to have an abortion are not 'self-indulgent, callous, irresponsible, or light-minded'; indeed, they are often quite the opposite (Hursthouse 2014b: 166).

Little (2014) takes a similar stance, arguing that abortion can be justified on grounds of 'decency' and the norms of 'responsible and respectful creation' and 'stewardship'. By this view, a woman might choose to abort a pregnancy – not because she is selfish or irresponsible or indecent, but because her circumstances do not permit her to provide love and care to a child, or to protect a child from a life of rejection and burdensome struggle. Here the worry is 'not that the child would have been better off never to have been born', but that, were the woman to continue her pregnancy, she would violate her integrity and commitment to responsible and respectful creation and stewardship of life (p 158). Little contends that due recognition needs to be given to the fact that gestation is 'not just any activity', and that burgeoning human life is not just 'tissue' but the valuable germination of human life (p 151). Moreover, there is a 'right way' to value this early human life and also to value what is involved with its development and, accordingly, why abortion is both 'morally sober and morally permissible' (p 151). She concludes that were abortion viewed in the more contextual terms of 'stewardship' rather than 'dominion', it could be properly situated as a 'sober matter, an occasion, often, for moral emotion such as grief and regret', not as an act of vice. Further, where there is grief and regret, this should be taken as a signal 'not that the action was indecent, but that decent actions sometimes involve loss' (p 158).

It could be objected, however, that the kinds of sacrifices a woman might ultimately be required to make by giving birth could be avoided by her allowing the unwanted child to be adopted. Indeed, many view the adoption option as a respectable way out of the abortion dilemma – even in cases involving severely disabled fetuses or severely disabled newborns. Thomson (1971), however, rejects the adoption option, arguing that it can be utterly devastating on relinquishing mothers. Although adoption practices have improved significantly over the past decade, adoption research continues to show that, for many women, the relinquishment of a child is a profound life experience that can have 'life-long emotional and interpersonal effects' (Madden et al 2018). It can also have a lifetime impact on adopted children, who may grow up 'wondering who they are' and spend a lifetime searching for their unknown biological parents. Although social processes (e.g. open adoptions, social media) have increasingly enabled adoptees to know/search for and locate their biological parents, adoption research has found that adoptees may nonetheless experience psychosomatic problems related to their adoption experience. In one study, for example, researchers found that adoptees were over-represented in clinical settings for externalising disorders (e.g. attention and learning difficulties, behaviour problems) (Wiley 2017).

In some countries, babies who are born out of wedlock (especially 'rape babies') can face a lifetime of shame and rejection (Doder 1993: 8). Babies conceived as a result of war rape are particularly vulnerable to being stigmatised, discriminated against, rejected, abandoned and even killed. In Rwanda, for example, children conceived as a result of war rape are referred to as 'devil's children' or 'sons of the enemy' (Banyanga et al 2017: 34). At the time of the Rwandan conflict (and in its aftermath) the pregnant mothers of these babies reportedly wanted to kill them after birth because 'they were not conceived in love' and 'they were ashamed of carrying the children of bad memories' (Banyanga et al 2017: 34). This shame was due not only to the fact that the children were 'illegitimate' or 'stood as reminders of sexual torture and national humiliation', but because they were perceived as carrying the 'bad blood' (violent genes) of their fathers and, as such, stood as 'potential future enemy combatants growing up within the community' (Banyanga et al 2017: 34).

In some countries, 'rape babies' have even been prevented by law from being adopted. After the Bosnia war, for example, it was reported that the government of the day prohibited adoption of the children of rape victims, in the hope that their natural mothers would one day accept them (Williams 1993: 8). Many infants were neglected, abandoned and even killed because of these policies (Banyanga et al 2017). As these examples show, the adoption option is not as straightforward as its advocates have perhaps assumed.

The liberal position

The third stance on abortion, the liberal position (see in particular Thomson 1971; Tooley 1972; Warren 1973, 1977, 1997, 2007, 2014), holds that abortion is morally permissible on demand. Michael Tooley (1972) argues, for example, that as fetuses are not persons they cannot meaningfully claim a right to life. He points out that the notion 'person', in this instance, is a purely moral concept, and that the unfortunate tendency by some to use it as if it were synonymous with the notions of '*human being*' and 'human life' is grossly misleading. Warren (1973) argues along similar lines. She contends that a fetus is not a human being and to claim that it is only begs the question. She points out that it is one thing to use *human* to refer 'exclusively to members of the species *Homo sapiens*', but quite another to use it in the sense of being 'a full-fledged member of the moral community' (Warren 1973: 53). In other words, it is one thing to be human in the *genetic* sense, but it is quite another to be human in the *moral* sense. These two senses are quite distinct, and care must be taken to distinguish between them. She concludes (Warren 1973: 53):[3]

> In the absence of any argument showing that whatever is genetically human is also morally human … nothing more than genetic humanity can be demonstrated by the presence of the genetic human code.

The consequence of this is unavoidable. It has yet to be demonstrated that the genetic humanity of fetuses alone qualifies them to have fully fledged membership of the moral community. Further, were this to be demonstrated convincingly, it then leaves unanswered the question of what moral status ought to be accorded human–animal chimeras – that is, other non-human species (e.g. pigs, sheep, mice, etc.) into which human genes have been cloned (see debate on the subject advanced by: Behringer 2007; Chan 2014; DeGrazia 2014; Fox 2005; Harvey & Salter 2012; Hui 2014; Piotrowska 2014). For example, ought a mouse or other animal into which human genes have been successfully planted (see Behringer 2007) be accorded the same moral status as a human fetus at least, if not a fully fledged human being? If genetic humanity is sufficient to accord moral humanity then human–animal chimeras ought also to be accorded moral status.

Judith Jarvis Thomson (1971) also argues that a fetus is not a person. She contends that it is nothing more than a 'newly implanted clump of cells' (p 48). In defence of this claim, she argues that a fetus is 'no more a person than an acorn is an oak tree' (p 48). The analogy can be extended further to show that, just as stepping on an acorn is significantly different from cutting down an oak tree, so too is aborting a fetus significantly different from killing an actual person.

FIGURE 10.1
Three positions on abortion

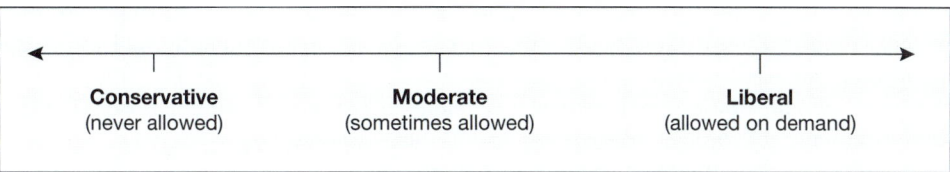

The conclusion of these and similar views is that, once it is admitted that a fetus is nothing more than a clump of genetically human cells, the abortion issue becomes a non-issue. It would make no more sense to speak of the right of a fetus to life than it would be to speak of some other piece of genetically human tissue's right to life – say a strand of human hair or a piece of human toenail (both of which are genetically human).

The three positions on abortion discussed so far can be expressed diagrammatically as shown in Fig. 10.1.

Abortion and the moral rights of women, fetuses and fathers

In considering further the above three positions on abortion, it can be seen that the abortion issue rests on two key points: (1) the moral status of the fetus, and (2) the moral rights of pregnant women to control their bodies and their lives (also referred to as '*reproductive autonomy*') (Greasley 2017). To recap, anti-abortionists argue that the human fetus is a human being, and therefore has a right to life at least equal to that of the mother's. Pro-abortionists, however, reject this view, arguing that, although a human fetus is genetically human, this in no way implies that it is morally a human being with a full set of rights claims. Neither, they argue, is a fetus a person. In defence of this position, pro-abortionists contend that in order for a fetus to be a person it must satisfy the moral criteria of *personhood* (which are very different from the criteria of fetalhood) – something that a fetus simply does not do. Let us consider this claim further.

The much-cited North American philosopher, Mary Anne Warren, has classically argued that, for an entity to be a person, it must satisfy a number of criteria, namely:

1. *consciousness (of objects and events external and/or internal to the being), and in particular the capacity to feel pain*
2. *reasoning (the developed capacity to solve new and relatively complex problems)*
3. *self-motivated activity (activity which is relatively independent of either genetic or direct external control)*
4. *the capacity to communicate, by whatever means, messages of an indefinite variety of types, that is, not just with an indefinite number of possible contents, but on indefinitely many possible topics*
5. *the presence of self-concepts, and self-awareness, either individual or racial, or both.* (Warren 1973: 55)

Warren admitted that there were numerous difficulties involved in formulating and applying precise criteria of personhood. Even so, it could be done. Commenting on the criteria she had formulated, Warren argued that an entity does not need to have all five attributes described, and that it is possible that attributes given in criteria 1 and 2 alone are sufficient for personhood, and might even qualify as necessary criteria for personhood. Given these criteria, all that needs to be claimed to demonstrate that an entity (including a fetus) is not a person is that any entity which fails to satisfy all of the five criteria listed is not a person. She concluded that if opponents of abortion deny the appropriateness of the criteria she has identified, she knows of no other arguments which would convince them, stating: 'We would probably have to admit that our conceptual schemes were indeed irreconcilably different, and that our dispute could not be settled objectively' (Warren 1973: 56).

Michael Tooley (1972), like Warren, also interpreted 'person' in rationalistic terms. He argued that in order for something to be a person it must have a serious moral right to life, and, in order to have a serious moral right to life, it must possess 'the concept of self as a continuing subject of experience and other mental states, and believe that it is itself such a continuing entity' (p 44). Since fetuses do not satisfy this basic 'self-consciousness requirement', as Tooley called it, they are not persons – they do not have a serious moral right to life, and therefore to kill them is not wrong.

More recently, in a revised version of her earlier work, Mary Anne Warren (2014 edn) has expanded on and refined the characteristics which she believes are central to the concept of personhood, namely:

1. *sentience – the capacity to have conscious experiences, usually including the capacity to experience pain and pleasure;*
2. *emotionality – the capacity to feel happy, sad, angry, loving, and so on;*
3. *reason – the capacity to solve new and relatively complex problems;*
4. *the capacity to communicate, by whatever means, messages of an indefinite variety of types; that is, not just with an indefinite number of possible contents, but on indefinitely many possible topics;*
5. *self-awareness – having a concept of oneself, as an individual and / or as a member of a social group; and finally*
6. *moral agency – the capacity to regulate one's own actions through moral principles or ideals.* (Warren 2014 edn: 140)

Although conceding that it is difficult to define these traits precisely, or to specify 'universally valid behavioural indications that these traits are present', Warren (1997: 84) nevertheless holds that these criteria of personhood are functional – pointing out that an entity 'need not have all of these attributes to be a person'. She explains:

> It should not surprise us that many people do not meet all the criteria of personhood. Criteria for the applicability of complex concepts are often like this: none may be logically necessary, but the more criteria that are satisfied, the more confident we are that the concept is applicable. Conversely, the fewer criteria are satisfied, the less plausible it is to hold that the concept applies. And if none of the relevant criteria are met, then we may be confident that it does not [apply]. (Warren 1997: 84)

Warren (1997: 2014) suggests that, in order to demonstrate that a fetus is not a person, all that is required is to claim that a fetus has none of the above six characteristics of personhood.

For some, the personhood argument does little to settle the abortion question. For example, it might be claimed that, even if it is true that a fetus is not a person, it nevertheless has the potential to become one, and therefore it has rights (see also Warren 1977). Thus abortion is still wrong on the grounds of the *potentiality* of the fetus (Glover 1977: 122) – or, to borrow from Warren's analogy cited earlier: even though an acorn is not an oak tree, it nevertheless has the potential to become one; therefore crushing an acorn is tantamount to chopping down an oak tree.

There are a number of difficulties with this view. First, the argument tends to presume that what is potential will in fact become actual. In the case of zygotes, however, this is quite improbable. As Engelhardt points out, only '40–50% of zygotes survive to be persons (i.e. adult, competent human beings)' (1986: 111). It might then be better, suggests Engelhardt, to speak of human zygotes as being only '0.4 probable persons'.

Second, the argument strongly suggests that it is not the fetus per se that is valued, but rather what it will become (Glover 1977: 122). It is difficult to interpret just what kind of moral demand this creates. As Glover (1977: 122) points out:

> *It is hard to see how this potential argument can come to any more than saying that abortion is wrong because a person who would have existed in the future will not exist if an abortion is performed.*

If we take the potentiality argument to its logical extreme, we are committed to accepting, absurdly, that contraception, the wasteful ejaculation of sperm, menstruation and celibacy are also morally wrong, since these too will result in future persons being prevented from existing (Warren 1977: 277).

The main unresolved question, however, is: 'Can a *potential* person be meaningfully said to have *actual* rights and, if so, can these rights meaningfully override the existing rights of actual persons?' or, to put this another way: 'Can a fetus (a potential person) have actual rights and, if so, can these meaningfully override the existing rights of its mother (an actual person)?' The crux of the dilemma posed here is whether the more immediate and actual rights of the pregnant woman should be recognised before the more remote and potential needs of the fetus, or vice versa.

One answer is that, given our understanding of the nature of moral rights and correlative duties, there is something logically and linguistically odd in ascribing rights to fetuses (non-persons), particularly during the pre-sentient stage. If we were to accept that non-sentient fetuses have moral rights, we would be committed, absurdly, to accepting that all sorts of other non-sentient things have moral rights – including human toenails, strands of hair or pieces of skin. For argument's sake, however, let us accept that the fetus does have moral rights and, further, that these can meaningfully conflict with the mother's moral rights. The question which arises here is: 'Which *fetal / maternal rights* are likely to conflict?'

The most obvious is the fetus's and the mother's common claim to a *right to life*. This is particularly so in cases where the mother's life would almost certainly be lost if the pregnancy were allowed to continue. In such situations it seems reasonable to claim that the mother's right to life must at least be as strong as the fetus's right to life. Further, since both stand to die unless the pregnancy is terminated, then surely it is better, morally speaking, that only one life is lost instead of two? It is difficult to see how anyone could reasonably and conscientiously choose an outcome which would see both the mother and the fetus die. Furthermore, as stated elsewhere in this book, morality does not generally require us to make large personal sacrifices on behalf of another, and thus it would be morally incorrect to suggest that the mother has a duty to sacrifice her life in defence of the fetus. In the case of life-threatening pregnancies, then, it seems reasonable to conclude that the pregnant woman's right to life has the weightier claim.

A second set of rights which may conflict is the mother's *right to have control over her body and life's circumstances* versus the fetus's *right to life*. It might be claimed, for example, that a woman's right to choose her lifestyle, career, economic circumstances, standard of health and similar override any claims the fetus might have to be 'kept alive'. The mother may then withdraw her 'life support' even if this means the fetus will die in the process (an unfortunate, but nevertheless unavoidable, consequence). Against this, however, it might still be claimed that the inconveniences and other psychological, physical or social ills caused by an unwanted pregnancy are still not enough to justify killing the fetus and violating its right to life (Brody 1982; Noonan 1983). The demand not to kill the fetus becomes even more persuasive when it is considered that there are alternatives available for helping to prevent or alleviate the ills of unwanted pregnancies, such as child welfare and other social security benefits, adoption, counselling, medication, or ectogenesis. Ectogenesis, which involves extracting the embryo or fetus and placing it in a surrogate or an artificial uterus, would essentially allow an extracorporeal pregnancy to occur (also called 'extrauterine fetal incubation' or EUFI) (Bulletti et al 2011: 126; see also Coleman 2004; Gelfand & Shook 2006; Yuko 2012). It should be noted that ectogenesis, described as the 'third era of human reproduction' (Abecassis 2016), is not as far-fetched as it might seem and can no longer be dismissed as 'just the stuff of science fiction'. Such 'theoretical devices' are already used in experimental animal science (Adinolfi 2004). For example, in 2017 it was reported that scientists had sustained the lives of lamb fetuses in a 'plastic womb' for between 105 and 115 days (Cohen 2017; Winter 2017). As Winter

(2017: 416) noted, reports of this experimental success 'invited inference' that human ectogenesis may soon be a reality. Although the technical problems remain formidable, some scientists contend that it is only a matter of time before efficient artificial uteri in humans will be available – especially for late-term fetuses where it would be easier to connect embryonic umbilical arteries and veins to equipment designed to pump, filter and nourish blood (Abecassis 2016; Adinolfi 2004; Bulletti et al 2011). Moreover, research dating back to the 1990s has already been carried out on 'maintaining uteri extracted from women outside of a woman's body', and implanting embryos into these wombs (Rowland 1992: 288–9). Aborted fetuses were 'kept alive for up to forty-eight hours' in these early research projects (Rowland 1992: 289; see also Caplan et al 2007; Coleman 2004; Gelfand & Shook 2006; Yuko 2012). In light of these alternatives (notwithstanding the complex ethical issues raised by ectogenesis in particular – for example, see Cohen 2017; Reiber 2010), some critics contend that the claim that a mother's rights ought to be given overriding consideration over those of the fetus becomes increasingly difficult to sustain (Langford 2008). Notwithstanding the ethical and legal concerns raised by ectogenesis, scientists are of the view that successful human ectogenesis will be achieved within the next two decades (Abecassis 2016). Commentators also foresee that, if achieved, human ectogenesis will radically change the parameters of the conventional abortion debate including rendering it a non-issue (Cohen 2017; Coleman 2005).

A third set of rights which might conflict is the mother's *right to health* (and to a quality of life) versus the fetus's *right to life*. In this instance, the mother's health and quality of life are threatened not by her pregnancy but by a progressive debilitating disease, such as Alzheimer's, Parkinson's or diabetes. The mother might, for example, contemplate getting pregnant for the sole purpose of growing tissue which can be harvested and transplanted into her brain or pancreas in an attempt to restore her health. The issue of fetal tissue transplantation has long been the subject of intense debate (Engelhardt 1989; Sandel 2004). Although governments are striving hard to prevent this type of scenario from occurring, there have already been cases of women getting pregnant and/or having abortions for the sole purpose of supplying fetal tissue for transplantation – if not for themselves, then for others especially a fetus's siblings (e.g. 'saviour sibling' or 'donor sibling' pregnancies / abortions) (Deech 2017; Morrow 1991; Raz et al 2017).

A fourth set of rights which may cause conflict involves not only the competing claims of a fetus and its mother, but also the *paternal rights* of the father (also called 'male abortion') (McCulley 1988). During the 1980s there were a number of legal cases (notably in the United Kingdom (UK), the United States (US), Canada and Australia) involving fathers undertaking legal action in an attempt to stop their (ex-)wives and (ex-)girlfriends from having abortions (AFP 1989; Beyer 1989; Leo 1983; Lowther 1988; McCulley 1988; PA 1987).

Court challenges brought by biological fathers against their partners have tended to be viewed with little sympathy from women who historically have been left alone with the burden and hardships of child rearing after the fathers of their children have long abandoned them. Some even worry that, if the paternity rights debate is allowed to progress to its logical extreme, it could have paved the way for rapists to prevent their victims from having abortions, and to press for access rights after the baby has been born.

To date, Australian courts have tended to deny the injunctions sought by biological fathers preventing their partners from having an abortion on the grounds that there is 'no rule in common law or statute which gives the father the right to be consulted about a termination' (Forrester & Griffiths 2015: 216). In the US, one Supreme Court stated that when a father and mother disagree on whether an abortion should go forward:

> The obvious fact is that [...] the view of only one of the two marriage partners can prevail. Inasmuch as it is the woman who physically bears the child and who is the more directly and immediately affected by the

pregnancy, as between the two, the balance weighs in her favor. (*Planned Parenthood of Central Missouri v Danforth* 1976: 72)

Abortion, politics and the broader community

As noted in the introduction to this discussion, the abortion issue is extraordinarily complex; it is also extremely political, as some spectacular overseas incidents have shown. For example, in 1990, Belgium was thrown into a constitutional crisis after King Baudouin, Belgium's reigning monarch, stepped down from his throne temporarily 'because his conscience would not let him sign a law legalising abortion' (Reuters 1990a: 7). As a result, the government had to take over the King's powers and pass the abortion law. It is reported that once the abortion law was passed the King's inability to reign ceased, and he resumed his position on the throne (Reuters 1990a: 7).

In the same year, it was reported that disagreement over abortion law threatened to 'derail a treaty on German unity' (Reuters 1990b: 7). The disagreement was primarily over whether 'West German women may take advantage of East Germany's liberal abortion laws after unification' (Reuters 1990b: 7).

In 1992, Ireland witnessed political uproar and large public demonstrations after the High Court banned a 14-year-old rape victim from travelling to Britain for an abortion (the girl had been raped repeatedly by a friend's father over a 1-year period) (Barrett G 1992a, 1992b; Holden 1994; Makri 2018). It was reported that many European constitutional lawyers considered the ban a breach of the Treaty of Rome, which had brought the European Community (EC) into being almost four decades earlier, and, among other things, 'permitted the right to free movement within the EC' (Barrett G 1992a). The situation reached crisis point when it was evident that the ban threatened the European Community's Maastricht Treaty on European political union, which Irish voters were due to vote on a few months later (Barrett G 1992c, 1992d, 1992e, 1992f; *Independent* 1992: 6).

In 2007, Ireland's abortion laws once again threatened to erupt into a political crisis when a pregnant 17-year-old began court proceedings to enable her to travel to Britain for an abortion. The teenager decided to have an abortion upon learning that the fetus she was carrying had a rare brain condition (anencephaly) and was not expected to live longer than a few days after being born (Bowcott 2007: 14). Although abortion was illegal in Ireland at the time (and the subject of a constitutional ban, overturned only in May 2018), it was permitted to be performed in cases where the risks to the mother were substantial. Neither the law nor the constitution allowed abortion to be performed on grounds of fetal abnormality, however, and it was this point that threatened to cause a constitutional crisis. The case is reported to have prompted 'fresh calls for constitutional reform' and for the provision of 'safe, free, and legal abortion in Ireland' (Bowcott 2007: 14). Other notable cases prompting calls for constitutional reform included the much-publicised case of Savita Halappanavar, who died on 28 October 2012 as a result of being refused an abortion for a non-viable pregnancy even though her life was at serious risk, and the 2014 case of 'Miss Y', a suicidal pregnant asylum seeker who revealed to authorities that her pregnancy was the result of being raped in her country of origin (Berer 2013; McCarthy et al 2018; Makri 2018; Quinlan 2017).

Abortion was also a major issue in the American presidential election of 1992, with the then presidential contenders Bill Clinton and Ross Perot both trying 'to lure pro-choice voters to their side' (Barrett L I 1992: 54). During the campaign, the Bush camp (whose law reforms saw the loss of civil rights protection for US abortion clinics (Denniston 1993) and the banning of abortion counselling at federally funded clinics (Toner 1993)) admitted publicly that anything raising the profile of the abortion issue was 'a problem for us' (Barrett L I 1992: 54).

The abortion debate in the US took a dramatic and historic turn in 1993, when an anti-abortion protester shot and killed a doctor during a pro-life demonstration outside a lawful abortion clinic (Rohter 1993: 7; see also Hadley 1996). Abortion rights groups took the shooting of the doctor as a 'symbol of the increasing harassment' of health workers involved in abortion work, which has since seen abortion clinics increasingly vandalised and destroyed by arsonists.

According to Robinson (2004) of Ontario Consultants on Religious Tolerance, since harassment and violence first began to be levelled at abortion clinics in the early 1970s, there have been literally tens of thousands of incidents directed against abortion clinic personnel. Citing US National Abortion Federation (NAF) figures, Robinson estimates that, in the 16-year period from 1989 to 2004, anti-abortion protesters were implicated in 24 murders and attempted murders; 180 (actual or attempted) bombings and arson attacks; 3349 incidents of invasion, assault and battery, vandalism, trespassing, death threats (including over 554 anthrax hoaxes), burglary and stalking; 11 448 instances of hate mail, harassing phone calls and bomb threats; 516 blockades; and 80 305 episodes of picketing across the US (Robinson 2004). Although the number of seriously violent crimes against abortion clinics (e.g. murders and attempted murders) has declined over the years, the NAF reports there has nonetheless been a steep rise in clinic invasions, obstructions and blockades by anti-abortion extremists emboldened by the current political environment (NAF 2017: 1). Specifically, for the period 2016–17, trespassing has more than tripled, death threats / threats of harm have nearly doubled and incidents of obstruction have risen from 580 to more than 1700 (NAF 2017: 1). It should be noted, however, that this situation is not unique to the US. Countries such as Australia, Canada, New Zealand and the UK have all had to grapple with anti-abortion protestation against women in need as well as abortion service providers. Women seeking an abortion in these countries often must run the gauntlet of anti-abortion protesters stationed outside reproductive health clinics handing out anti-abortion pamphlets, conducting 'pavement anti-abortion counselling' and harassing the women (and their partners) as they attempt to enter the clinic (Lowe & Hayes 2018; Regan & Glasier 2017; Sifris & Belton 2017; Whyte 2018). The problem of anti-abortion protestors stationed outside reproductive health clinics has become so serious that new legislation establishing 'safe access zones' (also called 'buffer zones') to protect women from harassment has had to be introduced (Lowe & Hayes 2018; Paxman 2017; Regan & Glasier 2017; Sifris & Belton 2017).

Australia has also experienced the politicisation of abortion, with a small number of politicians over the years attempting, unsuccessfully, to introduce legislation aimed at restricting abortion services for women. Arguably the most dramatic event to occur in Australia's abortion history, however, occurred in July 2001 when Steve Rogers, a security guard at the Fertility Control Clinic in East Melbourne, was fatally shot by a man intent on destroying the clinic (Dean & Allanson 2003). As already discussed in Chapter 5, this attack was the first of its kind in Australia and sparked fury and dismay at the vulnerability of abortion clinic personnel and the failure by law enforcement bodies to protect those attending and working at such clinics (Dean & Allanson 2003; Rees & Head 2001). Significantly, in 2006, another man attempted to kill – and was subsequently charged with threatening to kill – another security guard at the clinic, underscoring the risks and potential threats to the safety of abortion personnel in Australia (Nader 2007) and the tensions that exist between the right to access and the right to protest abortion (Dean & Allanson 2003). Also in 2009 a medical clinic in Mosman Park, Western Australia, was daubed with graffiti with the words 'Baby Killers' and subjected to an attempted firebombing using Molotov cocktails (Sapienza 2009).

Anti-abortion violence against individual workers and services continues in Western liberal democracies such as the US, UK, Canada, New Zealand and Australia. Occurring as a result of either strategic activism or one-off random attacks, anti-abortion violence includes, but is not limited to, stalking, assault, kidnapping, attempted murder, murder and the vandalism of property (including arson and bombing) (Wikipedia 2018e: http://www.wikipedia.org/wiki/Anti-abortion_violence).

Euthanasia

Euthanasia, like abortion, is also regarded as one of the most controversial bioethical issues to have captured the public's attention in Western liberal democracies. Like the abortion issue, it is unlikely to be resolved to the satisfaction of all concerned. A significant distinguishing feature of the euthanasia issue, however, is that, despite media-generated public opinion polls suggesting a global majority support for euthanasia, in reality it is a minority issue. As Johnstone (2013a) notes in her comprehensive critique of the politics of euthanasia, the actual practice of euthanasia affects only a small percentage of people – even in jurisdictions in which euthanasia has been legalised (e.g. the Netherlands). Moreover, the World Federation of Right to Die Societies (founded in 1980) has affiliated organisations in only 26 (13%) of the world's 195 recognised countries (https://www.worldrtd.net/). In light of this, as Johnstone (and others) have concluded elsewhere, 'the development and implementation of what has been termed "death policy" is neither a universal phenomenon nor a public policy imperative. Despite this reality, euthanasia is falsely promoted "as if" it is of universal importance and priority' (Johnstone 2013a: xvii).

Another distinguishing feature of the euthanasia issue is the extent to which pro-euthanasia activists have successfully used propaganda and 'dirty tricks fallacies' to advance their cause (Johnstone 2013a). Although anti-abortion campaigners have used similar devices, their efforts have tended to be less sophisticated and less well organised. As an examination of these devices has already been made elsewhere (see Johnstone 2013a), no further attention will be given to them here.

Euthanasia and its significance for nurses

Euthanasia and the so-called 'right to die' are not new issues for nurses. In Australia, one of the first articles addressing the subject was published as early as 1912 in the *Australasian Nurses Journal*. Reprinted from the *British Medical Journal*, the article contained concerns and viewpoints which remain current – including the question of whether euthanasia should be legalised.

Although euthanasia may not be a new issue for nurses in Australia, it has nevertheless become a more complex and significant one. For example, in 1996, Australia became the subject of international attention when it became the first country in the world to fully legalise active voluntary euthanasia. This followed the passage, in May 1995, of the Northern Territory's controversial *Rights of the Terminally Ill Act 1995 (NT)*, which came into effect on 1 July 1996. Almost 1 year later, however, the Act was overturned by the Australian Federal government – although not before five people had sought assistance to die under the Act. Recognising the possible implications of *Rights of the Terminally Ill Act* for members of the nursing profession, the Royal College of Nursing, Australia (RCNA) (now the Australian College of Nursing (ACN)) took the unprecedented step of releasing for comment a discussion paper entitled *Euthanasia: an issue for nurses* (Hamilton 1995). The RCNA received over 70 responses to this discussion paper from concerned and interested nursing organisations, groups and individuals from around Australia. The responses received represented nurses working in a variety of clinical areas and fields of nursing (including education) and reflected a wide diversity of knowledge, opinion, values and beliefs about euthanasia as well as the need for guidance on how best to respond the issue. Perhaps most confronting of all, however, was the emerging difficult question of whether the nursing profession should take a definitive stance in either supporting or opposing the legalisation of euthanasia and adopt a formal position statement clarifying its stance.

Recognising the complexity and perplexity of the issue, the RCNA subsequently commissioned, as part of its professional development series, a monograph entitled *The politics of euthanasia: a nursing response* (Johnstone 1996a). The purpose of this monograph was not to provide nurses with definitive answers to the difficult questions posed by the euthanasia debate. Rather, it was to advance a discussion that would enable nurses 'to formulate their own thinking and viewpoints on the subject and to be able to contribute to broader professional discussion on the whole issue of the right to die' (Johnstone 1996b: 22). In July 1996, the RCNA also issued its first position statement on voluntary euthanasia and assisted suicide – subsequently revised and reaffirmed respectively in 1999 and 2006 (RCNA 1996, 1999, 2006). This position statement primarily focused on clarifying the illegal status of euthanasia/assisted suicide in

Australia, acknowledging that there exists a diversity of moral viewpoints on the euthanasia issue, reminding nurses of their professional responsibility to be reliably informed about the ethical, legal, cultural and clinical implications of euthanasia and assisted suicide, and recognising and supporting the appropriateness of nurses taking a 'conscientious' position on the matter.

Significantly, in May 1996, less than 2 months before the *Rights of the Terminally Ill Act 1995 (NT)* came into effect, the then Nurses' Board of the Northern Territory took the unprecedented step of formulating and ratifying a formal position statement on euthanasia (see Nurses' Board of the Northern Territory *Position statement on the nurse's role in euthanasia*, included in full as Appendix 5 in Johnstone 1996a). This position statement was keyed to the *Rights of the Terminally Ill Act 1995 (NT)* and sought to clarify the role and function of nurses in relation to the Act's provisions. Specifically, the position statement supported:

- *the role of nurses assisting in the voluntary euthanasia of competent patients; and*
- *the rights of nurses to conscientiously refuse to participate in the euthanasia of patients.* (Johnstone 1996a: 36)

The position statement also outlined the obligations of nurses in regard to the ethical and legal aspects of euthanasia, employment policies, professional competence and education (Johnstone 1996a: 36–7).

Currently, with the notable exception of the Australian State of Victoria,[4] it is an offence in Australian jurisdictions 'to assist, encourage or aid a person to commit suicide or attempt to commit suicide' (Forrester & Griffiths 2015: 247). Thus, although the term 'euthanasia' as such is not a legally recognised word for the purposes of criminal law,[5] the term 'assisted suicide' (aiding someone to die) is (Forrester & Griffiths 2015: 244). Similarly in New Zealand, in which, as in Australia, there have been convictions for assisting the suicide of another.

Emboldened by the passage of the Victorian legislation, proponents of euthanasia / assisted suicide in Australia speculate that it will only be a matter of time before euthanasia and assisted suicide will be legal in all jurisdictions in Australia.

Definitions of euthanasia, assisted suicide and 'mercy killing'

Euthanasia

The term *euthanasia*[6] is generally used to refer to an instance in which a legally competent patient / client makes an informed and voluntary choice to have a medically assisted death, explicitly requests assistance to die and gives an informed consent for the actual procedure of euthanasia to be performed. In short, *the patient / client explicitly requests, and voluntarily consents to, a medical practitioner to administer a lethal substance (e.g. by intravenous injection) so as to bring about immediate death*. This form of euthanasia is also sometimes called *active voluntary euthanasia* because: (i) it involves *actively* bringing about death (e.g. by the deliberate administration of a lethal injection), as opposed to passive euthanasia encompassing *passively* bringing about death (e.g. by wilfully withholding or withdrawing clinically assisted nutrition and hydration), and (ii) it is chosen *voluntarily* – that is, in a manner that is free of coercive or manipulative influences (as opposed to being imposed under duress or when unable or incapable of giving a free and informed consent). Euthanasia of the active voluntary type is also sometimes referred to as 'consensual euthanasia'. This is generally contrasted with *non-voluntary euthanasia* (sometimes referred to as 'non-consensual euthanasia') as this type of euthanasia involves the act of killing a patient / client whose wishes cannot be known because of either immaturity, incompetence, or both.

Over the decades, the bioethics literature has variously drawn a distinction between six different types of euthanasia: (1) voluntary active euthanasia, (2) voluntary passive euthanasia, (3) involuntary active euthanasia, (4) involuntary passive euthanasia, (5) non-voluntary active euthanasia and (6) non-voluntary

FIGURE 10.2
Six categories of euthanasia

	Passive	Active
VOLUNTARY [Consensual]	Voluntary passive euthanasia	Voluntary active euthanasia
INVOLUNTARY [Non-consensual]	Involuntary passive euthanasia	Involuntary active euthanasia
NON-VOLUNTARY [Non-consensual]	Non-voluntary passive euthanasia	Non-voluntary active euthanasia

passive euthanasia. The six types of euthanasia just outlined can be expressed diagrammatically, as shown in Fig. 10.2.

In the case of *voluntary euthanasia*, as already stated, a fully competent patient makes an informed and voluntary decision to have a medically assisted death, asks for assistance to die and gives an informed consent for the actual procedure of euthanasia to be performed. *Involuntary euthanasia* (or non-consensual euthanasia), in contrast, involves the exact opposite – namely, killing a patient without the patient's informed consent and/or contrary to that patient's expressed wishes (where these are known or could be known). The involuntary killing of patients as part of the Nazi medicalised killing programs during World War II is an example of this. Non-voluntary euthanasia (also a form of non-consensual euthanasia) stands in contrast again and involves the act of killing a patient whose wishes cannot be known because of either immaturity or incompetency, or both. As McGuire (1987) explains, whereas the term 'involuntary' implies an action which is carried out against the wishes of the patient, 'non-voluntary' simply implies that there is no voluntariness – in the sense that the patient is not capable of either denying or giving consent (as in the case of the permanently comatose or brain-injured patient). In the case of the permanently comatose, McGuire contends, euthanasia would be 'neither voluntary nor involuntary, but is simply non-voluntary' (McGuire 1987: 12).

Despite the above categorisations, contemporary debate on the legalisation of euthanasia as a medical procedure primarily has as its focus just two forms: voluntary euthanasia and non-voluntary euthanasia. The reasons for this are threefold:

- The distinction between active and passive euthanasia is held to be unsustainable and effectively collapses once it is admitted that, whether actively administering a lethal substance or passively withholding a life-prolonging therapy (including food and fluids), the *intention* is still the same – namely, to hasten the foreseeable death of the patient.
- *Involuntary euthanasia* (euthanasia against a person's will) is regarded by proponents of active voluntary euthanasia as an act that could never be justified on moral grounds and hence as unconscionable and beyond the pale; accordingly there is nothing to debate (both proponents and opponents are agreed: involuntary euthanasia is wrong and impermissible).
- *Non-voluntary euthanasia* (euthanasia of entities without the capacity to request or consent to euthanasia – e.g. children and adults who are cognitively impaired, have a serious brain injury, etc.), in contradistinction to involuntary euthanasia, is regarded by proponents of active

voluntary euthanasia as an act that could be justified on moral grounds (e.g. the alleviation of unbearable and intractable suffering) and hence morally worthy of debate as to its moral permissibility or impermissibility.

Assisted suicide

The term '*assisted suicide*' (and variations thereof, e.g. physician-assisted suicide (PAS), medically assisted suicide (MAS), medically assisted death (MAD)) is sometimes used interchangeably with the term euthanasia, even though this is not, strictly speaking, correct. With assisted suicide, a qualified medical practitioner supplies the patient/client with the *means* of taking his/her own life (e.g. provides a prescription for a lethal dose of drugs), but, unlike in the case of euthanasia, it is the patient/client (not the doctor) *who acts last*. To put this another way, in the case of euthanasia it is the qualified medical practitioner who kills the patient/client, whereas in the case of assisted suicide the patient/client kills him- or herself. There is a presumption here that, because the patient is the person 'who acts last', assisted suicide is more defensible than and hence preferable to active euthanasia since:

- the willingness by the patient to action their own suicide 'gives compelling evidence of the patient's desire to die' (Dixon 1998: 29)
- the medical practitioner is able to gain some 'moral distance' and hence be exculpated from full moral responsibility for the act since his or her finger is 'not on the button' (Johnstone 1999a: 282).

A notable US example of assisted suicide can be found in the Oregon State's *Death with Dignity Act* (known as 'Measure 16'), which, upon coming into effect in 1997, legalised physician-assisted suicide in the form of prescribing a lethal dose of medication, but not active voluntary euthanasia (Magnusson 2002: 64). (Oregon has the distinction of being the first US state to legalise assisted dying (Parliamentary Library & Information Services, Department of Parliamentary Services 2017: 9).)

'Mercy killing'

A third terminology which has found usage in discussions on euthanasia is that of '*mercy killing*'. Although this term is also sometimes used interchangeably with the term 'euthanasia' it can nevertheless be distinguished from euthanasia on a contextual basis. Specifically, as Glick explains (1992: 81–2):

> Mercy killing is not the same as voluntary active euthanasia since many killings are committed without patient request or consent – typically an elderly husband shoots his terminally ill and unconscious or Alzheimer's disease-stricken wife. But the cases almost always exhibit wrenching long-term personal suffering and sacrifice and financial ruin … They evoke sympathy for both killer and victim and perpetuate interest in the legalisation [sic] of voluntary active euthanasia, which some believe might eliminate the compelling need that desperate people feel for killing their hopelessly ill spouses.

Views for and against euthanasia/assisted suicide

Like other controversial bioethical issues, euthanasia and assisted suicide have proponents and opponents. Attitudes towards them range from liberal and moderate acceptance to absolute conservative prohibition. It is to examining some of the various viewpoints for and against euthanasia and assisted suicide that this discussion will now turn.

Views in support of euthanasia

Those who support euthanasia typically take the view that it is morally wrong to allow people to suffer unnecessarily. Popular views traditionally advanced in support of euthanasia (and, in particular, in support of legalising it) fall under four main augmentative categories:

1. *arguments from individual autonomy and the right to choose*
2. *arguments from the loss of dignity and the right to the maintenance of dignity*
3. *arguments from the reduction of suffering*
4. *arguments from justice and the demand to be treated fairly.* (adapted from Beauchamp & Perlin 1978: 217).

A fifth and controversial category of argument raised in support of euthanasia is that, in some instances, patients have an altruistic 'duty to die' (Cooley 2007; Hardwig 2000, 2014) and, furthermore, that it might even be a violation of a person's 'freedom of conscience' not to respect this duty (Lewis 2001: 60–2).

Arguments from individual autonomy and the right to choose

It is generally accepted that people have a right to choose, and, as discussed in Chapter 3, the moral principle of autonomy demands that people's choices ought to be respected, even if we consider them to be mistaken or foolish. The only grounds upon which a person's autonomous choices can be justly interfered with are if they stand to impinge seriously on the significant moral interests of others. Proponents of voluntary euthanasia argue that the right to choose includes the right to choose death (reframed as 'the right to die'). Given the 'right to die', this means that others (including the state) should not interfere with a person's decision to die, and in some instances may even entail a positive duty to assist a person to die – as in cases where a person desires death but is physically unable to end his or her own life. Voluntary euthanasia is thus thought to be justified here on grounds of autonomy and the demand to respect a person's autonomous wishes.

Arguments from the right to dignity

Related to the demand to respect a person's autonomous choices is the further demand to respect and maintain a person's dignity. Advances in medical technology have increased the capacity of the medical profession to prolong a person's life using clinically assisted means. Its methods, however, are not always humane, and can seriously erode a person's self-concept, character, sense of self-worth and self-esteem, and the like. In instances of dignity violations euthanasia is a justified option.

Arguments from the reduction of suffering

Suffering may be defined as a state of severe distress that people experience when some crucial aspect of themselves, their being or their existence is threatened (Cassell 1991; Kahn & Steeves 1986). It is important to clarify that, although pain is a major cause of suffering, suffering itself is 'not confined to physical symptoms' (i.e. people can be suffering yet not be in physical pain) (Cassell 1991). Suffering may, for example, derive from other aspects of 'personhood' – including the cognitive, emotional, spiritual, social and cultural aspects of a person's identity – and not just their physical aspect. Moreover, when any one or a combination of these aspects is threatened, a person may simultaneously give cognitive, emotional, spiritual, social and other (cultural) meanings to that threat and respond accordingly.

Suffering is generally regarded as morally unacceptable and, as discussed in Chapter 3, morality demands that, where possible, people across the life span should be spared or prevented from suffering unnecessarily. In cases where patients' suffering is intense, protracted, unendurable and intractable, it seems cruel to deny them the choice of death as a means of release from their suffering. Euthanasia in these kinds of cases is said to be justified on grounds of 'prevention of cruelty' or 'mercy' (Beauchamp & Perlin 1978: 217). It is also thought to be justified on the grounds that people have the indisputable right to judge their suffering as unbearable, and the concomitant right to request euthanasia to end their unbearable suffering (see, for example, Admiraal 1991: 11). This, in turn, is grounded in the reality that, despite the achievements of modern medicine, doctors still cannot relieve all suffering (notwithstanding its highly subjective nature, making it difficult for clinicians to accurately access and treat 'suffering'

(Bozzaro & Schildmann 2018)). Due in no small way to disparities in pain management and palliative care across and even within different countries, people's pain states are also not always successfully managed, despite research showing marked improvements in pain management strategies (Are et al 2017).

Arguments from justice and the demand to be treated fairly

It is argued that everybody is entitled to be treated fairly and to share equally the benefits and burdens of life. To deny patients the option of being spared intolerable and intractable suffering is to treat them unfairly, and to make them carry a burden which others do not have to carry. Furthermore, to deny patients the right to die (i.e. in a manner and time of their choosing) is to impose unfairly on them the values of others. Only patients, or those intimately involved with them (e.g. family and friends), can judge what is in their own best interests. For others to deny patients the right to choose death is therefore to violate unfairly these patients' autonomy, dignity and entitlement to be spared the harms that will flow from experiencing intolerable and intractable suffering. Where euthanasia is the only thing that can end patients' intolerable and intractable suffering, it stands as a morally just alternative.

Arguments from altruism and the 'duty to die'

It is argued that in certain circumstances (such as in the case of old age, chronic illness, when medical treatment is futile, or when developing a 'rationality-eroding condition' such as dementia) it may be a person's *duty* to volunteer for euthanasia (Budić 2018; Cooley 2007; Hardwig 2014). Budić (2018), for example, states:

> *I see no reason in sustaining someone's biological life if that being will no longer live as a person with moral life, and at the same time they may contribute to loss or poor quality of life of others to whom they may pose a burden (p 112).*

One commentator argues controversially that it might also be a violation of a person's right to freedom of conscience to interfere with the exercise of their duty to die (Lewis 2001: 60–2).

In situations where a person's primary caregivers are burdened to the point where they cannot live their lives fully and are themselves beginning to suffer as a result of their burden of care, some argue that euthanasia is not only permissible, but required and 'simply the only loving thing to do' (Hardwig 2014: 104). In defence of this stance, Hardwig contends:

> *I may well one day have a duty to die, a duty most likely to arise out of my connections with my family and loved ones. Sometimes preserving my life can only devastate the lives of those who care for me. I do not believe I am idiosyncratic, morbid or morally perverse in believing this. I am trying to take steps to prepare myself mentally and spiritually to make sure that I will be able to take my life if I should one day have such a duty … Tragically, sometimes the best thing you can do for your loved ones is to remove yourself from their lives. And the only way you can do that may be to remove yourself from existence.* (Hardwig 2014: 104, 105)

Counter-arguments to views supporting euthanasia

People who are opposed to euthanasia tend not to be persuaded by these kinds of arguments. In responding to pro-euthanasia arguments, opponents tend to take two main approaches: (1) to assert a number of counter-claims and counter-arguments against the views put forward in support of euthanasia; and (2) to assert a number of distinctive arguments against euthanasia.

Autonomy and the right to choose death

The moral principle of autonomy is well established in Western moral thinking. Nevertheless, it is not without limits (see, for example, the comprehensive analysis of the limits of autonomy in assisted suicide by Campbell (2016)). Whether the principle of autonomy was ever meant to stretch so far as to impose a moral duty on others (e.g. a doctor or a nurse) to comply with a patient's request for euthanasia – to intentionally and actively assist that patient to die – is another question. If complying with a patient's request for euthanasia has the foreseeable consequence of harming or affecting prejudicially the significant moral interests of others (e.g. the doctors or nurses receiving the request, or the patient's family and friends), there is considerable scope for arguing that the doctors and nurses in question have no duty to perform euthanasia, no matter how autonomous the patient's request for it. Further, given the complex nature of the ethics and politics of euthanasia, it is rather simplistic to hold that euthanasia can be justified on the grounds of patient autonomy alone without taking into account other important moral considerations (including the autonomy interests of others) which might also have a significant bearing on a patient's choosing euthanasia / assisted suicide, and the supposed 'duty' of others to provide it (Johnstone 2013a).

Appeals to autonomy to justify euthanasia and assisted suicide are, however, problematic on another account. Paradoxically, acts of euthanasia / assisted suicide carried out in response to a patient's autonomous request destroy the very basis of their justification. According to Safranek (1998), whereas autonomy is necessary for the existence of a moral act, it is not sufficient to justify an act. As he explains (p 34):

> *The justification of the act will hinge on the end to which autonomy is employed: if for a noble end, then it is upheld; if depraved, then it is proscribed. It is not autonomy per se that vindicates an autonomy claim but the good that autonomy is instrumental in achieving. Therefore an individual cannot invoke autonomy to justify an ethical or legal claim to acts such as assisted suicide; rather he [or she] must vindicate the underlying value that the autonomous act endeavours to attain.*

Since autonomous requests for euthanasia and assisted suicide are socially threatening (they threaten human survival), it is appropriate that the autonomy of individuals requesting such threatening acts be circumscribed – at least until such time as it is clarified and agreed just what kinds of 'good' autonomy should be invoked to achieve (Safranek 1998: 34; see also Campbell 2016).

It is important to note here that autonomy discourse is extremely powerful, making challenges to it difficult. So successful has been the promotion of autonomy, and the assumed sovereign rights of individuals to exercise self-determining choices, that the imperatives of these things – especially in the case of euthanasia / assisted suicide – have come to seem 'so self-evident to all "right thinking people" that to question them seems almost perverse' (Moody 1992: 50). Those who do question them risk being publicly ridiculed and dismissed by opponents as ill-informed and 'illogical', or worse as being 'insulting' to people who are vulnerable and oppressed (Johnstone 2013a).

Dignity and the right to die with dignity

Dignity and dying with dignity does not necessarily entail choosing death over the clinically assisted prolongation of life. The demand to respect and maintain a person's dignity might equally entail respect for a person's autonomous wish that 'everything possible be done' to prolong or sustain her or his life – and to sustain a sense of hope that is fundamental to living that life meaningfully, even though (and when) dying. Here, it is important to understand that the ethical controversies surrounding the care of dying patients are not just about management at a technological, medical or institutional level. Rather, as Campbell (1992: 255) points out, they should also be seen 'as a sign of a deeper crisis of meaning in our culture', and as an indication of how impoverished our society has become in 'assessing the significance of suffering, dying and death as part of a whole human life'. Given this, as Campbell goes on to explain (p 255):

> *The emergence of the individual asserting inviolable rights to self-determination becomes intelligible in this void as a way to create meaning through a freely-chosen style of life and an authentic manner of death.*

One way to respond to this crisis of meaning is to 'provide compassionate presence to the sufferer', not to 'end the suffering by killing the sufferer' (Campbell 1992: 269, 276). Another is to deny altogether the philosophical bases for the so-called 'right to die' (Kass 1993).

The idea that euthanasia imbues death with dignity is problematic on another account – notably, that it stands as a contradiction in terms. As has been argued elsewhere, this is because 'there can be no dignity in death since the dignity or worth or self-esteem of an individual is rendered void by death' (Johnstone 2013a: 165). It is for this reason that 'dignity' per se can be neither promised nor delivered, either by the self ('self-deliverance') or by others (physicians/nurses) willing to provide assistance to die. Thus claims that euthanasia (or its counterpart, physician-assisted suicide) ipso facto 'endows a death with dignity' and that dignity 'depends on choice and control' cannot be sustained (Callahan 2009). In the final analysis, 'death can never be imbued with dignity since death itself calls into question the very meaning and value of human life' (Johnstone 2013a: 166).

Suffering and the demand to end it

Suffering is not just a medical problem; it is also an existential problem involving profound questions concerning the meaning and purpose of human life and destiny (Amato 1990; Bozzaro & Schildmann 2018; Campbell 1992; Klemke 1981; Neimeyer 2001; Spelman 1997; Starck & McGovern 1992). To 'end suffering by killing the sufferer' is, to borrow from Campbell (1992: 276), to misunderstand 'both suffering and ourselves in a way that threatens our moral integrity'. The 'suffering argument' also seems to beg and leave unanswered the question of whether death can (and does) *meaningfully* 'relieve' suffering; as pointed out elsewhere 'while euthanasia certainly kills the *sufferer*, this is not the same as *relieving suffering* per se since there is no longer a living being around to experience and give testimony to the relief that has ostensibly been bestowed' (Johnstone 2013a: 92).

Justice and the demand to be treated fairly

To deny patients the right to choose treatment – including the clinically assisted prolongation of 'hopeless life' – is as unjust as to deny patients the right to choose death. Denying patients' requests for 'everything possible to be done', where this conforms with their notions of dignity, meaning, value and quality of life, is to impose unfairly on them the values of others. As in the case for euthanasia, only patients (or those close to them) can judge what is in their best interests, and they must be permitted to make these judgments.

Altruism and the 'duty to die'

Not all agree that people with certain conditions have an altruistic 'duty to die'. Cholbi (2015: 607), for example, argues against the proposition that people with dementia or other 'rationality-eroding conditions' have a duty to die, on the following grounds: first, that there is no duty to self-destruct when anticipating the development of or developing a rationality-eroding condition such as dementia, and, second, that it is a mistake to assume that duties are owed to people only while they are free of a rationality-eroding condition, such as dementia.

Others argue that, in some circumstances, people may have a conscientious 'duty to live' in order to spare the pain of their grieving loved ones, who desire their ill loved one to live 'as long as possible'. Being dependent on others is not necessarily being a burden on them. Even if dependency does become burdensome – either for the dependent person or her/his carers – it is not clear how, if at all, this gives rise to a so-called 'duty to die'. At best, it may only substantiate 'our basic human predicament' that:

> the very experience of illness, and more fundamentally the process of aging that inevitably culminates in death, not only reveals our shared vulnerability and dependency, but also that we are all subject to some kind of ultimate powers beyond our control. Through our knowledge and technology we may aspire to a mastery of nature and the immortality of the gods, but we continually receive reminders of our dependency and finitude. From this it follows that any control we assert over our dying is already limited, and that dependency and dignity are not mutually exclusive. (Campbell 1992: 270)

At worst, to embrace a 'duty to die' may be to embrace an all-pervasive sense of pessimism and hopelessness which would blind people to understanding that 'the lives of even the terminally ill are precious and matter, right up to the last second of breath' (Mirin, reported by Gibbs 1993: 53). It may also risk blinding people to the fundamental insight which has been articulated so well by the late French philosopher and feminist Simone de Beauvoir (1987: 92) that, although all people must die, death is still an accident, and that, even if people know this and consent to it, death remains 'an unjustifiable violation' (de Beauvoir 1987: 92).

Specific arguments against euthanasia

Specific arguments commonly raised against euthanasia (and the need to legalise it) include:

- arguments from the sanctity-of-life doctrine
- arguments from prognostic uncertainty and misdiagnosis
- arguments from the risk of abuse
- arguments from non-necessity
- arguments from discrimination
- arguments from irrational or mistaken or imprudent choice
- the 'slippery slope' argument.

Arguments from the sanctity-of-life doctrine

A strong conventional argument raised against euthanasia draws on the tenets of the *sanctity of life*, a doctrine which derives from Roman Catholic moral theology. The basic premise of the sanctity-of-life doctrine is that, as human life is sacred and inviolable, nothing (not even intolerable and intractable suffering) can justify taking it. Sanctity-of-life arguments against euthanasia tend to take the following form:

1. human life is sacred, and taking it is wrong
2. euthanasia is an instance of taking human life, therefore
3. euthanasia is wrong.

Whether human life is sacred, and whether taking it is always wrong, is, however, a matter of long-standing philosophical controversy (Kuhse 1987b). If applied consistently, then any form of killing (including killing in self-defence, 'just wars' and state-sanctioned capital punishment for heinous crimes) would, under the sanctity-of-life doctrine, all be deemed morally wrong.

Arguments from prognostic uncertainty and misdiagnosis

An argument often used against euthanasia is that which speaks to the risks of prognostic uncertainty, misdiagnosis and the possibility of recovery. Doctors diagnosing life-threatening medical conditions are not infallible and can (and do) make mistakes. Furthermore, patients can sometimes recover spontaneously and unexpectedly from devastating and/or terminal illnesses — for reasons not always understood or accepted by medical scientists. A poignant example of this can be found in the case of the noted best-selling author of *The women's room*, Marilyn French. In 1992, French was diagnosed belatedly with metastasised oesophageal cancer. Her treating doctor at the time was extremely pessimistic about her prognosis, advising French that she had 'terminal cancer, that there was no hope for cure or remission, and that [she] was not to think of that' (French 1998: 34). Of this moment, French (1998: 34) writes:

> What was he saying? Hope, but not too much? Hope, but don't expect a cure? What was I to hope for, then? He emphasised that mental attitude was crucial to anything they did. I spoke up, assuring him that I had strong powers of concentration and that I wanted to hope … But he wasn't listening; he was talking over me. There was no hope for a cure, he said …

French, however, rejected the pessimism of her physician and simply 'decided' to survive. Accordingly she 'twisted' what medical information she had on oesophageal cancer to her purpose. For example, she seized on an article that stated 'one in five people treated with extreme measures survive non-metastasised esophageal cancer for five years' and decided those figures applied to her (despite her metastases). In French's words, 'I decided I had one chance out of five. I simply made it up' (French 1998: 35). By the end of that day, she had obliterated the word 'terminal' from her memory; and within a couple of days, she had increased her odds of survival to one in four and had 'repressed any sense that [she] was deluding herself' (French 1998: 35–6). After going through what French describes as a 'season in hell' involving years of pain, dread and severe illness, she reached 'a plateau of serenity' (French 1998: 237). At the time of writing an autobiographical account of her experience of survival (published in 1998), French stated that, although suffering from a number of symptoms related to the damage caused to her bodily systems by the intense radiotherapy and chemotherapy treatment she had received, she was feeling 'relatively well' and secure in the knowledge that the aches and pains she felt were not an indication of cancer (which had been cured).

There is also the possibility that new cures might be found for certain life-threatening conditions. For example, stem cell research and nanotechnology regenerative medicine research are heralding a new era of medicine, together with renewed hope for the remedial treatment (including permanent cures) of such conditions as spinal cord injuries, diabetes, Parkinson's disease and Alzheimer's disease. If a cure was found for the serious medical conditions from which people suffer (e.g. conditions that are incurable, progressive and will ultimately cause premature death) then people living with these conditions might, for example, not request assistance to die, as they are now doing.

Finally, an important example of how a misdiagnosis can misinform the choice of euthanasia as a 'treatment option' can be found in the much-publicised Australian case of Nancy Crick. Mrs Crick, a 69-year-old grandmother, died in a blaze of media publicity after having 'one last smoke, a sip of Bailey's Irish Cream liqueur and a drug overdose' (Griffith 2002: 4; see also Davies 2002; Hudson 2002: 1). Her death (witnessed by 21 relatives who were at her bedside) followed a campaign by pro-euthanasia supporters 'to allow Mrs Crick, who had suffered bowel cancer, the right to die at a time of her own choosing' (Franklin et al 2002: 1; see also Hudson 2002). The case took an unexpected turn after her death when a forensic pathology report following autopsy revealed no evidence of bowel cancer (Franklin et al 2002).

What is of concern about the euthanasia option (and what the above case highlights) is that once euthanasia is performed it cannot be reversed. Irreversible death in this instance is a catastrophic event that could otherwise have been prevented. The risk of error is thus unacceptable and overrides any other considerations which might favour euthanasia in a particular case.

Arguments from the risk of abuse

The possibility of euthanasia being abused is an argument frequently raised against euthanasia. Some people are especially concerned about legislation giving one group (notably doctors) the power to terminate life. Such power could be particularly problematic in contexts heavily influenced by coercive (negative) social and political processes. For those opposed to euthanasia, the risk of abuse is unacceptable and underscores the need to reject the moral permissibility (as well as the legalisation) of euthanasia.

An instructive example of how doctors might be seen as 'abusing' their lawful authority to perform euthanasia can be found in a 2013 Belgium case involving a 44-year-old female (born Nancy Verhelst) with a gender identity disorder who successfully sought euthanasia following botched sex-realignment surgery. Although the 44 year old (known as Nathan Verhelst after his sex-realignment treatment) was not terminally ill, he was deemed by his consulting doctors to be experiencing 'unbearable psychological suffering' and thus as meeting the criteria to be euthanised (Mortier 2013). The journalist reporting the case observed:

> *some doctors have discovered an easy way to dispose of some of their medical failures. They can kill them. Legally. […] Nancy Verhelst's doctors – her psychiatrist, urologist, gynaecologist, and cosmetic surgeon – had destroyed her life. But they weren't the ones who paid the price. She did.* (Mortier 2013: 1)

Arguments from non-necessity

Some contend that it is simply 'not necessary' to legislate or to support euthanasia. The reason commonly offered (particularly by those working in palliative care) is that the medical, nursing and allied health professions have been increasingly successful over the years in allowing patients to 'die with dignity'. Furthermore, euthanasia is not and should not be regarded as a substitute for the proper provision of palliative care services. Since patients who have access to proper palliative care are 'dying well' and are already having 'good deaths', why take the matter any further?

Arguments from discrimination

It is sometimes suggested that euthanasia entails blatant discrimination, notably by treating some lives as less worthy than others. Some disability advocates have been particularly troubled by the use of the criteria 'competent adults who are terminally ill or "severely disabled" [quotation marks original]' in physician-assisted suicide proposals and legislation (Scoccia 2010: 479). Others worry that, were euthanasia and assisted suicide to be legitimated, people with disabilities will be 'pressured to end their lives prematurely' (Wicks 2015: 3). Also of concern is that doctors may not have a clear understanding of the perspectives of people with disabilities relating to their health and care and may wrongly conclude that, in the case of treatment refusals (a common theme in disability care), euthanasia or assisted suicide is the only option (Tuffrey-Wijne et al 2018). By this view, just as any other act of discrimination is morally offensive, so too is euthanasia.

Arguments from irrational, mistaken or imprudent choice

It is sometimes argued that any person requesting euthanasia is not really exercising a rational or prudent choice, and that, for this reason, among others, an individual's request for euthanasia should not be taken seriously. One of the staunchest supporters of this view is the Vatican. In its 1980 *Declaration on euthanasia*, it states (1980: 7):

> *The pleas of gravely ill people who sometimes ask for death are not to be understood as implying a true desire for euthanasia; in fact it is almost always a case of an anguished plea for help and love.*

There is also the risk that a person's lawful representative might 'get it wrong'. Just as someone who is in unbearable and untreatable misery might make irrational or imprudent choices, so too might their proxies – who, even though well intended, might nevertheless be misguided in their beliefs and actions. For example, Professor Peter Singer, one of the world's most controversial philosophers and foremost advocates of euthanasia, has long argued that it is morally justifiable and even morally desirable (on utilitarian grounds) to kill severely disabled newborns and other 'non-persons' (e.g. children, adults and older people who, because of being brain injured or suffering from a severe organic brain disease such as end-stage Alzheimer's, are incapable of making rational and autonomous life choices) (Kuhse & Singer 1985; Singer 1993; Wikipedia 2018f). In 1999, however, it was reported that Professor Singer's beliefs about euthanasia and the grounds upon which euthanasia might be justified and/or morally required in certain cases were seriously challenged by a personal tragedy – notably, that of his mother becoming a 'non-person' (by his own definition) on account of developing advanced Alzheimer's disease (Churcher

1999). When asked whether his personal situation would cause him to abandon his beliefs, he is reported to have replied (Churcher 1999: 19):

> *I think this has made me see how the issues of someone with these kinds of problems are really very difficult. Perhaps it is more difficult than I thought before, because it is different when it's your mother.*

The question of whether a death request is necessarily the product of irrational or imprudent or mistaken choice, however, is likely to remain a matter of controversy (see also discussion on the ethics of suicide in Chapter 8).

'Slippery slope' argument

A core anti-euthanasia argument is the '*slippery slope*' contention. As in the case of the abortion debate, slippery slope arguments hold that, once the taking of human life is permitted under a given policy initiative, there will be a decline in society's moral standards and a slippery slope: it will not be long before the taking of life will be permitted under other policy initiatives. For example, if abortion is permitted today, infanticide will be permitted the next day, and euthanasia the next.

In the case of euthanasia, a slippery slope argument might be structured as follows: once euthanasia is allowed for consenting adults, eventually it will be permitted for unconsenting and non-consenting adults (e.g. those who are cognitively impaired, who have a catastrophic brain injury, who are believed to be permanently comatose), and then those who have not reached adulthood (e.g. infants and children). Likewise, once euthanasia is permitted for people with serious somatic life-threatening or life-ending illnesses, it will soon be permitted for people with less-serious and non-life-threatening or non-life-ending and non-somatic conditions. Then, once permitted for people who currently meet lawful criteria to be euthanised, eventually it will also be permitted for people who 'anticipate' meeting the criteria at some future point in time. Given this risk, euthanasia should never be justified.

There are many instructive examples of what might be construed as a slide down the slippery slope. Notable among these (and arguably among the first to receive public attention) is the 1991 Dutch case involving a psychiatrist who medically assisted the suicide of a female patient who was suffering emotionally but who was otherwise physically healthy; that is, she had no somatic illness (Klotzko 1995; Ogilvie & Potts 1994). Although deemed by her psychiatrist not to be suffering from a psychiatric illness, the patient was nevertheless regarded as being clinically depressed. The social history of this woman is as follows and worth quoting at length:

> *She was a 50-year-old social worker. She was also a painter in her spare time. She was divorced. She had been physically abused by her former husband for many years. She had two sons. One son, Peter, died by suicide in 1986, at the age of 20. She then underwent psychiatric treatment for a marriage crisis following his suicide. At the time, she strongly wished to commit suicide, but decided that her second son, Robbie, age 15, needed her as a mother.*
>
> *Her son, Robbie, died of cancer in 1991, at the age of 20. Before his death, she decided that she did not want to continue living after he died. She attempted suicide, but did not succeed. On July 13, 1991, she wrote to a social worker at the academic hospital where her second son died of cancer; she asked for a contact and for pills, so that she could kill herself. She had bought a cemetery plot for her sons, her former husband, and herself; her only wish was to die and lie between the two graves of her sons.* (Klotzko 1995: 240–1)

Subsequently, the patient wrote to Dr Boudewijn Chabot, a psychiatrist, requesting assistance to die. On 28 September 1991, Dr Boudewijn Chabot, after assessing the patient, provided her with a lethal dose of medication and remained with her while she swallowed the medication and died (Klotzko 1995: 239). He subsequently reported the death to the relevant authorities, following which he was prosecuted by the Supreme Court of the Netherlands. On 21 June 1994, in what has been described as a 'historic ruling', the Supreme Court of the Netherlands found Dr Chabot guilty, but declined to punish him. In reaching its verdict, the court rejected the contention that 'help in assistance with suicide to a patient where there is no physical suffering and who is not dying can never be justified' (Ogilvie & Potts 1994: 492). As Ogilvie and Potts report (p 492), the court:

> *explicitly accepted that euthanasia and assisted suicide might be justified for a patient with severe psychic suffering due to a depressive illness and in the absence of a physical disorder or terminal condition.*

Significantly, the court found that Chabot's guilt lay not in his providing a medically assisted death to his patient, but in his failure to obtain a second psychiatric opinion on the woman, and his failure to secure independent expert evidence that an 'emergency situation existed' – regarded as providing 'the normal mitigating defence in such cases' (Ogilvie & Potts 1994: 492).

Responses to the Chabot case have been mixed. Some have cited the case to underpin their sympathy for the view that (Ogilvie & Potts 1994: 493):

> *in severe and persistent depressive illness, when all appropriate physical treatments, including polypharmacy, electroconvulsive therapy, and psychosurgery, have apparently been exhausted, voluntary euthanasia may sometimes seem to be as justifiable an option as it does in intractable physical illness.*

Others, however, take the Chabot case as underscoring the fears of those advancing the slippery slope argument. As Ogilvie and Potts (1994: 493) point out, the Chabot case of '*psychiatric euthanasia*' has demonstrated that the 'slippery slope' exists. They conclude:

> *However well any legislation is hedged about with guidelines and protections against abuse, the slippery slope predicts an inevitable extension of those practices to other, more vulnerable, groups, such as those who are demented, mentally ill, chronically disabled, frail, dependent, and elderly – and perhaps even simply unhappy.*

Since the Chabot case, other examples have gradually emerged of the slippery slope leading to an 'inevitable extension' of euthanatic practices. For example, in the Netherlands, under its 2002 euthanasia laws, children of 12–18 years of age can legally request euthanasia; in addition, since 2005, the neonatal euthanasia of infants less than 1 year old has also been permitted under a policy known as 'The Groningen Protocol' (Brouwer et al 2018; Cuman & Gastmans 2017). There is now a move by several parent groups and Dutch paediatricians to extend the age criterion of *paediatric euthanasia* to include children who are between 1 and 12 years of age, arguing that the exclusion of this age group is unreasonable (Brouwer et al 2018).

Another example of 'a slide down the slippery slope' from adult euthanasia to child euthanasia can be found in the 2014 amendment of Belgian legislation making it 'the first country in the world to remove any age restrictions on euthanasia' paving the way for terminally ill children with a desire to end their lives to be euthanised (Cuman & Gastmans 2017; McDonald-Gibson 2014; Raus 2016; Samanta 2015). Belgium has also led the way in enabling *pre-emptive euthanasia* in cases of 'non-terminal conditions'. In 2013, for example, identical twins Mark and Eddy Verbessem were lawfully euthanised by their doctors. Born deaf, the 45-year-old brothers lived together and worked as cobblers. They learned, however, that they would soon go blind from glaucoma. Reported to be unable to bear the thought of 'never seeing one another again', the brothers successfully requested 'pre-emptive' euthanasia – euthanasia that pre-empted their actually developing the life-conditions they feared (Waterfield 2013).

The practice of pre-emptive euthanasia, which may also take the form of advance euthanasia directives, is not new. In the Netherlands, for example, advance euthanasia directives have long been permitted on grounds of a person's 'unbearable and hopeless suffering' (Hertogh 2009; Rurup et al 2006; van Delden 2004). In some cases, as in the Verbessem brothers case, the mere *anticipation* of suffering by a person together with his or her desire for death as a 'preemptive strike against the terrors of dying' has also been accepted as a circumstance under which euthanasia may be performed by a qualified medical practitioner (ten Have 2005: 163). 'Typical' cases put forward in debate about the feasibility of advance euthanasia directives have involved patients with dementia 'especially when they have become so demented that admittance to a nursing home is required' (van Delden 2004: 447; see also Johnstone 2013a).

Some argue that the evidence of 'good practices' sliding down the slippery slope is at best limited and that slippery slope arguments overall 'often make distinctly unhelpful contributions to debates over legalisation' (Lewis 2007: 205). This, however, is not entirely correct. A 2012 analysis by Canadian legal scholar Mary Shariff of the possible slippery slides in jurisdictions that have permissive assisted death laws has shown, for example, that there have been demonstrable shifts in the 'means, justification and logic' allowing euthanasia and assisted suicide to be made available to individuals. Shariff's comprehensive analysis shows that this shift encompasses allowing euthanasia / assisted deaths for those who:

- *have terminal or non-terminal conditions,*
- *have physical or non-physical illnesses,*
- *are conscious or unconscious,*
- *have competence or incompetence, or*
- *have reached or not reached adulthood.* (Shariff 2012: 147)

Arguably one of the most confronting slides down the slippery slope, however, has been the growing movement to allow people who are otherwise healthy but are simply 'tired of life' (also called 'life fatigue') to qualify for assisted deaths. For example, in an early article on the subject, Huxtable and Möller (2007) cite the Dutch case of Brongersma, an elderly man who was 'tired of life' and who had his suicide assisted by his general practitioner. Since this case was published there has been a burgeoning of literature on the subject arguing in favour of the extension of euthanasia laws to include 'life fatigue' as an eligibility criterion (see, for example, Bolt et al 2015; Florijn 2018; Miller 2016; van Wijngaarden et al 2015). As with the abortion debate, terminology is also emerging as an important issue. Of significance is the shift in using the term 'tired of life' to terms that might be regarded by some as less provocative – i.e. 'a sense that life is completed and no longer worth living' (see, for example, Florijn 2018; Miller 2016; van Wijngaarden et al 2015).

Closer to home, the Australian-based organisation *Exit International* (a self-described euthanasia advocacy organisation; see below) has been at the forefront of advocating the assisted deaths of 'healthy people' who have become tired of life ('life tired'). Its stance is dramatically depicted in the controversial iKandy Films documentary (directed by Janine Hosking and sold through Exit International) Mademoiselle and the doctor (2009). This documentary depicts the story of Lisette Nigot, a healthy 79-year-old woman who wanted to take her own life because she was 'tired of life'.

Another example of the slide down the slippery slope is the move to 'demedicalise' euthanasia, with its proponents calling for legislative reform that will allow non-physicians to provide the means of an assisted death for people with and *without* a medical diagnosis (Hagens et al 2017). Their advocacy for reform relates to three key areas, notably to remove legislative criteria mandating:

> *(1) the prerequisite of a medical condition in granting assistance in dying, (2) the role of the physician in distributing or administering the means to end life, and (3) the presence of the physician during the termination of life.* (Hagens et al 2017: 543)

Thus, whereas the compulsory involvement of physicians and a medical diagnosis were originally proposed (and have been promoted) as a 'rock solid' safety check in euthanasia legislation, it is now being framed as an unnecessary impediment to those not wishing to have physician assistance in dying and to those who do not have a medical diagnosis (Hagens et al 2017). A notable example of an organisation taking this position and which has already attracted media attention for its role in supporting people to achieve an assisted death without the direct involvement of medical practitioners is Exit International (https://exitinternational.net/). Founded in Australia in 1997, it now has affiliates in the UK, USA and the Netherlands.

Another challenge to the mandated involvement of physicians in assisted dying is the emerging role of nurse practitioners in this area. The most notable example of this can be found in Canada, where on 17 June 2016 royal assent was given to the *Medical Assistance in Dying (MAiD) Act* (Downie 2017; Lemmens et al 2018). Under the Act, medical assistance in dying is defined as:

(a) *the administering by a medical practitioner or nurse practitioner of a substance to a person, at their request, that causes their death; or*

(b) *the prescribing or providing by a medical practitioner or nurse practitioner of a substance to a person, at their request, so that they may self-administer the substance and in doing so cause their own death* (aide médicale à mourir). (MAiD 2016: Section 241.1).

The MAiD (2016) legislation is the first in the world that permits nurse practitioners to diagnose, obtain consent for, prescribe and administer assistance in dying (Stokes 2017). Nursing colleges and associations in Canada are reported as applauding the passage of the MAiD legislation. Given the new role of nurse practitioners in assisted dying it leaves open to question why the nomenclature of 'medical' assistance (versus nurse assistance) has been retained. It also leaves open the possibility of the pool of eligible healthcare professionals to provide assistance in dying being expanded to include others such as registered nurses and paramedics. This possibility is not far fetched considering recent legislative reforms in North Carolina apropos its *Restoring Proper Justice Act*. Under this Act the pool of eligible healthcare professionals to perform state executions of prisoners on death row has been expanded to include nurse practitioners, registered nurses and paramedics (Dodds 2017). Meanwhile, in the US state of New York, a proposed MAiD bill before the assembly is proposing to qualify nurse practitioners for involvement in medically assisted dying (Stokes 2017).

The doctrine of double effect

The *doctrine of double effect* is a Catholic doctrine developed by Catholic theologians that is appealed to when seeking to resolve the well-recognised dilemma posed by intolerable pain and the use of potentially lethal doses of narcotics as a means of suppressing pain. Although the Vatican prohibits euthanasia, it nevertheless permits the use of narcotics as a means of alleviating pain – and, furthermore, permits dosages that might suppress a patient's level of consciousness and even shorten a patient's life (Vatican 1980). There are, however, clearly defined conditions that must be met. First, there must be no other means of alleviating the patient's pain; in other words, potentially lethal doses of narcotics must never be prescribed except as a last resort. Second, the intention of using narcotics must be only to *alleviate pain*, and not to cause death. It is the second condition encompassing the intentionality of an act that finds its force in the doctrine of double effect.

The doctrine of double effect basically prescribes that it is always wrong to do a bad act for the sake of good consequences, but that it is sometimes permissible to do a good act even knowing it might have some bad consequences. To illustrate this doctrine, consider the case of a patient suffering intolerable and intractable pain. In this case, ending the patient's life would also result in ending the patient's intolerable and intractable pain. Whereas ending the patient's *pain* would be a 'good thing', ending the patient's *life* would not. Moreover, accepting the sanctity-of-life doctrine, deliberately ending an innocent patient's life would be a morally evil thing to do. Thus, in keeping with the doctrine: it would always be wrong to end an innocent patient's life (a bad act) in order to alleviate that patient's pain (a good consequence).

Given the 'good' of alleviating pain, however, giving the patient analgesia is morally permissible – even though this might have the foreseeable and unfortunate consequence of shortening the patient's life. This is permitted because, even though the act of narcotic administration is associated with the foreseen possibility of hastening death, ending the patient's life is *not the conscious intention behind the act*. In short, the decision and action of giving the narcotics was not done with 'murder in your heart'. To express the doctrine of double effect another way: it is always wrong to end patients' lives for the sake of alleviating their pain, but it is sometimes permissible to give potentially lethal doses of narcotics to alleviate pain, even though this might result in the patient's death – *as long as the patient's death is not the intended outcome*.

It is noteworthy that although primarily originating from Roman Catholic religious tradition, the doctrine of double effect has influenced secular legal reasoning in regard to end-of-life decision-making (McStay 2003: 53–6; Mendelson 1997: 112). One US legal commentator has even suggested that:

> *the double effect principle represents sound public policy to the extent that it allows physicians to provide adequate palliative care without engaging in clearly illegal conduct.* (McStay 2003: 54)

The doctrine of double effect has been the subject of much philosophical criticism, most notably on account of its over-reliance on what is called the foreseeability/intentionality distinction and the hypocritical manoeuvres used by some to 'hide, rather than reveal, their true intentions' (Watt 2017: 15). This distinction holds roughly that foreseeing that a bad consequence will occur as a result of a given act is not the same thing as intending that bad consequence. For example, foreseeing that a patient will die as a result of being given large doses of narcotics (or other medical regimen such as that used in palliative sedation) is not the same thing as intending to end that patient's life; therefore the person who administers the narcotic is not morally culpable.

Critics reject this, however, and argue that the distinction drawn here is misleading. They contend that foreseeing a bad consequence of an action is exactly the same as intending it, since the agent knows that a bad consequence is pending but deliberately refrains from preventing it. At the very least, intentions are relevant to determining the moral permissibility and impermissibility of given acts, just as they are to determining culpability in criminal law (Nelkin & Rickless 2016). There is also concern that the recent 'stretching' of double-effect reasoning in end-of-life cases 'requires ethical contortions about distinguishing intent and about treating death as a side effect' and, in so doing, moves a step closer to providing a 'shield to hide what is in effect assisted dying' (Duckett 2018: 36).

Palliative sedation

The issue of *palliative sedation* (PS) is believed to date back to the 1990s, when discussion first emerged in the scholarly literature about the practice of 'terminally sedating' dying patients in palliative care (Tännsjö 2004a, 2004b). The practice became the subject of debate for two reasons: first, because the methods in palliative care to control symptoms had improved substantially and thus it was no longer necessary to comatose patients with sedation in order to treat their refractory symptoms, and second, the system of 'terminal sedation' was being construed as 'euthanasia in disguise' or 'slow euthanasia', which many regarded as impermissible (Tännsjö 2004b: xiii). Some still hold the view that PS is merely 'slow euthanasia' and 'euthanasia in disguise' owing in no small way to the use of double-effect reasoning to justify its moral permissibility (discussed above) (Smith 2015).

The grounds on which palliative sedation is generally distinguished from euthanasia include:

> *(1) The intent of the intervention is to provide symptom relief; (2) the intervention is proportionate to the symptoms, its severity and the prevailing goals of care; (3) finally and most importantly, the death of the patient is not a criterion for the success of treatment.* (de Graeff & Dean 2007: 77)

The nature of PS and the clinical as well as philosophical bases on which it can be distinguished from euthanasia have been more comprehensively clarified since the 1990s and made the subject of guidelines, frameworks and regulations developed by various medical and palliative care associations around the world (for a detailed analysis of the distinction between PS and euthanasia as held by the world's various medical and palliative care associations, see Shariff & Gingerich (2018) and also: American

Medical Association 2008; Australian and New Zealand Society of Palliative Medicine (ANZSPM) 2017a, 2017b; Cherny et al 2009; Dean et al 2012; Royal Dutch Medical Association 2009).

Definition, purpose and intention of palliative sedation

Palliative sedation (a term that has superseded the less-appropriate and misleading term 'terminal sedation') has been variously defined as 'the monitored use of medications to reduce consciousness in order to relieve otherwise intractable suffering at the end of life in a manner ethically acceptable to patients, their families and healthcare providers' (Abarshi et al 2017: 223). Although there is no international consensus on the definition of PS, there is general agreement that it fundamentally involves:

> *(1) the use of (a) pharmacological agent(s) to reduce consciousness; (2) reserved for treatment of intolerable and refractory symptoms; and (3) only considered in a patient who has been diagnosed with an advanced progressive illness.* (Dean et al 2012: 870)

A 'refractory symptom', in turn, has been defined as 'a symptom that cannot be adequately controlled despite aggressive efforts to identify a tolerable therapy that does not compromise consciousness' (Cherny & Portenoy 1994 – cited in Schildmann et al 2015: 734). Palliative sedation is considered to be a 'last-resort' treatment in cases involving patients with refractory symptoms such as pain, dyspnoea, nausea and vomiting, delirium and terminal restlessness (ANZSPM 2017a; De Vries & Plaskota 2017; Gurschick et al 2015).

Although the 'prevalence, indications, monitoring, duration and choice of drugs' in PS (Maltoni et al 2013: 360), as well as the standards and guidelines for the practice and monitoring of PS, vary across and within different jurisdictions (see Abarshi et al 2017; Claessens et al 2008; Dean et al 2012; Maltoni et al 2013; Schildmann & Schildmann 2014; Schildmann et al 2015, 2018), it is nonetheless regarded as an 'important therapeutic intervention' (Bruera 2012: 1258) and an 'integral part of a medical palliative care approach' (Maltoni et al 2013: 360). Moreover, despite the variations in PS guidelines and the controversies these sometimes invite, there is nonetheless a consensus on the key purpose and intention of PS – namely: *to relieve refractory symptoms through reducing consciousness, not to hasten death* (Claessens et al 2008; de Graeff & Dean 2007; Dean et al 2012). As noted above, it is this *intention* (i.e. to alleviate the patient's refractory symptoms) that is taken as distinguishing PS from an act of *euthanasia* – the intention of which *is not to alleviate a patient's refractory symptoms but rather to end the patient's life*. Evidence in support of this conclusion can be found in Shariff and Gingerich's (2018) comprehensive analysis of termination-of-life (assisted death) laws, court determinations involving termination-of-life cases, and the position statements and guidelines of medical and palliative care associations from around the world. It concludes:

> *The preponderance of evidence reveals a critical difference between the practices of palliative care and termination of life [euthanasia]: between care that is directed toward a pain-free life, however long it may continue, and care directed toward the ending of pain and suffering through death (p 291).*

The administration of PS is proportional and individually tailored (known as 'proportionate palliative sedation' or PPS). For these reasons, palliative sedation can be highly variable in terms of 'depth of sedation, continuity, drug used, speed of instauration', with its most intense form being practised as 'deep continuous sedation' (DCS) (Imai et al 2018; Maltoni et al 2014). In keeping with this approach, three distinguishable levels of sedation may result:

- *Mild (somnolence): the patient is awake, but the level of consciousness is lowered.*
- *Intermediate (stupor): the patient is asleep but can be woken to communicate briefly.*
- *Deep (coma): the patient is unconscious and unresponsive.* (de Graeff & Dean 2007: 73–4)

In either case, a titrated regimen of drugs is used. Although regimens vary, the drug midazolam is considered the 'front-line choice' for initiating PS – primarily because 'it is easy to titrate, has rapid onset and offset (the latter being very important in cases of intermittent sedation), can be combined with other drugs used in palliative care, and has an antidote' (Claessens et al 2008: 320; see also Schildmann et al 2015, 2018). Other 'preferred drugs' (following the use of midazolam) are benzodiazepines, neuroleptics or sedating antipsychotics (Claessens et al 2008; de Graeff & Dean 2007; Dean et al 2012; Maltoni et al 2013). Significantly opioids tend not to be used for sedation purposes since, although these may cause drowsiness, they do not lead to a loss of consciousness (Claessens et al 2008: 330; see also Schildmann et al 2015, 2018).

When receiving PS, patients require close monitoring. In particular, clinical vigilance is required to ascertain whether the patient has, in fact, been relieved of suffering, that the desired depth of sedation and level of consciousness have been achieved, and whether the patient is suffering from any adverse side effects of the drugs administered (Dean et al 2012; Maltoni et al 2013). In addition, the emotional, spiritual and psychological state of family members and staff also need to be monitored and any distress noted, and managed appropriately (Bruinsma et al 2012; Dean et al 2012).

Of moral significance to practitioners is that, when correctly performed, PS – including deep continuous sedation – does not have a detrimental effect on survival rates; that is, it does not shorten life (Barathi & Chandra 2013; Claessens et al 2008; Maltoni et al 2012, 2013; Prado et al 2018). One study found that PS not only had no negative impact on the patients receiving it, but also that the patients actually survived longer than those who did not receive it (Prado et al 2018). The absence of its impact on survival rates is taken by some as refuting 'conceptual analyses that tend to equate palliative sedation with euthanasia' (Maltoni et al 2014) – that is, terminating life (Shariff & Gingerich 2018).

As palliative sedation neither negates the need for nor interrupts the administration of clinically assisted hydration, ethical issues associated with withholding or withdrawing clinically assisted nutrition or hydration (CANH, discussed below) are also sidestepped and are no more pressing than they are in non-sedated patient groups (Maltoni et al 2014). Moreover, there is a consensus that, as decisions to withhold or withdraw CANH from a patient receiving palliative sedation could have a life-limiting effect, these ought to be made *independently* of any decisions to administer palliative sedation (Claessens et al 2008; de Graeff & Dean 2007). These considerations have led some to conclude that, as palliative sedation does not shorten life (either actively through the provision of sedating drugs or passively through the unwarranted withdrawal of CANH), there is no ethical basis for restricting its use as a bona fide medical regimen (Berger 2010).

Palliative sedation in existential suffering

In recognition that people can also suffer refractory 'existential pain' (defined broadly as emotional or spiritual suffering) at the end of life, some writers have argued that palliative sedation should also be made available in such patients, on the basis that accords equal importance to the 'psychosocial and spiritual aspects of suffering' as that given to its physiological aspect (Sadler 2012: 195). The possible use of palliative sedation to treat existential suffering (e.g. refractory depression, death anxiety) is, however, highly controversial (Maltoni et al 2014; Rodrigues et al 2018; Sadler 2012). Underpinning this controversy is the problem that 'existential suffering' is not well defined, is based on philosophical theorisation rather than evidence and, related to these things, is vulnerable to being misdiagnosed and wrongly treated (Rodrigues et al 2018; Sadler 2012). Moreover, being more akin to the controversial practice of deep sleep therapy (DST) (Wikipedia 2018g), its justification as a therapeutic measure remains unfounded.

Nurses' attitudes and experiences

It is being increasingly recognised and demonstrated that nurses play an active and crucial role in the communication, administration and monitoring of palliative sedation (Abarshi et al 2014; Arevalo et al 2013; Claessens et al 2008; De Vries & Plaskota 2017; Engström et al 2007; Inghelbrecht et al 2011; Maltoni et al 2014). Specifically, as Inghelbrecht and colleagues (2011) point out:

Nurses usually remain at the bedside, administer drugs, look after the patient's comfort, monitor possible symptoms, and answer the questions and concerns of relatives. (Inghelbrecht et al 2011: 871)

In a systematic review of the literature on nurses' attitudes and practice of palliative sedation it was found that nurses tended to have a 'positive but cautious' attitude to the practice. Further, although nurses were generally willing to administer palliative sedation on the basis of its 'anticipated benefit in controlling unbearable symptoms and suffering', most nonetheless regarded it as a 'last resort' measure for the relief of refractory symptoms only — that is, not to hasten death (Abarshi et al 2014: 923). Some studies have found, however, that nurses are sometimes troubled emotionally by the practice of palliative sedation on account of their perceptions that its administration is tantamount (at least partially) to 'hastening death' (Arevalo et al 2013; Inghelbrecht et al 2011; Raus et al 2014; Sadler 2012; Woods 2004). The extent to which nurses have found the practice emotionally burdensome, however, has depended on a range of variables including 'their level of education, expertise and the roles they played per setting' (Abarshi et al 2014: 915) as well as the degree of emotional and causal 'closeness' or 'disengagement' they have felt in terms of being morally responsible for both the practice and outcomes of the sedation (Raus et al 2014).

Like others working in palliative care, some nurses have resolved their qualms about palliative sedation by appealing to the doctrine of double effect (discussed above), which they have found helpful in terms of justifying the distinction between 'palliative sedation' and 'euthanasia'. Others, however, have regarded appeals to the doctrine as problematic and unsustainable on account of the fact that the doctrine itself is problematic (i.e. as per the reasons discussed above). It is contended that once the nature, intention, practice and outcomes of palliative sedation are fully understood, it can be seen for what it is: a legitimate palliative care option that is morally defensible. Accordingly nurses need not feel emotionally burdened by its practice or their role in assisting with it (Gallagher & Wainwright 2007; Woods 2004).

Withholding or withdrawing clinically assisted nutrition and hydration

When seriously ill and/or nearing the end of their lives, many patients reach a point where they cannot take food and fluids 'naturally' — that is, voluntarily by mouth, with or without assistance, in order to satisfy their hunger and thirst. Because of this, their intake of food and fluids reduces. Reasons for this situation are varied but may include one or more of the following:

physical obstruction, anorexia/cachexia syndrome, generalised weakness, bowel obstruction, nausea, decreased levels of consciousness, loss of desire to drink or no specific cause may be identified. (Good et al 2014: 2)

When patients are unable or unwilling to take food and fluids, clinicians and proxies may be faced with the difficult decision of whether to withhold or provide the patient with *clinically assisted nutrition and hydration* (referred to by the acronym CANH). In the case of patients who voluntarily stop eating and drinking (referred to by the acronym VSED), decision-making in clinical contexts may be particularly fraught clinically, ethically and legally. This is because, theoretically, VSED (regarded as distinct from illness-associated anorexia–cachexia) does not require the involvement of a medical practitioner (Quill et al 2018a, 2018b; Wax et al 2018). With VSED a patient voluntarily *chooses* not to eat or drink even though physically able to do so (Mueller et al 2018; Rodriguez-Prat et al 2018; Wax et al 2018).

CANH may be delivered by several methods:

- *intravenous fluids* (noting that, although sufficient to sustain hydration, this route cannot deliver substantial nutrition)
- *parenteral nutrition* (the provision of a nutritional formula though a vein — e.g. central venous nutrition (CVN); types include total parenteral nutrition (TPN) and peripheral parenteral nutrition (PPN))
- *hypodermoclysis* (the subcutaneous infusion of fluids for minimal hydration purposes only)

- *nasogastric tubes* (for temporary feeding)
- *percutaneous endoscopic gastrostomy* (PEG) tubes (for long-term feeding)
- *jejunostomy tubes* (less often used for long-term feeding) (Ganzini 2006; Kozeniecki et al 2017).

CANH may be provided for two reasons: first, *to prolong life* (or at least to prevent the patient from experiencing a premature death) and, second, *to improve quality of life* – that is, alleviating the symptoms associated with the patient's declining condition (Cacciulanza et al 2018; Ganzini 2006; Good et al 2014; Hui et al 2015; Malia & Bennett 2011). There invariably comes a point, however, where the burdens of CANH outweigh the benefits, making it necessary for a decision to be made to either withdraw or withhold CANH as a treatment option. Even so, because of the strong emotional and cultural meanings attached to the intake of food and fluid as a 'basic' element of human comfort and survival, such decisions can be a source of emotional distress for families and care providers (Baillie et al 2018; del Río et al 2012). They can also invite moral controversy and intervention by the courts (English & Sheather 2017; Geppert et al 2010; Rady & Verheijde 2014; Richards & Coggon 2018; Willmott & White 2017). Right-to-life groups, for example, often equate the withdrawal of CANH with 'slow euthanasia' (Heuberger 2010) and may sloganeer the removal of a PEG tube as being tantamount to 'murder' (Ganzini 2006: 137).

Despite over three decades of established agreement about the 'appropriate use' of CANH, the issue of withholding or withdrawing nutrition and hydration from patients at the end stage of life remains highly contentious. During the early years of debate, there were two key points of view at issue:

1. hydration and nutrition should be administered ('artificially' or with clinical assistance if necessary) to patients *regardless of the terminal phase of their illness* (Craig 1994, 1996)
2. there should be a gradual reduction and eventual cessation or non-initiation of treatment as the patient's condition deteriorates (Ashby & Stoffell 1991, 1995).

Those who argued that hydration and nutrition should continue to be provided – even at the end stage of life – contended that if fluids were to be withheld or withdrawn from patients then the patients would inevitably enter into a state of dehydration, which, in turn, would result in 'circulatory collapse, renal failure, anuria and death' (Craig 1994: 140). In short, without hydration and nutrition, patients who are heavily sedated would die – whatever the underlying pathology (Craig 1994: 140). Furthermore, dehydration could lead to severe complications that may unacceptably alter the patient's quality of life while they are dying; such complications were identified to include: 'increased asthenia, nausea, postural hypotension, fever with no underlying infectious process, increased risk of bed sores, and constipation' as well as the 'accumulation of opioid metabolites, grand-mal seizures, and hyperalgesia' (Steiner 1998: 8, 12).

Another complication believed to be associated with dehydration was that of patients suffering from thirst and hunger during the terminal phase of their illness. On this, Craig argued (1994: 142):

> *It is widely assumed that a terminally ill patient is not troubled by hunger or thirst but this is difficult to substantiate as few people return from the grave to complain.*

Finally, some worried that doctors might 'get it wrong' (i.e. make diagnostic errors) and accordingly patients might not only die 'poorly', but needlessly. On this point Craig argued (1994: 140):

> *Diagnostic errors can also occur. A reversible psychosis or confusional state can be mistaken for terminal delirium, aspiration pneumonia for tracheal obstruction, obstruction [of the bowel] due to faecal impaction for something more sinister, and so on. The only way to ensure that life will not be shortened is to maintain hydration during sedation in all cases whereby inability to eat and drink is a direct consequence of sedation, unless the relatives request no further intervention, or the patient has made his/her wishes known to this effect.*

Despite – or perhaps because of – the growing body of research in recent years, these issues remain unresolved. For example, some continue to argue that failure to provide assisted hydration during the last days of life will give rise to a range of common complications such as: thirst, hunger, discomfort, agitation, delirium, urinary tract infections, kidney failure, cardiovascular collapse, and the diminished efficacy of drugs such as analgesics and sedatives otherwise administered to treat symptoms of distress (Rady & Verheijde 2014). In the case of the latter, distress can manifest as various spontaneous and reflex movements such as roving eye movements, chewing, teeth-grinding, tongue-pumping, groaning, facial grimaces, and crying, which maybe become more pronounced as the patient's condition deteriorates (Royal College of Physicians 2013: 5).

Others, however, argue to the contrary, reminding clinicians of the risk associated with certain methods of CANH – for example, in the case of enteral nutrition, this can include 'gastrointestinal issues (e.g. constipation, diarrhea, bloating, nausea, vomiting), pulmonary aspiration with or without pneumonia, [negative] drug–nutrient interactions, and clogged or dislodged tubes' (Kozeniecki et al 2017). One study has suggested that the use of PEG tubes in older populations can also lead to higher mortality rates, particularly in those with co-morbidities (Tabuenca et al 2018).

These views concur with earlier research which has shown that clinically assisted hydration (particularly intravenous infusions) can lead to a range of associated medical conditions and complications including: vital organ failure from fluid overload (this can lead to such conditions as pulmonary and cerebral oedema and their associated complications); infection and bacteraemia from catheter and cannulation sites; arterial perforation, thrombosis, cardiac arrhythmias, cardiopulmonary arrest and pneumothorax during/following insertion of central venous lines; and pulmonary emboli (Steiner 1998). Intriguingly, there is some suggestion that the 'risks' of dehydration during the actual death process may in fact be beneficial, with research suggesting that, due to their respective 'sedative properties', dehydration and ketosis are in effect mechanisms that help protect people against the 'potentially painful symptoms of dying' (Kozeniecki et al 2017: 263).

Although tools are being developed enabling the conduct of randomised feasibility trials of CAHN during the last days of life (Davies et al 2018), there remains a lack of high-quality studies examining the symptom benefits and/or adverse effects of CANH – including its impact on improving either the length or quality of life of those who are in the end stages of their lives (Good et al 2014; Hui et al 2015; Royal College of Physicians 2013). What evidence is available is regarded as being at best 'inconclusive' (Forbat et al 2017; Good et al 2014; Raijmakers et al 2011a, 2011b). Because of the lack of high-quality studies there is a related paucity of evidence-based guidelines to inform and guide CANH practices, particularly regarding the mode and quantity of hydration that should be administered during the last days of life (Forbat et al 2017). Even so, some still assert that the advantages of clinically assisted hydration, at least, outweigh the disadvantages in terms of its ease of application, low economic costs and fewer complications (e.g. infection) (Caccialanza et al 2018).

Disputes aside, CANH remains a substantial part of medical and nursing care. There is also some suggestion that the controversies over decisions about CANH may 'have less to do with ambiguous data, and more to do with differing judgments about the ethics of providing or withholding nutrition [and hydration] from patients with advanced illness or severe cognitive deficits' (Wolenberg et al 2013: 1052) and the point at which a decision ought to be made (i.e. when death is imminent). Whether this is so, only time will tell.

Position statements and the nursing profession

As the discussion thus far has shown, there are strongly warranted arguments both for and against the moral permissibility of abortion and euthanasia. These arguments range from *liberal* (always permitted), through *moderate* (sometimes permitted), to *conservative* (never permitted) positions – each of which is based on reasoned arguments. Despite this continuum of views, the nursing profession has nonetheless been pressured to take a definitive stance – often on the basis of public opinion – even though such a stance might not be able to be taken.

The issues of abortion and euthanasia are of significance to members of the nursing profession since each potentially involves the provision of nursing care. Whether professional nursing organisations *should* take a definitive stance on these issues is another matter, however – notwithstanding that even highly credentialled moral philosophers continue to disagree on the moral permissibility and impermissibility of these procedures. Possible options that are open to nursing organisations are to take either a partisan (clear for-or-against) stance or a non-partisan (neutral) stance.

Taking a partisan stance

It might be argued that, as a socially relevant profession, nurses must take a definitive stance favouring the moral permissibility and legalisation of abortion and euthanasia respectively – not least because public opinion has been shown to favour their legitimation as a matter of public policy. As discussed in Chapter 2 of this book, however, ethical issues are not matters to be resolved by appeals to public opinion alone. There must also be sound moral reasoning justifying any stance that is taken. Moreover, there are risks in taking a definitive stance. First, taking a definitive stance either way carries the risk of alienating and incurring the mistrust of constituents (e.g. members of the nursing profession, the diverse patient groups for whose care they share responsibility, and allied health workers among them) who hold counter-values and beliefs to those espoused. Second, taking a definitive stance risks nursing organisations being wrongly aligned with radical lobby groups whose extreme views and tactics are unconscionably divisive. If nurses were seen to be aligned with such groups, this too could risk the alienation and mistrust of constituents holding divergent views. Finally, taking a definitive stance risks eroding and undermining the foundational purpose of nursing organisations themselves, which have principally been formed to *develop and advance the profession of nursing* and its capacity to provide excellent nursing care across the life span. In short, it is not the *raison d'être* of professional nursing organisations to take a definitive stance on the issues either way; nor is it necessary. Attempts to coopt the nursing profession into taking a definitive stance on the issues at stake should be seen for what they are: political stunts aimed at dragging a *non-partisan* party into an unwanted dispute in order to give material advantage to a *partisan* party (Johnstone 2012c).

Taking a non-partisan (neutral) stance[5]

Another option open to the nursing profession is to take a non-partisan or *neutral stance* on these issues, akin to that generally associated with political or state neutrality (Johnstone 2012c). Underpinning the idea of political neutrality are values such as *equality* (encompassing the principles of egalitarian justice and equal respect), *individual autonomy* and *tolerance* (Laycock 1990; MacLeod 2008; Raes 1995; Sunstein 1992). Over the past two decades, these principles have been robustly challenged and tested in the context of political debate on same-sex marriage, abortion, pornography and surrogacy – each of which raises contentious issues about sexuality, morality, privacy, the nature and form of family, pluralism, autonomy, individual freedom, self-expression and choice (Wax 2007).

The principle of political or state neutrality has also been considered extensively in discourse on traditional peace operations thinking. Neutrality in this field has conventionally consisted in the 'observance of strict and honest impartiality, so as not to afford advantage in the war to either party' ('Lectric Law Library 2011). Although seemingly motivated by moral reasons, political neutrality largely evolved to 'allow states wishing to remain aloof from conflicts the freedom to carry out their policies and their nationals the freedom to trade' (Donald 2003: 418).

Arguably one of the most fruitful areas in which the notion of neutrality has been considered is the field of religious studies. In this context, neutrality has been defined in terms of an entity standing in relation to 'two or more parties which are themselves in tension, in such a way that the respective interests of those parties are not thereby materially affected' (Donovan 1990: 103). Donovan suggests that, by defining neutrality in these terms, it can be seen to be 'a relational concept, presupposing a particular kind of context' (p 103). This presupposition is crucial since neutrality cannot be meaningfully understood unless 'read' from within a particular kind of context. One reason for this is that *context* sets the normative baseline from which assessments of neutrality and partisanship can be measured (Sunstein 1992).

Donovan (1990) goes on to contend that, in highly value-laden fields like religious studies, neutrality may be pursued in three distinguishable modes: (1) observer-neutrality, (2) participant-neutrality, and (3) role-neutrality. The first of these, *observer-neutrality*, assumes that the observer stands detached on the sideline of a situation and serves as an onlooker only. As such, the observer refrains from any involvement in and contributes nothing to the situation at hand, other than making an 'accurate record of the facts' (p 104). Since onlooker observations are always interpreted subjectively, are profoundly influenced by external factors, often without the observer even being aware, and can be influenced by the mere presence of the observer ('the mere presence of an onlooker, however neutral his/her intention, may itself alter or distort the facts'), Donovan concludes that this stance exists as an *ideal* only and in reality is unrealisable (p 104).

The second form, *participant-neutrality*, seeks to overcome the limitations of observer neutrality 'by taking greater account of the complexities of actual situations' (Donovan 1990: 104). Donovan explains that, unlike the neutral *observer*, the neutral *participant* seeks to 'balance and adjust his/her participation in such a way as to avoid any material alteration of the balance of interests between the positions in question' (p 104). In reality, however, achieving such a balance may be extremely difficult and thus may be unsuitable for adoption as a methodological principle in value-laden disciplines. As Donovan (p 105) goes on to explain:

> *What may seem like impartiality or even-handedness from the participant's point of view may not have anything like a neutral effect for the parties themselves, given their different relative strengths, needs or interests.*

The third and final form, *role-neutrality*, which Donovan (1990: 106) contends is probably the 'paradigm case of neutrality in human affairs', refers to a special kind of participation that is clearly defined within a structure of rules and procedures (e.g. those of a committee, or law court). In this context, the contribution a role holder is expected to make is clearly defined by the rules and procedures governing the role. The role holder is obliged to follow these rules and procedures in the fulfilment of their role, which 'constitute the criteria as to their success or failure' (p 106). Donovan goes on to suggest that there are also three 'core internal standards' that help assure role-neutrality (p 106); these are: (1) the use of non-prejudicial language (e.g. avoiding prejudicial overtones, being sensitive to bias in terms and nomenclature used in the field), (2) suspension of belief and disbelief (also termed 'bracketing') so that full attention can be given to the matters under investigation without being side-tracked by the contentious and the dubious, and (3) attending to professional neutrality and personal bias (e.g. declaring one's vested interests and frankly acknowledging one's biases; this includes acknowledging the difficulties of both identifying and dealing with unconscious biases that may also affect a scholar's thoughts and sensitivities).

Despite the inherent difficulties of formulating a coherent theory and practice of neutrality, Donovan (1990) nonetheless concludes that not only is a neutral stance possible (at least in the form of role-neutrality), but it also is of fundamental importance both as a scholarly virtue and as a methodological prerequisite.

The above accounts of neutrality are germane to this discussion and stand to offer important insights into the nature, practice and possible implications of studied neutrality in the context of demands to formulate nursing organisation position statements on controversial ethical issues such as abortion and euthanasia. As has been shown, studied neutrality shares many features with (and is analogous to) political neutrality in that its purpose is to foster a culture of respect and to ensure that a non-partisan party in a dispute (in this case a professional nursing organisation) does not act in ways that give material advantage to opposing partisan camps.

In summary, studied neutrality is analogous to political neutrality. Its intended goals are to foster a respectful culture among people of diverse views and to guide action that does not afford material advantage to a partisan group on a given issue. Studied neutrality should not, however, be adopted as an end in itself. As Donovan reminds us, there are many reasons why neutrality is worth pursuing, including:

> *It helps free the subject from factional concerns or pressures. It ensures the widest possible range of relevant data, allowing world-wide comparisons and generalizations. It permits the reconsideration of established positions, the adoption of fresh points of view, the investigation of neglected or suppressed topics.* (Donovan 1990: 114).

Irrespective of the interest group pressure that has been placed on professional nursing organisations to take a definitive as opposed to a neutral stance on the issues in question, they and their memberships are entitled to resist such pressure. Whatever mitigating strategies are ultimately developed and operationalised, one thing is clear: professional nursing organisations have a stringent twofold role-neutral responsibility to the public. The first of these is to clearly define, advocate and assure the accessibility and sustainability of nursing care for all those who need it. The second responsibility is to maintain the integrity of and uphold the stated philosophy, principles and goals of nursing care and not get side-tracked by, or be dragged into, the warfare between other political interest groups.

As for those who have partisan interests in the abortion and euthanasia debates, they have a responsibility to bracket their interests and openly declare their personal biases and prejudices in public debate on the matter. This is not to silence dissent, or to suppress unwanted points of view. Rather, it is to ensure that a high degree of emotional and intellectual honesty is brought to the debate and that the decisions which are ultimately made are not an abdication of the public's interest in receiving excellent care across the life span.

The need for a systematic response

To date, there have been no universally agreed nursing positions on the ethics of either abortion or euthanasia. Different nursing organisations in different countries hold distinct and sometimes opposing views on these matters, and some have no published views on these matters at all. It is not surprising that there exists a diversity of moral opinion and viewpoints among members of the nursing profession about the 'rightness' and 'wrongness' of abortion and euthanasia. People generally hold differing views on these and related issues, and there is no reason why nurses should be any exception in this regard.

Coming to terms with the complex questions raised by the abortion and euthanasia debate requires a systematic response by both individual nurses and the broader nursing profession. Specifically, it requires nurses to gain knowledge and understanding of the profound ethical, legal, cultural, clinical and political dimensions of abortion and euthanasia, and the influence that these dimensions have on the profession and practice of nursing. Equally important, it requires peer support and understanding among nurses (especially those who hold conscientious objections to the procedures (Chavkin et al 2013)) and a recognition that these issues are not – and never have been – simple or clear-cut (Johnstone 2013a). In light of these considerations, if the profession is to take a formal position on these issues then, in order to be meaningful to members of the nursing profession, it must minimally reflect that each issue is morally controversial and politically divisive, that the diversity of opinion on these matters is likely to remain and unlikely to be resolved to everyone's satisfaction, and that nurses are likely to encounter this diversity of opinion during the course of their work. Further, any formal position taken must also remind nurses that they have a responsibility to ensure that they are reliably informed about the ethical, legal, cultural, political and clinical dimensions and implications of abortion and euthanasia procedures.

'The quandary of uncertainty' – one nurse's story

A few years ago I was participating in a panel discussion on euthanasia and assisted suicide which had been scheduled during a 1-day seminar on the topic. During the panel discussion (in which a number of distinguished guests participated) I noticed a young woman (a nurse) crying silently in the audience. Concerned about this young woman's obvious distress, I approached her during the morning tea break to ask if she wished to discuss with me what was troubling her. This she agreed to do. Upon hearing her story, I asked whether she would be willing to share her situation with the rest of the seminar participants once the proceedings recommenced after the morning tea break. This she also agreed to do. When the proceedings of the seminar recommenced, I had the opportunity to call on the young woman to share her feelings about the topic under discussion. She bravely faced her audience and related the following:

> *I am sitting here listening to you all. And I am so envious because you all seem to be so sure about where you stand on the [euthanasia] issue. You are either for or against it. But I do not have the benefit of such certainty. I simply do not know where I stand and this makes me feel very upset. You see, it is like this: I am a 'good Catholic girl', with a good Catholic education. My church tells me 'euthanasia is wrong' and that I must not support it. But then, I am also a nurse. I believe I am a good nurse and I believe in nursing. And my profession tells me I must support patients' rights – I must be an advocate for my patients' rights. And then there are my patients. Sometimes my patients want to die and ask for assistance to die. And I want to do what is right by them. And then there is me, the human being, torn between what my church tells me I should do, what my profession tells me I should do, and what my patients want me to do. I just feel so torn, because I really feel so uncertain about what is the right thing to do. I just don't know. I just don't know which side of the fence I should be on. And I feel that somehow maybe I am stupid or deficient because of this – especially when I listen to all of you here being so sure about the positions you are holding.*

With this courageous and frank admission came other admissions from other nurses in the audience; significantly, and contrary to superficial appearances, most of the nurses attending the seminar felt the way this nurse did, but had been unable to say so publicly. We then spent some time exploring the permissibility of feeling 'uncertain' about new and previously unexplored ethical issues, of taking the time necessary to consider other points of view and to explore possible answers to the difficult questions raised, and to ultimately reach a position on the issues identified that the person in question could 'live with'.

Some time later the nurse in question contacted me. She had reasoned the issue through and had reached a position about which she felt confident at both a personal and a professional level. What had helped her most in reaching this position was peer support, and the 'permission' her peers had given her to take the time she needed to 'think through' the issues at hand. She also particularly valued the opportunity the seminar had provided in regard to exposing her not just to the issues raised but also to the many different points of view expressed in response to them. Most important of all, though, she valued being able to share her story, and in this sharing to 'make visible' a problem that she was soon able to discover was not hers alone.

Conclusion

Nurses are not immune from the politics of either abortion or euthanasia. They also have an obvious stake in the outcomes of how these issues are treated at a political and public policy level. Accordingly they need to be more discerning than perhaps they have been in the past, be more cautious of public opinion polling, and advocate a level of intellectual honesty, transparency and public accountability in the debates on both of these issues that up until now has often been missing. This includes being able to recognise and resist media manipulation, which has the capacity to entice non-partisan bystanders into taking a partisan stance.

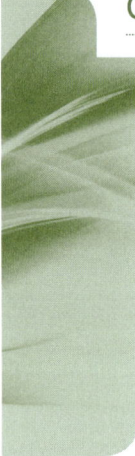

Case scenario 1

On 10 October 2008, following a highly charged emotional debate and historic vote in State Parliament, abortion was decriminalised in the Australian State of Victoria. For many observers, this reform was long overdue and simply brought the law into line with common practice in Victoria. It also meant that women who had abortions and the doctors who performed them no longer risked criminal prosecution, which if successful could carry a penalty of up to 10 years in jail. Others, however, were frankly dismayed by the reform, with some reportedly accusing those who supported the legislative reform as 'having blood on their hands' and being 'a disgrace to humanity', and warning 'there will be retribution' (Austin & Rood 2008: 4). Religious elites meanwhile reportedly threatened hospital closures, arguing controversially that, if passed, the new abortion laws would force doctors and nurses who were conscientiously opposed to abortion to 'break the law' (Zwartz 2008: 1). One Bishop went further and reportedly argued that 'nurses are in a particularly vulnerable position, since many would be under a duty to assist in an abortion if a doctor requests and determines it is an emergency'; he concluded, 'I do not believe that our community wants to force nurses, many of whom have a conscientious objection, to assist in late term abortions' (Prowse 2008: 1).

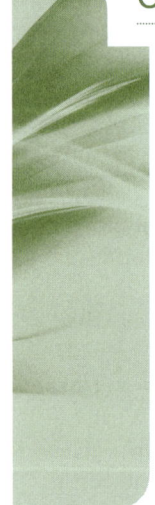

Case scenario 2

In its February 2018 issue of *On the record*, the Victorian Branch of the Australian Nursing Midwifery Federation (ANMF) commended the Victorian Government 'for introducing voluntary assisted dying legislation', which was passed by the Victorian Parliament on 29 November 2017 and due to come into effect mid June 2019. Victoria has become the only state in Australia to pass assisted dying legislation. The Australian Nursing and Midwifery Federation (ANMF) Victoria Branch confirmed that it had 'supported voluntary assisted dying since 1995 and believes the law is a safe and compassionate response to the voices of dying Victorians' (ANMF 2018: 6). The report in *On the record* clarifies that, under the legislation, nurses are permitted to conscientiously object to involvement in assisted dying procedures, but also points out that, under the nurses' code of conduct, 'nurses are obliged to respectfully inform the person and their employer of their conscientious objection and ensure the person has access to alternative care'; the report further clarifies that 'nurses must understand the limits of healthcare in prolonging life, recognise when efforts to prolong life may not be in a person's best interest and accept a person's right to refuse treatment' (ANMF 2018: 7). The ANMF's (Victorian branch) support for euthanasia is reflected in its policy on 'Voluntary euthanasia / assisted dying' (adopted in 1995 and reviewed February 2017) (ANMF 2017a) and also in the Federal ANMF's position statement on 'Assisted dying' (reviewed and re-endorsed November 2016) (ANMF 2016).

CRITICAL QUESTIONS

1. To what extent, if any, should nurses take note of public opinion polls or organisational policies and position statements on moral policy issues?
2. What, if any, formal position should the nursing profession adopt on the abortion and/or the euthanasia issue?
3. What justification might nurses claim to support the stance they take on the issue of abortion and/or euthanasia?

4   What processes might nurses use to accommodate, and where able reconcile, the possible competing requirements of the nursing profession, patients, society and their own beliefs concerning the ethics of abortion and/or euthanasia?
5   If opposed to either abortion or euthanasia, how should nurses manage their opposition in work-related contexts?

Endnotes

1   Taken from Johnstone, M-J (2013a) Alzheimer's disease, media representations and the politics of euthanasia: constructing risk and selling death in an ageing society. Ashgate, Farnham UK, Chapter 10, subsection: 'Morality policy' (p 178). Adapted for inclusion in this chapter.
2   Taken from Johnstone, M-J (2013a) Alzheimer's disease, media representations and the politics of euthanasia: constructing risk and selling death in an ageing society. Ashgate, Farnham UK, Chapter 10, subsection: 'Euthanasia politics' (p 177). Revised for inclusion in this chapter.
3   Copyright © 1973, The Monist, La Salle, IL 61301. All quotations from this work are reprinted with permission.
4   Victoria became the first state in Australia to legalise voluntary euthanasia after its *Voluntary Assisted Dying Bill 2017* was passed on 29 November 2017. This legislation is due to come into effect in June 2019 (Parliamentary Library and Information Services, Department of Parliamentary Services 2017). Further information available: https://www.parliament.vic.gov.au/publications/research-papers/download/36-research-papers/13834-voluntary-assisted-dying-bill-2017; see also Smith (2017).
5   According to Forrester and Griffiths (2015: 244) as the term 'euthanasia' is not recognised for the purposes of criminal law there is, in effect, 'no crime of euthanasia'.
6   The term euthanasia (from the Greek *eu* meaning 'easy', 'happy' or 'good', and *thanatos* meaning 'death') is commonly attributed to Greek thought and as meaning a 'good' or 'happy' death. Contrary to popular belief, the Greeks did not use the term euthanasia (or equivalents) to imply either 'a means or method of causing or hastening death' (Carrick 1985: 127). Rather, it was used in a somewhat metaphorical sense 'to describe the spiritual state of the dying person at the impending approach of death' (Carrick 1985: 127). Historical evidence also suggests that euthanasia, as we understand it today, was in fact prohibited in ancient medical circles (Carrick 1985: 81). The ancient Greek philosopher Plato (circa 428–348 BC), for example, is credited with suggesting that physicians who attempt to poison another 'must be punished by death', whereas the lay person who attempted such a thing should only be fined – indicating that physicians were regarded as having the greater burden of responsibility to refrain from causing death (Carrick 1985: 83). Carrick comments that if a person's life was terminated without his or her consent, normally this was treated as being a prima-facie case of homicide (Carrick 1985: 128).
7   Taken from Johnstone, M-J (2012c) Organisational position statements and the stance of 'studied neutrality' on euthanasia in palliative care. Journal of Pain and Symptom Management, 44(6): 896–907. Adapted for inclusion in this chapter.

CHAPTER 11

Professional judgment, moral quandaries and taking 'appropriate action'

KEYWORDS

appropriate action
appropriate disagreement
conscience
conscientious objection
ethics–quality linkage
moral conflict
patient safety
practical wisdom
preventive ethics
professional judgment
whistleblowers
whistleblowing

LEARNING OBJECTIVES

Upon the completion of this chapter and with further self-directed learning you are expected to be able to:
- Identify at least four key areas in which nurses might encounter a situation involving moral conflict.
- Discuss critically the nature and moral importance of nurses' professional judgment in morally conflicted situations.
- Discuss critically the nature of conscience and its role in guiding ethical nursing conduct.
- Outline five conditions that must be met in order for a claim of conscientious objection to be genuine.
- Examine critically arguments both for and against the view that nurses ought to be permitted to conscientiously refuse to participate in certain procedures in nursing and health care contexts.
- Define whistleblowing.
- Discuss the possible adverse consequences to nurses of blowing the whistle in health care.
- Examine critically the conditions under which whistleblowing in health care might be justified.
- Discuss critically the notion of 'preventive ethics'.
- Distinguish between a *reactive* and a *proactive* approach to ethical conflict in health care.
- Explain what is meant by the ethics–quality linkage.
- Outline the four-step process that might be used as a preventive ethics measure.
- Discuss the nature and role of 'appropriate disagreement' in regard to ethical issues in health care.

Introduction

At some time during the course of their professional practice, nurses will encounter situations in which they must take '*appropriate action*' in order to prevent or remedy a risk of harm being caused by another. Taking such action can involve either an individual or a collective initiative. Individual action may involve a nurse: refusing conscientiously to participate in a controversial medical or nursing procedure; reporting to an appropriate authority an instance of substandard practice, an impaired practitioner, an error, or some other troubling incident that poses a threat to patient safety (e.g. a health care provider practising beyond their scope of practice); seeking advice from a manager, clinical ethics committee or some other decision-making authority; or 'speaking out' in either a conference or some other public forum. On rare occasions, a nurse might decide to 'go public' and approach media outlets to have his/her concerns aired. Collective action, on the other hand, may involve groups of nurses embarking on an organised lobbying campaign aimed at particular target groups. Alternatively, as has become increasingly common around the world, it may involve industrial action – particularly in situations involving substandard working conditions that are placing patient safety at risk.

Whatever action is taken, it is never free of moral risk. There are many examples in the nursing, legal and bioethics literature (too numerous to list here) of nurses experiencing a range of hardships both personally and professionally because they took a stand on what they deemed to be an important professional or moral issue. For example, nurses who have gone public with patient safety concerns have sometimes been vilified and even lost their jobs for taking the actions they took (examples of which will be given in this chapter).

Despite the possible risks associated with taking appropriate action in response to a wrong-doing or a troubling moral issue, nurses nonetheless have both a moral and a professional obligation to take such action. There are, however, some misconceptions about the nature of this obligation, the options open to nurses for taking a stand, what kind of action they should take and even about whether it is right to take such action at all. Some nurses even fear that some of the options open to them are incompatible with their broader professional obligations *as nurses* and are therefore 'unprofessional'. In some instances this has caused significant inner personal conflict (emotional turmoil), and has served more to compound the moral problems they face in the workplace than to help resolve them.

This (and the following) chapter attempts to clarify some of the confusion surrounding various options open to nurses for taking a stand on a morally problematic issue. To this end, attention is given to briefly discussing the kinds of actions nurses might take, the bases upon which their actions might be justified, the kinds of quandaries that nurses might face when deciding whether to take a particular course of action or to 'stand back', and to show that, despite the quandaries associated with them, the options open to nurses might not only be compatible with professional nursing obligations, but may even be prima-facie professional nursing obligations in themselves. It is to discussing the particular options of conscientious objection and whistleblowing, and the possible option of taking a systems approach to preventing ethics conflicts in the workplace, that this chapter now turns. Before doing so, however, a point of clarification is required on dealing with *moral conflict* in the workplace and the role of professional judgment in deciding what is the 'right thing to do'.

Moral conflict and professional judgment

As discussed in Chapter 5 of this book, moral disagreements are an inevitable part of the health care landscape and are particularly pressing when they involve issues which people deem to be of high importance and which impinge on their personal moral values. Ethical conflicts are also 'a regular feature of our ethical lives' (Wong 1992: 763). Also, because they tend to involve people with whom 'continuing relationships are both necessary and desirable', every effort must be made to find a way either (i) to resolve them, or (ii) if this is not possible (e.g. resolution may be impossible in cases where opinion is deeply polarised) to accommodate the moral differences so that respectful working relationships can continue (Wong 1992). In regard to the latter, Wong (1992) explains:

> *Living with others in productive ways, despite our moral differences with them, can itself be morally valuable. It can be a particularly strong form of respect for persons, and being able to show this kind of respect is a sign of moral maturity. The willingness to live with others despite moral differences promotes cooperation on the moral ends that are shared.* (Wong 1992: 774)

Moreover, as also discussed in Chapter 5, nurses should not be afraid of moral disagreement since, as the history of moral philosophy has long demonstrated, disagreement is often the beginning of our moral thinking, not its end. It can also serve as a kind of 'quality assurance' when deciding moral issues as it provides an incentive to those who are arguing competing points of view to ensure (assure) the soundness of their reasoning and the justifications they are putting forward to support their respective stances. Some scholars even suggest that when faced with disagreement, rather than remain steadfast in their moral views, people should reduce the level of confidence they have in them and not merely assume that their views have reasonable unquestionable authority (Kappel 2018; see also the collection of essays in Christensen & Lackey 2013). At the very least, when confronted with moral disagreement, people should re-evaluate the basis on which they hold their own moral viewpoints (Frances 2013; Kappel 2018). One reason for this, it is contended, is that most people do not engage in sophisticated moral reasoning (conscientious reflection) about the issues they are arguing about; rather, they tend to draw intuitively on personal values and beliefs informed by the norms and culture in which they were raised (Kappel 2018). When encountering a morally troubling situation in the workplace, how, if at all, a nurse will and should ultimately respond to the situation will depend on whether she/he has correctly 'judged' what is going on, whether there is a 'case to be made' – for or against – taking action, what that action should be, all things considered, and when it should be taken.

Making 'correct' moral judgments

In the 'moral distress' literature (see discussion on moral distress in Chapter 5), it is commonly assumed that, when encountering a troubling moral issue, nurses have, from the start, *correctly judged what is the right thing to do* but are constrained from taking appropriate action. This, however, is a highly contentious point and one that warrants further examination (Johnstone & Hutchinson 2015). Given the moral importance of any decision to 'take a stand' and the reality that, in many instances, mistakes can be made about what the right course of action is in a given situation, nurses need to be clear about the nature of the judgment processes they are using to reach a point of view.

As previously discussed in Chapter 5, it was contended that, when faced with uncertainty and complexity, nurses are just as vulnerable as others to constructing idiosyncratic 'subjective interpretations of issues beyond their objective features' (Sonenshein 2007: 1026). It was further asserted that, like others, nurses approach situations with their own individual systems of ethics and predetermined stances on what they value and believe is right and wrong. Literature reviews on the subject of nurses' ethical reasoning and behaviour provide some evidence in support of this observation. Reviews by Dierckx de Casterlé and colleagues (2008) and Goethals and colleagues (2010), for example, have each respectively found that nurses tend to decide and justify their moral decisions by appealing to their *own personal values and experiences*, rather than by engaging in critical reasoning. Goethals and colleagues' review has further suggested that what often drives nurses' behaviour is not a considered select theoretical approach to ethical reasoning and behaviour, but rather personal convictions, religious beliefs, education, upbringing, intuition and feelings (Goethals et al 2010: 644). Although this review found that some nurses do engage in a more systematic approach to ethics, their approach was still problematic on account of their disposition to draw on a variety of ethical theories and principles and to apply these in idiosyncratic ways.

These findings concur with the findings of an earlier US study which found that the more years of experience nurse participants had the less inclined they were to use a critically reflective approach to their ethical decision-making in practice, relying instead on their own personal values (Ham 2004).

In light of these considerations, it is not at all clear that nurses' moral judgments will necessarily be 'correct' and thus it is inevitable that others, also acting on 'bounded personal ethics', will disagree with them. It is also highly probable that, while nurses might feel steadfast in their moral viewpoints, others (including patients and their families) might hold equally steadfast opposing views and feel just as rankled as do nurses when their personal values conflict with others and their viewpoints are not respected.

Common situations involving moral conflict

It is over three decades since Yarling and McElmurry (1986) identified the kinds of morally conflicted situations that nurses of the day commonly found themselves in when planning and delivering nursing care to patients. The situations identified included, but were not limited to: pain management, cardiopulmonary resuscitation (NFR / DNR) directives, withholding or withdrawing life-sustaining treatment, refusals of consent to treatment, professional control of client information, and harmful care by another practitioner. It was contended that ethical conflict dilemmas arose in these situations when nurses were forced to choose between the patients' interests, their own interests, moral integrity and professional survival. Cases in which patients' rights and wellbeing were threatened or violated by the actions of another (including 'the system') were seen as being particularly illustrative of the poignancy of the ethical conflicts nurses sometimes faced.

More recent research has suggested that, although the theorisation and practice of nursing ethics has developed substantially over the past 30 years, nurses continue to experience ethical conflict dilemmas in their employer organisations. For example, a small number of Canadian, Swedish, Pakistani and Polish studies have found that nurses experience ethical conflict and associated dilemmas with their employing organisations in four key areas:

- *resources* – both economic and human (encompassing a lack of time, a lack of staff, a lack of beds and the general impact these factors have on the work conditions of staff and on the quality and safety of patient care)
- *disagreement with organisational values, policies and rules* (e.g. early discharge of patients who lack social support)
- *conflict of interest* (between patients and health professionals, health professionals and health professionals, health professionals and health service organisations; 'professional secrecy' entailing a lack of transparency or openness of the organisations; ineffective or inappropriate actions taken by organisations – including 'turning a blind eye' to questionable practices)
- *lack of respect for professionals* (nurses not feeling respected, valued and supported by their organisations; lack of investment in nurses' professional development) (Gaudine et al 2011; Idrees et al 2018; Kälvemark et al 2004; Thorne 2010; Wlodarczyk & Lazarewicz 2011).

Whether nurses who have found themselves in the above kinds of situations have exercised wise and prudent judgments in dealing with them, however, remains an open question.

Professional judgment

Nursing competency standards, codes of conduct and codes of ethics all make clear that, when deciding and acting in nursing care contexts, nurses must use their *professional judgment*. The ICN Code of ethics for nurses (ICN, 2012a), for example, emphasises the role of judgment in nursing practice. For example, the Code prescribes that:

- *The nurse holds in confidence personal information and uses* judgement *in sharing this information (Element 1: Nurses and people, p 2)*

- *The nurse uses* judgement *regarding individual competence when accepting and delegating responsibility (Element 2: Nurses and practice, p 3).* [emphasis added] (ICN 2012a)

National nursing codes and standards contain similar statements. For example, in the preamble to the 'Domains, principles and values' section of the Nursing and Midwifery Board of Australia (NMBA 2018b: 4) *Code of conduct for nurses*, clarification is provided of the expectation that the principles outlined 'apply to all areas of practice, with an understanding that nurses will *exercise professional judgement* in applying them, with the goal of delivering the best possible outcomes [emphasis added]'. Likewise the Nursing Council of New Zealand (NCNZ 2012a: 44) *Code of conduct for nurses* recognises that, in the course of doing their work (in particular when performing health assessments), nurses must use their 'knowledge and judgement' when interpreting data. In regard to specific ethical issues, the NZ Code recognises that consumers have the right to consent to disclosures of information about themselves and that in 'the absence of consent' the nurses must make 'a judgement about risk to the health consumer or public safety considerations' (Principle 5.5); it also prescribes that nurses must declare 'any personal, financial or commercial interest which could compromise your professional judgement' (Principle 7.10).

Despite these and other codified expected behaviours, just what constitutes *professional judgment* and why, if at all, it is morally important tends to be assumed rather than made explicit. This is problematic since it may leave nurses unsure about what constitutes a bona fide professional judgment as opposed to a mere opinion when making moral decisions. It is here that some clarification of what constitutes professional judgment and its relationship to moral decision-making is warranted.

The nature and moral importance of professional judgment

Judgment has been variously defined as the 'ability to make considered decisions or arrive at reasonable conclusions or opinions on the basis of the available information' (*Oxford English dictionary* 2018 online), the 'faculty of being able to make critical distinctions and achieve a balanced viewpoint; discernment' (*Collins English dictionary* 2018 online) and the 'ability to judge, make a decision, or form an opinion objectively, authoritatively, and wisely, especially in matters affecting action; good sense; discretion: a person of sound judgment' (http://dictionary.reference.com/browse/judgment). The counterpart of judgment (as in 'against one's better judgment') is defined in terms of being 'contrary to what one feels to be wise or sensible' (*New Oxford dictionary of English* 2001: 989) and 'contrary to a more appropriate or preferred course of action' (*Collins Australian dictionary* 2011: 888).

Drawing on these basic definitions, professional judgment might be loosely defined as judgment based on a discerning and 'best use' of professional knowledge, values, experience etc., to make a decision. Although relying on professional knowledge, professional judgment involves substantially more than the application of mere 'technical knowledge' (Coles 2002: 5). Rather it encompasses what Coles (2002: 5) describes, quoting Carr (1995: 71), as the 'supreme intellectual virtue' of *practical wisdom* – a way of thinking that is inseparable from professional judgment. For Coles it is professional judgment and the practical wisdom that is inherent in it, which stands as the hallmark of professional practice and which distinguishes it from being 'merely technical work' (Coles 2002: 5).

Wisdom, regarded in philosophy as being one of the four cardinal virtues, may be defined as the ability to 'think and act utilizing knowledge, experience, understanding, common sense, and insight' (*Collins Australian dictionary* 2011: 1868). It has also been defined as encompassing a 'deep understanding and realization of people, things, events or situations, resulting in the ability to apply perceptions, judgements and actions in keeping with this understanding' (Wikipedia 2018h). At its most basic, however, wisdom may be defined simply as *making the best use of knowledge* – the opposite of which is *folly* (i.e. the state or quality of being foolish, stupid or rash).

Taking into account these basic definitions of judgment and wisdom, Coles (2002), with reference to the influential work of Carr (1995), argues that professional judgment occurs along a spectrum, notably:

- *Intuitive* – concerned with the immediate and the urgent; prompts the question: 'What *do* I do now?'
- *Strategic* – also concerned with the immediate and urgent and encompasses contemplation of a wider range of possibilities; prompts the question: 'What *might* I do now?'
- *Reflective* – concerned with situations of uncertainty and requires the time and capacity for deeper thought; prompts the question: What *could* I do now?
- *Deliberative* – concerned with situations occurring in professional practice that require *moral deliberation*; prompts the question: What *ought* I do now?

It is the last – deliberative judgment – which has particular relevance to the issue of moral decision-making in nursing care contexts.

According to Carr (1995: 284), the professional sees practice 'as involving competing moral ideals, moral conflicts and unresolvable dilemmas'. Drawing on this view, Fish and Coles (1998: 68, 284) contend that these competing moral ideals, conflicts and quandaries are 'endemic to practising as a professional'. It is a mistake, however, to think that the task of professional judgment is wholly to determine what is the 'right' course of action in morally conflicted situations since there may be no simple answers in some situations (Coles 2002: 4). Rather, it is to determine what is 'best' in the situation at hand. As Carr (1995: 71) explains:

> [Professional action] is not 'right' action in the sense that it has been proved correct. It is 'right' action because it is reasoned action that can be defended discursively in argument and justified as morally appropriate to the particular circumstances in which it was taken.

Professional judgment then may be taken as encompassing 'the nexus of expertise and wisdom' and it is this that sets it apart from more 'routinely technical work' (Hawse & Wood 2018). Practical wisdom is especially important since, as Zhu and colleagues (2016: 710) explain with reference to the ancient Greek philosopher Aristotle:

> Practical wisdom not only drives action that is intentional, it also uses tacit knowledge and experience, considers the long-term future, and incorporates a broad spectrum of ways of knowing and perspectives. In doing this, a wise person can generalize beyond what narrow expertise can, and know what to do in specific instances.

In light of these considerations it can be seen that, when encountering competing and conflicting moral points of view, it is not sufficient for nurses to rely on their own 'personally bounded ethics' or technical knowledge in deciding what is the right or best thing to do in the situation at hand. Rather they must use scrupulous professional judgment involving the entire spectrum of intuitive, strategic, reflective and deliberative thinking and ensure that, when deciding what to do, they do so on a foundation of practical and moral wisdom (moral praxis).

Conscientious objection[1]

Statements on *conscientious objection* and the circumstances in which it might be expressed are reflected in many nursing codes of ethics and related position statements. Their scope, however, varies; whereas some are broad reaching, others are more restrictive and focus narrowly on the areas of abortion and reproductive technology alone. For example, under the 'Professional behavior' section (Principle 4.4) of the Nurses and Midwifery Board of Australia (NMBA 2018a) *Code of conduct for nurses*, reference is made to situations in which conflicts of interest might arise and which 'might mean the nurse does not prioritise the interests of a person as they should, and may be viewed as unprofessional conduct'. It goes on to advise:

> To prevent conflicts of interest from compromising care, nurses must responsibly use their right to not provide, or participate directly in, treatments to which they have a conscientious objection. In such a situation, nurses

must respectfully inform the person, their employer and other relevant colleagues, of their objection and ensure the person has alternative care options (p 11).

Similarly, the Nursing Council of New Zealand (2012a) *Code of conduct for nurses* instructs nurses (Principle 1.9):

You have a right not to be involved in care (reproductive health services) to which you object on the grounds of conscience under section 174 of the Act. You must inform the health consumer that they can obtain the service from another health practitioner.

The UK Nursing and Midwifery Council (NMC), while recognising that there are occasions when nurses and midwives have a conscientious objection to a particular aspect of patient care, is more restrictive. In Section 4 of its Code it states that nurses and midwives who have a conscientious objection must 'tell colleagues, your manager and the person receiving care if you have a conscientious objection to a particular procedure and arrange for a suitably qualified colleague to take over responsibility for that person's care' (NMC 2015: 6). There are, however, only two recognised areas in which nurses have a lawful right to conscientiously object: abortion and reproductive technology (NMC https://www.nmc.org.uk/standards/code/conscientious-objection-by-nurses-and-midwives/). This restrictive stance is problematic, as will be considered shortly.

The 2017 revised edition of the Canadian Nurses Association *Code of ethics for registered nurses* is particularly worthy of note. Whereas other nursing codes primarily situate conscientious objection in the context of reproductive health, the Canadian code contains new content specifically addressing 'medical assistance in dying' in direct response to the passage of Medical Assistance in Dying (MAiD) legislation in 2017 (discussed in Chapter 10). In contradistinction to other nursing codes, the Canadian Code clearly defines conscientious objection – notably, as 'a situation in which a nurse informs their employer about a conflict of conscience and the need to refrain from providing care because a practice or procedure conflicts with the nurse's moral beliefs' (CNA 2017: 21). In Part 1, Section D ('Honouring dignity') of the Code, it is stated:

Nurses understand the law so as to consider how they will respond to medical assistance in dying and their particular beliefs and values about such assistance. If they believe they would conscientiously object to being involved with persons receiving care who have requested such assistance, they discuss this with their supervisors in advance. [emphasis original] (CNA 2017:13).

In addition, the Code contains a special section on 'Ethical considerations in addressing expectations that are in conflict with one's conscience' in which the steps for declaring a conflict in conscience are outlined (CNA 2017: 35–7). Finally, in contradistinction to other codes, the Canadian Code recognises a range of situations (not just those confined to reproductive health care contexts) in which a nurse might have conscientious objection. The Code clarifies:

Nurses may not abandon those in need of nursing care. However, nurses may sometimes be opposed to certain procedures and practices in health care and find it difficult to willingly participate in providing care that others have judged to be morally acceptable. Such situations include, but are not limited to, blood transfusions, abortion, suicide attempts, refusal of treatment and medical assistance in dying. (CNA 2017: 35).

Notwithstanding the provisions contained in these codes and other like statements, nurses have been 'conscientiously objecting' to workplace practices and related processes for years (e.g. by sidestepping a particular patient assignment, changing shifts, declining to work in a particular ward or area, or taking a 'sick day' off work). Their objections, however, have rarely gained public attention. It has only been in extreme situations, such as when a nurse has been dismissed from or denied employment, or has been threatened in some way, that issues involving conscientious objection have come to the attention of others outside of the unit or organisation where they have arisen. Those who have had the courage to formally voice their conscientious refusal to participate in certain medical procedures or organisational processes, or to carry out certain directives given by an employer or superior, have sometimes done so at great personal and professional cost, as the following examples will show. One of the most famous examples of this can be found in the much-cited United States (US) case of Corrine Warthen.

Corrine Warthen, a registered nurse of many years' experience, was dismissed from her employing hospital of 11 years for refusing to dialyse a terminally ill bilateral amputee patient. Warthen's refusal in this instance was based on what she cited as ' "moral, medical and philosophical objections" to performing this procedure on the patient because the patient was terminally ill and … the procedure was causing the patient additional complications' (Warthen v Toms River Community Memorial Hospital 1985: 205).

Warthen had apparently dialysed the patient on two previous occasions. In both instances, however, the dialysis procedure had to be stopped because the patient suffered severe internal bleeding and cardiac arrest (p 230). It was the complications of severe internal bleeding and cardiac arrest that she was referring to in her refusal. Her dismissal came when she refused to dialyse the patient for a third time.

Believing she had been wrongfully and unfairly dismissed, Warthen took her case to the Supreme Court, where she argued in her defence that the *Code for nurses* of the American Nurses' Association (ANA 2015) justified her refusal, since it essentially permitted nurses to refuse to participate in procedures to which they were personally opposed (p 229).

The court did not find in her favour, however, and she lost her case. In making its final decision, the court made clear its position on a number of key points (p 1985):

1. *An employee should not have the right to prevent his or her employer from pursuing its business because the employee perceives that a particular business decision violates the employee's personal morals, as distinguished from the recognised code of ethics of the employee's profession.* (p 233)
2. *[In support of the hospital's defence] it would be a virtual impossibility to administer a hospital if each nurse or member of the administration staff refused to carry out his or her duties based upon a personal private belief concerning the right to live … .* (p 234)
3. *The position asserted by the plaintiff serves only the individual and the nurses' profession while leaving the public to wonder when and whether they will receive nursing care.* (p 234)

Another notable example of the personal and professional cost a nurse can pay for taking a stand on an issue can be found in the case of Frances Free (also from the US). Free, an experienced registered nurse, was dismissed by her employer after she had refused to evict a seriously ill bedridden patient. Free's refusal (Free v Holy Cross Hospital 1987: 1190), in this instance, was based on grounds that to evict the patient would have been:

> in violation of her ethical duty as a registered nurse not to engage in dishonourable, unethical, or unprofessional conduct of a character likely to harm the public as mandated by the Illinois Nursing Act.

The female patient in question had been arrested for possession of a handgun. Meanwhile, an 'order' had been given for the patient to be transferred to another hospital. The police officer guarding the patient pointed out, however, that because of certain outstanding matters the other hospital would probably not accept the patient and it was likely that she would be returned to Holy Cross Hospital. Free communicated this information to the hospital's chief of security who responded by telling her that the patient was to be removed from the hospital 'even if removal required forcibly putting the patient in a wheelchair and leaving her in the park' which was across the road from the hospital (p 1189). Although Free disagreed with removing the patient, she gave the necessary instructions for the patient's transfer to the other hospital.

As part of the process of dealing with this situation, Free contacted the vice-president of her employing hospital to discuss the matter with him. It is reported that the vice-president 'became agitated, shouted and used profanity in telling Free that it was he who had given the order to remove the patient' (p 1189). After this incident, Free contacted the patient's physician who stated that 'he opposed the transfer' and instructed Free 'not to touch the patient but to document his order that the patient should remain at the hospital' (p 1189). After checking the patient and 'calming her down', Free received a telephone call 'ordering her to report to the office of the vice-president'. When she arrived at the vice-president's office Free was advised 'that her conduct was insubordinate and that her employment was immediately terminated' (p 1189). Free subsequently took court action arguing that her dismissal was 'unfair'. Free lost her case, however. Significantly, during the court proceedings, Free's actions were characterised 'as being of a *personal* as opposed to a *professional* nature and therefore as falling outside the scope of the Illinois Nursing Act' (Johnstone 1994a: 256).

These and more recent examples demonstrate that the issue of conscientious objection by nurses warrants attention (see, for example, three cases circa 2005–15 involving midwives respectively from Scotland, Croatia and Sweden who conscientiously objected to participating in abortion work; each of the midwives involved faced 'hostile reactions from colleagues, professional associations and managers' with two of the cases being escalated to be dealt with by the court system (Fleming et al 2018)). In particular, the cases considered demonstrate the need for attention to be given to clarifying the nature and authority of conscience, distinguishing between genuine and bogus claims of conscientious objection, and determining the kinds of policy and protective legislation there should be in regard to those who conscientiously refuse to perform or to participate in morally controversial medical and/or nursing procedures. As well as this, attention needs to be given to the question of: 'When, if ever, can an employer or manager decently direct nurses to perform tasks which they are conscientiously opposed to performing?' Similarly, 'Are nurses morally obliged to follow the policy and position statements of their professional associations if these stand to violate their personal moral integrity?' An additional question is: 'Can nurses decently refuse to assist with tasks which others do not regard as morally problematic – particularly if such refusals result in restricting patient access to the treatment and care they are seeking?' These and other key concerns raised by the conscientious objection debate are addressed in the following sections.

The nature of conscience explained

The *Oxford English dictionary* (2014 online) defines 'conscience' as:

> the internal acknowledgment or recognition of the moral quality of one's motives and actions; the sense of right and wrong as regards things for which one is responsible; the faculty or principle which pronounces upon the moral quality of one's actions or motives, approving the right and condemning the wrong.

The *Collins English dictionary* (2018 online) defines 'conscience' as a 'sense of right and wrong that governs a person's thoughts and actions'. These definitions, however, are inadequate to answer questions concerning the legitimacy and power of conscience as a bona fide moral authority. In short, although they help to describe what conscience is, these definitions say nothing about whether individuals should always obey their conscientious senses of right and wrong, or whether others can reasonably be expected to respect another's conscientious claims. In order to find answers to these and related questions, a philosophical analysis is required, and will now be advanced.

Philosophical accounts of conscience fall roughly into three categories: as *moral reasoning*, as *moral feelings* and as a combination of *moral reasoning and moral feelings* (see Beauchamp & Childress 2013; Hume 1888; Kant 1930; Mill 1962; Rawls 1971).

Conscience as moral reasoning

Conscience as reasoning takes 'extended consciousness' encompassing the gathering of knowledge, rational moral principles and reason as the source of one's moral convictions (Damasio 1999: 232). Conscientious judgments, by this view, are really critically reflective moral judgments concerning right and wrong (Broad 1940; Garnett 1965). Rational insight can be either religious or non-religious in nature, depending on what a person's worldviews are. Either way, a rational conscience typically manifests itself as 'a little voice inside one's head saying what one should and should not do' — also called 'the "voice" of conscience' (Benjamin 2004: 513) — or, to put this in moral terms, it tells us what our moral obligations and duties are. Statements of conscientious objection then are, by this view, merely statements of moral duty which individuals recognise and commit themselves to fulfil. Whether the duties or obligations identified impose overriding or absolute demands, or only prima-facie demands on the individual, is, however, another matter and one that is considered shortly.

Conscience as moral feelings

There are two possible versions of a 'moral feelings' account of conscience — emotivist and intuitionist. Both consist of a tendency to spontaneously experience either emotions or intuitions 'of a unique sort of approval of the doing of what is believed to be right and a similarly unique sort of disapproval of the doing of what is believed to be wrong' (Garnett 1965: 81).

It is generally recognised that these feelings are significantly different from the sorts of feelings we might have when, for example, looking at a beautiful painting (aesthetic approval) or an awful painting (aesthetic disapproval), or eating a favourite food (the feelings of mere liking) or smelling an awful smell (feelings of mere disliking), or witnessing an act of remarkable human achievement (feelings of admiration) or an act of extraordinary human failure (feelings of disdain). By contrast, in the case of wicked acts or the violation of duty, conscience may manifest itself in strong and distinguishable feelings of moral loathing, disgust, shame, remorse or guilt (see Greenspan 1995), or, as Beauchamp and Childress (1989: 387) suggest, the unpleasant feelings of 'a loss of integrity, wholeness, peace, and harmony'. To borrow from Fletcher (1966), conscience can manifest itself as 'a sharp stone in the breast under the sternum, which turns and hurts when we have done wrong' (p 54). In the case of virtuous acts, conscience may manifest itself as strong feelings of reassurance or moral goodness (Fletcher 1966: 54; Kant 1930: 130), or, as Beauchamp and Childress (1989: 387) suggest, as feelings of integrity, wholeness, peace and harmony. Either way, moral feelings instruct individuals on what they ought and/or ought not to do. As with the account of conscience based on reason, statements of conscience emerge as statements of obligation and duty.

Conscience as moral reason and moral feelings

The concept of conscience as a combination of reason and feelings basically involves an integrated response to 'moral catalysts' in the world. It does not rely on 'blind emotive obedience', as Kordig (1976) calls it, nor on an exclusive and blind devotion to reason. Rather, it relies on the mutually guiding and instructive forces of both moral sensibilities and moral reasoning. This account of conscience is, arguably, the most plausible of the three given, and is thus the one that underpins this discussion.

How conscience works

Now that we have briefly examined the essential nature of conscience, the next question is: 'How does conscience function as a moral authority?'

Contentious convictions can be exercised in one or both of two ways: 'to avoid doing what is apparently evil or engage in doing what is apparently good' (Murphy & Genuis 2013: 348). In either case, conscience functions as a personal (internal) sanction and as a personal moral authority for decision-making (Beauchamp & Childress 2013). Claims of conscience typically identify individual people with their self-chosen or autonomously chosen standards and principles of conduct (Nowell-Smith 1954: 268). Further, they commit individual people to act in accordance with those principles. In other words, claims of conscience commit the individual person to act morally (Timms 1983: 41). Thus, when conscience is said to be 'personal' or 'one's own', all that is being claimed is that a particular set of autonomously chosen moral standards has authority over a particular person – not, as is sometimes mistakenly thought, that the person has a unique and different set of moral standards from everybody else, and thus is a kind of 'moral freak'.

Conscience can be appealed to both as a kind of 'reviewer' or 'judge' of past acts, and as an 'authority on' or as a 'guide to' future acts. Whether conscience is appealed to as judge or guide, however, it is important to understand that conscience is not morality itself, nor is it the ultimate standard (or even a standard) of morality. Rather, as Gonsalves (1985: 55) explains, it is:

> *only the intellect itself exercising a special function, the function of judging the rightness or wrongness, the moral value, of our own individual acts according to the set of moral values and principles the person holds with conviction.*

Or, as Beauchamp and Childress explain (2013: 42), it is 'a form of self-reflection about whether one's acts are obligatory or prohibited, right or wrong, good or bad, virtuous or vicious'.

The above views make it plain that statements of conscience are not statements of a unique moral faculty or of unique moral standards. Rather, they are statements of a particular application of adopted moral standards. Conscientious objection, by this view, essentially translates into a case of moral disagreement in regard to which moral statements apply and what one's moral duty is in a particular situation. If this is so, the case for respecting a conscientious objector's claims becomes compelling – particularly in instances where there are no clear-cut moral grounds for settling a specific disagreement (e.g. responding to a patient's request for euthanasia).

The problem remains, however, that consciences are fallible and can make mistakes (Seeskin 1978). As Nowell-Smith (1954: 247) points out, some of the worst crimes in human history have been committed by people acting on the firm convictions of conscience. Hitler, for example, believed he was fulfilling a supreme moral duty by purging the German race of its 'Jewish disease' (Kordig 1976). Others also point out that, in some instances, what appears to be a claim of conscience may be nothing more than a claim of prudence, self-interest or convenience. This invariably raises the question: 'Should I always obey my conscience?' Further to this, claims of conscience can be insincere or counterfeit, raising the additional questions of: 'How can I distinguish between genuine and bogus claims of conscientious objection?' and 'Should I always respect another's conscientious claims?' It is to answering these questions that this discussion now turns.

Bogus and genuine claims of conscientious objection

Whether a claim of conscience should ever be permitted and under what circumstances is a matter of controversy and is emerging as a deeply polarising issue – particularly in regard to whether conscientious objection should ever be permitted in health care contexts (see, for example, the debate progressed in the special issues of the *American Journal of Bioethics* (June and December issues 2007), *Bioethics* (January issue 2014), the *Cambridge Quarterly of Healthcare Ethics* (January issue 2017) and the *Journal of Medical Ethics* (April issue 2017) respectively, as well as articles published at random in other journals). Controversy aside, and accepting for argument's sake that there are grounds for permitting conscientious objection, one of the key issues concerns how to *prove* whether claims of conscientious objection are 'genuine' and 'reasonable', and whether standards of justification for permitting or refusing claims of conscientious objection can ever be satisfactorily met. In an attempt to address this problem, various criteria for distinguishing between bogus and genuine (reasonable) claims of conscience have been devised, noting that at a minimum 'they cannot involve empirical falsehoods, objectively discriminatory attitudes or unreasonable normative beliefs' (Liberman 2017: 495). Neither can they rest on mere dislikes and aversions or arbitrary points of view (Uberoi & Galli 2017). It is to considering possible criteria for distinguishing genuine from bogus claims of conscientious objection that this section now turns.

It is contended here that, for a conscientious objection to be genuine, it must satisfy at least five conditions.

1. It must have as its basis a *distinctively moral motivation*, as opposed to the motivations of mere self-interest, prudence, convenience or prejudice. By this is meant:
   (i) that the action has as its aim the maintenance of sound moral standards, and the achievement of a desired moral end (Garnett 1965)
   (ii) that the person performing the act sincerely believes in the moral characteristics of the action in question, and sincerely desires to do what is right (Broad 1940: 75; Childress 1979: 334), and
   (iii) that the desire to do what is right is sufficient to override considerations of fear, cowardice, self-interest and prejudice.

2. It must be performed on the basis of *autonomous, informed and critically reflective choice*. By this is meant:
   (i) that the action must be the individual's 'own' – that is, it is autonomous and not the product of coercion or manipulation, and
   (ii) that the action has been carefully considered – that is, that the person has taken into account all the relevant factual as well as ethical information pertaining to the situation at hand, possible alternatives to the action being contemplated, and predicted moral outcomes of the action once it is taken (Broad 1940: 75).

3. It should be appealed to only *as a last resort* – that is, in defence of one's moral beliefs and integrity. A claim of conscientious objection is a last resort when all other means of achieving a tolerable solution to a given moral problem have failed. Here conscientious objection is justified on grounds analogous to those justifying self-defence, which permit people to use reasonable force in order to preserve their integrity (in this case, their moral integrity) (Machan 1983: 503–5).

4. The conscientious objector must admit that *others might have an equal and opposing claim of objection*. For example, a nurse refusing on conscientious grounds to assist with an abortion procedure must be prepared to accept that the aborting surgeon may feel obliged as a matter of conscience to go ahead with the abortion. To quote from Broad: 'What is sauce for the conscientious goose is sauce for the conscientious ganders who are his [sic] neighbours or his [sic] governors' (Broad 1940: 78).

5. *The situation in which it is being claimed must itself be of a nature which is morally uncertain* – that is, there are no clear-cut moral grounds upon which the matter at hand can be readily and satisfactorily resolved, and competing views can be shown to be equally valid.

If these criteria are accepted, then the task of distinguishing bogus from genuine claims of conscientious objection becomes easier. To illustrate this, consider two types of situations in which nurses might claim conscientious objection: (i) the lawful but morally controversial directives of an employer or manager; and (ii) a conflict of personal values between a nurse and a patient.

Conscientious objection to the lawful but morally controversial directives of an employer/manager

Nurses as employees are compelled by the principle of employment law to obey the lawful and reasonable directives of an employer or manager. The problem is, however, that nurses might not always agree morally with the lawful directives they have been given, and thus may sometimes find themselves in the uncomfortable position of having to perform acts which violate their reasoned moral judgments.

Situations involving nurses' conscientious refusal to follow lawful but morally questionable directives invariably pose the age-old question of whether an individual can, all things considered, be decently expected to follow morally controversial or morally bad, although legally valid, laws – or, in this case, lawful directives.

The problem of legal–moral conflict is not new to philosophy. Questions of, for example, what is the proper relationship of morality to law, what is to count as a good legal system, or whether individuals ought to be compelled to obey immoral laws, have long been matters of philosophical controversy. Hart, an Oxford scholar and professor of jurisprudence, for example, argued over half a century ago that existing law must not supplant morality 'as a final test of conduct and so escape criticism' (Hart 1958: 598). He also argued that the demands of law must be submitted to the scrutiny and guidance of sound morality before they can be justly enforced (Hart 1961).

In answer to the question of whether an employer or manager can decently direct a nurse to perform a task or procedure to which he/she is genuinely opposed on conscientious grounds, the short answer is no.

It might be objected that permitting conscientious objection is not conducive to the efficient running of hospitals and other health services. There is, however, little to support this kind of claim. In the case of military service, for example, it has been found that objectors are rarely amenable to threats and usually make unsatisfactory soldiers if coerced, and that in fact there are generally not enough objectors to frustrate the community's purpose (Benn & Peters 1959: 193). There is room to suggest that something similar is probably true of objectors in nursing. As many examples in the nursing literature have shown, nurses have preferred to resign and risk dismissal than perform acts which they find morally offensive. Further to this, those nurses who have been coerced have not wholly complied with given orders. It is also unlikely that conscientious objection by nurses would occur en masse, or be in sufficient number to obstruct the efficient running of the hospital system.

Conscientious objection and the problem of conflict in personal values

The ICN *Code of ethics for nurses* (2012a: 2) states that 'the nurse's primary professional responsibility is to people requiring nursing care'. It further states (p 2) that: 'In providing care, the nurse promotes an environment in which the human rights, values, customs and spiritual beliefs of the individual, family and community are respected'. Sometimes, however, a nurse may find it genuinely difficult to respect a person's (or a family's or a community's) values, customs and spiritual beliefs, and for this reason may decline to be involved in caring for such entities. Consider the following cases.

Case 1

A registered nurse working in a general medical ward was assigned a male patient who was known to be an orthodox Muslim. Upon learning of the man's religion, the nurse refused to care for him, stating that she could not accept the attitudes of Muslim males towards women, and that if she cared for him she would be as good as condoning his (and his community's) views.

Case 2

A registered nurse working in an infectious diseases unit was assigned a male patient in the end stages of AIDS. Upon learning that the patient was a homosexual and prior to his illness had been actively involved in the gay community, the nurse refused to accept the assignment. The nurse argued that as a Christian he could not condone homosexuality, and therefore it would be against his religious beliefs to care for the patient.

> **Case 3**
> A registered nurse working in a country hospital was asked to admit and care for a patient injured in a fight. When she recognised the patient as a member of a family who had been engaged in a feud with her own family for years, she declined to care for him. She stated as her reason that, were she to care for the man, she would be violating the loyalties she owed to her own family.

All three registered nurses in the cases just given may have each had sincere motivations behind their refusals to care for the patients in question. What is not so clear, however, is whether these motivations have a *moral* basis. For instance, their refusals to care for these patients seem to be based more on, for example, non-moral personal dislike, prejudice, fear, disdain or mere disapproval than on sincere moral motivation and the desire to achieve morally desirable ends. Second, it is not clear whether, by refusing to care for these patients, the nurses will preserve their moral integrity. Lastly, the professional requirement to care for the patients in question is not itself morally controversial – at least not in the same way that, for example, a request to assist with euthanasia would be.

Although it may be imprudent to compel the nurses in these cases to care for the patients assigned to them, it is not immediately apparent that it would be unethical to do so. It might be concluded then that their refusals can, at least from a moral perspective, be justly overridden. Nevertheless, there may still exist pragmatic grounds for permitting their refusals. If they cannot be relied upon to give adequate care, for example, it might be better to allow their refusal. If their prejudices and personal feelings are of such a nature as to seriously cloud their professional judgments and indeed their ability to care and engage in an effective therapeutic relationship, it may be that they should not be allocated the patients in question. The matter should not rest there, however. The nurses in question will need to account for their actions and, in keeping with professional standards of conduct, undertake professional development including further education (e.g. on cultural diversity and inclusiveness, dealing with conflict, professionalism and professional ethics).

Conscientious objection and policy considerations

The question remains of whether legislative and policy provisions should be made for conscientious objection in health care contexts. In answering this question the following considerations apply. First, forcing nurses to act against their reasoned or conscientious judgments is to undermine their moral authority and also to unjustly violate their integrity as morally responsible and accountable professionals.

Second, it is generally recognised that if people are forced constantly to violate their conscience then their conscience will gradually weaken and lose its authority (Kant 1930). This in turn makes it easier for individuals to avoid fulfilling their perceived moral duties and acting in accordance with their autonomously chosen moral standards. As a result, there is likely to be a general breakdown in compliance with moral rules and principles, and a general erosion of individual moral responsibility and accountability.

Third, it is generally accepted that moral duty is mainly concerned with the prohibition and avoidance of behaviour that is intolerable (Urmson 1958: 214). If fulfilling one's supposed duty does not avoid or prevent intolerable results, it seems reasonable to question whether in fact it was one's duty in the first place. As with the case of supererogatory acts (i.e. acts above the call of duty, such as those performed by saints and heroes), care must be taken to distinguish those deeds which can be reasonably expected of 'ordinary' persons (or 'ordinary' nurses) from those which it would merely be nice of 'ordinary' persons (nurses) to perform, but which could never be reasonably expected of them. On this point, Urmson (1958: 213) argues: 'a line must be drawn between what we can expect and demand of others and what we can merely hope for and receive with gratitude when we get it'.

Fourth, those who coerce others to act against their conscience erroneously presume that coercion vitiates moral responsibility. This, however, is not so. Just as more-sophisticated claims of duty cannot be escaped or deceived, nor can claims of conscience. It is a mistake to hold that, if a person is forced to perform an act to which they are conscientiously opposed, they are less morally culpable for that act, and that they will feel less morally guilty for having performed it. What users of force fail to understand is that an instance of moral violation still stands, regardless of whether it has been caused by an act of coercion or an act of free will.

Fifth, nurses are and can be held independently accountable and responsible for their actions. Given this, it is a mistake to hold that nurses have an unqualified duty to obey the directives of an employer or manager.

Lastly, it is ultimately more desirable than not to have a health care system comprised of conscientious nurses. Nurses comprise more than 50% of the total health care workforce. Since most of us cannot be saints, but can be conscientious, we need to preserve and cultivate conscientiousness (Garnett 1965: 91; Nowell-Smith 1954: 259). Only by doing this can we be assured of achieving and maintaining some sort of moral order in health care domains. As Seeskin (1978) argues, 'we have no guarantee that our deliberations will be perfect or our moral sensibilities adequate' (p 299); it is for this reason, among others, that conscience and moral conscientiousness should be given a place among the moral virtues. We might be condemned as fanatics if we hold conscience to be infallible, but if we do not at least acknowledge its ultimateness in the scheme of moral reasoning, we might be guilty of moral negligence and moral irresponsibility (Kordig 1976; Seeskin 1978).

Despite those who insist otherwise (see debate in the special issues of the journals mentioned earlier), 'conscience matters' and is worthy of protection (Sepper 2012; Trigg 2017; Wicclair 2011). This warrant becomes especially pressing when it is considered that a clinician with a conscience (doctor, nurse, pharmacist) is not just a 'health worker' compelled to do a job but, as Harris and colleagues (2018: 563) point out, also 'a social, economic, and political agent, responding to, and exerting, social and political pressures'– something which policies on conscientious objection usually fail to take into account and which 'are themselves created in the context of similar pressures'. This does not mean that conscientious objection should be given 'blanket protection'. However, it does mean, as Wicclair (2000: 227) has concluded in an influential essay on the subject, that 'there is a need for a more nuanced understanding and analysis of the relevant moral interests and values' at stake.

Conscientious objection stands as a site of conflicting rights. This has seen the emergence of debate on three conflictual positions (see, for example, Fleming et al 2018; Sepper 2012; Trigg 2017; Uberoi & Galli 2017; Wicclair 2011; and the special issues (mentioned earlier) of the *American Journal of Bioethics*, *Bioethics*, the *Cambridge Quarterly of Healthcare Ethics* and the *Journal of Medical Ethics*). Significantly, these positions mirror the respective positions (e.g. conservative, moderate and liberal) that may be taken on the issues that are the focus of a conscientious objection claim (e.g. abortion, euthanasia / assisted dying discussed in the previous chapter). These positions may be characterised as follow:

- *Conservative view* – which has been termed by Wicclair as the 'incompatibility thesis' and is based on the assumption that 'conscience-based refusals to provide legal and professionally permitted goods and services within the scope of a practitioner's competence are incompatible with the practitioner's professional obligations' (Wicclair 2011: 33). In this view, conscientious objection can never be justified and thus should never be allowed (the rights of patients supersede the conscience claims of health care providers; those who decline services on conscientious grounds should be disciplined, dismissed and even deregistered in a manner commensurate with that of other negligent failures; alternatively, those with conscientious objections should leave or not even enter the profession at all – e.g. 'quit nursing').

- *Moderate view* – which Wicclair has termed the 'compromise view' and holds that 'the exercise of conscience is compatible with fulfilling one's core professional obligations' (Wicclair 2011: 34). By this view, conscientious objection is justified and permissible in clearly defined circumstances but limited on grounds of service delivery; this position controversially encompasses an 'obligation to refer' cases of requests for abortion, euthanasia and the like to other providers who are not conscientiously opposed to the procedures in question. The obligation to refer, however, is controversial, with some regarding it as being as tantamount to complicity in the acts in question and hence as morally culpable.
- *Liberal view* – which Wicclair has termed 'conscience absolutism' and is based on the assumption that 'there are no ethical constraints on the exercise of conscience by health care professionals' and that 'health care professionals generally do not have an obligation to perform any action, including disclosure and referral, contrary to their conscience' (Wicclair 2011: 34). Conscientious objection, by this view, is regarded as a human right and, as such, is both justified and permissible not least on grounds of preserving an agent's moral integrity, which they have a right to defend. It is also justified on grounds of the value of 'moral diversity' and allowing different moral viewpoints to be expressed and considered (Fleming et al 2018; Sepper 2012; Trigg 2017; Uberoi & Galli 2017; Wicclair 2011; and special issues of the journals referred to earlier).

These three positions, which have been robustly debated in the literature (too numerous to list here) are likely to become the subject of increasing attention in the future as jurisdictions around the world enact legislation that falls within the domain of 'moral politics' – for example, abortion, euthanasia and medically assisted dying, organ transplantation, rationing of health care resources, and the like. Moreover, as the three cases discussed by Fleming and colleagues (2018) show, there can be a serious mismatch between 'conscience clauses' (policies and legislation that espouse to safeguard the right of practitioners to conscientious objection) and the reality that practitioners often face and are forced to live with upon exercising a right to conscientious objection (see also Sepper 2012). It will be recalled that the three midwives referred to earlier faced 'hostile reactions from colleagues, professional associations and managers'. It is significant that not only were they not supported, they were alienated by their peers and member associations, who spoke out against them (Fleming et al 2018). These and similar cases have worrying implications for the rights of nurses and others ostensibly protected by 'conscience clauses' in euthanasia / assisted dying legislation. Just what is to count as a 'reasonable objection' and 'reasonable accommodation' under such legislation and related policies is unclear and yet to be tested (Sepper 2012; Trigg 2017). Also of concern is the possible risk to nurses where a liberal view on conscientious objection might be imposed – which, to some extent, it already is by virtue of the requirement for objected cases to be referred to another practitioner. Just how 'easy' making referrals will be for nurses – particularly as morally controversial practices become 'normalised' – is yet to be verified. It is not far-fetched to imagine, for example, that in the future, just as nurses have been rebuked, disciplined and ostracised for refusing to assist with abortion work, so too will they face such responses for refusing to assist with or refer patients for euthanasia / assisted dying.

In its position statement on *Conscientious objection*, the federal Australian Nursing and Midwifery Federation (ANMF 2017) makes clear that colleagues who exercise their right to make a conscientious objection should be supported and 'not placed in situations that may compromise their religious, moral and ethical beliefs'. It also clarifies that 'discriminatory or adverse action should not be taken against any nurse, midwife or assistant in nursing voicing a conscientious objection either in an application for, or during employment' and that 'in health and aged care facilities nurses and midwives should have access to counselling and support services to meet their needs in their workplaces' (ANMF 2017). How well this stance will be upheld in practice remains to be seen and is likely to be tested in the not too distant future.

The above considerations have important implications for legislators and policy-makers (including those in nursing organisations and nurse regulating authorities) attempting to respond to the conscientious objection problem. For example, even if nurses' consciences are mistaken, on balance there are moral benefits to be gained by permitting their conscientious objections — not least, the benefits of fostering moral sensitivity and moral responsibility in the workplace. A second implication is that, if nurses are not permitted to object conscientiously, then health care contexts may be morally worse off by virtue of thwarting their conscientious practice. There is much to support the view that a health care system comprised of morally conscientious and sensitive nurses would be much better than one without such nurses. This seems to support the conclusion that genuine conscientious objection is not only morally permissible, but also, in the ultimate analysis, may even be morally required. For a conscientious objection policy to be effective and reliable, however, at least two minimal requirements must be fulfilled.

First, conscientious objectors must demonstrate that their claims are sincere. A given proof need not be religious in nature, nor necessarily absolute. As we have seen throughout this book, it is not always inconsistent for nurses (or others) to have a 'moderate' position on the moral permissibility of certain procedures, such as abortion and euthanasia / assisted suicide. Thus, it would not necessarily be inconsistent of nurses to, say, support abortion and to participate in most abortion procedures at their place of employment, yet nevertheless be opposed to a 'particular case' of abortion where the procedure in question fails to satisfy certain autonomously chosen moral standards. The same applies in the case of euthanasia / assisted suicide. Conscientious objection policies, then, must recognise and make provision for the moderate's position, and accept that sometimes conscientious objectors might refuse to assist with a type of procedure they have previously assisted with, such as abortion.

A second minimal requirement is that employers must carry the burden of proof that no alternative is available when not permitting nurses to refuse, on conscientious grounds, to assist with a given procedure. It is difficult to accept that a claim of conscientious objection cannot be accommodated in cases where nurses have used rightful means in expressing a conscientious refusal — that is, superiors have been given advance notice of an intention to refuse, reasons for refusal have been made explicit, replacement or other attending personnel have not been unduly compromised, other interests of comparable moral worth have not been sacrificed and patients have not been stranded. Where an employer does not accept a nurse's genuine conscientious objection claims, serious questions need to be asked about whether the employer has sincerely tried to find viable alternatives which would make it possible for conscientiously objecting nurses to withdraw from situations they deem morally troubling or intolerable.

Whistleblowing in health care

The International Council of Nurses (ICN) holds that 'patient safety is fundamental to quality health and nursing care' and that all nurses have a fundamental responsibility to 'address patient safety in all aspects of care', including (but not limited to) 'informing patients and others about risk and risk reduction', 'advocating for patient safety' and 'reporting adverse events to an appropriate authority promptly' (ICN 2012a: 1). In keeping with contemporary principles of human error management, the ICN explains:

> *Early identification of risk is key to preventing patient injuries, and depends on maintaining a culture of trust, honesty, integrity, and open communication among patients and providers in the health care system. ICN strongly supports a system-wide approach, based on a philosophy of transparency and reporting — not on blaming and shaming the individual care provider — and incorporating measures that address human and system factors in adverse events.* (ICN 2012a: 1)

The ICN position statement reflects a longstanding stance of the nursing profession, which historically has been at the forefront of the development and implementation of processes aimed at preventing practice errors, injuries and threats to *patient safety*. For instance, although not widely recognised, Florence Nightingale was among the first of the modern health professionals to advocate a system approach to human error management in hospitals (Johnstone & Kanitsaki 2006b). In her classic book *Notes on nursing* (first published in 1859, and still in print today) Nightingale laments the 'fatal accidents' she had observed directly or known of and which, in her opinion, would not have happened had there been in existence an 'organised system of attendance' notably of qualified nurses. She writes:

> *If you look into the reports of trials or accidents, and especially of suicides, or into the medical history of fatal cases, it is almost incredible how often the whole thing turns upon something which has happened because 'he', or still oftener 'she', 'was not there' […] The person in charge was quite right not to be 'there', he was called away for quite sufficient reason, or he was away for a daily recurring and unavoidable cause: yet no provision was made to supply his absence. The fault was not in his 'being away', but in there being no management to supplement his 'being away'.* (Nightingale 1980 edn: 22–3)

She goes on to state:

> *Upon my own experience I stand, and I solemnly declare that I have seen or known of fatal accidents, such as suicides in delirium tremens, bleeding to death, dying patients being dragged out of bed by drunken Medical Staff Corps men, and many other things less patent and striking which would not have happened in London civil hospitals nursed by women. The medical officers should be absolved from all blame in these accidents. How can a medical officer mount guard all day and all night over a patient (say) in delirium tremens? The fault lies in there being no organised system of attendance […] Were a trustworthy woman in charge of the ward, or set of wards, the thing would not, in all certainty, have happened.* (Nightingale 1980 edn: 29)

Notwithstanding Florence Nightingale's insights and innovations, and the nursing profession's history of patient safety advocacy, it has never been easy for nurses to fulfil their responsibilities associated with preventing practice errors, injuries and threats to patient safety and quality of care (Johnstone & Kanitsaki 2006b; Roberts 2017; Watson & O'Connor 2017). As the nursing literature (too numerous to list here) and the examples given in the following sections amply demonstrate, fulfilling the responsibilities associated with upholding patient safety has not been without significant moral and legal risk to nurses, raising important questions concerning the ethics of committing, communicating and correcting nursing errors in practice domains.

As noted above, in keeping with the requirements of *The ICN code of ethics for nurses* (ICN 2012a) and *Position statement: patient safety* (ICN 2012b), nurses have a stringent responsibility to 'take appropriate action to safeguard individuals, families and communities when their health is endangered by a co-worker or any other person' (ICN 2012a: 4). The codes of ethics and professional conduct ratified by other peak nursing organisations (e.g. the Nursing and Midwifery Board of Australia, the New Zealand Nursing Council, the Nursing and Midwifery Council (UK), the American Nurses Association and the Canadian Nurses Association) have also taken a stance that obligates nurses to take appropriate action (including reporting to an external authority) to safeguard individuals when placed at risk by the incompetent, unethical or illegal acts of others – including 'the system'. For example, under Principle 2 of the NMBA (2018) *Code of conduct for nurses*, nurses are required to 'document and report concerns if they believe the practice environment is compromising the health and safety of people receiving care' and to do so in 'a timely manner' (NMBA 2018: 6, 7). Likewise, the NCNZ (2012a) *Code of conduct*. Standard 6.9 of the NZ Code clarifies the responsibility of nurses to:

> *Intervene to stop unsafe, incompetent, unethical or unlawful practice. Discuss the issues with those involved. Report to an appropriate person at the earliest opportunity and take other actions necessary to safeguard health consumers.* (NCNZ 2012a: 29)

Fulfilling these codified obligations and taking action to produce an 'appropriate response' are not, however, straightforward processes and, as the examples given below demonstrate, can have painful consequences.

The Moylan case (Australia)

In 2002, the *Australian Nursing Journal* carried a feature article detailing the story of Kevin Moylan, a senior psychiatric nurse, who experienced a 6-year 'journey into hell' after he exposed the poor-quality practices at a psychiatric clinic in the Australian state of Tasmania (Armstrong 2002: 18–20). Moylan's ordeal began after he reported a range of workplace safety issues to hospital management. His concerns included what he believed to be the legal and ethical abuse of patients, inadequate training of staff and the provision of incompetent services, and serious problems with workplace health and safety – including:

> *the employment of a temporary psychiatrist who was not registered, police reluctance to provide support to protect staff from dangerous patients, and the sexual harassment of patients.* (Armstrong 2002: 19)

The employment of the unregistered psychiatrist caused Moylan particular concern and provided the catalyst for him deciding that he 'could not remain silent as patients were diagnosed, prescribed medication, and given electro-convulsive therapy by someone he considered a "fraud"' (Armstrong 2002: 19). The workplace safety issues provided a further catalyst for action after these 'reached a critical level when Kevin [Moylan] himself was attacked by a patient' (p 19). Significantly, when Moylan reported his concerns, rather than 'being praised and rewarded for his advocacy role' he was reportedly 'isolated and intimidated into silence' (p 19).

Concerned about the lack of response to the issues he had reported, Moylan decided to take the matter further and wrote to the then Tasmanian Minister for Health outlining his concerns. In a chain of circumstances remarkably similar to the *Pugmire case* (cited below), a copy of the letter was delivered to the Tasmanian Shadow Minister for Health who subsequently raised the matter in parliament, and named Moylan as the 'whistleblower'. Unfortunately, this single act of naming removed Moylan's anonymity and privacy and, in his own words, 'changed his life forever' (Armstrong 2002: 19). Over the next 6 years he lost his home, his farm, his livelihood and his health. Although the psychiatric clinic was eventually closed and Moylan received some compensation, his lost health, reputation and livelihood remain largely unaddressed. Now a campaigner against what he calls the 'suppression of dissent in the system', Moylan reflects:

> *I have been threatened, isolated, intimated and abused […] My actions were motivated by a desire to see justice done. I tried to protect my patients, but no-one protected me.* (quoted in Armstrong 2002: 19)

As a consequence of not being protected, at the time the *Australian Nursing Journal* report was published, Moylan was suffering from a post-traumatic stress disorder (PTSD) and unable to work. He was reported as having 'nothing left but his car and his dog' (Armstrong 2002: 19).

The Pugmire case (New Zealand)

In 1993, Neil Pugmire, a registered psychiatric nurse, wrote in confidence to the then Minister of Health outlining concerns he had about the *Mental Health (Compulsory Assessment and Treatment) Act 1992* (New Zealand) and its failure to provide for the compulsory detainment of patients whom responsible mental health professionals strongly believed were 'very dangerous' (Liddell 1994: 14). To support his concerns, Pugmire used as an example a named patient whom mental health professionals thought was 'highly likely' to commit very serious sexual crimes against young boys. This concern was based on admissions by the named patient (who, 7 years previously, had attempted to rape and strangle two boys) that he had continual feelings of 'wanting to commit sexual acts with little boys' (p 15). The Minister, however, reputedly took the position that 'mental health legislation should not be used to justify the detention of difficult or dangerous individuals' (p 14). Dissatisfied with this response, Pugmire sent a copy of his letter to a member of the opposition, Mr Goff (p 14). In a chain of events, similar to those that occurred in the Moylan case (referred to above), Mr Goff subsequently released the letter publicly, but with the patient's name deleted. However, the patient's name was eventually revealed by other sources thus breaching his confidentiality. Consequently, Pugmire was suspended by his employer for 'serious misconduct' involving the 'unauthorised disclosure of confidential patient information' (p 16).

The Bardenilla case (US)

In 1988, in what has been described as 'one of the most influential whistleblowing incidents ever to be initiated by a nurse during the [20th] century', Sandra Bardenilla, a registered nurse, was awarded damages for wrongful dismissal (involuntary resignation) from her place of employment (*American Journal of Nursing* 1988: 1576; Anderson S 1990: 5–6; Fry 1989b: 56). Bardenilla lost her employment as a result of reporting her concerns about two physicians whom she believed had directed 'unethical and potentially illegal nursing care to a comatose patient who later died' (Fry 1989b: 56).

It is reported that, during the course of attempting to have the matter addressed, Bardenilla was 'sharply criticised and accused of overstepping her role as a nurse' (Fry 1989b: 56). Bardenilla was instructed by her director of nursing to 'be quiet and to apologise' to the physicians concerned (Fry 1989b: 56). She was also advised to 'adopt a more realistic attitude about the hospital system, and she was warned against taking her concerns outside the hospital' (Veatch & Fry 1987: 176). Bardenilla did not accept these directives, however, and resigned from her position instead. Following her resignation, she formally reported the two physicians to the local county health department who initiated an investigation into the matter (*American Journal of Nursing* 1988: 1576; Veatch & Fry 1987: 176). Following the investigation into the death of the patient, the two attending physicians were charged with murder. Although the physicians were both subsequently acquitted of the charges against them, 'the case had a strong influence on subsequent termination-of-treatment decisions across the US' (Fry 1989b: 56). The consequences to Bardenilla, however, were extremely burdensome at both a personal and professional level. As Sara Fry notes (1989b: 56), although Bardenilla eventually received financial compensation for her employment losses, she nevertheless:

> received a great deal of recrimination as a result of her actions. While she received the support of many individual nurses, she did not receive formal professional support or find re-employment an easy matter. She suffered personal harm and the matter dragged through the courts for a long time.

The MacArthur Health Service case (Australia)

In 2002, four nurses met with the then New South Wales (NSW) Minister for Health to draw to his attention certain management and clinical practices that they believed were placing patients' safety at risk – and had allegedly already resulted in patient deaths – at two hospitals that were part of the MacArthur Health Service (MHS) in NSW. These nurses, together with three other nurses who later came forward in the formal investigation that was to follow, had between 13 and 30 years' nursing experience, and included clinical nurse specialists and nurse unit managers. As one report put it:

> Their professional experience enabled them to identify deficiencies in patient care and to alert the management of the hospital to problems. (Health Care Complaints Commission (HCCC) 2003: 2)

The Health Minister referred the matter to the Director-General of the NSW Department of Health; the Director-General, in turn, made a formal complaint to the NSW Health Care Complaints

Commission who then formally investigated the matter. The Commission's investigation included an analysis of 47 specific clinical incidents that had occurred between June 1999 and February 2003, in the emergency departments, the intensive care unit (of one hospital), the operating suite (of one hospital) and on the medical wards of both of the hospitals involved. Significantly, 'the evidence obtained about the incidents strongly supported the allegations by the nurse informants about the standard of care' (HCCC 2003: 4). Some examples of the clinical incidents verified are:

- *no surgical review of a patient with very poor blood supply to her foot – an urgent surgical problem (an ischaemic foot), for more than two days;*
- *unacceptable delay in triage of a severely ill newborn baby;*
- *a patient with severe chest pain was discharged from [sic] an emergency department when a bed with a cardiac monitor could not be found – she died a few hours later;*
- *a critically ill cardiac patient who was in shock was left untreated in [an] emergency department for many hours;*
- *failure to diagnose a patient with serious post-birth infection (puerperal sepsis) in the emergency department;*
- *a delay of over 12 hours in the transfer of a critically ill woman;*
- *post-operative intra-abdominal infection not diagnosed for four days;*
- *an agitated psychotic patient who waited unsupervised in an emergency department for five hours and subsequently absconded.* (HCCC 2003: 4)

The nurses' 'whistleblowing' actions in this case resulted in their suffering significant hardship at both a personal and professional level. For instance, in the days, weeks and months following their action, they were vilified and isolated by some of their colleagues ('because of the criticism of the health service brought about by the investigation' that followed after their allegations were made public). All four of the nurses were also disciplined by the health service – one of whom was suspended. Of these nurses, two were disciplined after they had apparently 'intervened' on the behalf of a child patient in the operating theatres. Following an investigation into this particular matter, the health service recommended that the nurses be disciplined 'over the way they had addressed a medical officer' (HCCC 2003: 5).

The matter did not end with the HCCC's investigation, however. In what arguably stands as one of the most significant nurse whistleblowing cases to occur in Australia, following the release of the Commission's report the then NSW Health Minister sacked the head of the NSW HCCC and announced a new inquiry – to be headed by an eminent barrister at law (Johnstone 2004b). This sacking came amid claims that the Commission's report did not go far enough in holding people accountable (Johnstone 2004b). In addition to the sacking of the Commission's head, two doctors were suspended, nine other doctors were referred to the NSW Medical Board for investigation and possible disciplinary action, and disciplinary action was initiated against four senior administrative staff at the health service (Saunders 2003a, 2003b). Also, an investigation was commenced into two further allegations – notably, that the former Minister for Health threatened and bullied two of the nurses who first went to him with their allegations, and that crucial documents pertinent to the allegations had been shredded at the two hospitals involved (Saunders 2003a, 2003b).

Despite having their concerns validated and receiving an apology from the Minister for Health as well as the MacArthur Health Service (a subsequent inquiry into the disciplinary action taken by the Service concluded that there was no evidence linking the disciplinary action to the whistleblowing – the action was ostensibly taken on other grounds) (see Hindle et al 2006: 49), the nurses' careers and lives were changed forever. Meanwhile questions raised in the news media about the nurses' 'real' motivations in this case remain unanswered and continue to cast doubt on the nurses' integrity in this case.

The Bundaberg Base Hospital case (Australia)

In 2003, Dr Jayant Patel, a general surgeon based in the US, was appointed as a surgical medical officer (and subsequently promoted to Director of Surgery) at Bundaberg Base Hospital in the Australian state of Queensland. Over a 2-year period between 2003 and 2005, Dr Patel operated on approximately 1000 patients, of whom 88 died and 14 suffered serious complications (Van Der Weyden 2005). During this period, Toni Hoffman, the nurse in charge of the intensive care unit at the hospital, had serious misgivings about Dr Patel's practice and repeatedly raised her concerns about patient safety and Patel's treatment of patients with the relevant hospital officials and other authorities – none of whom took her concerns seriously (see also Thomas 2007). Hoffman is reported to have spoken to 'the police, the Queensland coroner and up to 12 other officials about patient deaths before she went to a state lawmaker', and authorities started to take her concerns seriously with an official inquiry into the matter being called (Reuter's Health 2005).

The events that followed the inquiries led to resignations of the Queensland Minister for Health and the Director-General of Queensland Health, the General Manager and Director of Medical Services of the Bundaberg Base Hospital, and the suspension of the Director of Nursing (Dunbar et al 2007). A clinical review, meanwhile, found that Dr Patel had 'directly contributed' to the deaths of eight patients and 'may have exhibited an unacceptable level of care in another eight patients who died' (Van Der Weyden 2005: 284). The review also reportedly found that although 'in the comfortable majority of cases examined, Dr Patel's outcomes were acceptable ... [he] lacked many of the attributes of a competent surgeon' (Van Der Weyden 2005: 284). Despite these findings, Dr Patel was able to leave Australia before investigations into his conduct were completed and any measures taken to hold him accountable for his actions (Dunbar et al 2007).

The ramifications for Toni Hoffman of being a 'whistleblower' have been far reaching (Jones & Hoffman 2005). In a published conversation with the editor of the *Australian Journal of Advanced Nursing* about the case, Hoffman describes her 'aloneness', fear and sense of threat she felt she was under:

> *I went alone to see the Member of Parliament for my area. I was very fearful; I did not know what he was going to do [...] I have been threatened by telephone and out in the community. I have been vilified on the stand and had to 'cop it'. This situation was far worse than I had ever imagined.* (Hoffman, in Jones & Hoffman 2005: 5)

It has also been revealed from various sources, including the Australian Broadcasting Corporation's *Australian story* 'At death's door' (ABC 2005), that she was warned by senior medical officers and executives at the hospital that she could face disciplinary action and could even lose her job and serve jail time if she went public with her concerns (Australian Private Hospitals Association 2007). Despite eventually being fully vindicated for her actions and her advocacy for patient safety at Bundaberg (in recognition of what she did, she was made Australian of the Year Local Hero 2006), in her own words, the entire affair has had 'a huge personal toll' (Australian Private Hospitals Association 2007).

It should perhaps be clarified that whistleblowing in health care and by nurses in particular is a rare event. Even so, when such events do occur, the consequences can be dire – despite the operationalisation of policies and laws ostensibly designed to protect whistleblowers from retaliation. Here questions arise of: 'Why is whistleblowing problematic?' and 'What, if anything, can be done to improve the status quo?' It is to answering these questions that the remainder of this discussion now turns. Before proceeding, however, some clarification is required on what the term 'whistleblowing' refers to.

The notion of whistleblowing/whistleblowers

The term '*whistleblowing*', like other terms used in bioethics, is a contested notion. For the purposes of this discussion, however, it may be taken as a colloquial term that is used to refer to:

> *The voluntary release of non-public information, as a moral protest, by a member or former member of an organization outside the normal channels of communication to an appropriate audience about illegal and/or immoral conduct in the organization or conduct in the organization that is opposed in some significant way to the public interest.* (Boatright 1993: 133)

Citing Elliston and colleagues (1985), Vinten (1994: 256–7) argues that, in order for an act to count as whistleblowing, the following conditions must be met:

- *an individual performs an action or series of actions intended to make information public;*
- *the information is made a matter of public record;*
- *the information is about possible or actual, non-trivial wrongdoing in an organization;*
- *the individual who performs the action is a member or former member of the organization.*

Vinten (1994) further clarifies that whistleblowing disclosures lack authorisation, and can apply to both internal and external whistleblowing (see also Coyne 2003; Dougherty & Weber 2004; McDonald 2002; Rosen 1999). Others contend that whistleblowing reports are also usually made to a person in a position of authority (i.e. who has the power to stop the wrong), or to some other entity who, if not having the direct power to stop the wrong, nevertheless is perceived to have the capacity to exert pressure on those who do have the power to stop the wrong – for example, the media (Jackson et al 2010a, 2010b; Rosen 1999). More recent works have affirmed these defining characteristics of whistleblowing and its key purposes of making public the illegal, immoral or illegitimate activities, or activities that are contrary to the public interest, in order to effect change (Watts & Buckley 2017).

A key reason people resort to whistleblowing is to cause other people to pay attention and to take action immediately. Like the siren of an ambulance or a police car, or the fire alarm in a building, the sound of the 'whistleblower' seeks to alert people immediately to the fact 'that something is either happening or is about to happen [and] there is a need to pay attention to the alarm that has been sounded' (Erlen 1999: 67). Erlen (p 67) explains:

> *Just as the ring of the alarm clock arouses people from sleep, so, too, does an act of whistleblowing. While other sounds and their respective messages do not always signal danger or caution, whistleblowing within the context of a health care situation says that something is seriously wrong.*

The act of whistleblowing

In an influential and highly cited article on the subject, Near and Miceli (1985) suggest that the act of whistleblowing follows a four-step decision-making process. First, the whistleblower must decide 'whether the activity observed is actually wrongful' (i.e. whether it is illegal, immoral or illegitimate, or contrary to the public interest); second, the whistleblower must decide whether to report the activity; third, the organisation must decide if, when and how it will respond to the reported activities – noting that it may decide not to respond at all; and finally, the organisation must decide if, when and how it will respond to the whistleblower (see also Watts & Buckley 2017).

Deciding to 'go public'

The notion of 'nurse whistleblower' has been defined as 'a nurse who identifies an incompetent, unethical or illegal situation in the workplace and reports it to someone who may have the power to stop the wrong' (Ahern & McDonald 2002: 305). A key question facing members of the nursing profession is: 'Are there situations in which nurses *should* "blow the whistle" – including "going public" with their concerns?' The short answer to this is 'yes, no, maybe' – depending on the circumstances at hand and whether there are genuinely no other avenues for having the situation addressed.

Nursing codes and standards make clear that, if and when encountering a situation in which the care of individuals is being – or is at risk of being – endangered by a co-worker or any other person, nurses have a stringent responsibility to take 'appropriate action'. The issue here is not *whether* nurses should take action, but rather what *kind* of action they should take.

In situations involving an exceptionally serious failing that, in turn, is placing the public or the public interest at serious risk, and no other means exist for having the situation remedied, it is understandable that a nurse (or nurses) might consider whistleblowing as an option (Erlen 1999; King & Scudder 2013). Even so, every effort should be made first to try and correct the situation internally before 'going public' (Rosen 1999: 41). There are two reasons for this: first, as the examples given above have shown, there are significant risks associated with whistleblowing; second, given the developments in clinical governance and clinical risk management over the past three decades, more-effective processes are now in place in health care organisations across the globe that are enabling staff to raise issues of safety and quality within their organisations without having to resort to the extreme measure of whistleblowing (Johnstone 2004b). Consider the following.

Risks of whistleblowing

As the Moylan, Pugmire, Bardenilla, MacArthur Health Service and the Bundaberg Base Hospital cases have each shown, whistleblowing can be a traumatic (and costly) method of 'putting to right a wrong' (Lee 2002). Rather than seeing a whistleblower's report as an opportunity to improve the system and protect those whose interests have been placed at risk by questionable practices, an organisation whose conditions have been exposed may take a defensive stance and seek, instead, to protect itself (Erlen 1999). Equally troubling is that whistleblowing offers 'no guarantee that the individual or the system will make the necessary changes to improve the situation' (Erlen 1999: 69; see also Bjørkelo 2013).

Whistleblowing always upsets the status quo and accordingly is commonly perceived as 'rocking the boat' (Erlen 1999) – something which, in bureaucratic organisations, is generally regarded as taboo. Thus, even though a nurse might have done the 'right thing', whistleblowing can nevertheless result in him/her being portrayed as a disloyal 'troublemaker' and a 'Judas', and stigmatised and shunned accordingly (Erlen 1999; Rosen 1999). More seriously, *whistleblowers* can also be subjected to soul-destroying retaliation (including denigation and marginalisation) by their employers, their co-workers and even future employers; it can also result in deregistration by nurse regulating authorities (Ahern 2018; Eisenstadt & Pacella 2018; Jackson et al 2014; Kenny et al 2018; Lim et al 2017; Vandekerckhove & Phillips 2017).

Bjørkelo's (2013) exposé of retaliatory behaviours against whistleblowers shows that such behaviours can involve either singular or repeated acts, and can be either *formal* (e.g. unfavourable work evaluations by a manager) or *informal* (e.g. social ostracisation by co-workers) in nature (Bjørkelo 2013). Common unfavourable behaviours in either case can involve: trying to discredit whistleblowing nurses, intimidating them by overly scrutinising the standards of their practice, involuntarily changing their work allocation or location, changing their job title (e.g. demotion), threatening to terminate or actually terminating their jobs, bullying (undermining them and engaging in personally offensive behaviour), and taking legal action against them for defamation (Ahern 2018; Bjørkelo 2013; Eisenstadt & Pacella 2018; Erlen 1999; Jackson et al 2014; Kenny et al 2018; Lim et al 2017; Rosen 1999; Vandekerckhove & Phillips 2017). Furthermore, given that whistleblowing tends to be a protracted process (Vandekerckhove & Phillips 2017) this retaliation can continue long after the situation has been corrected (Rosen 1999). In sum, as the experience of Stephen Bolsin (the UK anaesthetist who famously blew the whistle on problems in paediatric cardiac surgery at the United Bristol Healthcare Trust (UBHT)) warns: speaking out *outside* of an organisation will always make a whistleblower unpopular *inside* that organisation (Bolsin 2003: 294).

Nurses who blow the whistle can also experience serious and significant adverse effects on their physical and mental health as a result of their experience (it will be recalled that Kevin Moylan was left suffering from PTSD as a result of his ordeal). As has been found the case with other whistleblowers, the problems experienced can include (but not be limited to): anxiety, depression, stress-induced lethargy, flash-backs, intrusive thoughts, sleep disturbances, nightmares, headaches, backaches, weight loss / gain, increased substance use (e.g. drugs and alcohol intake, smoking), immunosuppression (manifesting as lingering colds, influenza), gastrointestinal problems, cardiac symptoms, anger, disillusionment, fear, poor self-esteem, and the breakdown of family and other personal relationships (including dislocation of family life, separations and divorce) (Ahern 2018; Bjørkelo 2013; Jackson et al 2010b, 2014; Kenny et al 2018; McDonald 2002; Park & Lewis 2018; Peters et al 2011; Wilkes et al 2011).

Whistleblowing and clinical risk management

Health care systems around the world have implemented clinical governance and clinical risk management processes as part of a global strategy aimed at improving safety and quality in health care and reducing the incidence and impact of preventable adverse events. The World Health Organization (WHO Patient Safety: http://www.who.int/patientsafety/en/) has been at the forefront of this global strategy (see also WHO 2005a, 2005b, 2006a). A key feature of this global agenda is the almost universal recognition that:

> *Safety is everyone's responsibility. Almost everyone working in health care cares about patient safety, in the sense of wanting to do their best for patients. However patient safety needs to be embedded in the culture of health care, not just in the sense of individual high standards, but of a widespread acceptance of a systematic understanding of risk and safety and the need for everyone to actively promote patient safety.* (Vincent 2001: 6)

An essential feature of effective clinical governance is having robust and safe incident reporting systems. As the World Health Organization (WHO) (2005b: 3, 7) has contended in its draft *Guidelines for adverse event reporting and learning systems*:

> *Reporting is fundamental to detecting patient safety problems [...] Some believe that an effective reporting system is the cornerstone of safe practice and, within a hospital or other health-care organization, a measure of progress towards achieving a safety culture. At a minimum, reporting can help identify hazards and risk, and provide information as to where the system is breaking down. This can help target improvement efforts and systems changes to reduce the likelihood of injury of future patients.*

This stance derives from the recognition that, when a mistake is made, admitting and promptly reporting the error to an appropriate authority is the 'right thing to do'. This is because hiding errors can have serious adverse consequences at both a moral and a practical level. At a moral level, hiding of errors (especially those that are clinically significant) may result in:

- *otherwise avoidable harms to patients*; that is, on account of:
  - depriving the relevant parties (doctors, nurses, patients and their loved ones) of information that is otherwise necessary to correct the error that has been made, including the provision of effective post-error care and treatment;
  - depriving the patient (and his / her surrogates) of their entitlement to make informed choices and to provide informed consent to ongoing post-error remedial cares and treatments;
  - imposing on patients and their loved ones an unjust burden of suffering on account of a hidden error not being remedied;
- the nurse–patient fiduciary / trust relationship being seriously undermined and ipso facto the good standing and reputation of the nursing profession as a whole (notably on account of the agreed ethical and professional practice standards of the profession concerning patient safety reporting requirements being violated). (Johnstone & Kanitsaki 2006a: 371–2)

On a practical level, if errors are left unreported then hospital incident data collected may be unreliable and hence misleading, resulting in lost opportunities for valuable 'lessons to be learned' from the mistakes that were made (Johnstone & Kanitsaki 2006b). Without complete data sets, it will not be possible to get a picture of the true nature and frequency of a problem which, if left unchecked, may result in future, otherwise-avoidable, harmful errors occurring (WHO 2005b, 2014c).

Clinical governance and clinical risk management frameworks are enabling staff within the health care sector to raise issues within their organisation both formally and informally as part of their everyday practice and responsibility for ensuring patient safety and quality in health care (Tarrant et al 2017). As these frameworks have become embedded in the culture of health care organisations, and incident reporting becomes accepted as the cornerstone of patient safety (Pham et al 2013; WHO 2005b), the identification and management of risks to safety and quality have become 'normalised' thus reducing the need for staff to have to resort to the extreme measure of whistleblowing. Professional accountability, trust in the incident-reporting system, and a culture of 'learning from error' have also contributed to improved risk management and reporting behaviours (Hewitt et al 2017; Tricarico et al 2017). Even so, challenges remain as research continues to find that staff fear repercussions from incident reporting, or refrain from reporting because of lacking confidence that 'anything will be done' (Hewitt et al 2017; Pham et al 2013; Tricarico et al 2017).

Reporting incompetent, illegal and/or unethical practices in health care is now a codified professional requirement and a professional responsibility (to be discussed in more detail in Chapter 12). Given this, it is curious why making reports concerning such behaviour is still sometimes labelled 'whistleblowing'. As Robbins (1983) points out, reporting improprieties on the part of colleagues, co-workers or associates is not *whistleblowing*, but rather a matter of *professional ethics*. It is also a democratic act of 'truth telling in the workplace' (after Mansbach 2009). Accordingly there is room to contend that the term 'whistleblowing' is not only an unfortunate misnomer (wrong name), but also that it has no place in a contemporary health care system striving to foster a culture of safety and respect (Leape et al 2012). Likewise for the term 'whistleblower': this term is misleading and serves little more than to damn as immoral the acts of those who have had the moral courage to report the immoral acts of others.

Whistleblowing as a last resort

Some contend that whistleblowing has made an important contribution to patient safety and may even have a place in maintaining 'best standards' (Jones & Kelly 2014; Kelly & Jones 2013). Given the risks of 'going public', however, whistleblowing should only ever be considered as a last resort – that is, after all other avenues have been exhausted and attempts to progress open communication about patient safety concerns have gone unheeded.

The risks and benefits of engaging in such action must also be considered carefully. As with any moral decision-making, any nurses contemplating 'going public' should first carefully assess the situation and ensure that they have access to all the relevant facts of the matter (this may include seeking advice from other colleagues or a supervisor). It is important that nurses also have 'back-up' support to assist dealing with the aftermath of their actions should they need it (see Miller 2013). Finally, careful consideration must be given to the moral consequences of such an act and how best to achieve the desirable moral outcomes intended.

Preventing ethics conflicts[2]

Since the early 2000s, growing patient safety concerns have seen the development of a global patient safety movement aimed at reducing the incidence and impact of preventable adverse events in health care. This movement has resulted in health service providers and managers taking a *proactive* rather than a *reactive* approach to promoting a culture of safety in health care organisations around the world. Commensurate with this development (and in recognition of the fundamental linkage between ethics and the quality and safety of patient care) there has been a resurgence of interest in what is called '*preventive ethics*' in health care and 'preventing the predictable' (Pena 2015).

The idea of 'preventive ethics' dates back to the early 1990s and the burgeoning field of bioethics in which increasing attention was being given to ethical issues in the clinical setting (Forrow et al 1993). At that time, the limits of clinical ethics were being recognised, as was the problem that 'waiting until a conflict arises makes resolution of ethical quandaries more difficult' (Forrow et al 1993: 287). Recognising that clinical ethics 'do not arise suddenly, but they develop predictably over time', Forrow and colleagues (1993: 292) proposed a preventive ethics approach as a means to help expand the contributions of clinical ethics and shift attention away from the mischaracterisation of moral conflicts in health care as 'discrete ethical problems' requiring crisis management.

The ethics–quality linkage

Proponents of preventive ethics have recently revitalised the proposal of Forrow and colleagues (1993) and called for a system-orientated preventive approach to ethical issues in health care. This approach is similar to that which has been adopted to help reduce the incidence and impact of preventable *clinical* adverse events in hospitals. Highlighting what has been termed the '*ethics–quality linkage*' (Nelson et al 2010: 526), proponents contend that, by stakeholders collaboratively developing protocols that include 'a clear system for determining the appropriate management of common ethical conflicts that are grounded in ethical principles, patient safety goals and adherence to the organization's mission' (Nelson et al 2008: 20), staff members will be assisted to 'do the right thing'. They go on to suggest that anticipating and preventing ethics conflicts in this way will be more effective than the conventional 'reactive approach' which has long proven to be unsatisfactory because of focusing on complex and catastrophic isolated clinical ethics cases that, once manifest, are near impossible to resolve.

To progress a preventive approach to ethical conflict in health care, a four-step process encompassing the following has been recommended:

1. *identifying recurring ethical issues (e.g. limiting patient rights, DNR directives, informed consent issues, confidentiality and privacy, patient safety concerns, and others)*
2. *studying the issues*
3. *developing an ethical practice protocol, and*
4. *propagating the protocol into the culture of the organisation.* (Nelson et al 2008: 17)

Based on their knowledge and experience of the health care system, as well as their codified obligations as ethical professionals, nurses have an obvious and important role to play in establishing and advancing this four-step process.

Appropriate disagreement

The patient safety movement is principally concerned with reducing the incidence and impact of preventable *clinical* adverse events and promoting patient safety in health care. Even so, as Nelson's proposal suggests there are valuable lessons that can be learned and applied to improving what might be termed here the *moral safety* of health care (Johnstone & Hutchinson 2015). By developing mechanisms for reducing the incidence and impact of 'preventable moral harms' in clinical settings and fostering a 'culture of moral safety', the health care environment can emerge as a safe place that is free of preventable threat to the significant moral interests of those who frequent it. Accepting this, however, there is one notable point of difference that warrants acknowledgement: *the role of 'appropriate' disagreement on ethical issues in the workplace*.

As suggested earlier in this chapter (under the discussion on professional judgment), disagreement on ethical issues in health care contexts is not only inevitable, but ought to be encouraged as a means of 'quality-assuring' the ethical decisions that are made and the processes for making them. Moreover, it is important to understand that moral disagreements in practice need not be the cause of distress. This is because consideration of other points of view can enrich people's moral thinking and experience, can help them to think about old problems in new ways, and can also help them to identify and respond to previously unrecognised problems. This process must, however, remain discretionary and not inadvertently encapsulate rules that could see ethical issues take on a legal form (a risk also with national consensus statements involving ethical issues). If this were to happen, the whole intention and purpose of a preventive ethics approach would be seriously undermined.

Conclusion

Conscientious objection, whistleblowing and preventive ethics mechanisms are all important processes that nurses can use when seeking to fulfill the requirements to 'take appropriate action' in order to prevent or remedy a harm in health care contexts. Being able to use these processes in a just and effective way, however, requires nurses to have sound professional judgment, knowledge and understanding of ethics and its application to and in nursing care contexts, moral wisdom and a willingness to take 'moral risks' in the interests of achieving desired moral outcomes.

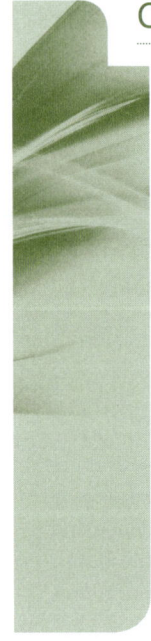

Case scenario 1

In 2012, two Catholic midwives engaged in court action in an attempt to have their right to conscientiously abstain from abortion work protected after allegedly being 'forced' by their employer to supervise staff participating in terminations (BBC News 2012; see also Fleming et al 2018). While not required to directly participate in abortions, both midwives, who were 'labour ward coordinators', were nonetheless required to delegate, supervise and support staff assigned to care for patients undergoing pregnancy terminations. The midwives had reportedly 'given notice of their conscientious objection under the abortion legislation many years ago', but became concerned after termination work was transferred to the labour wards under their supervision (BBC News 2012). The midwives lost their case, however. The judge hearing the case did not agree that their religious rights had been violated, arguing that both midwives were 'sufficiently removed from direct involvement as [...] to afford appropriate respect for and accommodation of their beliefs'. She went on to clarify that the midwives' right of conscientious objection 'was not unqualified and they had agreed to take up the roles of labour ward coordinators, although they now took objection to the job content'. Meanwhile, in a response to the court decision, a spokeswoman for the health board responsible for the midwives' employment reportedly stated:

> We are fully supportive of staff who hold a position of conscientious objection and make every effort to accommodate them, however at the same time we have an unequivocal duty of care to ensure the safety of our patients and as such we must balance this responsibility with the rights of the conscientious objector. (BBC News 2012)

Case scenario 2

In 2011, a nursing student working as a personal care worker in an aged care facility became aware of the death of a 76-year-old female resident, whom she reportedly saw from a window lying face down in a pond located in the facility's courtyard. The student suspected a cover-up when she learned that the family had been told the woman, who suffered from dementia, had died of a 'heart attack' (Lamperd 2013). Although a doctor had been called to certify her death, information was not given that the woman had been found face down in the pond. By the time the family had arrived, staff at the home had dried the woman's body, changed her clothes and had laid her out on her bed (Lamperd 2013). When staff members were allegedly threatened with dismissal if they discussed the circumstances of the elderly woman's death, the student sought advice from the Victorian State Branch of the Australian Nursing and Midwifery Federation (ANMF). The next day, when she arrived for work, she was sacked (Lamperd 2013).

In response to the student's concerns, the ANMF notified the coroner on the student's behalf. Concerned about a 'potential cover up', the ANMF also reported details of the incident to the Police, who were already aware of the matter having been also notified by the Coroner. CCTV footage later confirmed that the elderly resident had lain motionless in the pond for 50 minutes before staff noticed her body (Lamperd 2013). The ANMF also later notified the Federal Department of Health and Ageing and liaised with the Director of the Commonwealth Government aged care complaints scheme.

In a letter to the editor of the *Sunday Herald*, a Melbourne-based tabloid which had omitted details of the ANMF's involvement in the matter, the ANMF unequivocally affirmed 'the need to report accidental and suspicious deaths to the Coroner'. It also highlighted the need 'for laws to protect aged care nurses and personal care workers who bravely speak out on behalf of patients, their families and the community' (Gilbert 2013: 9). It also reiterated that 'the cover up and the distressing impact on [the woman's] family was an important story about events that should not have happened in a nursing home and should never happen again' (Gilbert 2013: 9).

CRITICAL QUESTIONS

1. With regard to Case scenario 1, is it reasonable for staff who are opposed to abortion work to seek employment in organisations that provide abortion services?
2. Reflecting on the abortion issue in general, in what circumstances might a nurse validly claim a 'right' to refuse to provide advice on and/or assist with abortion work and, conversely, a 'duty' to refuse?
3. Some critics are claiming that conscientious objection in reproductive health is 'unworkable', 'frequently abused' and threatens to have 'harmful impacts on women's health care and rights' and therefore should not be permitted.[3] They go even further and controversially contend that conscientious objection in reproductive health 'is not actually *Conscientious Objection*, but *Dishonourable Disobedience*'.[3] Do you agree or disagree with this stance? Give reasons for your answers.
4. Reflecting on Case scenario 2, what would you have done if you had found yourself in the same circumstances as the nursing student depicted in this case?
5. If, after reporting your concerns to an appropriate authority, nothing was done about the matter, what would you do? Would you 'blow the whistle'?
6. If you decided to 'blow the whistle' what steps would you take to ensure you were doing the 'right thing'?

Endnotes

1. An earlier version of the discussion of conscientious objection was presented as a paper entitled 'Conscientious objection and professional obligation – a contradiction in terms?' at Nursing Law and Ethics, 2nd Victorian State Conference, Dealing with dilemmas, Monash University, 5 May 1989 (organised by the School of Nursing, Phillip Institute of Technology, now RMIT University). The paper has been substantially revised for publication in this text.
2. The original was published in the *Australian Nursing and Midwifery Journal*, © 2014 ANMF. Revised for inclusion in this chapter, with permission.
3. Fiala C & Arthur J H (2014) 'Dishonourable disobedience' – why refusal to treat in reproductive healthcare is not conscientious objection. *Woman – Psychosomatic Gynaecology and Obstetrics*, 1: 12–23.

CHAPTER 12

Professional obligations to report harmful behaviours: risks to patient safety, child abuse and elder abuse

KEYWORDS

child abuse
child maltreatment
child protection
child protection services
elder abuse
elder maltreatment
impaired conduct
mandatory and voluntary reporting
notifiable conduct
protective interventions
redressing elder abuse
violence

LEARNING OBJECTIVES

Upon the completion of this chapter and with further self-directed learning you are expected to be able to:

- Define 'notifiable conduct' as set out in legislative provisions regulating health practitioners.
- Distinguish between 'notifiable conduct' and 'health-impaired conduct' as set out in legislative provisions regulating health practitioners.
- Discuss critically four principles that might be appealed to for guiding decisions about whether to make a notification to a practitioner regulating authority.
- Discuss critically the ethical requirements for reporting wrongdoing by a registered practitioner or student to a practitioner regulating authority.
- Define child abuse.
- Discuss critically the significance of child abuse and its prevention as a moral issue.
- Explore possible ethical issues associated with the identification and prevention of child abuse.
- Examine critically the moral responsibilities of nurses and the broader nursing profession in regard to the mandatory and voluntary notification of child abuse.
- Define elder abuse.
- Discuss critically the significance of elder abuse and its prevention as a moral issue.
- Explore ethical issues commonly associated with the identification and prevention of elder abuse.
- Examine critically the moral responsibilities of nurses and the broader nursing profession with regard to intervening and preventing elder abuse.
- Discuss critically the similarities and differences between child abuse and elder abuse.

Introduction

At some stage during the course of their work, nurses will encounter a situation in which they may be required either by law or by professional conduct standards to report to an 'appropriate authority' (either internal or external to their employer organisation) the harmful behaviour of another, or intervene in some other way to prevent the harm that might be caused by the behaviour in question. In either case, even though making a notification or initiating some other *protective intervention* is the 'right thing to do', it is not necessarily an easy thing to do – not least because of the moral quandaries that a nurse contemplating a protective intervention might experience in the process. This chapter discusses some of the ethical issues associated with requirements to report 'wrongdoing' or to initiate a protective intervention. Three key requirements will be considered: (i) reporting the notifiable and/or health-impaired conduct of practitioners and students to a practitioner regulating authority; (ii) reporting known or suspected cases of child abuse and neglect to a child protection agency; and (iii) engaging in a protective intervention in cases of elder abuse and neglect.

Reporting notifiable and health-impaired conduct of practitioners and students

Most jurisdictions in Western democracies have legislative provisions requiring health professionals (including nurses) to report to a practitioner regulating authority (in the case of nurses, a nursing board or council) any conduct or health impairment that is reasonably believed to place the safety of the public at serious risk.

Legal requirements to report wrongdoing

As noted in the previous chapter, reporting sources of risk and actual incidents resulting in patient harm is widely recognised as being the 'cornerstone of safe practice and, within a hospital or other health care organisation, a measure of progress towards achieving a safety culture' (World Health Organization (WHO) 2005b: 7). Reporting, however, is not restricted to notification solely of clinical incidents or adverse events. It can also include notifications of 'disruptive behaviour' defined as 'any behavior that can undermine a culture of safety'– for example, 'any inappropriate behavior, confrontation, or conflict ranging from verbal abuse to physical or sexual harassment that can potentially negatively impact patient care' (Rosenstein 2017: 62).

In Australian jurisdictions since 1 July 2010, registered health practitioners (including nurses), employers of practitioners, and education providers have been mandated under the Australian *Health Practitioner Regulation National Law Act* (2009) (referred to hereon in as the 'National Law') to report to the Australian Health Practitioner Regulation Agency (AHPRA) any 'notifiable conduct' or 'notifiable impairment' as defined in Section 140 of the National Law (AHPRA 2014). For the purposes of the Act, *'notifiable conduct'* is taken to mean any conduct whereby the health practitioner has: practised while intoxicated by alcohol or drugs, engaged in sexual misconduct in connection with the practice of their profession, practised while suffering from an impairment that places the public at risk of substantial harm, or practised the profession in a way that constitutes a significant departure from accepted professional standards (National Law, Section 140). The relevant section of the Act is reproduced in Box 12.1.

'Impairment', in turn, is taken to mean conduct in relation to a person (i.e. practitioner or student) and where the person has a physical or mental impairment, disability, condition or disorder (including substance abuse or dependence) that detrimentally affects or is likely to detrimentally affect their capacity to practise their profession, or, in the case of students, their capacity to undertake clinical training as part

> **BOX 12.1 Definition of 'notifiable conduct'**
>
> **Division 2 Mandatory Notifications**
> 140. Definition of notifiable conduct
> In this Division –
> **notifiable conduct**, in relation to a registered health practitioner, means the practitioner has –
> (a) practised the practitioner's profession while intoxicated by alcohol or drugs; or
> (b) engaged in sexual misconduct in connection with the practice of the practitioner's profession; or
> (c) placed the public at risk of substantial harm in the practitioner's practice of the profession because the practitioner has an impairment; or
> (d) placed the public at risk of harm because the practitioner has practised the profession in a way that constitutes a significant departure from accepted professional standards.
>
> •••••••••••••
> (*Health Practitioner Regulation National Law Act 2009*, Section 140, p 100, current as at 9 June 2018)

> **BOX 12.2 Definition of 'impairment'**
>
> **5. Definitions**
> In this Law –
> **impairment**, in relation to a person, means the person has a physical or mental impairment, disability, condition or disorder (including substance abuse or dependence) that detrimentally affects or is likely to detrimentally affect –
> (a) for a registered health practitioner or an applicant for registration in a health profession, the person's capacity to practise the profession; or
> (b) for a student, the student's capacity to undertake clinical training –
>   (i) as part of the approved program of study in which the student is enrolled; or
>   (ii) arranged by an education provider.
>
> •••••••••••••
> (*Health Practitioner Regulation National Law Act 2009*, Schedule 5, Part 1 Preliminary, pp 13–14, current as at 9 June 2018)

of the approved program of study, or arranged by an education provider (National Law, Schedule 5). The relevant section of the Act is reproduced in Box 12.2.

In addition, the National Law contains provisions for making *voluntary notifications* 'for behaviour that presents a risk but does not meet the threshold for notifiable conduct' (AHPRA 2014: 5). Under these provisions, a voluntary notification about a registered health practitioner may be made to AHPRA on a number of grounds, including: where the practitioner's professional conduct, knowledge and skill are, or may be, of a lesser standard than that which might reasonably be expected by the public or the practitioner's professional peers; the practitioner is not, or may not be, a 'fit and proper person' to hold registration in the health profession; the practitioner has contravened the Law, or a condition of practice given by the practitioner's registration board; or the practitioner has improperly obtained registration by providing false or misleading information. The relevant section of the Act is reproduced in Box 12.3.

Under these provisions, a voluntary notification about a student can also be made to AHPRA on the grounds that the student has been charged with, found guilty and convicted of an offence that is punishable by 12 months imprisonment or more; has, or may have, an impairment; or has contravened

> **BOX 12.3 Grounds for voluntary notification**
>
> **Division 3 Voluntary Notifications**
> 144. Grounds for voluntary notification
>
> (1) A voluntary notification about a registered health practitioner may be made to the National Agency on any of the following grounds –
>   (a) that the practitioner's professional conduct is, or may be, of a lesser standard than that which might reasonably be expected of the practitioner by the public or the practitioner's professional peers;
>   (b) that the knowledge, skill or judgment possessed, or care exercised by, the practitioner in the practice of the practitioner's health profession is, or may be, below the standard reasonably expected;
>   (c) that the practitioner is not, or may not be, a suitable person to hold registration in the health profession, including, for example, that the practitioner is not a fit and proper person to be registered in the profession;
>   (d) that the practitioner has, or may have, an impairment;
>   (e) that the practitioner has, or may have, contravened this Law;
>   (f) that the practitioner has, or may have, contravened a condition of the practitioner's registration or an undertaking given by the practitioner to a National Board;
>   (g) that the practitioner's registration was, or may have been, improperly obtained because the practitioner or someone else gave the National Board information or a document that was false or misleading in a material particular.
>
> ....
> (*Health Practitioner Regulation National Law Act 2009*, Schedule, Part 8 Health, Performance and conduct, pp 103–104, current as at 9 June 2018)

a condition of the student's registration or an undertaking given by the student to a National Board. The relevant section of the Act is reproduced in Box 12.4.

It is important to note that the threshold for making a notification to AHPRA is high and must be based firmly on a 'reasonable belief' (as opposed to a mere suspicion) that the behaviour in question meets the criteria for 'notifiable conduct' or 'notifiable impairment'. To assist those contemplating making a notification, the Australian Health Practitioners Regulation Agency (AHPRA) has devised the following principles:

> 1. *A belief is a state of mind.*
> 2. *A reasonable belief is a belief based on reasonable grounds.*
> 3. *A belief is based on reasonable grounds when,*
>   (i) *all known considerations relevant to the formation of a belief are taken into account including matters of opinion and*
>   (ii) *those known considerations are objectively assessed.*
> 4. *A just and fair judgement that reasonable grounds exist in support of a belief can be made when all known considerations are taken into account and objectively assessed.* (AHPRA 2012: 6)

Further clarifying the nature of what constitutes a 'reasonable belief', AHPRA explains:

> *A reasonable belief requires a stronger level of knowledge than a mere suspicion. Generally it would involve direct knowledge or observation of the behaviour which gives rise to the notification, or, in the case of an*

> **BOX 12.4** Voluntary notifications about students
>
> **Division 3 Voluntary Notifications**
> 144. Grounds for voluntary notification
> (2) A voluntary notification about a student may be made to the National Agency on the grounds that –
>   (a) the student has been charged with an offence, or has been convicted or found guilty of an offence, that is punishable by 12 months imprisonment or more; or
>   (b) the student has, or may have, an impairment; or
>   (c) that the student has, or may have, contravened a condition of the student's registration or an undertaking given by the student to a National Board.
>
> •••••••••••••
> (*Health Practitioner Regulation National Law Act 2009*, Section 144, p 173, current as at 9 June 2018)

employer, it could also involve a report from a reliable source or sources. Mere speculation, rumours, gossip or innuendo are not enough to form a reasonable belief. (AHPRA 2014: 6)

Forming a reasonable belief and deciding to act on it, in turn, requires both professional judgment (discussed in Chapter 11) and moral justification (discussed in Chapter 3). To help guide the decision-making processes, the AHPRA (2014) published a set of guidelines pertinent to the kinds of notifications that health practitioners (including nurses) are required to make. These include examples of decision guides for significant departure from accepted professional standards and for impairment in relation to practitioners and students respectively (https://www.ahpra.gov.au/notifications/make-a-complaint/mandatory-notifications.aspx).

In New Zealand, under the *Health Practitioners Competence Assurance Act* (2003) similar provisions exists requiring health practitioners to make notifications of practice that 'may pose a risk of harm to the public by practising below the required standard of competence' and/or when a practitioner has an 'inability to perform required functions due to [a] mental or physical condition' (Section 3).

Professional requirements to report wrongdoing

Some nurses might worry that making a notification, even though a legal requirement, is a breach of professional ethics. This might be especially so in cases where making a notification requires breaching privacy and confidentiality (discussed in Chapter 7), or violating the nurse–patient relationship (e.g. in instances where the nurse being reported is also a patient). Nurses might also experience a profound quandary where the legal mandate to make a notification involves and would violate an important interpersonal relationship (e.g. in instances where the nurse needing to be reported is a spouse or intimate partner, a relative, a close friend and/or a trusted and highly valued colleague).

As mandated reporting requirements are fundamentally based on the moral imperative to prevent or mitigate harm to the public, making either a mandatory or a voluntary notification is not generally considered to be a breach of professional ethics or a departure from accepted ethical standards of conduct (AHPRA 2014: 5). Moreover, as nursing codes of conduct in Australia, New Zealand and elsewhere make clear, reporting to an appropriate authority behaviours such as those described in the Australian National Law (AHPRA 2014) is not only a legal obligation, but, in clearly defined instances, also a moral one. Consider the following.

The codified moral obligation of nurses to report to an 'appropriate authority' any conduct or behaviour that places others at risk of serious harm is well established. For example, *The ICN code of ethics for nurses* (ICN 2012a) states (Element 4: Nurses and co-workers, p 3):

The nurse takes appropriate action to safeguard individuals when their care is endangered by a co-worker or any other person.

Other national nursing codes and standards take a similar stance, with appropriate action described as including but not limited to questioning, reporting and intervening to redress an instance of questionable behaviour.

The codified obligation to 'take appropriate action' is not unique to the cultural context of Australia. The Nursing Council of New Zealand (NCNZ 2012a), the UK Nursing and Midwifery Council (NMC 2015), the Canadian Nurses Association (2017) and the American Nurses Association (ANA 2015) have each articulated similar requirements in their respective codes of ethics and conduct.

Interestingly, most codes and guidelines stop short of addressing *how* a nurse should respond in instances where he/she has an intimate personal relationship with the nurse needing to be reported – for instance, the notifiable or *impaired conduct* at issue is being exhibited by a spouse or intimate partner, an immediate relative, a close friend, and/or a trusted and highly valued colleague with whom the nurse is on a close collaborating professional relationship (e.g. co-researcher). Not only is the nurse faced with a conflict of obligation in such situations, but he/she also risks significantly damaging and possibly even destroying irrevocably the personal relationship(s) in question. This is so even if an intended or actual notification is well intended, and made in good faith and without malice, and in the hope of, say, getting the partner, relative or good friend assistance to 'get back on track' professionally.

In the USA, some states exempt the reporting of 'spouses by spouses' and nurses who are in a professional–client relationship (Buppert & Klein 2008: 6). Most also limit the reporting requirement to 'directly observed incidents' – that is, not 'confiding' disclosures made to an intimate partner or spouse (Buppert & Klein 2008: 6). Despite the obvious conflict of interest involved in partner reports, the Australian National Law and related guidelines are, however, silent on this matter. Controversially, exemptions are not made for treating practitioners (e.g. a medical practitioner, psychologist, dentist, nurse or chiropractor) who are treating other registered practitioners – although, at the time of writing, this was under review. In a discussion paper 'Mandatory reporting under the Health Practitioner Regulation National Law', the Australian Health Ministers Advisory Council (AHMAC) has proposed a change to the National Law to allow an exemption for treating practitioners – clarifying, however, that if the amendment goes ahead, 'the employers and other registered health practitioners who are not treating practitioners, such as colleagues, would continue to be under an obligation to report notifiable conduct' (AHMAC 2017: 4).

The possibility of making spouse-by-spouse/friend-by-friend notifications conditional or voluntary seems not to have been considered. For example, decisions to make notifications could be made using a modified version of what Hickson and colleagues (2007) have described in another context as a 'complementary approach to professionalism'. This approach involves the following steps:

> *informal conversations for single incidents, nonpunitive 'awareness' interventions when data reveal patterns, leader-developed action plans if patterns persist, and imposition of disciplinary processes if the plans fail.*
> (Hickson et al 2007: 1040)

In the case of spouse-by-spouse/friend-by-friend reporting, this could be made conditional on a reporting nurse first going *directly to the wrongdoer/health-impaired practitioner* to have an informal conversation (e.g. 'I have observed you do X, can we talk about this and the option of you making a self-report to the Board to get help'; or 'I have observed you do X, if you do this again I will have no option but to make a notification'). This would also have the effect of being a 'non-punitive awareness intervention' (what might be termed colloquially as a 'wake-up call' for the wrongdoer/health-impaired practitioner to acknowledge 'they have a problem' and to take personal responsibility for their own actions).

'No blame' culture and patient safety

Some nurses might also worry that reporting errant practitioners to an appropriate authority goes against the principles of human error management, which have been widely adopted and operationalised in health services locally and globally. There is some foundation to this concern, although, in recent years, the basis upon which such concerns might have rested has since been called into question for the reasons given below.

In 2002, in response to growing international concerns about the alarming incidence of preventable adverse events in health care, patient safety was, for the first time, situated as 'a worldwide endeavour, seeking to bring benefits to patients in countries rich and poor, developed and developing, in all corners of the globe' (Donaldson 2002: 112). This endeavour was informed by the influential publication of the US Institute of Medicine's *To err is human* (Kohn et al 2000). In the intervening years, health services around the world have embraced a 'no blame' model in their approach to managing human error and attempts to reduce the incidence and impact of preventable adverse events in their organisations. This model has been adopted in good faith and in response to a well-argued need to shift away from what had traditionally been a punitive hospital culture of 'naming, blaming and shaming' individuals who, due to their human fallibility (including 'forgetfulness, inattention or moral weaknesses') made an honest mistake; this approach has been termed the 'person approach' by safety scientists (Reason 2000). In its place, an alternative approach was proposed – the 'system approach', which, unlike the person approach, 'concentrates on the conditions under which individuals work and tries to build defences to avert errors or mitigate their effects' (Reason 2000: 768). Whereas the *person approach* singled out individuals to blame when things went wrong, the *system approach* focused on the weaknesses and failures of 'the system' (not individuals), which enabled what James Reason (2000: 769) famously called a 'trajectory of accident opportunity' that brings hazards into 'damaging contact with victims'. In this approach, when things go wrong, the question to ask is not '*Who* messed up?' but 'What contributed to the system failing?' As Reason argues, if the same system weaknesses and conditions persist (e.g. poor storage and labelling of drugs), the same errors (e.g. medication errors) will continue to be made regardless of who it is at the interface of the patient–provider relationship.

A key objective in encouraging the organisational cultural change from a 'person approach' to a 'system approach' was to encourage errant practitioners to report their mistakes voluntarily and to increase voluntary incident reporting generally. It was held that, once reported, a careful analysis of the adverse events in question could be made, and staff and their employer organisation afforded an important opportunity to learn from their mistakes and put in place processes that would help prevent their reoccurrence (Reason 2000). Safe reporting, in this instance, was thus seen to be not only of practical value, but also quintessential to achieving patient safety outcomes because, as Bagian and colleagues (2001: 524) put it: 'You can't fix what you don't know about'.

Although initially resulting in a productive cultural change in health care organisations, the 'no blame' approach had an unintended consequence: it saw professional accountability for poor behaviour shift away from individual practitioners to 'the system'. The poor behaviours in question included practitioners': *intentional and routine rule violations* (i.e. knowingly disregarding rules or procedures, including wilfully 'cutting corners' and the 'normalisation of deviance' – for example, routine failures in everyday practice to perform hand hygiene (Goldman 2006), or failures by staff to don personal protective equipment to prevent the transmission of infectious agents (Krein et al 2018)), *reckless conduct* (involving a 'conscious disregard of substantial and unjustifiable risk') and *negligence* (failing to exercise due care) (Banja 2010; Marx 2001). Concerned about the risks posed to patient safety by 'repeat offenders' and 'bad apples' – defined as 'individuals who repeatedly display incompetent or grossly unprofessional behaviours' (Shojania & Dixon-Woods 2013: 529) – proponents of the new patient safety movement started to experience disquiet about the 'system approach' and seriously questioned whether the right balance had been achieved between 'system failure' and 'personal accountability' (Goldman 2006; Levitt 2014; O'Connor et al 2011; Shojania & Dixon-Woods 2013; Wachter & Pronovost 2009; Walton 2004; Wong & Ginsburg 2017). While recognising that every safe industry has its 'transgressors' (Wachter & Pronovost 2009: 1402), the growing tradition of what some described as the 'lax enforcement of safety rules' was perceived to have led many clinicians to ignore them (Wachter & Pronovost 2009: 1403). Recognising the need for the early identification, management and, where able, the remediation of 'problem clinicians', the imperative to reinstate individual accountability as a cornerstone of patient safety thus gained traction.

An important step towards identifying problem clinicians and reinstating personal accountability is the mechanism of internal reporting. Although research has suggested that clinicians cannot be relied upon to report 'poor conduct or performance', internal reporting nonetheless stands as an important mechanism for weeding out 'bad apples' (Shojania & Dixon-Woods 2013: 529). To be effective, however, other more robust mechanisms for improving an organisation's patient safety culture need also to be in place. Drawing on Walton's (2004) clarion call for finding the 'right' balance between individual accountability and patient safety, the following three processes warrant consideration, notably that:

- *professionalism in the workplace becomes part of the safety agenda*
- *methods for managing and responding to intentional violations by individuals in the workplace are devised and operationalised (this should include 'building in sanctions for routine violations and rewards for workplace compliance')*
- *clinicians are taught not only about the inevitability of mistakes but also how best to respond to them.*
(Adapted from Walton 2004: 164)

Attitudes and experiences of reporting patient safety concerns

As noted above, reporting patient safety concerns is the right thing to do. This is because hiding of patient safety concerns can have serious adverse consequences at a moral and a practical level. For instance, the hiding of clinical errors, substandard or unethical practice may result in otherwise preventable harm to patients on account of the relevant parties being deprived of information that is otherwise necessary to effect the prevention or mitigation of possible adverse outcomes. This, in turn, risks undermining the fiduciary / trust relationship between stakeholders both within and outside of a given agency and ipso facto its otherwise good standing and reputation in the community. Despite these risks, research has shown that clinicians (including nurses) have mixed attitudes to and experiences of fulfilling this professional obligation to report, with instances of adverse events, substandard or inadequate care, unethical or 'poor' behaviours by staff towards patients and co-workers, and health-impaired practice tending to be substantially under-reported (Bismark et al 2014, 2016; Firth-Cozens et al 2003; Malmedal et al 2009; Monroe & Kenaga 2010; Roberts 2017; Weenink et al 2014). Despite the radical shift in attitude and organisational culture that has occurred in recent years, notably from a 'name, blame and shame' culture to a 'just culture' (Dekker 2012), research suggests that practitioners remain reluctant to make notification even when legally mandated to do so (Bismark et al 2014, 2016; Spittal et al 2016). There is a particular reluctance to report disruptive behaviour (unprofessional conduct) even though it is known that such behaviour can adversely affect patient safety (Bismark et al 2016; Wong & Ginsburg 2017). In their analysis of the outcomes of notifications to AHPRA, for example, Spittal and colleagues (2016: 9) found that notifications concerning the health, conduct or performance of a health practitioner were 'a rare event'.

Robust comparative research on this subject is not available (mostly because of researchers confusing or conflating 'regular' internal incident reporting with 'irregular' whistleblowing events, their using vignettes and hypothetical case scenarios instead of interviewing or surveying nurses who *actually made reports*, and various methodological weaknesses – including small samples, poor response rates, and nurses choosing not to participate). Even so, there are sufficient studies to suggest that, where nurses feel certain and confident, and that their concerns are well founded (i.e. they have 'proof'), they tend to have a strong attitude towards reporting poor care and behaviour (Firth-Cozens et al 2003; King & Scudder 2013; Moumtzoglou 2010; Weenink et al 2014).

Research also suggests that most nurses who have *actually* made internal reports of substandard care did not have a negative experience. A study by Firth-Cozens and colleagues (2003: 334), for example, found that most of the nurses surveyed ($n=342$) did not have a negative experience and, furthermore, that 'almost all would report again in such circumstances'. Nonetheless, a minority ($n=19$, or 27%) of the nurse respondents reported experiencing stress and, in one case, victimisation by a ward manager (e.g. 'not being given holidays or off duty when requested') (Firth-Cozens et al 2003: 333). Several participants in that study also reported 'disillusionment' on grounds of 'no action being taken' in response to their reports, or, in some instances, being made the subject of counter-accusations.

A study by King and Scudder (2013: 626) meanwhile has found that, when faced with reporting a colleague, nurses experience a struggle between maintaining 'their own ethical standards and personal survival within the social system of their nursing environment'. Of the 238 registered nurses who participated in this study, 30% ($n=71$) reported having directly observed a wrongdoing and, of these, 90% ($n=64$) reported the incident. Concurring with the study by Firth-Cozens and colleagues (2003), the King and Scudder study also found that only a minority ($n=67$, or 28%) of respondents reported a negative experience upon reporting a wrongdoing. Significantly, the main reasons given for making the reports were a perceived threat to the wellbeing of patients as well as a 'strong sense of personal and professional ethics' (King & Scudder 2013: 633).

The moral motivations behind peer-reporting by registered nurses were similarly identified in an earlier study by King. In a study of 372 nurses, King (2001: 10) found that the nurses' decision to report a peer was strongly influenced by their perceptions of *intentionality* of the wrongdoing, the *severity* of the wrongdoing and the *blatancy* of the wrongdoing – especially in the case of unethical conduct. Decisions not to report, in contrast, were primarily influenced by the nurses' perception that the wrongdoing was not intentional; in these instances, rather than report the wrongdoing, the nurses tended to confront the wrongdoer directly. Other factors previously identified by King and colleagues have been the *individual characteristics of the observer* (e.g. personal ethics), *situational factors* (e.g. severity of the wrongdoing) and *organisational issues* (e.g. compliance or non-compliance with policy and procedure) (King 1997; King & Hermodson 2000). Research by King and colleagues has also found that nurses who are 'newcomers' to an organisation, who are unfamiliar with the correct reporting procedures, who perceive themselves as powerless to bring about effective change, who fear reprimand and/or who perceive the climate of their employer organisation as being retaliatory are less likely to report a wrongdoing than are others (King & Hermodson 2000: 320).

Another relatively unacknowledged factor influencing whether nurses will report a wrongdoing is 'interpersonal closeness' – including friendships and other close interpersonal relationships with colleagues (King 1997). In an early study by King, involving the survey of 261 registered nurses employed at an acute care non-profit hospital in a large metropolitan city, respondents indicated that they were less likely to report a close friend's wrongdoing to an immediate supervisor, but would report the conduct to an administrator (King 1997). Reasons for this were speculated to be twofold: 'First […] reporting a close friend would likely foster the perception of disloyalty or betrayal, resulting in the loss of a friend. Second, employees within the organisation may perceive the betrayal as grounds to ostracize the person' (King 1997: 430).

Although limited, research on reporting a *health-impaired* (as opposed to an errant or unethical) practitioner has yielded mixed results. Although nurses have an obligation to report peer substance abuse and other impairments to a nurse regulating authority, many are reluctant to do so (Monroe & Kenaga 2010). Even so, a small US study involving 120 nurses found that the psychologically validated estimate of the odds of a nurse reporting a co-worker for substance use while at work were 5 to 1 (92.5% / 20.4%) (Beckstead 2005: 329). Despite a suggested reluctance to report, one recent US study by Cook (2013) has found that, of the 119 nurses surveyed, nearly all indicated that they would report a nurse colleague who was impaired by alcohol (99%), illegal drugs (99%) or prescription medicine (98%). Significantly, respondents also indicated that they were 'willing to trust their recovering colleagues' and strongly agreed that nurses in recovery 'should be allowed to return to the healthcare profession' (Cook 2013: 21; see also Miller et al 2015). This study is limited, however, as the survey had as its focus what the nurse participants *believed* they would do (e.g. 'I would report a nurse …') rather than what they had *actually done* in a practice context (e.g. 'I reported a nurse …').

In a small study by Monroe and Kenaga (2010) it was found that nurses were also generally reluctant to *self-report* their own health-impaired practice. The main reason for this was fear of reprisal (including deregistration and termination of employment) even though the nurses in question were in need of help and despite the fact that nurse regulating agencies having in place remediation or 'alternative discipline' programs (Monroe & Kenaga 2010).

In Australian vernacular, reporting a colleague could be construed as being tantamount to 'dobbing in a mate' – something that, culturally, is generally regarded as being outside the boundaries of decency. In cases of 'mateship', spouse by spouse, and other intimates making notifications, irrespective of the mandatory reporting requirements and the moral justifications that might underpin an obligation to report, making a notification might nonetheless be deemed by notifiers to be intrusive of the private sphere of their personal relationships and, all things being equal, insufficient to override personal loyalties and the personal relationship ethics underpinning these loyalties. What moral weight ought to be given to the 'loyalties' in question, however, is open to question.

Loyalty has been equated with 'dutifulness'. As Ladd (1967: 98) has classically argued:

> *Loyalty includes fidelity to carrying out one's duties to the person or group of persons who are the object of loyalty; but it embraces more than that, for it implies an attitude, perhaps an affection or sentiment, towards such persons. Furthermore, at the very least, loyalty requires the complete subordination of one's own private interests in favour of giving what is due, and perhaps also the exclusion of other legitimate interests.* (quoted in Ewin 1992: 404–5)

Notwithstanding judgments about what objects (persons, groups, causes) are worthy of a person's loyalty, as Ewin (1992: 411) points out, one of the things about loyalty is that 'it appears to involve as part of itself a setting aside of good judgment, at least to some extent'. What is at issue in professional contexts, however, is the demand to *invoke* good judgment (not set it aside) and to complement this with sound moral justification (discussed in Chapter 3 of this book). It is also fundamentally about 'doing the right thing' and somehow finding the 'right balance' between competing loyalties where these are in play.

Whether loyalties to a particular person, group or cause are deemed 'good' or 'bad' it is understandable that a nurse might feel compelled to 'set aside good judgment' and to exclude 'other legitimate interests' when faced with the obligation to mandatorily report a wrongdoing or an instance of health-impaired practice by a spouse or a 'mate'. The failure to take into account the 'split loyalties' that a nurse in such a situation might have is a significant oversight in legislative provisions and guidelines on mandatory reporting and one that stands in need of being redressed.

Interestingly, the issue of resolving the possible tensions that might exist between personal loyalties and 'doing what is right' is not new, with recorded debate related to the subject dating back to the Ancient Greek Socratic dialogues, notably Plato's *Euthyphro* (circa 399 BC). In this dialogue (Book IV,

Sections 4–5), Euthyphro reveals that he (Euthyphro) has brought a murder charge against his own father for allowing one of his workers to die (Plato 1886 edn: 7–9; see also 2003 edn: 11–12). The worker had, in a drunken rage, killed a slave belonging to one of the family's estates. Not sure what to do, Euthyphro's father bound and gagged the worker and left him in a ditch while he sent a messenger to seek advice from a seer in Athens on what he should do. While waiting for the messenger to return, Euthyphro's father totally neglected the worker 'thinking that he was a murderer, and that it would be no great matter, even if he were to die' (IV-4) (Plato 1886 edn: 7). It was under the conditions of being bound, starving and exposed to the cold that the worker died.

Euthyphro's family was astonished and indignant that he sought to prosecute his father for murder, an act which they regarded as 'unholy' ('It is unholy for a son to prosecute his father for murder') (IV-4) (p 8). Against Euthyphro's stance, the family argued that the father 'did not kill the man at all' and that 'even if he had killed him over and over again, the man himself was a murderer' (IV-4) (p 7). Underscoring this indignation was that, in Athenian law, only relatives were permitted to sue for murder, thus Euthyphro's actions were 'unnecessary'. Euthyphro was, however, unmoved by these assertions, arguing that 'holiness means prosecuting the wrong doer […] whether he be your father or your mother or whoever he be' and that 'unholiness means not prosecuting him' (V-5) (p 9). Euthyphro further defends his decision to bring the murder charges against his father, arguing (IV-4) (p 7):

> *What difference does it make whether the murdered man was a relative or a stranger? The only question that you may ask is, did the slayer slay justly or not? If justly, you must let him alone; if unjustly, you must indict him for murder, even though he share your hearth and sit at your table. The pollution is the same, if you associate with such a man, knowing what he has done, without purifying yourself, and him too, by bringing him to justice.*

Euthyphro brought the charges ostensibly on grounds that it was the 'pious' (supremely right and virtuous) thing to do since, regardless of the fact that the offender was his father, to kill someone without justification deserves to be punished. Socrates, however, is not taken by this argument and questions how much justification is 'enough' to distinguish pious from impious actions.

Although the *Euthyphro* is primarily concerned with attempts to define piety and holiness, it nonetheless provides a useful frame for examining the question under consideration here, namely: 'When, if ever, is it "right" for a spouse, partner, close friend, etc. to report a wrongdoing to a regulating authority?' and 'What is to count as a *reasonable justification* for making a decision either for or against making a notification?' A Socratic irony also emerges in this instance, notably: *'Is reporting an instance of wrongdoing by an intimate "right" because it is required by law, or does the law require the reporting of a wrongdoing by an intimate because it is right?'*

To date, the attitudes and experiences of nurses reporting patient safety concerns and the related ethical issues they have faced in fulfilling their obligations in relation to both *mandatory and voluntary reporting* requirements is an area that is under-investigated. Meanwhile, nurses have a responsibility to check the mandatory reporting requirements (and possible exceptions) of the jurisdictions in which they work and also to be familiar with their national codes of conduct and ethics relating to these requirements. Ultimately, however, the decision to report a wrongdoing must be based not only on a blind obedience to law, but also on sound professional judgment and moral justification.

Reporting child abuse and elder abuse

There is arguably no greater issue that brings into focus the pressing tensions that can exist between the ethical, legal and clinical dimensions of nursing, or that tests the relevance and applicability of the common ethical theories and codes guiding professional nursing conduct, than legal requirements to report to a designated authority (e.g. a person, government department, or other protective agency) known or suspected cases of child abuse. Also testing the integrity of professional ethics are situations involving the abuse of elderly people. Although many jurisdictions currently do not have specific laws criminalising 'elder abuse' or mandating a requirement to report known or suspected cases of elder abuse (unless occurring in an aged care facility), the abuse of older people – as of any adult person – may nonetheless constitute a criminal act (e.g. physical assault, sexual assault, stalking, neglect, unlawful confinement, fraud, theft, domestic violence, etc.) requiring protective intervention, including making a report to the police.

Children and elderly people (in particular older people who are frail and/or dependent on others for care) are amongst the most vulnerable members of society. Although it should be otherwise, because of generally being unable to defend and protect themselves, children and dependent elderly people are particularly at risk of abuse and neglect by those who are more powerful than them – including their primary carers. Authorities have come to recognise that, unless intervention and help is offered by benevolent others, the abuse and neglect of children and elderly people rarely stops. It is for this reason that jurisdictions in common-law countries around the world have introduced various mechanisms, ranging from abuse identification and prevention units, to guardianship regimens (particularly for those with impaired decision-making capacity) and mandatory and voluntary reporting laws, in an attempt to prevent and reduce the well-documented harms that the abuse and neglect of children and elderly people cause.

Whether acting on a mandated or on a voluntary basis, making a notification to a designated protection or law enforcement authority is not necessarily an easy course of action to take; nor is it free of moral risk. Despite the possible moral risks and quandaries associated with intervening to prevent or stop abuse and neglect, this issue has received surprisingly little attention in either the mainstream bioethics or the nursing ethics literature. Because of this oversight, nurses may not be as familiar as they need to be with the ethical issues associated with making notifications of child abuse to protection authorities, or intervening to protect the elderly such as by notifying a geriatric assessment team, general practitioner, guardianship board or a law enforcement agency. Thus, in the remainder of this chapter, attention will be given to examining briefly the ethical issues commonly associated with the shared responsibility that nurses have to co-participate in processes aimed at reducing the incidence and harmful impact of the abuse and neglect of children and dependent elderly people in society.

Child abuse and neglect

Internationally there has been the growing recognition that child maltreatment and its harmful consequences can and ought to be prevented (WHO & International Society for the Prevention of Child Abuse and Neglect (ISPCAN) 2006). As the United Nations (UN) has made clear:

> *no violence against children is justifiable, and all violence against children is preventable ... whether accepted as 'traditional' or disguised as 'discipline'.* (Pinheiro 2006: 3)

In keeping with this stance, common-law countries around the world have enacted *child protection* legislation mandating the notification of known or suspected cases of child abuse and neglect to designated child protection authorities (Mathews & Kenny 2008). Over the past three decades, nurses have been increasingly named in legislative provisions mandating the notification to a relevant protection authority known or suspected cases of child abuse and neglect (Johnstone 1999b; Nayda 2005). A key reason for this is that, while practising in a professional capacity, nurses (especially those working in paediatrics, maternal and child health care, emergency departments, critical care units, mental health, primary care clinics and community care) might come into contact with children who are at risk of maltreatment, or who have actually been abused and neglected.

Defining child abuse

Child abuse and neglect are both forms of *child maltreatment* – literally the 'wrong handling' of children. Even so, the term *'child abuse'* might be described as a 'contested notion' on the grounds that historically it has been the subject of various definitions and interpretations, something that has also made meaningful comparative research into its incidence and impact difficult (Price-Robertson et al 2013).

Contemporary academic interest in child abuse and neglect dates back to the 1960s and the publication of Kempe and colleagues' (1962) landmark article 'The battered-child syndrome' published in the *Journal of the American Medical Association* (Corby et al 2012). It was to take another decade, however, before the first international conference on child abuse was held (this occurred in 1976 in Geneva) (Fogarty & Sargeant 1989). Despite the growing academic and professional interest in the subject, it was to be a further two decades before a working definition of child maltreatment was to be formally adopted, notably:

> *Child abuse or maltreatment constitutes all forms of physical and/or emotional ill-treatment, sexual abuse, neglect or negligent treatment or commercial or other exploitation, resulting in actual or potential harm to the child's health, survival, development or dignity in the context of a relationship of responsibility, trust or power.* (WHO 1999: 15)

During the process of formulating and adopting this definition, there also emerged a much greater – and long overdue – appreciation of child abuse constituting an act of violence, which in turn has been defined as:

> *The intentional use of physical force or power, threatened or actual, against another person or against oneself or a group of people, that results in or has a high likelihood of resulting in injury, death, psychological harm, maldevelopment or deprivation.* (WHO 2002a: 5)

It is important to clarify that experiences of child maltreatment rarely occur in isolation. As Price-Robertson and colleagues (2013: 1) note, 'different forms of abuse often co-occur, and trauma often develops over prolonged periods'. In recognition of the need to better understand and to measure the interrelatedness of child maltreatment experiences (including the impact of these experiences and their sequelae accumulating over time), two key frameworks have been developed:

- *multi-type maltreatment* – which provides a theoretical framework for the inclusion of five forms of maltreatment in a single measure (i.e. sexual abuse, physical abuse, psychological maltreatment, neglect, and witnessing family violence); and
- *polyvictimisation* – which focuses not only on different forms of maltreatment, but also on broader experiences of victimisation, such as bullying and exposure to neighbourhood conflicts (Price-Robertson et al 2013: 2).

Over the past two decades the problem of child maltreatment has gained increasing visibility at an international level. Nonetheless, as the WHO (2006b: 1) points out, even with developments in human rights, law, forensic medicine and public health, the visibility and preventive action that child maltreatment requires 'is far from sufficient'.

Incidence of child abuse

Throughout recorded history, children have suffered *violence* (been menaced, maimed and murdered) at the hands of adults (Corby et al 2012; Johnstone 1999b). Today, the abuse of children constitutes one of the world's most longstanding and tragic public health issues (WHO 2002a: 59, 60–5; WHO & ISPCAN 2006). Child abuse continues to occur in epidemic proportions and, despite global efforts to redress it, its incidence and negative impact continue to be under-recognised, under-reported and poorly addressed by governments across the globe (WHO 2002a; see also Pinheiro 2006; WHO & ISPCAN 2006). Due to a lack of reliable data, it is difficult to provide reliable estimates of the global incidence of child maltreatment. Nonetheless, based on the currently available evidence, ISPCAN estimates that five children die every day because of being maltreated, with many more suffering lifelong physical and mental health consequences (https://www.ispcan.org/). ISPCAN further estimates that over 1 billion children worldwide experience violence annually.

The above figures do not take into account the exploitation of children as labourers or soldiers. In the case of child labour, although data is incomplete, according to the most recent estimates 85 million children aged 5–17 years and 38 million children aged 5–14 years have been engaged in hazardous work (Avis 2017). For the purposes of these estimates 'hazardous work' (regarded as one of the worst forms of child labour) has been defined as including 'any activity or occupation that, by its nature or type, has or leads to adverse effects on the child's safety, health and moral development' (Avis 2017: 7). More specifically, as Avis (2017: 7) further explains:

> *hazardous work is work in dangerous or unhealthy conditions that could result in a child being killed, injured and / or made ill as a consequence of poor safety and health standards and working arrangements.* (Avis 2017: 7).

In war-torn countries, children (mostly in the 15–17-year-old age group) are also often forcibly conscripted as soldiers. It is estimated, for example, that approximately '300,000 children are being used in armed conflict around the world at any given time' (Avis 2017: 12). The vast majority of these are recruited in African and Asian-Pacific regions.

Children are also exploited in sex and drug trafficking work. It is estimated, for example, that 1.8 million children (of both sexes) are exploited for prostitution and pornography, and 600 000 children have been engaged in illicit work – mostly drug production and trafficking (Avis 2017).

In Australia, for the period 2016–17, a total of 168 352 (1 in 32) children were reported to have received *child protection services* (i.e. investigation, care and protection order and / or were in out-of-home care) (AIHW 2018: vii). During the same period, Aboriginal and Torres Strait Islander children were reported as being seven times as likely as non-indigenous children to have received child protection services (AIHW 2018: vii).

In New Zealand (NZ), approximately 150 000 reports related to children are made annually to the Ministry for Vulnerable Children (https://www.unicef.org.nz/in-new-zealand/child-abuse). UNICEF NZ reports that, on average, 'a New Zealand child dies every five weeks as a result of violence', with children under 12 months old making up the majority of this statistic. Of these, 90% have been killed by a parent or family member (https://www.unicef.org.nz/in-new-zealand/child-abuse).

Redressing child abuse

The causes and consequences of child maltreatment are complex and unforgiving. In recognition of this, and the need to engage in a collaborative approach to the prevention, intervention and postvention of child maltreatment, governments and protection authorities have sought to take a systematic, multisectorial approach comparable to that used in public health (sometimes referred to as the 'public health model') (WHO 2006a: 3). In keeping with this approach, child protection policies and programs have as their focus:

- *implementing measures to prevent violence against children;*
- *detecting cases and intervening early;*
- *providing ongoing care to victims and families when maltreatment occurs;*
- *preventing the recurrence of violence.* (WHO 2006a: 3)

Commensurate with this approach, in 2009, the Council of Australian Governments (COAG) endorsed the *National framework for protecting Australia's children 2009–2020* (COAG 2009). Underpinned by the principles of the *United Nations Convention on the Rights of the Child*, the framework aims to ensure that 'Australia's children are safe and well' and achieve a 'substantial and sustained reduction in child abuse and neglect in Australia over time' (p 11). To this end, the *National framework* has six broad supporting outcome areas:

1. *Children live in safe and supportive communities.*
2. *Children and families access adequate support to promote safety and intervene early.*
3. *Risk factors for child abuse and neglect are addressed.*
4. *Children who have been abused or neglected receive the support and care they need for their safety and wellbeing.*
5. *Indigenous children are supported and safe in their families and communities.*
6. *Child sexual abuse and exploitation is prevented and survivors receive adequate support.*
   (COAG 2009: 11)

Under this framework, protecting children and promoting their safety and wellbeing is positioned as being 'everyone's responsibility' (COAG 2009: 12). It is hoped that, by everyone providing support in these six broad areas, the rights of all children 'to be safe and to receive loving care and support' and 'to receive the services they need to enable them to succeed in life' will be realised (COAG 2009: 6).

Elder abuse and neglect

Conceptualisations of *elder abuse* have shifted dramatically since legislated protective social welfare services for vulnerable older adults were first introduced in the 1930s (Jackson 2016a). In the decade following the 'discovery' of child abuse ('baby battering') in the 1960s,[1] 'granny battering'[2] was also identified and gained recognition (Jackson 2016a). Whereas previously elder abuse had been regarded by authorities as a 'private matter' involving interpersonal violence, it slowly became recognised as a 'family (domestic) violence issue' (WHO 2008: vii) and ultimately a criminal justice issue (Jackson 2016a).

Despite these seismic shifts in attitudes and understandings of elder abuse, many jurisdictions around the world today, including common-law countries, still do not have specific 'elder law' or 'elder abuse' legislation aimed at protecting vulnerable elderly people. According to the World Health Organization only around 40% of the world's countries have reported enacting laws to prevent elder abuse; furthermore, enforcement of these laws is often inadequate (WHO 2014d: 24). In addition, less than a third of countries (around 26%) reported 'implementing campaigns aimed at educating professionals to recognize the signs and symptoms of elder abuse and improve their problem-solving and case management skills on a larger scale', and only 23% reported 'implementing public information campaigns on elder abuse' (WHO 2014d: ix). These reports might help to explain why the medical and other health professions have generally been slow to recognise elder abuse as a serious (public) health issue, despite the phenomenon of 'granny battering' being described in contemporary geriatric medicine in the mid 1970s (Baker 1975: ix).

In recent years there has been growing concern, nationally and internationally, that, as the population ages, life expectancy increases and carer relationships change, the incidence and severity of elder maltreatment is likely to escalate (WHO 2008). This concern has led to calls for evidence-based national plans of action to be developed for the prevention of elder abuse (WHO 2014d). In the Australian context this call has underscored recognition of 'the need for a national approach to elder abuse and to provide a coordinating framework for state and territory initiatives as well as those at the Commonwealth level' (ALRC 2017: 61).

Today, elder abuse is recognised as being a fundamental human rights issue, not least because of the violation of human rights that it entails (ALRC 2017; Kaspiew et al 2016; WHO 2002b, 2014d). By framing elder abuse as a human rights issue, obligations are now imposed on others (including health care professionals) to take positive action aimed at enabling the proper protection of older people who are risk of maltreatment.

Defining elder abuse

Elder abuse and neglect are both forms of *elder maltreatment* – literally the 'wrong handling' of older people (defined as persons 65 years and older).

Today, there are a number of accepted definitions (Kaspiew et al 2016). The most commonly cited definition, however, comes from the *Toronto Declaration on the Global Prevention of Elder Abuse* (devised at an expert meeting sponsored by the Ontario Government in Toronto, 17 November 2002), which defines elder abuse as:

> a single or repeated act, or lack of appropriate action, occurring within any relationship where there is an expectation of trust which causes harm or distress to an older person. It can be of various forms: physical, psychological / emotional, sexual, and financial or simply reflect intentional or unintentional neglect. (WHO 2002c: 3)

Although definitions of elder abuse vary, most make reference to 'harm' and provide descriptors of what are regarded as 'core categories' of abuse – namely: physical abuse, psychological or emotional abuse, financial abuse, sexual assault and neglect (ALRC 2017: 42). Brief descriptions of the core types of abuse that feature in elder abuse prevention policies and plans are given below:

- *Physical abuse* – 'non-accidental acts that result in physical pain, injury or physical coercion' (DoH 2012: 1); this includes all kinds of physical violence, including kicking, hitting, punching, pushing, shoving, shaking, slapping and physical restraint (including confinement in their own home); it can also include physical neglect (e.g. 'leaving the older person confined to bed in soiled sheets') (Ellison et al 2004: 279).
- *Verbal abuse* – the conscious use of threatening or denigrating language by a perpetrator; this can include 'any form of verbal communication of a threatening or intimidating nature or any form of verbal communication of a belittling or degrading nature which diminishes [an older person's] sense of well-being, dignity or self-worth' and which may also lead that older person to 'fear for his or her safety' (adapted from the Canadian Centre for Elder Law 2011: 28).
- *Psychological and / or emotional abuse* – behaviours (both verbal and non-verbal) that are designed to intimidate the older person and which foster in them feelings of isolation, deprivation, shame and powerlessness; these behaviours characteristically involve 'repeated patterns of behaviour over time, and are intended to maintain a hold of fear over a person' (DoH 2012: 1). Such behaviours can include: the use of threatening or denigrating language; isolating the older person from family, friends and other social contacts; making the older person feel disempowered, ashamed and/or that they are entirely dependent upon their carers and 'stuck in an abusive situation from which they cannot extricate themselves' (Ellison et al 2004: 278).
- *Financial or economic abuse* – the 'illegal use, improper use or mismanagement of a person's money, property or financial resources by a person with whom they have a relationship implying trust' (DoH 2012: 1); this can include stealing money or assets from the older person (e.g. 'stealing Nan's pension'), getting the older person to sign over their life savings to the perpetrator, using manipulation or standover tactics to get money from or to pressure the older person to assign an enduring power of attorney to the perpetrator (who then siphons off the money for his or her own use), or using manipulation or standover tactics to pressure the older person to change a will in favour of the perpetrator (Ellison et al 2004: 271).
- *Sexual abuse or assault* – 'unwanted sex acts where the older person's consent is not obtained, or where consent was obtained through coercion' (DoH 2012: 1); offences can include rape,

indecent assault and sexual harassment as well as 'sexually exploitive or shaming behaviour, such as leaving an aged person undressed' (Ellison et al 2004: 280).
- *Social isolation* – the 'forced isolation of older people, with the sometimes additional effect of hiding abuse from outside scrutiny and restricting or stopping social contact with others, including attendance at social activities' (DoH 2012: 1); this can include isolating the older person from contact from family, friends and other social contacts by monitoring or restricting access to phone calls and other social communication media.
- *Neglect* – the 'failure of a carer or responsible person to provide life necessities, such as adequate food, shelter, clothing, medical or dental care, as well as the refusal to permit others to provide appropriate care (also known as abandonment)' (DoH 2012: 1); this can include a carer's or service provider's failure 'to act in some way that has a detrimental effect on the older person's health or welfare' – this can include failures to medicate, or over-medication (Ellison et al 2004: 280).
- *Any combination of the above* (Ellison et al 2004; see also ALRC 2017; Canadian Centre for Elder Law 2011; OPA & QLS 2010; WHO 2008).

Definitions also describe the 'variation in the nature of the relationships within which abuse may occur, including those with adult children, spouses, other family members, friends, carers or institutions' (Ellison et al 2004: 302–3).

Incidence of elder abuse

Due to a lack of reliable data (only a few developed nations have undertaken prevalence studies), the actual global incidence of elder abuse is difficult to estimate. Where prevalence studies on elder abuse have been conducted, estimates range from between 1% and 35% of older people experiencing some kind of maltreatment (WHO 2008: 1). As already discussed in Chapter 6 of this book, a systematic review of prevalence studies published between 2002 and 2015 has concluded that the overall prevalence of elder abuse globally is 15.7%, with 1 in 6 older people (141 million) being affected (Yon et al 2017). These figures may, however, be an underestimate; as noted by WHO (2008), available figures may represent 'only the tip of the iceberg' as elder abuse may be under-reported by as much as 80%. Possible reasons for this underreporting have been identified to include: 'the isolation of older people, the lack of uniform reporting laws, and the general resistance of people – including professionals – to report suspected cases of elder abuse and neglect' (WHO 2008: 1). A lack of awareness of the various forms that elder mistreatment can take and of the 'proper course of action to pursue when mistreatment is suspected' has also been identified as a contributing factor (Falk et al 2012: 1; see also ALRC 2017; Garma 2017; Kaspiew et al 2016). The hidden nature of elder abuse and cultural taboos surrounding the issue is another factor (DoH 2012). In the case of seniors who have experienced financial abuse, 'feelings of shame and embarrassment' have been identified as factors contributing to high levels of underreporting (Kaspiew et al 2016: 32). Regardless, elder abuse stands as a major public health issue across all regions and countries – including low-, middle- and high-resource nations (Australia, Canada, New Zealand, UK and the USA among them).

Redressing elder abuse

There is no 'quick fix' to the problem of elder abuse. As the Australian Victorian State Government Department of Health (DoH 2012: 5) has correctly observed:

> *Elder abuse prevention and response is complex, requiring a multifaceted approach that involves a combination of information and community education, service responses and legal interventions. Service responses include coordinated support from health and community service agencies, criminal and civil justice remedies, and complaint and compliance mechanisms.*

Significantly, most jurisdictions in common-law countries (including Australia and New Zealand) have shied away from enacting laws mandating the reporting of elder abuse to a designated protection agency and other protective mechanisms (e.g. making elder abuse a specific civil or criminal offence), preferring instead to operationalise community awareness programs and multi-agency advisory units and support programs (ALRC 2017; Kaspiew et al 2016). For example, in its approach to elder abuse prevention and response, the Department of Health of the Victorian State Government in Australia has focused on:

> *developing and delivering a range of concurrent activities within existing resources that lead to the following outcomes:*
>
> - *increased community awareness of elder abuse*
> - *empowerment of older people – through an increased awareness of their legal, financial and societal rights, and the provision of avenues for advice and support*
> - *active engagement by professionals – through an increased ability to identify and respond to elder abuse*
> - *coordinated multi-agency support –* provided by relevant services to older people experiencing elder abuse. (DoH 2012: 5)

In the case of abuse occurring in aged care facilities, complaints can be made to (and advice obtained from) the Aged Care Complaints Commissioner, which 'provides a free service for anyone to raise their concerns about the quality of care and services being delivered to people receiving aged care services subsidised by the Australian Government' (https://agedcare.health.gov.au/programs/aged-care-complaints-commissioner).

It is notable that some jurisdictions outside of Australia have taken a more proactive response to elder abuse, including enacting mandatory reporting laws. For example, in the USA, the *Elder Abuse Victims Act of 2009* was passed by the House of Representatives on 11 February 2009. The purpose of the Act is to:

> *protect seniors in the United States from elder abuse by establishing specialized elder abuse prosecution and research programs and activities to aid victims of elder abuse, to provide training to prosecutors and other law enforcement related to elder abuse prevention and protection, to establish programs that provide for emergency crisis response teams to combat elder abuse, and for other purposes.* (Open Congress 2009: 1)

In the same year, the *Elder Justice Act of 2009* was also introduced and passed into law by US President Obama on 23 March 2010. The aims of this legislation are to:

> *enhance the social security of the Nation by ensuring adequate public–private infrastructure and to resolve to prevent, detect, treat, intervene in, and prosecute elder abuse, neglect, and exploitation, and for other purposes.* (OPA & QLS 2010: 22)

In Canada, legislation has been enacted in each state and province to protect vulnerable older adults from abuse (OPA & QLS 2010: 25). Other non-legal mechanisms are also gaining traction in Canadian jurisdictions. For example, older Canadians have begun 'authorising their banks to monitor their accounts for unusual transactions' (OPA & QLS 2010: 22). If the bank detects any unusual transactions, it may raise its concerns with the account holder; it can also warn them against fraud. At the time of writing, similar provisions were being explored in the cultural context of Australia, with bankers themselves calling for 'urgent financial protections to prevent abuse of elderly Australians' (Doran & Henderson 2018). This call is strongly supported by the findings of the ALRC (2017 – see Recommendation 9.1). Other authors have also called for mechanisms to be put in place to combat what has been termed 'inheritance impatience' whereby adult children or grandchilden 'help themselves' to an elderly person's financial assets (Webb & Somes 2017).

Not all agree that a criminal justice response will be effective. For example, drawing on the US experience, Jackson (2016a, 2016b) argues that, although there is political appetite to punish perpetrators, it will have only a minimal if any deterrent effect. Moreover, even where mandatory laws have been enacted, prosecutions are uncommon, difficult to execute and rarely succeed (Jackson 2016b). This may be due to an inability to meet the very high level of evidence that is required to meet the threshold for and sustain a criminal prosecution (ALRC 2017).

Ethical issues associated with protecting children and elderly people from abuse

Despite involving age groups at opposite ends of the life span continuum, child abuse and elder abuse share several features in common. For example, as can be readily demonstrated, both:

- occur in all cultures and at all socio-economic levels (high and low alike)
- are recognised as being epidemic in nature
- commonly occur at the hands of someone known to the child or older person (e.g. a trusted primary carer, family member, professional, friend or neighbour)
- can be and are perpetrated by either individuals or institutions (i.e. individual abuse and neglect / institutional abuse and neglect)
- have been poorly addressed historically because of being hampered by cultural taboos – including taboos against interfering with the private sphere of the family home (NB. This derives from the principle of the sovereignty of the individual, discussed in Chapter 7. It will be recalled that the principle of the sovereignty of the individual finds expression in the idea of the sovereignty and sanctity of the family home; by this view, the family home should be kept free of the unwanted interference of others, including 'the state')
- have seen victims suffer preventable harm because of the moral passivism of others – i.e. involving a tendency among onlookers to avoid 'getting involved' and looking the other way (the 'bystander effect')
- have been neglected as fundamental human rights issues warranting attention by health care providers, policy-makers and governments.

Although the maltreatment of children and dependent elderly people share the above similarities, there are also some notable differences; these include:

- in the case of children, abuse and neglect may be perpetrated by their parents; in the case of elderly people, the abuse may be perpetrated by their children
- in the case of abuse and neglect, children have always been treated differently under law compared with adults, and have generally had their interests treated as being subordinate to those of adults; in the case of elderly people, the law does not regard them differently from any other adult. The presumption is made that, as older people have 'the right to access all the current laws available', it is their decision and choice whether to take legal action in order to achieve a legal remedy
- getting the issue of child abuse and neglect recognised and addressed as a human rights issue is often hampered because of the punishment of children being 'dressed up' (framed) and justified as being 'merely discipline', not punishment (Johnstone 1999b); in the case of older people, getting the issue recognised and addressed as a human rights issue has been hampered because of it having been construed as a 'private domestic matter' (OPA & QLS 2010).

Irrespective of these similarities and differences, the ethical issues associated with the maltreatment of children and elderly people – and in particular the bases of the moral imperatives of making notifications of known or suspected cases of abuse and neglect to relevant protection authorities – are much the same.

Why the maltreatment of children and elderly people constitutes a moral issue

The maltreatment of children and elderly people constitutes a significant moral problem and, as such, demands a substantial moral response. Reasons for this are outlined below.

As previously considered in Chapter 5, it is generally accepted that something involves a (human) moral / ethical problem where it has as its central concern:

- the promotion and protection of people's genuine wellbeing and welfare (including their interests in not suffering unnecessarily)
- responding justly to the genuine needs and significant interests of different people
- determining and justifying what constitutes right and wrong conduct in a given situation.

Adjunct to these concerns is an additional consideration – namely, that people have a moral responsibility to not cause unnecessary harm to others and, where able, ought to come to the aid of those who are suffering and in distress. As Amato (1990) notes in his *Victims and values: a history and a theory of suffering* (p 175):

> *There is an elemental moral requirement to respond to innocent suffering. If we were not to respond to it and its claims upon us, we would be without conscience and, in some basic sense, not completely human. And without compassion for others and passion for the causes on behalf of human wellbeing, what is best in our world would be missing.*

These considerations apply equally in the cases of both child and elder abuse. As can be readily demonstrated, the problem of child and elder maltreatment fundamentally concerns:

- promoting and protecting the wellbeing and welfare of children and elderly people at risk of harm because of the abuse and neglect by more powerful others
- protecting children and elderly people from this harm requires a careful calculation and balancing of the needs and interests of 'different people' – for example, the children and elderly people themselves, their primary caregivers (who are often, although not always, the perpetrators) and others (e.g. family, friends) who may also have an important relationship with the child or elder person, prospective notifiers (who may themselves sometimes experience negative outcomes – including violence and abuse – as a result of their interventions aimed at protecting children or elderly people at risk), society as a whole and, not least, future generations (who may find themselves unwitting participants in the sequelae of intergenerational abuse)
- determining and justifying the 'rightness' and 'wrongness' of intervening or not intervening when cases of the maltreatment of children or elderly people are known or suspected.

Underscoring the maltreatment of children and elderly people as a moral problem is a number of other important considerations revolving around the extraordinary vulnerability of children generally and dependent elderly people in particular. As already stated, children and dependent elderly are among the most vulnerable members of our community. For the most part, they are unable to protect themselves from the harms imposed on them by people more powerful than themselves. Invariably children and dependent elderly people have to rely on others for help if their wellbeing and welfare are to be safeguarded since, as has long been recognised, without intervention and help offered by others the abuse and neglect rarely stop.

The ethical implications of maltreating children and elderly people

Whether driven by legal obligation or moral commitment, or both, a health care professional's decision to report (or not report, as the case may be) instances involving the maltreatment of children or elder people never occurs in a moral vacuum and is never free of moral risk. Even in the face of clinical evidence and the threat of legal or professional censure for non-compliance with reporting requirements, there is always room to question: 'Should I report this particular case of known or suspected child abuse or elder abuse?' Underpinning this question are the additional questions of: 'What are the possible consequences to the child or elder person of my reporting or not reporting this case?', 'What are the possible consequences to the child's or elder person's family/caregivers of my reporting or not reporting this case?' and 'What are the possible consequences to me of my reporting or not reporting this case?' Possible answers to these questions will depend, in varying degrees, upon an effective harm/benefit analysis of the situation.

The moral demand to report child and elder maltreatment

A key feature of the maltreatment of children and elderly people concerns the risk of non-accidental and culpable harm that it poses to these entities' genuine welfare and wellbeing. These risks are not merely speculative or imaginary, but substantive and known through an increasing body of professional literature on the subject, the supportive findings of research, the findings of established commissions of inquiry into allegation of child sexual abuse and, not least, by the maltreated children and elderly people themselves who are increasingly coming forward to share their experiences by making their 'stories' public. It is this consequence of preventable harm that makes the maltreatment of children and elderly people morally objectionable. Understanding this, however, requires at least a rudimentary understanding of the notion of 'harm', the way it is linked to human welfare and wellbeing, and why it is morally compelling both not to cause harm and to prevent harm to others.

The notion of harm and its link with the moral duty to prevent child and elder abuse

As previously considered in Chapter 3, harm may be taken as involving the invasion, violation, thwarting or 'setting back' of a person's significant welfare interests to the detriment of that person's wellbeing (Feinberg 1984: 34; see also Beauchamp & Childress 2013). Wellbeing, in turn, can include interests in:

> *continuance for a foreseeable interval of one's life, and the interests in one's own physical health and vigour, the integrity and normal functioning of one's body, the absence of absorbing pain and suffering or grotesque disfigurement, minimal intellectual acuity, emotional stability, the absence of groundless anxieties and resentments, the capacity to engage normally in social intercourse and to enjoy and maintain friendships, at least minimal income and financial security, a tolerable social and physical environment, and a certain amount of freedom from interference and coercion.* (Feinberg 1984: 37)

The test for whether a person's interests and wellbeing have been violated or thwarted rests on 'whether that interest is in a worse condition than it would otherwise have been in had the invasion not occurred at all' (Feinberg 1984: 34). For instance, if a person (e.g. an infant, child or elderly person) is left psychogenically distressed (e.g. emotionally unstable, anxious, depressed and/or suicidal) as a result of his/her experiences of being maltreated, our reflective common sense tells us that this person's interests have been violated and the person him/herself 'harmed'. As the American philosopher Joel Feinberg (1984: 37) explains, the violation of a person's welfare interests renders that person 'very seriously harmed indeed' since 'their ultimate aspirations are defeated too'.

It is generally recognised in contemporary bioethical thought that people ought not to cause harm to or impose risks of harm on others. It is also accepted that people have a moral obligation to prevent harm to others if this can be done without sacrificing other important moral interests (Beauchamp & Childress 2013). By this view, acts which violate the interests of others, or fail to prevent the interests of others being violated, are prima facie morally wrong. The abuse of children and elderly people – and the failure to prevent it – clearly violates the interests of children and elderly people and renders them seriously harmed. It is the profound risk of the harmful consequences of the maltreatment, and the preventability of these consequences, that makes intervention by benevolent others morally compelling. Failure to prevent this harm is not only morally wrong, but unconscionable.

In the case of child abuse and neglect, it is now well documented and recognised that the negative physical and mental health effects of child maltreatment can be life-long, extending even into old age. Over the past decade, research and systematic reviews have consistently revealed that individuals who have experienced maltreatment as children are at an increased risk of developing major mental health issues (including depression, mood and anxiety disorders, suicidality and post-traumatic stress disorder (PTSD)), chemical dependency (on drugs, alcohol, tobacco), somatic disorders, chronic pain, psycho-social impairment, crime and recidivism, and general interruptive 'life stress' (Chen et al 2010; Goddard & Pooley 2018; Jones et al 2018; Jonson-Reid et al 2012; Nelson et al 2018; Paras et al 2009; Patten et al 2015; Powers et al 2014; Sachs-Ericsson et al 2009, 2017; Springer et al 2007; Steine et al 2017; Webb et al 2007; Wegman & Stetler 2009). Adding to this is substantial lifetime economic costs of child maltreatment including survivors' 'diminished capacity to productively engage in education and employment over the long term' (McCarthy et al 2016: 221; see also Fang et al 2012).

In the case of elder abuse and neglect, the negative effects of elder maltreatment can result in increased morbidity (in both physical and psychological health conditions), increased mortality (particularly those who have experienced caregiver neglect and financial exploitation), reduced quality of life (exacerbated by feelings of loneliness), loss of property and security, and increased risk of hospital admission and institutionalisation (Burnett et al 2016; Dong & Simon 2013; Dong et al 2011; Garma 2017; Podnieks & Thomas 2017; Schofield et al 2013; Wong & Waite 2017; Yon et al 2017). Of further concern, the negative psychological effects of elder abuse (e.g. anxiety, depression, irritability, feelings of extreme loneliness, post-traumatic stress disorder) may endure for the remainder of the older person's life, destroying their capacity to enjoy their twilight years (Anetzberger 2004, 2012). Compounding these outcomes, social support may not be effective in moderating their impact (Wong & Waite 2017).

Considerations against reporting the maltreatment of children and elderly people

Arguably the most contentious ethical issue in both the child abuse and elder abuse debate is whether the reporting of abuse and neglect should be made *mandatory* – that is, made the subject of legislative provisions compelling designated persons (e.g. doctors, nurses, psychologists, physiotherapists) to report certain kinds of abuse and neglect to a government protection authority or other protective services (e.g. the police). Some worry that public policy requirements to report the abuse and neglect of children and elderly people may not (and do not) always achieve their intended moral outcomes (ALRC 2017; McTavish et al 2017; Raz 2017). This concern is underscored by a lack of evidence regarding the efficacy of mandatory reporting and the risks associated with increases in reporting depleting already stretched resources in the field (McTavish et al 2017; Raz 2017). On this point, Raz (2017: 2) argues that, although the introduction of mandatory reporting may be 'good politics' (particularly in the aftermath of high-profile cases demanding action), it may not be 'good policy'. Considering these concerns, calls have been made for a moratorium on expanding mandatory reporting laws until they have been thoroughly evaluated via pre- and post-outcome studies (Raz 2017).

The grounds for concern have mostly been utilitarian in nature, involving a calculation of harms and benefits to: (1) the professional–client relationship, (2) the families of the children and elderly people who have allegedly been maltreated and, lastly, (3) the allegedly abused and neglected children and elderly people themselves (Lantos 2004; Ploeg et al 2009; Schmeidel et al 2012). These considerations are not unproblematic, however, and are themselves vulnerable to criticism. Consider the following.

The professional–client relationship

Requirements to report the abuse and neglect of children and elderly people have been viewed as being problematic primarily on grounds that they threaten the sanctity of the professional–client relationship by eroding professional discretion about: (1) duties of confidentiality and (2) how best to deal with maltreatment cases. A related concern has been that reporting requirements can also shift and extend the boundaries of responsibility of the professional–client relationship. This is seen as potentially creating an intolerable tension between the possibly competing and conflicting interests of all stakeholders in question. For example, it could create for an attending health professional the moral dilemma of how best to uphold the interests of an abused client without also violating the interests of the perpetrator who may also be a client, and vice versa. It may well be that, in the end, it is not possible for the health professional to uphold the interests of both clients equally, prompting the question: 'What should I do?'

Consequential to the shift in boundaries of responsibility, there is also a commensurate change in role for the health professional – namely from that of clinician / healer / therapist to that of 'statutory protector' whose primary role is surveillance. For some, this assumed role of 'statutory protector' not only conflicts with their primary therapeutic role but also threatens the therapeutic sanctity of the professional–client relationship, which begs the question of the moral acceptability of health care professionals functioning as the 'arm of the state'.

The issue of mandatory reporting can become particularly pressing in the case of elder abuse where, for example, an abused adult client refuses to consent to a protective intervention. In such situations, the health care professional is faced with the dilemma of which moral interest to uphold: 'the client's right to self-determination' (autonomy and dignity) or 'the client's right to safety and a mistreatment-free life' (Lithwick et al 2000: 108).

In Australia, concern about respecting the autonomy and dignity of the abused elderly (and those at risk of abuse) has been considered at length by the Australian Law Reform Commission (ALRC), which in 2016 was commissioned to undertake an inquiry into *Protecting the rights of older Australians from abuse*. In its final report, the ALRC concluded that professionals 'should not be required to report all types of elder abuse', arguing:

> Older people must not be treated like children [...]. Elder abuse is a broad category, and older people should generally be free to decide whether to report abuse they have suffered to the police or a safeguarding agency or to not report the abuse at all. (ALRC 2017, footnote 14.189, p 415)

This conclusion was based on various submissions made to the ALRC during its inquiry and which had emphatically objected to the introduction of mandatory reporting on grounds of 'the need to respect [older] people's autonomy' – regarded by many as 'the' key issue (ALRC 2017, footnote 9.58, p 308). Accordingly, in its final report, the ALRC made the following recommendation:

> Adult safeguarding laws should provide that the consent of an at-risk adult must be secured before safeguarding agencies investigate, or take any other action, in relation to the abuse or neglect of the adult. However, consent should not be required:
>
> (a) in serious cases of physical abuse, sexual abuse, or neglect; or
>
> (b) if the safeguarding agency cannot contact the adult, despite extensive efforts to do so; or
>
> (c) if the adult lacks the legal capacity to give consent, in the circumstances. (ALRC 2017, Recommendation 14-4)

Families

Requirements to report maltreatment have also been criticised and rejected on grounds that these stand to undermine the 'liberal rights' (to privacy and self-determination), welfare interests and wellbeing of families. The risk of this happening is seen to be especially high in cases where health care professionals are 'overly zealous', incompetent or impaired in performing their assessments of allegedly abused children or elder people and in reporting their findings to protection services. For example, in the case of child abuse, health care professionals may be lacking in the necessary skills, or may make the wrong judgments or, because of their own unresolved personal issues, just not be able 'to come to terms fully with any abuse' (Renvoize 1993: 152; see also McTavish et al 2017). In the case of nurses, for example, research suggests that insufficient knowledge about the manifestations of child maltreatment and a lack of confidence hampered their reporting experience in 'keeping children safe' (Fraser et al 2010; Lines et al 2017).

In the case of elder abuse, personal biases and a reluctance to become entangled in 'complex and intransigent family dynamics' (Jackson & Hafemeister 2013: 255) may also cloud a professional's judgment, leading to mistakes being made and preventive interventions botched. Although research on this issue is limited, studies nonetheless suggest that health professionals' personal experience of interacting with elderly people and family caregiving, and the quality of their own relationships, may influence significantly their perceptions of abuse – including whether an abusive instance was 'abuse' or merely a one-off aberration (Fitzpatrick & Hamill 2010: 4).

In light of these failings, some critics contend that, in the ultimate analysis, reporting requirements could result in families being left irreparably damaged – particularly if misjudgments have been made.

Maltreated children and elderly people

Perhaps among the most serious and troubling criticisms of all is the view that requirements to take protective action and report the abuse and neglect of children and elderly people may, paradoxically, cause further harm to the abused themselves. In the case of children, the 'harmfulness' of the intervention is thought to derive from, and be compounded by, a number of processes:

- through children being separated (sometimes prematurely) from their parents/primary caregivers and surrendered to 'ambiguous substitute family arrangements' (Giovannoni 1982: 108; Miller & Weinstock 1987: 162). In some cases, the environment of a substitute family or foster caregiver may be worse than that of the family of origin (McTavish 2017)
- where separation and removal damage the child–parent/guardian relationship, not least through 'interfering with the ability of abusing parents to deal with their problems and reintegrate their families' (Miller & Weinstock 1987: 162). Further, if protective interventions (e.g. making notification to a child protection authority, court action) are unsuccessful, this could result in an abused child being returned 'unprotected to an unbelieving family which might scapegoat them and blame them for all the disruption' (Renvoize 1993: 152); in such instance, the abuse may not only continue but also be intensified (McTavish 2017)
- where protective services simply fail mistreated children, for example:
  - where referrals and protective interventions are handled poorly (investigations may be delayed or be ineffective; children may be returned to violent and abusive homes and thus committed to a life of re-abuse, crime and/or death (Fogarty 1993; MacNair 1992; McTavish 2017))
  - where mechanisms for securing child protection may themselves be traumatic and abusive (legal processes (including police involvement and court proceedings) are, for example, characteristically intrusive and adversarial in nature; media coverage is characteristically intrusive and can be harmfully 'exposing' and adversarial in nature) (Lewin 1994)
  - where protective services are inadequate to meet the needs of mistreated children, resulting in increasing numbers of children being drawn into a child protection system that is 'incapable of caring for them properly' (e.g. as can occur in the case of a protective system plagued by budgetary constraints) (Fogarty 1993: 7; see also McTavish 2017; Raz 2017).

It is likewise in the case of elder abuse. Reports to and interventions by adult protection services might not always achieve their desired moral outcomes: relationships with offending family members might be inadvertently destroyed, abuse may reoccur and even be accentuated if a protective intervention fails and the elderly person is returned to their original living arrangements, or the maltreated elderly person may suddenly find themselves being placed into a nursing home or under the authority of an appointed guardian against their will (Anetzberger 2012; Groh & Linden 2011; Ploeg et al 2009). Compounding the problem, elderly people are often reluctant to report abuse, or to cooperate with an adult protection service if a report is made by another (Jackson & Hafemeister 2013). The reasons for this are complex, some of which are briefly considered below.

Elderly people are often in a dependent relationship with a relative or caregiver, which can make it extremely difficult for them to take protective action themselves or to accept the protective interventions of another. For example, in some cases, an elderly person may 'choose to remain in an abusive relationship rather than risk destroying the relationship with the offending family member or caregiver by using a punitive or enforcement approach' (Groh & Linden 2011: 128). An important factor influencing this stance is that the abused elder may feel 'ashamed that a relative has been abusing them' (Groh & Linden 2011: 128). In other contexts, elderly people may decline protective intervention simply because of a 'dislike of the idea of having strangers in the house'; on this point, Lithwick and colleagues explain, many older people believe that 'it is the duty of the family to take care of them rather than paid professionals' (Lithwick et al 2000: 108). In the case of spousal abuse, the problem is even more complex. As Lithwick and colleagues (2000: 107) note:

> *After a lifetime together, it can be difficult for spouses to face the need for major changes in the nature of their relationship, even more so if the suggested intervention involves placement (in cases where cognitive and / or physical impairment suggest it).*

In the case of elderly people who have no family or children, one research study has suggested that they may be less equivocal about involving law enforcement – although there is a caveat to this: they tend to prefer that the perpetrator 'receive some form of treatment that was not forthcoming outside of the criminal justice system' (Jackson & Hafemeister 2013: 272).

Whether involving the maltreatment of children or of elderly people, there is an ever-present risk that, rather than promoting and protecting the welfare and wellbeing of children and elderly people who have been maltreated, reporting requirements might thwart, intrude upon, set back, invade and even violate these moral entitlements. In short, reporting requirements used as a protection intervention may have the unintended consequence of ultimately being more harmful than the abuse and neglect itself.

Response to the criticisms

The question remains, however, of whether reporting known and suspected cases of the abuse and neglect of either children or elderly people does stand to 'adversely' affect the nature and boundaries of the professional–client relationship, the 'deserving' interests of families and, not least, the interests of maltreated children and elderly people – and, if so, what might the moral implications of this be? It is to briefly considering these questions that the remainder of this chapter will now turn.

The problem of maintaining confidentiality

Reporting the maltreatment of children or elderly people, unless consented to by both the abuser and the abused (provided they have capacity to give consent), almost always involves a breach of confidentiality and privacy. A key reason that health care professionals are reluctant to breach confidentiality relates to a fear that, if perpetrators cannot rely on or trust professional caregivers to keep secret abuse-related information disclosed in the professional–client relationship, then they (the perpetrators) may be discouraged from seeking help to remedy their abusive behaviours. In effect, legitimised reporting laws could 'drive people underground' (Goddard 1996; MacNair 1992; Schmeidel et al 2012). It is not clear, however, that this fear is sufficient to justify maintaining confidentiality in favour of an abusing adult. There are a number of reasons for this. The first of these concerns the very nature of the moral demand to maintain confidentiality itself.

Traditionally, as discussed in Chapter 7, the rule of confidentiality has demanded that information gained in the professional–client relationship ought to be kept secret even when its disclosure might serve a greater public good. Over time, however, real-life examples and moral theorising have repeatedly shown that treating the rule of confidentiality as being *absolute* is morally unjust, indefensible and unreasonable (Bok 1978). At best, maintaining confidentiality should be treated as only a prima-facie obligation. What this means is that although, as a general rule, confidentiality ought to be maintained in the professional–client relationship, there may sometimes be stronger moral reasons for overriding this obligation. An example here would be where an abusing adult discloses to an attending health care professional his/her intention to deliberately injure a child or elder parent. A decision to disclose this information in order to warn and protect the intended victim would be justified on grounds that it could help to prevent an otherwise-avoidable harm from occurring.

Superficially, the disclosure of privileged information in the above example might appear to be in breach of a disclosing client's 'rights' to confidentiality. However, confidentiality was never meant to stretch so far as to compel an attending health care professional to lie or to protect those who have no right to impose their malevolence on innocent victims (Bok 1978: 148). Borrowing from Bok (1978: 155), 'only an overwhelming blindness to the suffering of those beyond one's immediate sphere' could justify the maintenance of absolute confidentiality in the case where innocent others are at risk of being harmed. Further, clients' moral entitlements to have certain information about themselves kept secret are forfeited where the maintenance of confidentiality about the case stands to impinge seriously on the moral interests and wellbeing of innocent others. In this instance, morally constrained discretionary breaches of confidentiality are ethically justified.

In the case of maltreated children and elderly people, there exist strong moral grounds for justifiably overriding an obligation of confidentiality that might otherwise be due to a perpetrator, and for discretionary disclosures to be made to appropriate people. In regard to the 'possible harm' that discretionary disclosures may cause to abusers (e.g. driving perpetrators 'underground' and discouraging them from seeking help; causing them to feel hurt, embarrassed and stigmatised; dismembering families; and so forth), this is not sufficient to justify the maintenance of absolute confidentiality. One reason for this is: it is not clear that discretionary disclosures will necessarily harm the welfare interests of perpetrators. The aim of protective interventions (of which legitimated reporting is a form) is to *protect the abused, not to punish abusers* and to be *curative and remedial rather than punitive* (Corby et al 2012; Fogarty 1993; Lewin 1994; Miller & Weinstock 1987; O'Brien 2010; Scott & O'Neil 1996). Thus disclosures that are made to appropriate people stand not only to benefit an abused child or elderly person, but also to set in motion a process that could potentially assist the perpetrator as well. If the perpetrator is genuinely accepting of responsibility for his/her abusive behaviour, and is committed to rehabilitation, then the problem of competing demands to maintain confidentiality can be overcome by the health care provider negotiating the discretionary disclosure of privileged information gained in the professional–client relationship. If, however, a perpetrator is unwilling to accept responsibility for his/her abusive behaviour and is unwilling to give permission for a discretionary breach of confidentiality to the relevant authorities, the health care professional has an overriding moral obligation (and in some jurisdictions, is legally mandated) to take the action necessary to protect the interests of an at-risk child or elderly person. Discretionary breaches of confidentiality are morally justified in these instances.

The problem of being 'the arm of the state'

It might be argued that reporting requirements could exacerbate the problem of the maltreatment of children and elderly people in another way – namely, by facilitating its 'over-reporting' (including a proliferation of false allegations being made about its incidence). Were health care professionals seen to be spearheading this 'over-reporting' through their surveillance role, this could result in a loss of community trust in service providers and ultimately 'the system', which, in turn, could work against an effective overall societal response to child and elder maltreatment.

It is not clear, however, whether community trust in health care professionals would be eroded by a proliferation in reporting cases of maltreatment. For one thing, a proliferation in the reporting of the maltreatment of children and elderly people may not necessarily be spurious. An increase in reporting could be directly linked to a genuine increase in the actual incidence of abuse (which can be demonstrated by a high rate of substantiation of received notifications), which, in turn, can be further linked to increased professional and community awareness of what constitutes child and elder abuse and its unacceptability. Thus, while being perplexed by an increase in the reporting of the maltreatment of children and/or elderly people, the community might nevertheless be reassured that 'the system' is working and that children and vulnerable elderly people are being protected from unnecessary harm. Contrary to the claims made above, it might be a *failure* by health care professionals to report cases of the maltreatment of children and elderly people that risks undermining community confidence in their services, and not the reverse.

Preserving the integrity of the professional–client relationship

Requirements to report the abuse and neglect of children and elderly people do not necessarily threaten the sanctity or integrity of the professional–client relationship (O'Brien 2010; Ploeg et al 2009; Wekerle 2013). If disclosures are handled in a morally, legally and clinically informed, culturally and clinically competent and sensitive manner, this need not involve a collapse of the boundaries between matters of clinical competence and legal and moral prescription/proscription. On the contrary: legal and moral prescriptions/proscriptions concerning preventive action in cases of the maltreatment of children and elderly people can strengthen the bases and boundaries of clinical competence by reminding health care professionals always to consider carefully the precise impact that their acts and omissions can have on the lives of others, and to remain vigilant in regard to their capacity to harm as well as benefit those in their care.

Upholding the interests of families

It is acknowledged that when engaging in an intervention aimed at protecting children and elderly people from abuse and neglect, there is an ever-present risk that mistakes will sometimes be made. But the risks of *failing to intervene* are equally if not more onerous. By not taking protective action in instances of the maltreatment of children and elderly people, there is a risk that those who have been abused and neglected will be left forgotten and invisible. In the case of child abuse and neglect, there is an additional risk that, without intervention, the sequelae of the mistreatment could continue to wreak havoc generation after generation (Bartlett et al 2017; Fergusson et al 2006; Goddard & Pooley 2018; Narayan et al 2017). Appropriate intervention to prevent child abuse (of which reporting may be the first step) can make a significant contribution to breaking the cycle of intergenerational violence (including 'learned helplessness' which may predispose future generations being victimised as adults), which unless interrupted can result in not only the next generation of children being affected (Fergusson et al 2006; Oliver 1993; Renner & Slack 2006), but also their grandparents. As Fitzpatrick and Hamill (2010: 4) have observed:

> in a significant number of elder abuse cases, there is a demonstrated history of prior abuse […] In families characterized by conflicted relationships, abuse may be seen as an extension of that relationship.

It needs to be remembered that a key aim of interventionist strategies is to protect the abused, 'not to punish the abusers', and, where able, to offer dysfunctional adults and families remediation. Thus appropriate interventions stand not only to benefit the children or elderly people who have been abused or neglected, but also to set in motion a process that could potentially assist and benefit perpetrators as well.

The importance of a supportive socio-cultural environment in abuse prevention

In her influential and highly cited work *Trauma and recovery: the aftermath of violence – from domestic abuse to political terror*, the American psychiatrist Judith Herman (1992: 9) persuasively argues that:

> In the absence of strong political movements for human rights, the active process of bearing witness inevitably gives way to the process of forgetting. Repression, dissociation, and denial are phenomena of social as well as individual consciousness.

Applied in the context of child and elder abuse, there is room to suggest that, without a strong political movement for upholding the rights of children and the elderly, the process of bearing witness (to child and elder mistreatment) will likewise give way to a communal forgetting. The risk of forgetting is particularly great in an environment which is not supportive of nor encourages personal moral initiative and individual acts of benevolence (moral action) aimed at genuinely assisting and protecting children and elderly people who are at risk.

There are not, of course, any 'quick-fix' solutions to the problem of how best to protect children and elderly people from abuse and neglect. But there is considerable scope to suggest that a lot more could be done at an individual, familial, group, community and state level to improve the status quo. Health care professionals have a particularly important role to play on account of their being in a prime position to discern and provide evidence of instances of the abuse and neglect of children and elderly people, and to intervene to prevent these instances from continuing. Through their informed and morally judicious interventions, health care professionals could, in turn, make a significant difference to the lives and welfare interests of both the abused and those who abuse them. Reporting requirements should, therefore, be seen not as an intrusion or a violation of the professional–client relationship, but as an opportunity to provide support and care to injured and distressed human beings.

A system of protection is only as good as the people who are charged with – and who are willing to accept – the responsibilities of upholding it. All health care professionals have an obligation to become sufficiently informed about the clinical, legal, cultural and ethical dimensions of child and elder abuse to enable them to participate competently in protection processes. To this end, improving the education of health care professionals about the maltreatment of children and elderly people and related protection issues will enable them to be better prepared to deal with cases that come to their attention. But, as Judith Herman (cited above) makes plain, commitment and education may not be enough; there also needs to be a supportive social environment and a deeply ingrained cultural commitment to preventing the harms of child and elder maltreatment across the board.

Conclusion

Children should not have to bear 'silent and unacknowledged witness to their own suffering in many ways throughout their lives' (Valent 1993: 4). Neither should elderly people. Everyone has a moral responsibility (irrespective of the law) to break the culture of silence and enduring taboos that surrounds the abuse and neglect of children and elderly people and which has been so effective in invalidating, marginalising and rendering as invisible its untoward effects. Unless this responsibility is accepted and acted upon at an individual and private level, children and elderly people will remain at risk of the otherwise-avoidable harms caused by their being abused and neglected by others – including those who are supposed to care *for* and *about* them. To fail in this responsibility is not only to fail those who are among the most vulnerable members of our society, but also to fail ourselves and the community as a whole in which we share membership.

The abuse and neglect of children and elderly people does not affect only children and elderly people, it affects us all. It is, therefore, up to each and every one of us (as co-participating members of a moral community) to do what we can in order to prevent its harmful incidence and impact. Preventing the harms that flow from the maltreatment of children and elderly people is not merely a charitable cause which people can choose to either support or not support; rather, it is an obligation which is supported by the deepest of ethical considerations and which is binding on all of us. The ultimate question, then, is not one of *whether* we ought to intervene to protect children and elderly people from the incidence and negative impact of abuse and neglect, but how we may *better* intervene and achieve the desired moral outcomes of this intervention.

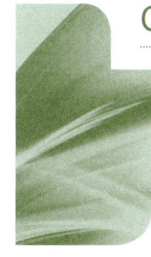

Case scenario 1[3]

You are a registered nurse working in a large metropolitan hospital. You observe a registered nurse who is employed in a new graduate program struggle with her work. Specifically, you observe that she experiences 'major problems' in managing time, administering medications and managing many other aspects of nursing care – including complying with accepted standards of care. Based on various behaviours you have observed, you also suspect that the registered nurse has some kind of 'personality disorder' and, at times, seems to you to be depressed.

Case scenario 2[4]

You are a registered nurse working in a paediatric unit. You have been assigned to care for a 12-year-old girl by the name of Christine who has been admitted for observations and investigation of a recent and severe bout of undifferentiated abdominal pain. Shortly after Christine's admission, while assisting her to have a shower, you notice bruising on her arms and back. After asking her gentle probing questions, Christine confides in you that her mother beats her regularly. She further confides that the bruises on her arms and back are the result of a particularly vicious beating her mother had given her recently using a wooden coat hanger. She also discloses that some weeks earlier she had taken an overdose of aspirin to 'try and make her mother stop beating her', but that all her mother had done at the time was to laugh at her and tell her 'how stupid she was' and sent her to her room to 'sleep it off'. Christine then begs you not to tell anyone, pleading, 'If my mother finds out that I've told anyone, she will beat me up. It will be much worse for me.'

Concerned for Christine's wellbeing and mindful of your statutory duty to report known or suspected cases of child abuse, you decide to seek advice from Christine's consultant paediatrician. On doing so, the paediatrician tells you: 'Christine is my patient, not yours. You are not to take this matter any further.'

Case scenario 3

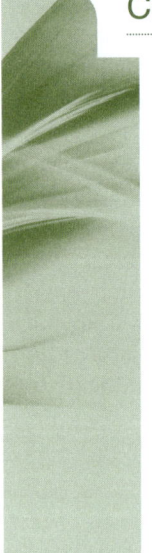

You are a registered nurse living in a neighbourhood which has a relatively high number of older people living in it. An elderly neighbour, an 82-year-old widow who lives alone in her small two-bedroom home of over 50 years, walks every day to the local shops and is often seen sitting in her front yard when the weather permits. Over time, neighbours begin to observe that the woman has seemingly 'disappeared' and ponder among themselves 'What has happened to her?' They note that this disappearance has coincided with the elderly woman's granddaughter and three school-aged great-grandchildren coming to live with her. It is assumed that 'things must be OK', because the granddaughter is a 'nurse' who works in a local aged care facility. One neighbour, however, is concerned and resolves to 'find out for sure'. When an opportunity arrives, she approaches the granddaughter to inquire after her grandmother. This inquiry is met with a swift and rude response of: 'Mind your own business!' Subsequently, another neighbour (an elderly pensioner who had been acquainted with the grandmother for years) decides to 'see for herself'. Upon observing the children walking to school and the granddaughter (in a nurse's uniform) driving off to work, she walks over to the house and knocks loudly on the front door calling out the name of the elderly woman, asking 'Are you there "Nan"?' To this she receives an unexpected response: 'I'm here. I'm here. My granddaughter has locked me in. Can you get me out? Please get me out'. Distressed and perplexed by what she has discovered, the neighbour approaches you for advice on what to do. She also reveals that 'Nan' has said that her granddaughter has 'taken over the house'.

CRITICAL QUESTIONS

1. What are your moral and legal responsibilities in these cases?
2. In regard to the first case scenario, would you report your concerns to a practitioner regulating authority (e.g. a nurses board or council)? On what grounds would you make your decision?
3. In regard to the second case scenario, what are your obligations? For instance, are you obliged to uphold Christine's request for confidentiality to be maintained? Are you also obliged to honour the paediatrician's directive in this case?
4. In regard to the third case scenario, what advice would you give to the concerned neighbour?
5. What actions should and would you take?

Endnotes

1. The term 'baby battering' is credited with having been termed by Kempe and colleagues (1962).
2. The term 'granny battering' is believed to have first been used in an editorial (Burston 1975) published in the *British Medical Journal*.
3. Adapted from Nurses and Midwives Board of New South Wales (2010) *Professional conduct: a case book of disciplinary decisions relating to professional conduct maters*, 2nd edn. Nurses and Midwives Board of New South Wales, Sydney, p 472.
4. Reprinted with permission from Johnstone M & Crock E (2015) Dealing with ethical issues in nursing practice. In: E Chang & J Daly (eds) *Transitions in nursing: preparing for professional practice*, 4th edn. Churchill Livingstone / Elsevier, Sydney.

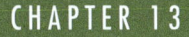

Nursing ethics futures – challenges in the 21st century

KEYWORDS

antimicrobial resistance (AMR)
climate change
health equity movement
health inequalities
health inequities
multidrug-resistant bacteria
nursing ethics futures
pandemic influenza
public health emergencies

LEARNING OBJECTIVES

Upon the completion of this chapter and with further self-directed learning you are expected to be able to:
- Identify at least five 'whole-of-world' scenarios that are going to give rise to ethical challenges for nurses and that will extend 'beyond the bedside'.
- Discuss critically the moral challenges posed respectively by:
  – public health emergencies
  – climate change
  – pandemic influenza
  – antimicrobial resistance (AMR)
  – inequities in health and health care.
- Discuss critically how, if at all, the nursing profession can be appropriately prepared to respond justly and effectively to the moral challenges posed by 'whole-of-world' scenarios such as those listed above.
- Explore and describe the kinds of strategies the nursing profession could develop and/or contribute to in order to ensure that, when faced with public health emergencies or health care disasters, the needs of society are upheld in a just, accountable and transparent manner.

Introduction

Nursing has long been positioned as a profession on which society depends. In keeping with this stance it is appropriate that nurses, both individually and collectively, take time to reflect on the kinds of ethical problems they will be likely to encounter in the future and on whether they are as adequately prepared as they need to be in order to be able to respond ethically to what lies ahead.

As I have argued previously (Johnstone 2009b), past futurist thinking about *nursing ethics futures* has tended to focus on conventional issues such as the expansion of medical knowledge and developments in medical technology, continued health care reform, and the transformation of the profession in relation to these developments. Issues typically identified have included:

- advancing patients' rights in health care
- patient advocacy
- ongoing cultural shifts and changes in attitude towards end-of-life care (e.g. 'Not For Treatment' directives, euthanasia/assisted dying, advance care planning)
- the growth and use of technology in caring
- 'genomic' medicine – often accompanied by alarmist warnings of threats to the privacy and confidentiality of genetic information, and of genetic discrimination and exclusion of people from society and health care (i.e. in a manner such as that portrayed in the 1997 US science fiction movie *Gattaca* (Johnstone 2009b)).

The identification of these and related issues has typically been followed by a rehearsal of the 'usual' arguments about professional accountability and responsibility. Although these issues are important, they will not be the most pressing issues that nurses will have to grapple with over the next few decades. As this chapter will attempt to show, there will be other (more) pressing ethical issues that the nursing profession will face in the future and that need to be anticipated. Of particular concern are the health-care-related ethical issues raised by public health emergencies, which may be driven by the threats to public health posed by climate change, pandemic influenza and antimicrobial resistance, and the sobering problem of local and global inequities in health and health care. Also of concern is whether conventional nursing ethics will be up to the task of guiding and motivating nurses to behave in ways that meet society's needs. It is to briefly considering these issues and their possible moral implications for the nursing profession that this final chapter will now turn.

Public health emergencies[1]

A public health emergency is defined by the World Health Organization (WHO) as:

> *an occurrence or imminent threat of an illness or health condition, caused by bio terrorism, epidemic or pandemic disease, or (a) novel and highly fatal infectious agent or biological toxin, that poses a substantial risk of a significant number of human fatalities or incidents or permanent or long-term disability.* (WHO (nd) http://www.who.int/hac/about/definitions/en/ - current 10 June 2018)

For a public health emergency to 'exist', government authorities must formally declare 'a state of public health emergency' so that state regulations can be suspended and the functions of state agencies changed so that appropriate responses can be operationalised.

'Emergency preparedness', in turn, is defined as consisting of:

> *all activities taken in anticipation of a crisis to expedite effective emergency response. This includes contingency planning, but is not limited to it: it also covers stockpiling, the creation and management of standby capacities and training staff and partners in emergency response.* (Inter-Agency Standing Committee 2007: 40)

Over the past decade, questions concerning the 'emergency preparedness' of countries, communities and citizens have received increasing attention as the lessons learned from an array of widely reported public health emergencies (e.g. those caused by hurricanes, bush fires, catastrophic flooding, earthquakes, tsunamis and the unprecedented outbreak in 2014 of the Ebola virus disease in western Africa) have highlighted 'gaps in ethics guidances' on how best to decide and act in emergency ultra-scenarios.

From an ethical standpoint, public health emergencies are challenging because they call into question and contradict 'many of the values we hold dearest, such as providing each patient with the best available care' (Stroud et al 2010: 51). Accordingly, fundamental ethical guidances and preparedness for dealing with ethical issues that may arise during public health emergencies are required. This is because, as Stroud and colleagues explain:

> *if we don't act in accordance with our ethical principles, the repercussions both for individuals and the society after the fact will be enormous. They are fundamental because our ethical principles serve as the foundation of our laws. They are fundamental because people will only act and sacrifice if they believe they are operating in an ethical system, and that individuals are being treated with fairness and transparency in the full view of the law. In addition, they are fundamental, quite frankly, because many of the decisions contemplated will be made with imperfect information – they will be best guesses. Those guesses, in the absence of firm evidence, will need to be made based on a shared ethical construct.* (Stroud et al 2010: 51)

The outbreak in 2003 of the severe acute respiratory syndrome (SARS), the 2009 swine flu epidemic and the 2014 outbreak of the Ebola virus disease in western Africa have each served to provide an important catalyst for raising probing questions about how prepared the world is to respond ethically to what has been termed in the public health literature the 'three Rs' of public health emergencies – notably: *rationing* (e.g. of vaccines, medications), *restrictions* (on people's liberties / access to and from health care services) and *responsibilities* (of health care professionals to continue providing care and treatment even when doing so places them, their families and others close to them at risk) (Wynia 2007; see also Reid 2005; Singer et al 2003). They also provided a catalyst for reflecting on the 'tragic choices' encompassing the ethical tradeoffs that will invariably have to be made in 'ultra-scenarios'. As Campbell and colleagues have warned, when disaster strikes:

> *At progressively more extreme levels, the decisions will be increasingly harsh; morally agonizing to those who must make and execute them – but in the end, morally deadening.* (Campbell et al 2007: 77)

There are at least three looming scenarios which are posing threats and challenges to the public's health and health security but which authorities and the health professions (including nursing) have yet to substantively prepare for from an ethical standpoint: climate change, pandemic influenza and the 'slow pandemic' of antimicrobial resistance (AMR), which some scientists regard as being more threatening than climate change (*Telegraph Reporter* 2014). Adding to the complexity of these scenarios and compounding their harmful impact is the problem of health inequalities, particularly those associated with the immediate and long-term impact of the austerity measures imposed on countries following the global financial crisis circa 2007–09. These will each be considered under separate subheadings below.

Climate change[2]

Images of the catastrophic damage left in the wake of widely reported extreme weather events across the globe stand as graphic harbingers of what lies ahead as the world's climate changes. Regardless of the political disagreements over what 'the' ultimate cause of climate change is, there is a near-global consensus among the world's scientists that the climate is warming and that this change in climate involves harm – to human beings, to other species (many of which face being wiped out) and to the environment. It is the harms (preventable and otherwise) that are projected to occur in the near and distant futures (and that are already occurring) that place climate change firmly within the domain of ethics. Moreover, as Gardiner (2010: 87) correctly points out, 'at a most general level [...] we cannot get very far in discussing why climate change is a problem without invoking ethical considerations'. He further contends:

> *If we do not think that our own actions are open to moral assessment, or that various interests (our own, those of our kin and country, those of distant people, future people, animals, and nature) matter, then it is hard to see why climate change (or much else) poses a problem.* (Gardiner 2010: 87)

Some might counter that 'science has all the answers' and that it is 'drawing a long bow' characterising climate change as an ethical issue, or that the ethical dimensions of climate change are serious enough to warrant attention. Such a stance is, however, misguided. As the discussion in the previous chapters of this book has shown, ethics as a discipline fundamentally involves concern for others and, in particular, the prevention of harm and suffering to innocent others. Climate change at its most basic level threatens preventable harm to many entities. Although scientific research can tell us *what* is going on, it cannot tell us what we *should* do about it. This is because deciding what we 'should' do requires not only a grasp of the facts of the matter, but also a grasp of the values pertinent to the decisions that will ultimately need to be made – including what we value, what we think is 'right', how we justify our judgments of right and wrong, whose interests should count, who we are and who we want to be (Gardiner 2010, 2011; Garvey 2008).

Climate change is a 'burgeoning public health concern' that is already contributing to health disparities in vulnerable populations (Kreslake et al 2018). As noted by Kreslake and colleagues (2018), climate change has serious and significant implications for 'chronic health conditions; nutrition and food security; food, water, and vector borne diseases; and social disruption, injuries, displacement, and death associated with extreme weather' (Kreslake et al 2018: 568). It is also raising the possibility of what Dyer (2008) has called 'climate wars' whereby regions and nations enter into a 'desperate struggle for advantage and survival' and are ultimately drawn into conflict over acute and permanent crises in food and water supplies. A major casualty of these events will undoubtedly be the health security of people and whole nations.

In response to growing local and global concerns about the public health impacts of climate change, the nursing literature and nursing organisations are increasingly giving attention to the issue, believing it to be 'one of the largest threats to human health that the planet has ever experienced' (Sullivan-Marx & McCauley 2017: 593; see also Adlong & Dietsch 2015; Anderko 2017; Angelini 2017; Australian Nursing and Midwifery Federation (ANMF) 2015; Leffers & Butterfield 2018; New Zealand Nurses Organisation (NZNO) 2016). This has included drawing attention to the issue of 'climate justice' – a notion that refers to 'the ethical and human rights issues that occur as a result of climate change', including the unequal distribution of the burdens of climate change (e.g. in terms of health, food and water security) imposed on vulnerable populations (Nicholas & Breakey 2017: 609). A notable example of this emerging trend can be found in the publication of a collection of essays in the November 2017 special issue of *Image: Journal of Nursing Scholarship* (the official journal of the Sigma Theta Tau International (STTI) Honor Society of Nursing) in which critical attention is given to addressing the issue of 'Climate change, global health, and nursing scholarship' (Sullivan-Marx & McCauley 2017). Despite this emerging trend in the nursing literature, important questions remain such as: 'Is nursing ethics up to the task of guiding what Garvey (2008: 114) terms a "morally adequate" response to the moral challenges posed by climate change?', 'Or will nursing ethics, like other ethical perspectives, require a fundamental paradigm shift in order to cope with the moral demands that lay ahead (after Jamieson 2010)?'

The nursing profession has yet to make more than a rhetorical response to the ethics of climate change, the window of opportunity for which is narrowing. Responding to the ethics of climate change will, however, not be easy on account of its involving what Gardiner (2011) has famously termed 'the perfect moral storm' (after the Hollywood film of the same title), which he describes as involving the unusual convergence of a number of serious, and mutually reinforcing, problems (or 'storms') that undermine our ability to behave ethically (Gardiner 2011: 77). The intersecting 'storms' in this instance include: (i) a serious global asymmetry of power whereby some (i.e. the more powerful) may take undue advantage of others; (ii) an intergenerational power imbalance whereby current generations may affect the prospects of future generations, but not vice versa; and (iii) the problem of theoretical inadequacy whereby conventional moral theories are simply ill-equipped to deal with the kinds of problems posed by long-term futures (Gardiner 2011).

The nursing profession has the intellectual and emotional resources to 'unpack' the issues at stake and to develop a robust understanding of and a nursing-focused response to each of the three intersecting problems which Gardiner has described. Using an adaption of Garvey's (2008: 114–18) 'criteria of moral adequacy', the profession can begin by collectively examining and describing its:

- *historical responsibility* (encompassing consideration of nurses' individual and collective responsibilities locally and globally, to current and future generations, to other species and to the environment)
- *present capacities* (including an honest analysis of the role of nurses and what is required in prudential and ethical terms for the sustainable delivery of essential nursing services)
- *sustainability* (taken as implying 'meeting the needs of the present without compromising the ability of future generations to meet their own needs')
- *processes for procedural fairness* (these must minimally be reasonable, open and transparent, inclusive, responsible and accountable).

Scoping the moral adequacy of the nursing profession's response to the ethics of climate change will not only enable enlightened ethical reflection on the world's current predicament, but will also assist nurses to identify what can and should be done in order to ensure the sustainability of essential nursing services, in both the immediate and the distant future.

Pandemic influenza

In May 2009, the world awoke to the news that a 'swine flu' pandemic was possibly emerging. As the number of suspected and confirmed cases of the flu increased, so too did the levels of anxiety among governments and people as fears mounted that this could be the 'ultra-scenario' that pandemic influenza experts have been warning about for years (McKibbin & Sidorenko 2006). Meanwhile, GPs and emergency departments were reportedly becoming swamped by people exhibiting flu-like symptoms. In some instances health services were stretched to capacity as health care professionals themselves had to be quarantined because either they or a close family member had come into contact with someone infected by the virus.

The recorded history of pandemic influenza dates back to the 5th century BC, with experts suggesting that there have probably been between three and ten human influenza pandemics since this time (McKibbin & Sidorenko 2006: 3). In the 20th century, virologically confirmed human pandemics of the disease were the Spanish H1N1 influenza pandemic (1918–19), the H2N2 Asian influenza (1957–58) and the H3N2 Hong Kong influenza pandemic (1968–69) (McKibbin & Sidorenko 2006: 4). A characteristic feature of all three pandemics was a shift in the age distribution of associated deaths; notably, the mortality rate tended to be higher among previously healthy young adults.

The Spanish influenza pandemic of 1918–19 (which killed more people than World War I) is regarded as being 'the most deadly contagious calamity in human history' (Markel et al 2007: iii). Reportedly over 500 million people (one-third of the world's population) were infected, with an estimated 40–100 million people (3%–5% of the world's population) dying from the virus – a rate that was 5–20 times higher than expected (Johnson & Mueller 2002; Taubenberger & Morens 2006). To this day, the Spanish influenza pandemic stands as 'an ominous warning to public health' (Taubenberger & Morens 2006: 15), with experts cautioning that the big question is not *if* there will be another 'ultra' scenario pandemic (i.e. like the Spanish pandemic) but *when*. Warning of its inevitability, Taubenberger and Morens (2006: 21) point out that:

> Even with modern antiviral and antibacterial drugs, vaccines, and prevention knowledge, the return of a pandemic virus equivalent in pathogenicity to the virus of 1918 would likely kill > 100 million people

worldwide. A pandemic virus with the (alleged) pathogenic potential of some recent H5N1 outbreaks could cause substantially more deaths.

Envisaging a range of possible scenarios (mild, moderate, severe and ultra), other experts warn that 'even in a mild pandemic' an estimated 1.4 million lives would be lost at a cost to the world's economy and GDP of around 0.8% (or $US 330 billion); in the case of an 'ultra' scenario an estimated 142.2 million lives would be lost at a cost to the world's economy and GDP of around $US 4.4 trillion (McKibbin & Sidorenko 2006: iii).

As it turned out, the emergence of swine flu epidemic did not become the 'ultra' pandemic scenario many feared it could become. Even so, it prompted a number of important questions: ' "What if" things had been worse?', 'What if swine flu had progressed rapidly to the "ultra-scenario" that experts have been warning about for years?', 'How prepared "really" are government agencies, the health care professions and the community at large for dealing not just with the practical aspects of managing a pandemic (e.g. keeping the infrastructure of society functioning), but also with the morally agonising choices that would have to be made?' and, more importantly, 'How prepared are individual countries and the world at large for dealing ethically with the consequences that are likely to arise from catastrophic disasters generally (whether of a natural, technological or human cause) and their implications for health care services?'

2018 marked the 100th anniversary of the Spanish influenza pandemic (circa 1918–19). This anniversary prompted experts in the field to reflect on how well prepared (if at all) the world is for the next influenza pandemic (Belser & Tumpey 2018; Medina 2018; Zhang & Webster 2017). Of particular concern were the characteristic features of influenza pandemics – notably their capacity to emerge suddenly, unexpectedly and with little warning (Belser & Tumpey 2018; Medina 2018), the capacity of the viruses responsible to 'rapidly acquire mutations that evade our most recent vaccine formulations' (Belser & Tumpey 2018: 255), and the inability of scientists to predict 'if and when a particular viral subtype will acquire pandemic ability' (Zhang & Webster 2018: 111). Scientists also reflected on the processes compounding the continuous and real threat of a new influenza pandemic emerging – namely: the growth in human population, the rapid development of megacities in the developing world, and the 'unprecedented level of global trade and travel' – all of which will enable the rapid and wide transmission of the disease (Osterholm 2017). Global travel is a particularly worrying factor. For example, it has been estimated that there were more than 4 billion international travellers in 2017, with global air travel expected to double by 2036 (https://www.travelpulse.com/news/airlines/global-air-passenger-traffic-soared-in-2017.html).

In addition to the above, scientists have reflected on the moral as well as the practical lessons learned from the recent outbreaks of other highly contagious and dangerous diseases such as those caused by the Ebola, Chikungunya and Zika viruses (Gostin & Ayala 2017) and the risk of what Quick and Fryer (2018: 57) have described as 'the triple threat: bioterror, bio-error and Dr Frankenstein', described below.

Bioterror, which involves the deliberate and malicious use of harmful microbial agents as a terrorist weapon, is defined by the US Centers for Disease Control and Prevention (CDC) as the use of biological agents (microbes or toxins) 'as weapons to further personal or political agendas' (CDC 2017). The CDC (2017) further explains that acts of bioterrorism can 'range from a single exposure directed at an individual by another individual to government-sponsored biological warfare resulting in mass casualties'. Bioterrorism is not a new phenomenon and has been used as a weapon of war throughout history, with one of the earliest recorded events dating back to AD1155 (Quick & Fryer 2018: 60).

Bio-error refers to the mistakes and accidents that can and do occur even in the world's highest-level biosafety laboratories, including research laboratories that hold repositories of highly dangerous and deadly organisms (Quick & Fryer 2018: 67). As these laboratories are not 'fool proof' and human beings are prone to error, mistakes can be made with catastrophic consequences to both individual and public health.

Finally, there are the risks associated with scientists playing 'Dr Frankenstein' (i.e. 'playing God'), particularly those involved in genetic sequencing (Quick & Fryer 2018: 69). On this issue, Quick and Fryer (2018: 71) ask: 'What kind of research jumps over the line of acceptability?' and conclude, 'It's a stop-and-think question, and an old one' for which security checks may not be the answer.

Reflecting on the outbreaks of Ebola, Chikungunya, Zika and other diseases caused by these viruses, Gostin and Ayala (2017: 3) provide the sobering reminder that while scientists 'cannot tell us which epidemics will strike […] they can predict with assuredness that dangerous infectious disease threats will materialize, based on historical trends and currently circulating pathogens'. They go on to contend that 'despite the certainty and magnitude of the threat, the global community has significantly underestimated and underinvested in avoidance of pandemic threats' (Gostin & Ayala 2018: 3). There is scope to add that authorities have also significantly underestimated the ethical issues that will arise during pandemics and have underinvested in anticipating and developing a sound ethics framework for dealing with the quandaries that will inevitably emerge.

Antimicrobial resistance

Antimicrobial resistance (AMR) is a broad term that refers to the 'resistance of a microorganism to an antimicrobial drug that was originally effective for treatment of infections caused by it' (WHO 2014e: 1). Resistant microorganisms include bacteria, fungi, viruses and parasites that are no longer susceptible to antimicrobial drugs, such as antibacterial drugs (e.g. antibiotics), antifungals, antivirals and antimalarials (WHO 2014e, 2014f). When people become infected with microorganisms resistant to antimicrobial drugs, they are unable to be treated with standard treatments since these will not be effective. Moreover, if infection persists, there is a risk of this spreading to others thereby exacerbating the incidence and impact of antimicrobial resistance.

Of particular global concern in the 21st century are drug-resistant bacteria that cause common infections. In recognition of this, the WHO Assistant Director-General, Health Security, provides the following stark warning:

> *A post-antibiotic era – in which common infections and minor injuries can kill – far from being an apocalyptic fantasy, is instead a very real possibility for the 21st century.* (Fukuda 2014: ix)

For over six decades, antibacterial drugs have been the front-line defence against infections – irrespective of where they were acquired. However, due to their widespread acceptance and (mis)use in humans and non-humans over the decades, their effectiveness has gradually declined. Commensurate with this decline has been the failure, since the 1980s, to discover any completely new classes of antibacterial drugs to which most common pathogens are susceptible (WHO 2014e, 2014f).

Today patients with infections caused by drug-resistant bacteria are already at an increased risk of 'worse clinical outcomes and death, and consume more health care resources, than patients infected with the same bacteria not demonstrating the resistance pattern in question' (WHO 2014e: xii). An everyday example of this can be found in the high percentage of hospital-acquired infections caused by the highly resistant bacteria methicillin-resistant *Staphylococcus aureus* (or MRSA) or other multidrug-resistant Gram-negative bacteria (WHO 2014e: 1). These bacteria are responsible for the global incidence of such common drug-resistant infections as urinary tract infections, pneumonia and bloodstream infections. Another increasingly worrying trend is the emergence of multidrug-resistant tuberculosis – both as a primary and as an opportunistic disease (e.g. in people whose immune system is already compromised, such as with HIV/AIDS, rendering them more susceptible to the disease). For example, WHO (2018d) reported that in 2016 there were approximately 600 000 new cases of multidrug-resistant tuberculosis (MDR-TB), with 117 countries worldwide reporting at least one case of extensively drug-resistant tuberculosis (XDRTB) at the end of 2015 (Chan 2017; WHO 2016). Other 'apocalyptic' bacteria (first seen in India in 2009) are the *carbapenem-resistant Enterobacteriaceae* (or CRE), a group of gut bacteria (including the common microbe *Escherichia coli*) that are resistant to carbapenems – the 'antibiotics of last resort' to treat severe community-acquired and hospital-acquired infections (WHO 2014d: xi).

The WHO has designated AMR as a 'political priority' alongside climate change and air pollution (Chan 2017: 140). In 2016 the UN General Assembly held its 'first high-level meeting on antimicrobial resistance and adopted a far-reaching political declaration' aimed at mobilising a global effort to combat the problem (Chan 2017: 142). In addition, WHO has assumed a proactive role as a 'guardian of public health' regarding this issue. This role, as described by the WHO, involves 'tracking rapidly evolving threats, quantifying the harm to health, and sounding the alarm' (Chan 2017: 136). In keeping with this role, WHO also works 'to raise political awareness and extend advice on the best protective strategies for safeguarding public health', which often requires establishing collaboration with multiple non-health sectors (Chan 2017: 136).

The emergence and spread of drug-resistant bacteria and other microbial organisms has drawn attention to the 'three Rs' of public health emergencies referred to above. In particular, it raises profound moral questions about: *rationing* (of antibiotics and other antimicrobial drugs to those who 'really' need them and in whom they are most likely to be effective), *restrictions* (on people's liberties / access – noting that, as in the case of influenza pandemics, 'coercive social distancing' may be necessary – i.e. isolating patients and contacts, closing schools, and closing some businesses in order to prevent the spread of cross-infection; third-party notifications may also be required (MacKenzie 2009; Selgelid 2008)), and *responsibilities* (e.g. health care professionals' 'duty to treat' at the risk of acquiring occupational AMR infections; the 'responsible' prescription, administration and monitoring of antibiotics and other antimicrobial drugs; avoiding 'medically futile' treatment) (Marcus et al 2001).

The problem of drug-resistant bacteria and other microbial organisms is now recognised as a major public health issue. Although not as acute as an influenza pandemic, the moral quandaries associated with this global problem are much the same. In recognition of this, the WHO (2014e, 2014f) has called for concerted and coordinated action to help minimise the spread of drug-resistant antibiotics and to tackle generally microbial resistance. Of particular note is its call to 'preserve the efficacy of existing drugs' and 'prescribing and dispensing antibiotics *only when they are truly needed*' (WHO 2014e: 1).

Inequalities in health and health care

In 1978, at the International Conference on Primary Health Care held in Alma-Ata, Kazakhstan (formerly the Kazakh Soviet Socialist Republic), the 'Alma-Ata Declaration' was adopted. The Declaration expressed the need 'for urgent action by all governments, all health and development workers, and the world community to protect and promote the health of all the people of the world' (WHO 1978: 1). At the foundation of the Declaration were the principles of primary health care, which was seen by its proponents 'as the way to overcome gross health inequalities between and within countries' (Lee 2003: 4).

Positioned as a clarion call to action, the Declaration became the catalyst for a 'health for all' movement (Lee 2003: 4). While the ideal of 'health for all' emerged as a slogan for the movement, as former WHO Director-General Jong-Wook Lee explained, it was much more than this: *it was also an organising principle for the movement* – 'everybody needs and is entitled to the highest possible standard of health' (Lee 2003: 4).

In 1979, in a move that effectively endorsed the Alma Ata Declaration, the 32nd World Health Assembly (WHA) adopted resolution WHA32.30 and launched the *Global strategy for health for all by the year 2000* (WHO 1981). In the same resolution, the WHA invited Member States of WHO 'to act individually in formulating national policies, strategies and plans of action for attaining this goal, and collectively in formulating regional and global strategies' using the WHO's Executive Board's *Global strategy for health for all by the year 2000*, which had been based on the Alma-Ata Declaration (WHO 1981: 7). It was strongly believed and envisaged that this strategy would be foundational to all the world's people achieving a level of health that would enable them to lead socially and economically productive lives (WHO 1981). As the year 2000 approached, however, it soon became clear that the ambitious goal of 'health for all by the year 2000' would not be realised. Thus, in 1998, a new global health policy 'health for all in the 21st century' was released. This document incorporated additional elements not considered in Alma-Ata and sought to confirm the goals of 'health for all' as:

- *To attain health security for all*
- *To achieve global health equity*
- *To increase healthy life expectancy*
- *To ensure access for all to essential health care of good quality*. (WHO 1981, 1998)

Meanwhile, in the year 2000, frustrated by a lack of progress made to achieve the goals of the Alma-Ata Declaration, and the deepening *health inequalities* around the world, 1453 delegates from 92 countries met at Dhaka, Bangladesh, for the First *People's Health Assembly* (People's Health Movement (2000), online: http://phmovement.org/the-peoples-charter-for-health/). This meeting led to the founding of the 'People's Health Movement' (PHM) and the drafting of the *People's charter for health*. Now available in 40 languages, the *People's charter for health* stands as 'the most widely endorsed consensus document on health since the Alma Ata Declaration' (People's Health Movement, online at http://phmovement.org/the-peoples-charter-for-health/). Taking as its slogan 'Health for all now!', the Charter provides 'a statement of the shared vision, goals, principles and calls for action that unite all the members of the PHM coalition' (People's Health Movement, online).

Despite these and associated initiatives, inequalities in health and health care remained stubbornly recalcitrant. Lamenting the situation, in 2003, WHO Director-General Jong-Wook Lee warned that the world's 'healthier future' was in serious jeopardy:

> *Today's global health situation raises urgent questions about justice. In some parts of the world there is a continued expectation of longer and more comfortable life, while in many others there is despair over the failure to control disease although the means to do so exist. [...] A world marked by such inequities is in very serious trouble. We have to find ways to unite our strengths as a global community to shape a healthier future.* (Lee 2003: 3)

In 2010, echoing the sentiments of her predecessors, WHO Director-General Dr Margaret Chan renewed calls for 'deliberate policy decision' and associated action; she wrote:

> *Decades of experience tell us that this world will not become a fair place for health all by itself. Health systems will not automatically gravitate towards greater equity or naturally evolve towards universal coverage. Economic decisions within a country will not automatically protect the poor or promote their health. Globalization will not self-regulate in ways that ensure fair distribution of benefits. International trade agreements will not, by themselves, guarantee food security, or job security, or health security, or access to affordable medicines. All of these outcomes require deliberate policy decisions.* (Chan 2010: 2)

Endorsing the WHO's latest publication, *Equity, social determinants and public health programmes* (WHO 2010, edited by Blas & Kurup), Chan goes on to challenge all to consider the 'sheer magnitude' of people's unmet health needs and the related compelling need to consider 'fresh – sometimes daring – proposals', such as those set out in the publication, in order to redress the health inequities that are so apparent (Chan 2010: 2).

Calls to 'close the gap' in health inequalities continue. Portrayed as a 'life and death' social justice issue (and one that is quite literally 'killing people'), stakeholders are reminded that *health inequities* affect 'the way people live, their consequent chance of illness, and their risk of premature death' (Commission on Social Determinants of Health (CSDH) 2008: ii). This view is not new.

It has long been recognised that the health of people rests on a complex array of conditions and processes, not merely access to health care. For instance, it is known that the public's health is deeply rooted in social, cultural, economic and political circumstances and that, if the health of people is to be achieved, these conditions need to be understood and considered (Anand et al 2004; Daniels 2006; McMurray 2007; Mann et al 1999; Wilkinson & Marmot 2003). It is also known that, to achieve the goal of health, people need to be situated in a 'strong, mutually supportive and non-exploitative community' (WHO 1995: 4). Over the past four decades this knowledge has seen cycles of public attention given to such things as poverty, unemployment, poor housing, racial discrimination, homophobia, cultural dispossession, social isolation and the impact these conditions have had on the health of people. But, as commentators observed as early as 1975:

> *this attention and interest rapidly wane when it becomes clear that solving these problems requires painful costs that the dominant interests in society are unwilling to pay. Our public ethics do not seem to fit our public problems.* (Beauchamp 1976: 20)

Inequities in health should be neither tolerated nor 'explained away'. As succinctly stated by the Commission on Social Determinants of Health (CSDH):

> *It does not have to be this way and it is not right that it should be like this. Where systematic differences in health are judged to be avoidable by reasonable action they are, quite simply, unfair. It is this that we label health inequity. Putting right these inequities – the huge and remediable differences in health between and within countries – is a matter of social justice. Reducing health inequities is, for the Commission on Social Determinants of Health [...] an ethical imperative.* (CSDH 2008: vii)

In 2014, in an address to graduates of the AT Still University (ATSU), School of Osteopathic Medicine, renowned US futurist Dr Clem Bezold identified the growing *health equity movement* as the 'next civil rights movement'. He warned, however, that:

> *This goal to achieve health equity is no small thing in human history. Like movements to abolish slavery, to end segregation and oppression, to give women equal rights, and to protect the environment – the health movement will take time.* (Bezold 2014: 2)

Just how much time it will take to reduce health inequities and inequalities will depend, in no small way, on how committed governments, the business sector, communities and indeed the health care sector are to 'eliminating unfair and avoidable differences in health conditions among racial, economic and neighborhood groups' (Bezold 2014: 2). The Global Financial Crisis (or 'GFC') of 2007–09, which resulted in the collapse of large financial institutions and led to the 2008–12 global recession and which, in turn, contributed to the European sovereign-debt crisis, provides some salutatory lessons on the question of health inequity and what Kentikelenis and colleagues (2014: 751) have termed the 'health hazards of austerity', an example of which follows.

During the years 2009–12, as part of the austerity measures it adopted, the Greek government slashed funding to the country's health care and social services. Unlike Iceland and Finland, which had 'ring fenced' health and social budgets when dealing with the GFC, the Greek government drastically cut funds for such things as hospital operating costs (cut by 26%), pharmaceutical supplies, prevention and treatment programs for illicit drug use, mosquito-spraying programs and mental health services (Kentikelenis et al 2014). These cuts all had a flow-on effect to the not-for-profit sector, which had to scale back operations, shut down or reduce staff. Worryingly, state funding for mental health reportedly decreased by 20% between 2010 and 2011, and by a further 55% between 2011 and 2012, which severely constrained the capacity of the country's mental health services to cope with an estimated 120% increase in use over the past 3 years (Kentikelenis et al 2014: 750). The aged care sector has also been seriously affected by the austerity measures, which saw a significant increase in the inability of most older people 'to obtain care' (Kentikelenis et al 2014: 749).

Both the immediate and long-term health consequences of these austerity measures have proved to be dire. As Kentikelenis and colleagues reported (2014):

- as a result of cutbacks to street work programs for injecting drug users, the number of new HIV infections rose from 15 in 2009 to 484 in 2012
- cutbacks in mosquito-spraying programs have seen the re-emergence of locally transmitted malaria 'for the first time in 40 years'
- cuts in pharmaceutical funding have resulted in shortages of medicines and medical equipment, with some medicines becoming unobtainable
- cuts to mental health services are seeing a substantial deterioration in the mental health of people, with the prevalence of depression increasing from 3.3% in 2008 to 8.2% in 2011, and an estimated 36% increase in people attempting suicide
- cuts to perinatal and maternal and child health services have also had a dramatic impact on maternal and child health, with a reported 21% rise in still births between 2008 and 2011, the reversal of a long-term fall in infant mortality, which rose by 43% between 2008 and 2011, and a rise in the proportion of children suffering from malnutrition.

Meanwhile, government officials reportedly rejected claims that 'vulnerable groups (e.g. homeless or uninsured people) have been denied access to health care, and claim that those who are unable to afford public insurance contributions still receive free care' (Kentikelenis et al 2014: 751). The negative and long-lasting impact of austerity measures on health, both locally and globally, continue to be researched and documented (Basu S et al 2017; Carney & Kenworthy 2017; Ruckert & Labonté 2017; Stuckler et al 2017). Of particular concern is the enduring two-pronged impact of austerity mechanisms on health; as noted by Stuckler and colleagues (2017: 18) these encompass direct and indirect 'social risk effects' (manifest as 'increasing unemployment, poverty, homelessness and other socio-economic risk factors') and direct 'health care effects' (manifest through 'cuts to health care services, as well as reductions in health coverage and restricting access to care').

Interestingly, the effects of Greece's austerity measures on people's health are predicted to have another more insidious long-term consequence: stress-related genetic changes, which may threaten the health of future generations for years to come.

Social determinants of health and stress have long been recognised as a predictor of morbidity and mortality. However, the mechanisms underpinning both the short- and long-term effects of social stresses on health have not been well understood, until now. Researchers in the burgeoning field of social genomics, for instance, are increasingly suggesting that there exists a high risk of what has been termed 'austerity's toxic genetic legacy' when people are faced with extreme social stress such as that caused by austerity (Coghlan 2013).

Social genomics is credited with fostering a significant 'paradigm shift in thinking on gene–environment interactions' as new evidence emerges showing that 'social–environmental factors can substantially alter the expression of literally hundreds of genes', yielding new insights into 'how social conditions shape complex phenotypes and susceptibility to disease' (Slavich & Cole 2013: 343). For example, studies are beginning to demonstrate how acute social stressors and neurocognitive pathways may be implicated in increasing people's susceptibility to disease via the gene regulation of an individual's physiology and immune system (Tung et al 2012). Diseases with an inflammatory component (e.g. cardiovascular disease and depression) are particularly susceptible to influences of the social environment (Slavich & Cole 2013; Slavich et al 2010).

The results of these and similar studies are regarded as providing 'new theoretical and computational modelling frameworks that link human molecular genetics to genomic evolution and gene–culture coevolution' (Slavich & Cole 2013: 343). They are also heralding a potentially new era of moral accountability as findings make it increasingly difficult to ignore the interconnectedness between human beings and their social environment and the morally culpable impact this stands to have on current and future generations. On this point, as Slavich and Cole conclude:

> *For although as adults we are often physically separated from those around us, our presence in different social groups means that we are transcriptionally connected, giving rise to a human metagenome that has implications for collective health and behavior.* (Slavich & Cole 2013: 343)

The negative health impact of austerity measures and the health and social injustices these have imposed on vulnerable populations are a nursing concern. The nursing profession has long subscribed to social justice as a given in health care and as the foundation of public health. It also has a rich and distinctive history of promoting health care justice for the individuals, groups and communities it serves (Johnstone 2011). Social justice as a representative idea of contemporary nursing is expressed through various visions and mission statements that commit the nursing profession 'to lead our societies toward better health' (ICN 2007: 1) and to advocate for human rights 'especially those related to access to essential health care and patient safety' (ICN 2011a).

For justice to 'truly' serve as a representative idea of nursing, however, nurses like other health professionals, need to 'go beyond the "binding of wounds"' and 'the tradition of remaining morally and politically neutral' (Summerfield, 2000: 234). They need fundamentally to activate for social reform as well as public recognition and reparation of the harmful health consequences of injustices that those whose vulnerability is exacerbated by austerity measures bear often silently, alone and without recompense (Johnstone 2011).

Emergency preparedness

Like others (government agencies, policy-makers and bioethicists among them), the nursing profession has been slow to anticipate, plan and prepare for the ethical quandaries of public health emergencies. As even a cursory search of the nursing literature will show, the nursing profession has not really begun to imagine the ethical challenges it will confront when called upon to respond to the emergency health and social care needs of a public devastated by local and 'whole-of-world' disasters, such as an ultra-pandemic scenario and the spread of *multidrug-resistant bacteria*. Although an increasing number of studies are being published on nurses' anticipated and actual experiences of providing care in public health emergencies, few have examined the ethical issues that nurses actually encountered in these situations or how prepared they are to deal with the ethical quandaries they may have to face during public health emergencies in which they may become involved (Johnstone & Turale 2014).

The converging scenarios and catastrophic consequences imposed by influenza and other pandemics, the growing spread of drug-resistant microbial infections, climate change and other crises (e.g. global financial crises, failings in cybersecurity[3]) are likely to place unprecedented and overwhelming demands on the health care system and the individuals comprising it. For example, as indicated earlier, climate change will see a significant increase in illness and deaths from frequent and severe heat waves, vector-borne diseases and other extreme weather events. The interconnected scenarios posed by pandemic influenza, the spread and health impact of multidrug-resistant bacteria, climate change and other scenarios (such as that posed by the unprecedented outbreak and spread of Ebola virus disease (see Kieny et al

2014; Quammen 2014) will increasingly give rise to unprecedented moral quandaries in health care. As demand for health care services rapidly exceeds supply, nurses and allied health care professionals will quickly discover that, contrary to what they have become accustomed to, they will not be able to treat and care for everybody equally in every situation. Especially confronting will be the reality that, what would ordinarily be regarded as unethical under normal circumstances will become ethical 'under the emergency rules activated by the trigger' (Berlinger & Moses 2007). These realities will, in all likelihood, be exacerbated in situations involving infectious diseases (such as Ebola virus disease) that are highly contagious, have a high morbidity and mortality rate (complicating the processes of diagnosis, treatment and prevention), have an acute onset, progress rapidly, are associated with a high level of both individual and community susceptibility, evoke in people widespread fear and panic, and stand to have a substantially negative socioeconomic impact (Selgelid et al 2006; Smith et al 2006). Coupled with widespread fear and panic amongst the public, fuelled in no small way by mass news media reporting (see Hooker et al 2012), the practical and moral consequences, both immediate and long term, are likely to be dire.

It has already been anticipated that, in ultra-scenarios caused by catastrophic events, health care professionals and the public at large must expect that:

- accepted standards of care will be altered (termed 'altered standards of care', it has been suggested that this will be necessary if the catastrophic collapse of health care is to be averted)
- (in the case of influenza and other pandemics) patients will be removed from life supports without their consent (there simply will not be time to follow the 'usual procedures')
- patients will die without their loved ones being present (if in a quarantined or disaster zone, people will not be able to get to their loved ones)
- 'palliative disaster care' will become the only option for many people (patients without access to critical care will receive 'comfort care' only – provided, of course, there are sufficient palliative care services available)
- other treatable conditions will not be able to be treated
- euthanasia as a policy-directed triage option may become a reality
- pastoral care nursing may, in many cases, be all that can be offered (e.g. when a drug-resistant microbial infection is out of control) (Johnstone & Turale 2014).

Worryingly, many countries still lack a comprehensive, clearly articulated, agreed-upon ethical framework for guiding policy, planning and decision-making in public health emergencies. So too does the nursing profession. Although some countries (e.g. Canada, New Zealand, the United Kingdom and the USA) have developed ethical frameworks for responding to pandemic influenza (WHO 2007d), these documents fall short of providing guidance in 'all hazards' ultra-scenarios.

There is a pressing need – and only a small window of opportunity – to redress this oversight. The health care professions and the broader community need to come together to explore and agree on the ethical values (e.g. solidarity, altruism, justice) and ethical framework that is necessary to guide a just response to the disaster scenarios that lay ahead. Moreover, this needs to happen now while we still have 'choices' and there is time to prepare. The underpinning moral imperatives of this are clear; as noted by the Toronto-based Joint Centre for Bioethics Pandemic Influenza Working Group (2005: 4):

> SARS showed there are costs from not having an agreed-upon ethical framework, including loss of trust, low morale, fear and misinformation. SARS taught the world that if ethical frameworks had been more widely used to guide decision-making, this would have increased trust and solidarity within and between health care organisations. SARS gave the world an advance warning of the need for ethical frameworks for decision making during other communicable disease outbreaks, such as a flu pandemic.

The Working Group further noted that:

> If ethics are clearly built into pandemic plans in an open and transparent manner, and with buy-in from multiple sectors of society, the plans carry greater trust, authority and legitimacy. Advance discussions on such issues can help to address fears of the unknown. People will be more likely to cooperate and accept difficult decisions made by their leaders for the common good. (Joint Centre for Bioethics Pandemic Influenza Working Group 2005: 3)

A useful resource and starting point for this initiative can be found in the World Health Organization (WHO 2007d) *Ethical considerations in developing a public health response to pandemic influenza*. The stated purpose of this document is to 'assist social and political leaders at all levels who influence policy decisions about the incorporation of ethical considerations into national influenza pandemic preparedness plans' (WHO 2007e: 2). This document, however, also has the capacity to assist nursing leaders to plan for and prepare members of the profession to navigate the moral quandaries and obligations that inevitably lie ahead when a human influenza or other pandemic, antimicrobial resistance or other public health emergency arisees.

Conclusion

The capacity of nurses to respond ethically to future 'whole-of-world' events is going to require a much greater readiness than that supplied by a textbook rehearsal of arguments about moral agency, accountability and responsibility. It is also going to require: collaboration with other disciplines (the issues briefly considered in this chapter are far too big to be addressed by nursing *alone*); thinking *centuries* not just decades ahead, anticipating and preparing for the ethical issues that these 'whole-of-world' problems will give rise to; and working with people to help overcome their 'deep indifference' or 'paralysing fear' about the future (as Brooks (2009: 25) has noted, it is notoriously difficult to inspire people to prepare for a potential crisis that either 'has never happened before or may not happen for decades to come', or, that is so terrifying they cannot bear to even begin thinking about). Ethical readiness will also require the deep internalisation and practice of the ideals of *moral wisdom*, *decency*, *altruism* and *justice*, without which human survival will not be possible.

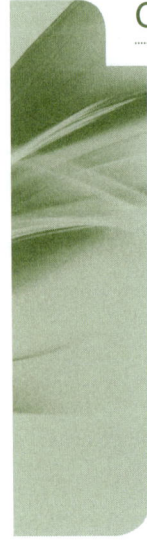

Case scenario 1

In 2003, during the outbreak of SARS in Canada, a registered nurse with 17 years' experience was 'drafted' into a special SARS team. When drafted, the nurse gained the impression that if she refused to join the team 'this might lead to dismissal' (Sibbald 2003: 141). Concerned that the hospital did not have adequate measures 'to protect her, and by extension her 3 children and immunocompromised mother, who is recovering after a kidney transplant' she refused to join the team (p 141). She further asserted that 'If it was just myself, I would join [the team]. But can the hospital guarantee that I [won't] get sick, or my kids and mother?' Upon announcing her refusal the head nurse reportedly told her 'not to come in for her regular shift the next day' (p 141). It was later reported that, under Ontario's Occupational Health and Safety Act, the nurse was permitted to refuse to work when the 'physical condition of the workplace ... is likely to endanger' – which in this case it was (p 141). In response to the case, a bioethicist also contended that:

> There is a threshold beyond which health care workers aren't obliged to take personal risks. We don't expect firefighters to jump into a burning pit, or police officers to throw themselves in front of a bullet ... How health care workers define this threshold is an intensely personal decision ... but obviously, it has serious implications for our collective response to a problem like SARS. (Singer, quoted in Sibbald 2003: 141)

Case scenario 2[4]

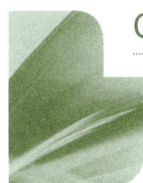

In 2005, in the aftermath of Hurricane Katrina, allegations were made that a number of 'mercy killings' had occurred at the Memorial Medical Centre in the city of New Orleans. As inquiries progressed, it was revealed that four non-ambulatory patients had been 'euthanised' apparently to prevent their needless suffering in the face of having 'no realistic chances of surviving in a stranded, incapacitated hospital' (Curiel 2006: 2067). In July of the following year, a New Orleans physician and two nurses were arrested and charged with second-degree murder in relation to the patients' deaths, sparking public debate on whether the killings were 'murder or mercy'.

It was eventually revealed that none of the four patients in question were expected to die immediately from natural causes, were in pain, or had consented to the lethal dose of drugs they were given. They did, however, have several characteristics in common: they were poor, black, old (61–90 years of age) and dependent on their professional caregivers. Another thing in common was that all were the subject of a consented 'DNR' (Do Not Resuscitate) directive – although, as one observer noted, no one had warned them that in case of a natural disaster the hospital staff would interpret DNR to mean 'Do Not Rescue'.

Case scenario 3

In 2013, at the Australian Nursing and Midwifery Federation (ANMF) National Biennial Conference, an agenda was set for the Federation which included commitments to lobby government for *social justice* (including human rights) and *political issues* (including defending 'universal health care for all' and opposing the 'privatization of public health services') (*Australian Nursing and Midwifery Journal* (ANMJ) 2013–14: 20–21).

CRITICAL QUESTIONS

1. In regard to the first case scenario, despite her fears and misgivings, should the RN have nonetheless agreed to join the SARS team? Should she have been reported to and censured by the local Nurses Board for refusing to join the SARS team? (Whether yes or no, give reasons for your answer.)
2. At what point (at what 'threshold') is it reasonable (or unreasonable) to expect a nurse to place her own personal wellbeing or the wellbeing of her family 'at risk' because of her work?
3. In regard to the second case scenario, were the nurses 'right' or 'wrong' to assist with euthanising the patients? (Give reasons for your answer.)
4. In your view, were the nurses adequately prepared to make such a life-and-death decision in a disaster, and if not, what could have prepared them?
5. With reference to the ANMF agenda in the third case scenario, or any one of the scenarios given in this chapter, develop a strategy for engaging the nursing profession to better prepare for the moral quandaries and challenges that lay ahead and to take action to remedy the harmful sequelae that may occur.

Endnotes

1. This discussion is an expanded version of Johnstone M-J (2013d) Climate change. *Australian Nursing Journal*, 20(8): 24. (Reprinted with permission.)
2. This discussion is an expanded version of Johnstone M-J (2009b). Health care disaster ethics: a call to action. *Australian Nursing Journal*, 17(1): 27. (Reprinted with permission.)

3. Cybercrime in health care has become a universal challenge, with public health institutions across the globe (including those in Australia, the UK and the USA) increasingly facing threats (Ahmed & Barkat Ullah 2018; Coventry & Branley 2018; Krisberg 2017; Kruse et al 2017; Martin G et al 2017). Breaches in cybersecurity have the capacity to severely disrupt both public health services and the critical infrastructures of society (e.g. energy systems, water supply systems, the transportation system, sewerage management) which are essential to maintaining the public's health (Kruse et al 2017). While ransomware poses significant challenges and costs to health services, the more serious issue is the theft of patients' medical records. This is because these records contain patients' personal data – e.g. name, birthdate, Medicare numbers) for which there is a high demand in the black market – i.e. by those engaged in identity theft (Ahmed & Barkat Ullah 2018). Equally troubling is the risk of false data being injected into the system, which, as Ahmed and Barkat Ullah (2018) correctly argue, could lead to the dangerous consequences of wrong diagnoses being made, loss of 'real-time' monitoring during surgical procedures, wrong or unwanted treatment being administered, and thus preventable harmful events occurring including deterioration in a patient's health condition and/or even death. There is also a risk of implanted devices being hacked – such as pacemakers (Hamlyn-Harris 2017) and connected diabetes devices – which, quite simply, could kill a patient (Klonoff 2015). The capacity of cybercrime to severely disrupt public health should not be underestimated.

4. Taken from Johnstone M-J (2008) Questioning nursing ethics. *Australian Nursing Journal*, 15(7): 19. (Reprinted with permission.)

Bibliography

Abarshi E A, Paapavasiliou E S, Preston N, Brown J & Payne S (2014) The complexity of nurses attitudes and practice of sedation at the end of life: a systematic literature review. *Journal of Pain and Symptom Management*, 47(5): 915-25

Abarshi E, Rietjens J, Robijn L on behalf of EURO IMPACT, et al (2017) International variations in clinical practice guidelines for palliative sedation: a systematic review. *BMJ Supportive and Palliative Care*, 7: 223-9

Abecassis M (2016) Artificial wombs: the third era of human reproduction and the likely impact on French and US law. *Hastings Women's Law Journal*, 27: 3-27

Abimbola K (2013) Culture and the principles of biomedical ethics, *Journal of Commercial Biotechnology*, 19(3): 31-9

Adams S (2013) *NHS 'bans' GPs from carrying out minor operations on patients who smoke unless they promise to quit*, Mail Online. Available: http://www.dailymail.co.uk/news/article-2436944/NHS-bans-GPs-carrying-minor-operations-patients-smoke-unless-promise-quit.html

Addelson K (1994) *Moral passages: toward a collectivist moral theory*. Routledge, New York

Adinolfi M (2004) The artificial uterus. *Prenatal Diagnosis*, 24(7): 570-2

Adlong W & Dietsch E (2015) Nursing and climate change: an emerging connection. *Collegian*, 22(1): 19-24

Admiraal P V (1991) Is there a place for euthanasia? *Bioethics News*, 10(4): 10-23

Affara F A (2000) When tradition maims. *American Journal of Nursing*, 100(8): 52-61

Affara F A (2002) Female genital mutilation is a human rights issue of concern to all women and men. *International Nursing Review*, 49(4): 195-7

AFP (1989) Toronto Court has rethink to allow women's abortion. *Australian*, 13 July: 8

Ahern K (2018) Institutional betrayal and gaslighting. *Journal of Perinatal and Neonatal Nursing*, 32(1): 59-65

Ahern K & McDonald S (2002) The beliefs of nurses who were involved in a whistleblowing event. *Journal of Advanced Nursing*, 38(3): 303-9

Ahmed M & Barkat Ullah A S S M (2018) False data injection attacks in healthcare. In: Y L Boo, D Stirling, L Chi, L Liu, K-L Ong & G Williams (eds) *Data mining: 15th Australasian Conference, AusDM 2017 Melbourne, VIC, Australia, August 19–20, 2017, Revised selected papers*. Springer Nature, Singapore, pp 192-202

Alao A, Soderberg M, Pohl E L & Lolaalao A (2006) Cybersuicide: review of the role of the internet on suicide. *Cyberpsychology and Behaviour*, 9(4): 489-93

Allen R E (ed) (1966) *Greek philosophy: Thales to Aristotle*. Free Press, New York

Allmark P (1995) Can there be an ethics of care? *Journal of Medical Ethics*, 21(1): 19-24

Amato J A (1990) *Victims and values: a history and theory of suffering*. Praeger, New York

American Institutes of Research (2004) *Cultural competency and nursing: a review of current concepts, policies and practices*. Report prepared for the Office of Minority Health, Department of Health and Human Services, Washington, DC

American Journal of Nursing (1988) Court backs nurse fired for questioning an MD. *American Journal of Nursing* 88(11): 1576

American Medical Association (2008) Sedation to unconsciousness in end-of-life care. In: *Report of the Council on Ethical and Judicial Affairs, CEJA Report 5-A-08*. Online. Available: https://www.ama-assn.org/sites/ama-assn.org/files/corp/media-browser/public/about-ama/councils/Council%20Reports/council-on-ethics-and-judicial-affairs/a08-ceja-palliative-sedation.pdf

American Nurses Association (ANA) (2015) *Code of ethics for nurses with interpretative statements*. Buppert, Silverspring, MD.

Amering M, Denk E, Griengl H, Sibitz I & Stastny P (1999) Psychiatric wills of mental health professionals: a survey of opinions regarding advance directives in psychiatry. *Social Psychiatry Psychiatric Epidemiology*, 34(1): 30-4

Amore K (2016) *Severe housing deprivation in Aotearoa/New Zealand: 2001–2013*. He Kainga Oranga/Housing & Health Research Programme, University of Oatgo, Wellington. Online. Available: http://www.healthyhousing.org.nz/wp-content/uploads/2016/08/Severe-housing-deprivation-in-Aotearoa-2001-2013-1.pdf

Amore K, Viggers H, Baker M G & Howden-Chapman P (2013) *Severe Housing Deprivation: The problem and its measurement*. Official Statistics Research Series, 6. Statistics New Zealand, Wellington. Online. Available: http://www.healthyhousing.org.nz/wp-content/uploads/2016/08/Severe-housing-deprivation-in-Aotearoa-2001-2013-1.pdf

Anand S, Peter F & Sen A (eds) (2004) *Public health, ethics, and equity*. Oxford University Press, Oxford

Andaya E & Mishtal J (2017) The erosion of rights to abortion care in the United States: a call for a renewed anthropological engagement with the politics of abortion. *Medical Anthropology Quarterly*, 31(1): 40-59

Anderson S (1990) Patient advocacy and whistleblowing in nursing: help for the helpers. *Nursing Forum*, 25(3): 5-13

Anderson W T (1990) *Reality isn't what it used to be: theatrical politics, ready-to-wear religion, global myths, primitive chic, and other wonders of the postmodern world*. Harper San Francisco, New York

Anderko L (2017) Climate change and public health: nurses can make a difference. *Public Health Nursing*, 34: 99-100

Andorno R (2016) Is vulnerability the foundation of human rights? In: A Masferrer & E García-Sánchez (eds) *Human dignity of the vulnerable in the age of rights*. Ius Gentium: Comparative Perspectives on Law and Justice book series, vol. 55. Springer International, Switzerland, pp 257-72

Anetzberger G J (2004) *The clinical management of elder abuse*. Hawthorne Press, New York

Anetzberger G J (2012) An update on the nature and scope of elder abuse. *Generations – Journal of the American Society on Aging*, 36(3): 12-20

Angelini K (2017) Climate change, health, and the role of nurses. *Nursing for Women's Health*, 21(2): 79-83

Antony M G (2017) How moral disengagement facilitates the detention of refugee children and families. *Journal of Ethnic and Migration Studies*. doi: 10.1080/1369183X.2017.1419860 [Epub ahead of print]

Appelbaum L (2001) The influence of perceived deservingness on policy decisions regarding aid to the poor. *Political Psychology*, 22(3): 419-42

Appelbaum P S (1991) Advance directives for psychiatric treatment. *Hospital and Community Psychiatry*, 42(10): 983-4

Appelbaum P S (2004) Psychiatric advance directives and the treatment of committed patients. *Psychiatric Services*, 55(7): 751-2

Appelbaum P S (2006) Commentary: Psychiatric advance directives at a crossroads – when can PADs be overridden? *Journal of the American Academy of Psychiatry and Law*, 34(3): 395-7

Appelbaum P S (2007) Assessment of patients' competence to consent to treatment. *New England Journal of Medicine*, 357(18): 1834-40

Appelbaum P S & Grisso T (1995) The MacArthur Treatment Competence Study. I: Mental illness and competence to consent to treatment. *Law and Human Behavior*, 19(2): 105-26

Arabi Y M, Al-Sayyari A A & Al Moamary M S (2018) Shifting paradigm: from "No Code" and "Do-Not-Resuscitate" to "Goals of Care" policies. *Annals of Thoracic Medicine*, 13: 67-71

Are M, McIntyre A & Reddy S (2017) Global disparities in cancer pain management and palliative care. *Journal of Surgical Oncology*, 115(5): 637-41

Arevalo J J, Rietjens J A, Swart S J, Perez R S G M & van der Heide A (2013) Day to day care in palliative sedation: survey of nurses' experiences with decision making and performance. *International Journal of Nursing Studies*, 50: 613-21

Armstrong A E (2006) Towards a strong virtue ethics for nursing practice. *Nursing Philosophy*, 7(3): 110-24

Armstrong A E (2007) *Nursing ethics: a virtue-based approach*. Palgrave / Macmillan, Basingstoke, Hants

Armstrong F (2002) Blowing the whistle: the cost of speaking out. *Australian Nursing Journal*, 9(7): 18-20

Armstrong N (2018) Overdiagnosis and overtreatment as a quality problem: insights from healthcare improvement research. *BMJ Quality and Safety*, 27(7): 571-5. doi: 10.1136/bmjqs-2017-007571

Arnold R & Sandy A (2012) Left to die a lonely death as bodies of mother, son found in Enoggera. *Courier-Mail*, 2 March. Online. Available: http://www.news.com.au/national/left-to-die-a-lonely-death-story-e6frfkp9-1226287006838

Aroskar M A (1986) Are nurses' mind sets compatible with ethical practice? In: P L Chinn (ed) *Ethical issues in nursing*. Aspen Systems, Rockville, Maryland, pp 69-79

Asch D, Hansen-Flaschen J & Lanken P (1995) Decisions to limit or continue life-sustaining treatment by critical care physicians in the United States: conflicts between physicians' practices and patients' wishes. *American Journal of Respiratory Critical Care Medicine*, 151: 288-92

Ashby M & Mendelson D (2003) Natural death in 2003: are we slipping backwards? *Journal of Law and Medicine*, 10(3): 260-4

Ashby M & Stoffell B (1991) Therapeutic ration and defined phases: proposal of ethical framework for palliative care. *British Medical Journal*, 302 (1 June): 1322-4

Ashby M & Stoffell B (1995) Artificial hydration and alimentation at the end of life: a reply to Craig. *Journal of Medical Ethics*, 21(3): 135-40

Ashworth A (2002) Responsibilities, rights and restorative justice. *British Journal of Criminology*, 42(3): 578-95

Åstedt-Kurki P, Paavilainen E, Tammentie T & Paunonen-Ilmonen M (2001) Interaction between family members and health care providers in an acute care setting in Finland. *Journal of Family Nursing*, 7(4): 371-90

Athanassoulis N (2013) *Virtue ethics*. Bloomsbury, London

Atkinson J (2004) Ulysses' crew or Circe? – the implications of advance directives in mental health for psychiatrists. *Psychiatric Bulletin*, 28(1): 3-4

Atkinson J (2007) *Advance directives in mental health: theory, practice and ethics*. Jessica Kingsley, London

Atkinson J, Garner H, Patrick H & Stuart S (2003) Issues in the development of advance directives in mental health care. *Journal of Mental Health*, 12(5): 463-74

Atkinson J, Garner H & Gilmour W (2004) Models of advance directives in mental health care: stakeholder views. *Social Psychiatry Psychiatric Epidemiology*, 39(8): 673-80

Atkinson R L, Atkinson R C & Hilgard E R (1983) *Introduction to psychology*, 8th edn. Harcourt Brace Jovanovich, New York

Atkinson S, Bihari D, Smithies M, Daly K, Mason R & McColl I (1994) Identification of futility in intensive care. *The Lancet*, 344 (29 Oct): 1203-6.

Austerlic S (2009) *Cultural humility and compassionate presence at the end of life*. Markkula Centre for Applied Ethics. Online. Available: http://www.scu.edu/ethics/practicing/focusareas/medical/culturally-competent-care/chronic-to-critical-austerlic.html

Austin Health (2006a) *Respecting patient choices: final evaluation of the community implementation of the Respecting Patient Choices Program*. Austin Health, Melbourne

Austin Health (2006b) *Respecting patient choices: report on the evaluation of the national implementation of the Respecting Patient Choices Program*. Austin Health, Melbourne

Austin Health (2011) *Respecting patient choices "Making health choices" Steering Committee submission DR803 to Productivity Commission Inquiry into Caring for Older Australians*. Online. Available: https://www.pc.gov.au/inquiries/completed/aged-care/submissions/subdr0803.pdf

Austin P & Rood D (2008) Abortion reform clears last hurdle. *Sydney Morning Herald*, 11 October. Online. Available: http://www.smh.com.au/national/abortion-reform-clears-last-hurdle-20081010-4yds.html

Australian and New Zealand Society of Palliative Medicine Inc (ANZSPM) (2017a) *Guidance document: Palliative sedation therapy*. ANZSPM, Canberra. Online. Available: http://www.anzspm.org.au/c/anzspm

Australian and New Zealand Society of Palliative Medicine Inc (ANZSPM) (2017b) *Position statement: the practice of euthanasia and physician assisted suicide*. ANZSPM, Canberra. Online. Available: http://www.anzspm.org.au/c/anzspm

Australian Broadcasting Corporation (ABC) (2002) *Media Watch* Tampering with Defence PR, 22 April. Online. Available: http://www.abc.net.au/mediawatch/stories/220402_s2.htm

Australian Broadcasting Corporation (ABC) (2005) *Australian story* 'At death's door' (Toni Hoffman). Australian Broadcasting Commission, Sydney [video recording]. Online. Available: http://www.abc.net.au/austory/content/2005/s1402495.htm

Australian Bureau of Statistics (ABS) (2011) *2050.0.55.002 – Position paper: ABS review of counting the homeless methodology*. ABS, Canberra.

Australian Bureau of Statistics (ABS) (2012a) *4922.0 – Information paper – a statistical definition of homelessness, 2012*. Online. Available: http://www.abs.gov.au/AUSSTATS/abs@.nsf/Latestproducts/4922.0Main%20Features32012?opendocument&tabname=Summary&prodno=4922.0&issue=2012&num=&view=#

Australian Bureau of Statistics (ABS) (2012b) *2071.0 – Reflecting a nation: stories from the 2011 census, 2012–2013*. Online. Available: http://www.abs.gov.au/ausstats/abs@.nsf/lookup/2071.0main+features852012-2013

Australian Bureau of Statistics (ABS) (2016) *3303.0 – Causes of death, Australia 2016*. ABS, Canberra. Online. Available: http://www.abs.gov.au/ausstats/abs@.nsf/mf/3303.0/

Australian Commission on Safety and Quality in Health Care (ACSQHC) (2010) *Australian safety and quality framework for healthcare*. ACSQHC, Sydney.

Australian Commission on Safety and Quality in Health Care (ACSQHC) (2013) *Safety and quality of end of life care in acute hospitals: a background paper*. ACSQHC, Sydney

Australian Commission on Safety and Quality in Health Care (ACSQHC) (2015) *National consensus statement essential elements for safe and high-quality end-of-life care*. ACSQHC, Sydney. Online. Available: https://www.safetyandquality.gov.au/wp-content/uploads/2015/05/National-Consensus-Statement-Essential-Elements-forsafe-high-quality-end-of-life-care.pdf

Australian Commission on Safety and Quality in Health Care (ACSQHC) (2017) *National safety and quality health service standards*. ACSQHC, Sydney

Australian Commonwealth Government, Department of Social Services. *myagedcare*. Online. Available: http://www.myagedcare.gov.au/

Australian Consumers' Association (1988) *Your health rights*. Australasian Publishing Company and Australian Consumers' Association, Sydney

Australian Government Department of Health (2008) *National mental health policy*. Commonwealth of Australia, Canberra.

Australian Government Department of Health (2010) *National standards for mental health services 2010*. Commonwealth of Australia, Canberra

Australian Government Department of Health (2011) *National carer strategy (2011)*. Commonwealth of Australia, Canberra

Australian Government Department of Health (2012) *Mental health statement of rights and responsibilities*. Australian Government Publishing Service, Canberra

Australian Government Department of Health (2013) *A national framework for recovery-oriented mental health services: guide for practitioners and providers*. Commonwealth of Australia, Canberra

Australian Government Department of Health (2017) *Fifth national mental health and suicide prevention plan*. Commonwealth of Australia, Canberra. Online. Available: http://www.coaghealthcouncil.gov.au/Portals/0/Fifth%20National%20Mental%20Health%20and%20Suicide%20Prevention%20Plan.pdf

Australian Health Ministers Advisory Council (AHMAC) (2011) *A national framework for advance care directives*. AHMAC, Canberra

Australian Health Ministers Advisory Council (AHMAC) (2013) *A national framework for recovery-oriented mental health services: guide for practitioners and providers*. Commonwealth of Australia, Canberra

Australian Health Ministers Advisory Council (AHMAC) (2017) *Discussion paper: mandatory reporting under the Health Practitioner Regulation National Law*. AHMAC, Canberra.

Australian Health Practitioner Regulation Authority (APHRA) (2012) *Legal practice note: reasonable belief (10 August)*. APHRA, Canberra

Australian Health Practitioner Regulation Agency (AHPRA) (2014) *Guidelines for mandatory notifications*. AHPRA, Canberra

Australian Human Rights Commission (2008) *Homelessness is a human rights issue*. Human Rights Commission, Sydney. Online. Available: https://www.humanrights.gov.au/publications/homelessness-human-rights-issue

Australian Human Rights Commission (AHRC) (nda) *Direct discrimination*. AHRC, Sydney. Online. Available: https://www.humanrights.gov.au/quick-guide/12030

Australian Human Rights Commission (AHRC) (ndb) *Indirect discrimination*. AHRC, Sydney. Online. Available: https://www.humanrights.gov.au/quick-guide/12049

Australian Indigenous HealthInfoNet (2017) *Summary of Aboriginal and Torres Strait Islander health status 2016*. Australian Indigenous Health*InfoNet*, Perth, WA: 16

Australian Institute of Health and Welfare (AIHW) (2015) *The health of Australia's prisoners 2015*. Cat. no. PHE 207. AIHW, Canberra

Australian Institute of Health and Welfare (2017a) *Mental health services – in brief 2017*. AIHW cat. no. HSE 141, AIHW, Canberra. Online. Available: https://www.aihw.gov.au/getmedia/3ac11554-817d-4563-ad97-46bc6a90bee5/20502.pdf.aspx?inline=true

Australian Institute of Health and Welfare (AIHW) (2017b) *Australia's welfare 2017*. Australia's welfare series no. 13. AUS 214. AIHW, Canberra

Australian Institute of Health and Welfare (AIHW) (2018) *Child protection Australia 2016–17*. Child welfare series no. 68. Cat. no. CWS 63. AIHW, Canberra

Australian Law Reform Commission (ALRC) (2014) *Equality, capacity and decision making in Commonwealth laws* (ALRC Report 124). ALRC, Sydney. Online. Available: https://www.alrc.gov.au/publications/supported-and-substitute-decision-making

Australian Law Reform Commission (ALRC) (2017) *Elder abuse – a national response*. Final report (Report 131). ALRC, Sydney

Australian Medical Association (2016) *AMA code of ethics (revised 2016)*. AMA, Barton, ACT. Online. Available: https://ama.com.au/sites/default/files/documents/AMA%20Code%20of%20Ethics%202004.%20Editorially%20Revied%202006.%20Revised%202016.pdf

Australian Nursing and Midwifery Federation (ANMF) (2015) *Position statement: climate change*. ANMF, Melbourne

Australian Nursing and Midwifery Federation (Federal Office) (2016) *Position statement: Assisted dying*. ANMF (Federal), Melbourne

Australian Nursing and Midwifery Federation (Victorian Branch) (2017a) *Policy: Voluntary euthanasia / assisted dying*. ANMF (Vic Branch), Melbourne

Australian Nursing and Midwifery Federation (Federal Office) (2017b) *Position statement: Conscientious objection*. ANMF (Federal), Melbourne

Australian Nursing and Midwifery Federation (ANMF) (Victorian Branch) (2018) ANMF commends voluntary assisted dying laws. *On the Record*, February: 6-7

Australian Nursing and Midwifery Journal (ANMJ) (2013–2014) ANMF Members set the agenda. *Australian Nursing and Midwifery Journal*, 21(6): 20-1

Australian Private Hospitals Association (2007) *Protecting patients the priority – Toni Hoffman*, 14 August

Aveyard H (2004) The patient who refuses nursing care. *Journal of Medical Ethics*, 30(4): 346-50

Avis W (2017) *Data on the prevalence of the worst forms of child labour. K4D Helpdesk Report*. Institute of Development Studies, Brighton, UK

Ayres S (1991) Who decides when care is futile? *Hospital Practice*, 26 (30 September): 41-53

Baehr A, Peña J C & Hu D J (2015) Racial and ethnic disparities in adverse drug events: a systematic review of the literature. *J Racial and Ethnic Health Disparities*, 2: 527-36

Bagian J, Lee C, Gosbee J, DeRosier J, Stalhandske E, Williams R & Burkhardt M (2001) Developing and deploying a patient safety program in a large health care delivery system: you can't fix what you don't know about. *Journal of Quality Improvement*, 27(10): 522–30

Baier K (1978a) Deontological theories. In: W T Reich (ed) *Encyclopedia of bioethics*. The Free Press, New York, pp 413-17

Baier K (1978b) Teleological theories. In: W T Reich (ed) *Encyclopedia of bioethics*. The Free Press, New York, pp 417-21

Bailey Z D, Krieger N, Agénor M, Graves J, Linos N & Bassett M T (2017) Structural racism and health inequities in the USA: evidence and interventions. *The Lancet*, 389: 1453-63

Baillie J, Anagnostou D, Sivell S, Van Godwin J, Byrne A & Nelson A (2018) Symptom management, nutrition and hydration at end-of-life: a qualitative exploration of patients', carers' and health professionals' experiences and further research questions,. *BMC Palliative Care*, 17(1): 60. Open access: doi: 10.1186/s12904-018-0314-4

Baily M (2011) Futility, autonomy and cost in end-of-life care. *Journal of Law, Medicine and Ethics*, 39(2): 172-82

Bain P G, Vaes J & Leyens J P (eds.) (2013) *Advances in understanding humanness and dehumanization*. Taylor & Francis, Hoboken, NJ

Baker AA (1975) Granny-battering. *Modern Geriatrics*, 5(8): 20-4

Balcombe J (2016) Lessons from animal sentience: towards a new humanity. *Chautauqua Journal*: 1, Article 5 (17 pp). Online. Available: https://encompass.eku.edu/tcj/vol1/iss1/5

Baltussen R, Mitton C, Danis M, Williams I & Gold M (2017) Global Developments in Priority Setting in Health. *International Journal of Health Policy Management*, 6(3): 127-8

Bandman E L & Bandman B (1985) *Nursing ethics in the life span*. Appleton-Century-Crofts, Norwalk, CT

Bandura A (1986) *Social foundations of thought and action: a social cognitive theory*. Prentice-Hall, Englewood Cliffs, NJ

Bandura A (1990) Selective activation and disengagement of moral control. *Journal of Social Issues*, 46(1): 27-46

Bandura A (1999) Moral disengagement in the perpetration of inhumanities. *Personality and Social Psychology Review*, 3(3): 193-209

Bandura A, Barbaranelli C, Caprara G V & Pastorelli C (1996) Mechanisms of moral disengagement in the exercise of moral agency. *Journal of Personality and Social Psychology*, 71(2): 364-74

Banja J (2010) The normalization of deviance in healthcare delivery, *Business Horizons*, 53(20): 139-48

Banner N F (2012) Unreasonable reasons: normative judgements in the assessment of mental capacity. *Journal of Evaluation in Clinical Practice*, 18: 1038-44

Banyanga J A, Björkqvist K & Österman K (2017) The trauma of women who were raped and children who were born as a result of rape during the Rwandan genocide: cases from the Rwandan Diaspora. *Journal of African Studies and Development*, 3(4): 31-9

Barathi B & Chandra P S (2013) Palliative sedation in advanced cancer patients: does it shorten survival time? A systematic review. *Indian Journal of Palliative Care*, 19(1): 40-7

Barker P J, Reynolds W & Ward T (1995) The proper focus of nursing: a critique of the "caring" ideology. *International Journal of Nursing Studies*, 32(4): 386-97

Barrett G (1992a) Parents of girl in abortion row to appeal against ban. *The Age*, 22 February: 7

Barrett G (1992b) Pressure for change in Irish abortion ban. *The Age*, 24 February: 8

Barrett G (1992c) Ireland abortion law poll likely. *The Age*, 20 February: 9

Barrett G (1992d) Abortion ruling is threat to EC treaty. *The Age*, 21 February: 8

Barrett G (1992e) Court rules against Ireland on abortion. *The Age*, 31 October: 8

Barrett G (1992f) Election, abortion vote in Ireland. *The Age*, 26 November: 7

Barrett L I (1992) Abortion: the issue Bush hopes will go away. *Time Magazine*, 13 July: 54–5

Barry V (1982) *Moral aspects of health care*. Wadsworth, Belmont, CA

Barsky A J, Saintfort R, Rogers M P, Borus J F (2002). Nonspecific medication side effects and the nocebo phenomenon. *Journal of the American Medical Association*, 287(5): 622-7

Bar-Tal D (1989) Delegitimization: the extreme case of stereotyping and prejudice. In: D Bar-Tal, C Graumann, A W Kniglanski & W Stroebe (eds.) *Stereotyping and prejudice: changing conceptions*. Springer-Verlag, New York, pp 169-88

Bar-Tal D (1990) Causes and consequences of delegitimization: models of conflict and ethnocentrism. *Journal of Social Issues*, 46(1): 65-81

Bartlett J D, Kotake C, Fauth R & Easterbrooks M A (2017) Intergenerational transmission of child abuse and neglect: do maltreatment type, perpetrator, and substantiation status matter? *Child Abuse and Neglect*, 63: 84-94

Bastian B, Laham S M, Wilson S, Haslam N & Koval P (2011) Blaming, praising, and protecting our humanity: the implications of everyday dehumanization for judgements of moral status. *British Journal of Social Psychology*, 50(3): 469-83

Bastian B, Jetten J, Chen H, Radke H R M, Harding J F & Fasoli F (2012) Losing our humanity: the self-dehumanizing consequences of social ostracism. *Personality and Social Psychology Bulletin*, 39(2): 156-69

Bastos J L, Harnois C E & Parides Y C (2018) Health care barriers, racism, and intersectionality in Australia. *Social Science and Medicine*, 199: 209-18

Basu G, Phillips Costa V & Jain P (2017) Clinicians' obligations to use qualified medical interpreters when caring for patients with limited English proficiency. *American Medical Association Journal of Ethics*, 19(3): 245-52

Basu S, Carney M A & Kenworthy N J (2017) Ten years after the financial crisis: the long reach of austerity and its global impacts on health. *Social Science and Medicine*, 187(August): 203-7

Battin M P (1982) *Ethical issues in suicide*. Prentice Hall, Englewood Cliffs, NJ

Battin M P (1996) *The death debate: ethical issues in suicide*. Prentice-Hall, Upper Saddle River, NJ

Battin M P & Mayo D (1980) *Suicide: the philosophical issues*. Peter Owen, London

Bauman Z (1993) *Postmodern ethics*. Blackwell, Cambridge, MA

Bauman Z & Donskis L (2013) *Moral blindness: the loss of sensitivity in liquid modernity*. Polity Press, Cambridge, Cambs

Baxter A, Patton G, Scott K, Degenhardt L & Whiteford H (2013) Global epidemiology of mental disorders: what are we missing? *PLoS One*, 8(6): e65514

Bayer R, Gostin L O, Jennings B & Steinbock B (2006) *Public health ethics: theory, policy and practice*, Oxford University Press, New York

Bayles M D (1981) *Professional ethics*. Wadsworth, Belmont, CA

BBC News (2012) *Catholic midwives lose abortion 'conscientious objection' case*. Online. Available: http://www.bbc.com/news/uk-scotland-glasgow-west-17203620

BBC News (2018) *Supreme Court rejects NI abortion law case* (7 June). Online. Available: https://www.bbc.com/news/uk-northern-ireland-44395150

Beals A R (1979) *Culture in process*. Holt, Rinehart & Winston, New York

Beauchamp D & Steinbock B (eds) (1999) *New ethics for the public's health*. Oxford University Press, New York

Beauchamp D E (1976) Public health as social justice. In: W Teays & L Purdy (eds) *(2001) Bioethics, justice, and health care*. Wadsworth, Belmont, CA, pp 20-3 (reprinted from *Inquiry*, 13: 1-14, with permission of the Blue Cross and Blue Shield Association. *Inquiry*, 13: 1-14)

Beauchamp T (1978) Paternalism. In: W T Reich (ed) *Encyclopedia of bioethics*. Free Press, New York/Collier Macmillan, London, pp 1194-201

Beauchamp T (1980) Suicide. In: T Regan (ed) *Matters of life and death: new introductory essays in moral philosophy*. Random House, New York, pp 67-108

Beauchamp T (2004) Paternalism. In: S Post (ed) *Encyclopedia of bioethics*, 3rd edn. Library Reference, USA, pp 1983-9

Beauchamp T L & Childress J F (1983) *Principles of biomedical ethics*, 2nd edn. Oxford University Press, New York

Beauchamp T L & Childress J F (1989) *Principles of biomedical ethics*, 3rd edn. Oxford University Press, New York

Beauchamp T L & Childress J F (1994) *Principles of biomedical ethics*, 4th edn. Oxford University Press, New York

Beauchamp T L & Childress J F (2001) *Principles of biomedical ethics*, 5th edn. Oxford University Press, New York

Beauchamp T L & Childress J F (2013) *Principles of biomedical ethics*, 7th edn. Oxford University Press, New York

Beauchamp T L & Perlin S (1978) *Ethical issues in death and dying*. Prentice Hall, Englewood Cliffs, NJ

Beauchamp T L & Walters L (eds) (1982) *Contemporary issues in bioethics*, 2nd edn. Wadsworth, Belmont, CA

Becker E 1971 *The birth and death of meaning*, 2nd edn. The Free Press, New York

Becker E (1973) *The denial of death*. Free Press / Simon & Schuster, New York

Becker E (1975) *Escape from evil*. The Free Press, New York

Beckstead J S (2005) Reporting peer wrongdoing in the healthcare profession: the role of incompetence and substance abuse information. *International Journal of Nursing Studies*, 42(3): 325-31

Beecher H (1966) Ethics and clinical research. *New England Journal of Medicine*, 274(2), June: 1354-60

Begley A M (2006) Facilitating the development of moral insight in practice: teaching ethics and teaching virtue. *Nursing Philosophy*, 7(4): 257-65

Behringer R R (2007) Human-animal chimeras in biomedical research. *Cell Stem Cell*, 1(3): 259-62

Bekoff M & Pierce J (2009) *Wild justice: the moral lives of animals*, University of Chicago Press, Chicago

Belcher J L R, DiBlasio F A, Siegfried L D & Turnquist A G (2017) Overcoming medication refusal using a patient-centered approach. *Social Work in Mental Health*, 15(6): 690-704

Bell J, Mok K, Gardiner E & Pirkis J (2018) Suicide-related internet use among suicidal young people in the UK: characteristics of users, effects of use, and barriers to offline help-seeking. *Archives of Suicide Research*, 22(2): 263-77

Belser J A & Tumpey T M (2018) The 1918 flu, 100 years later. *Science*, 359 (6373): 255

Benedetti F, Lanotte M, Lopiano L & Colloca L (2007) When words are painful: unravelling the mechanisms of the nocebo effect. *Neuroscience* 147: 260-71

Benhabib S & Dallmayr F (eds) (1990) *The communicative ethics controversy*. MIT Press, Cambridge, MA

Benjamin M (2001) Between subway and spaceship ethics: practical ethics at the outset of the twenty-first century. *Hastings Center Report*, 31(4): 24-31

Benjamin M (2004) Conscience. In: S G Post (ed) *Encyclopedia of bioethics*, 3rd edn. Macmillan Reference USA, New York, pp 513-17

Benn S I (1971) Privacy, freedom, and respect for persons. *Nomos* 13. In: J R Pennock & J W Chapman (eds) *American Society for Political and Legal Philosophy: Privacy*. Artherton Press, New York, pp 1-21

Benn S I & Peters R S (1959) *Social principles and the democratic state*. George Allen & Unwin, London

Benner P (1991) The role of experience, narrative, and community in skilled ethical comportment. *Advances in Nursing Science*, 14(2): 1-21

Benner P (ed) (1994) *Interpretive phenomenology: embodiment, caring, and ethics in health and illness*. Sage, Thousand Oaks

Benner P & Wrubel J (1989) *The primacy of caring*. Addison-Wesley, Menlo Park, CA

Bentham J (1962) An introduction to the principles of morals and legislation (reprinted from 1789 edition) In: M Warnock (ed) *Utilitarianism*. Fontana Library / Collins, London, pp 33-77

Berer M (2013) Termination of pregnancy as emergency obstetric care: the interpretation of Catholic health policy and the consequences for pregnant women. *Reproductive Health Matters*, 21(41): 9-17

Berger J T (2010) Rethinking guidelines for the use of palliative sedation. *Hastings Centre Report*, 40(3): 32-8

Berghmans R & van der Zanden M (2012) Choosing to limit choice: self-binding directives in Dutch mental health care. *International Journal of Law and Psychiatry*, 35: 11-18

Bergman A L, Christopher M S & Bowen S (2016) Changes in facets of mindfulness predict stress and anger outcomes for police officers. *Mindfulness*, 7(4): 851-8

Berlinger N & Moses J (2007) The five people you meet in a pandemic and what they need from you today. *Bioethics Backgrounder*, The Hastings Center. Online. Available: http://www.thehastingscenter.org

Berry J & Munro I (2002) 'Remorseless' recluse gets life. *The Age*, 20 November. Online. Available: http://www.theage.com.au/articles/2002/11/19/1037697662403.html

Berwick D & Kotagal M (2004) Restricted visiting hours in ICUs. *Journal of the American Medical Association*, 292(6): 736-7

Better Health Channel (2018) *Gay and lesbian discrimination*. Online. Available: https://www.betterhealth.vic.gov.au/health/HealthyLiving/gay-and-lesbian-discrimination

Beyer L (1989) The globalization of the abortion debate. *Time Magazine*, 21 August: 60-1

Beyrer C & Pizer H F (eds) (2007) *Public health and human rights: evidence-based approaches*. Johns Hopkins University Press, Washington, DC

Bezold C (2014) *Being the 21st century physician – a futurist's commencement speech*. Online. Available: http://www.altfutures.org/pubs/Newsletters/2014/June2014-B.html

Biddle L, Donovan J, Hawton K, Kapur N & Gunnell D (2008) Suicide and the internet. *British Medical Journal*, 336: 800-2

Bielby P (2014) Ulysses arrangements in psychiatric treatment: towards proposals for their use based on 'sharing' legal capacity. *Health Care Analysis*, 22: 114-42

Biggs S (2014) Adapting to an ageing society: the need for cultural change. *Policy Quarterly*, 10(3): 12-16

Bioethics Committee, Canadian Paediatric Society (2005) Use of anencephalic newborns as organ donors. *Paediatrics and Child Health*, 10(6): 335-7

Bioethics News (1985) Request to die. *Bioethics News*, 5(1): 2.

Birbal R, Maharajh H D, Birbal R, Clapperton M, Jarvis J, Ragoonath A & Uppalapati K (2009) Cybersuicide and the adolescent population: challenges of the future? *International Journal of Adolescent Medical Health*, 21(2): 151-9

Bishop A H & Scudder J R (1990) *The practical, moral and personal sense of nursing: a phenomenological philosophy of practice*. State University of New York Press, Albany

Bismark M M, Spittal MJ, Plueckhahn TM, Studdert D M (2014) Mandatory reports of concerns about the health, performance, and conduct of health practitioners. *Medical Journal of Australia*, 201: 399–403

Bismark M M, Mathews B, Morris J M, Thomas L A & Studdert D M (2016) Views on mandatory reporting of impaired health practitioners by their treating practitioners: a qualitative study from Australia. *BMJ Open*, 6: e011988. doi: 10.1136/bmjopen-2016-011988

Biton V & Tabak N (2003) The relationship between the application of the nursing ethical code and nurses' work satisfaction. *International Journal of Nursing Practice*, 9(3): 140-57

Bjørkelo B (2013) Workplace bullying after whistleblowing: future research and implications. *Journal of Managerial Psychology*, 28(3): 306-23

Bjorklund P & Lund D M (2017) Informed consent and the aftermath of cardiopulmonary resuscitation: ethical considerations. *Nursing Ethics*, Jan 1: 969733017700234. Doi: 10.1177/0969733017700234 [Epub ahead of print]

Blackburn S (1984) *Spreading the word*. Clarendon Press, Oxford

Blackhall L, Murphy S, Frank G, Michel V & Azen S (1995) Ethnicity and attitudes toward patient autonomy. *Journal of the American Medical Association*, 13(274): 820-5

Blacksher E & Stone J R (2002) Introduction to "vulnerability" issues of theoretical medicine and bioethics. *Theoretical Medicine and Bioethics*, 23(6): 421-4

Blas E & Sivasankara Kurup A (eds) (2010) *Equity, social determinants and public health programmes*. World Health Organization, Geneva

Blum L (1988) Moral exemplars: reflections on Schindler, the Trocmes, and others. *Midwest Studies in Philosophy*, 13, pp 196-221

Blumenthal-Barby J & Burroughs H (2012) Seeking better health care outcomes: the ethics of using the "nudge". *American Journal of Bioethics*, 12(2): 1-10

Boatright J (1993) *Ethics and the conduct of business*. Prentice-Hall, New Jersey

Bok S (1978) *Lying: moral choice in public and private life*. Vintage Books, New York

Bok S (1980) *Lying: moral choice in public and private life*. Quartet Books, London

Bolsin S (2003) Whistle blowing. *Medical Education*, 37: 294–6

Bolt E E, Snijdewind M C, Willems D L, van der Heide A & Onwuteaka-Philipsen B D (2015) Can physicians conceive of performing euthanasia in case of psychiatric disease, dementia or being tired of living? *Journal of Medical Ethics*, 41(8): 592-8

Bolton M B (1983) Responsible women and abortion decisions. In: S Gorovitz, R Macklin, A L Jameton, J M O'Connor & A Sherwin (eds) *Moral problems in medicine*, 2nd edn. Prentice Hall, Englewood Cliffs, NJ, pp 330-8

Borckardt J J, Grubaugh A L, Pelic C G, Danielson C K, Hardesty S J & Frueh B C (2007) Enhancing patient safety in psychiatric settings. *Journal of Psychiatric Practice*, 13(6): 355-61

Bortolotti L & Widdows H (2011) The right not to know: the case of psychiatric disorders. *Journal of Medical Ethics*, 37: 673-6

Bosslet G T, Pope T M, Rubenfeld G D, Lo B, Truog R D, Rushton C H, Curtis J R, et al (2015) An official ATS/AACN/ACCP/ESICM/SCCM policy statement: responding to requests for potentially inappropriate treatments in intensive care units. *American Journal of Respiratory and Critical Care Medicine*, 191(11): 1318-30

Bosslet G T, Lo B & White D B (2017) Resolving family-clinician disputes in the context of contested definitions of futility. *Perspectives in Biology and Medicine*, 60(3): 314-18

Bowcott O (2007) Ireland torn as pregnant teen seeks right to travel for abortion. *The Age*, 3 May. Online. Available: http://www.theage.com.au/news/world/ireland-torn-as-pregnant-teen-seeks-right-to-travel-for-abortion/2007/05/02/1177788225120.html

Bowden P (1994) The ethics of nursing care and 'the ethic of care'. *Nursing Inquiry*, 2: 10–21

Bowen T (2005) When can treatment be withdrawn from a patient? *Defence Update MDA National*, 5 March: 13

Bower M, Conroy E & Perz J (2018) Australian homeless persons' experiences of social connectedness, isolation and loneliness. *Health and Social Care*, 26(2): e241-e248

Boyd R & Richerson P (eds) (2005) *The origin and evolution of cultures*. Oxford University Press, New York

Boyle J (1994) Radical moral disagreement in contemporary health care: a Roman Catholic perspective. *Journal of Medicine and Philosophy*, 19(2): 183-200

Bozzaro C & Schildmann J (2018) "Suffering" in palliative sedation: conceptual analysis and implications for decision-making in clinical practice. *Journal of Pain and Symptom Management*, 56(2): 288-94. doi: 10.1016/j.jpainsymman.2018.04.003

Bozzo A (2018) A challenge to unqualified medical confidentiality. *Journal of Medical Ethics*, 44: 248-52

Brach C & Fraserirector I (2000) Can cultural competency reduce racial and ethnic health disparities? A review and conceptual model. *Medical Care Research and Review*, 57 (suppl 1): 181-217

Braithwaite J (1999) Restorative justice: assessing optimistic and pessimistic accounts. *Crime and Justice*, 25: 1-127

Brandt R (1959) *Ethical theory*. Prentice Hall, Englewood Cliffs, NJ (see in particular Chapter 4, 'The use of authority in ethics')

Brandt R (1978) The morality and rationality of suicide. In: T Beauchamp & S Perlin (eds) *Ethical issues in death and dying*. Prentice Hall, Englewood Cliffs, NJ, pp 122-33

Brandt R (1980) The rationality of suicide. In: M Pabst Battin & D Mayo (eds) *Suicide: the philosophical issues*. Peter Owen, London, pp 117-32

Broad C D (1940) Conscience and conscientious action. *Philosophy*, 15(58): 115-30

Broad J B, Gott M, Kim H, Boyd M, Chen H & Connolly M J (2013) Where do people die? An international comparison of the percentage of deaths occurring in hospital and residential aged care settings in 45 populations, using published and available statistics. *International Journal of Public Health*, 58(2): 257-67

Brockman J (ed) (2013) *Thinking: the new science of decision-making, problem-solving, and prediction*. Harper-Perennial, New York

Brody B (1982) The morality of abortion. In: T L Beauchamp & L Walters (eds) *Contemporary issues in bioethics*, 2nd edn. Wadsworth, Belmont, CA, pp 240-50

Brody B (1986) *Should there be a distinctively Jewish medical ethics? Isaac Frank Memorial Lecture*. Kennedy Institute of Ethics, Georgetown University, Washington, DC, ICC Auditorium, 2 June

Bromberger B & Fife-Yeomans J (1991) *Deep sleep: Harry Bailey and the scandal of Chelmsford*. Simon & Schuster, Sydney

Brooks M. 2009. Gone in seconds. *New Scientist*: 2700 (21 March): 31-5

Brouwer M, Kaczor X, Battin M P, Maeckelberghe E, Lantos J D & Verhagen E (2018) Should pediatric euthanasia be legalized? *Pediatrics*, 141(2): e20171343. doi: 10.1542/peds.2017-1343

Brown M, Ruberu R & Thompson C H (2014) Inadequate resuscitation documentation in older patients' clinical case notes. *Internal Medicine Journal*, 44(1): 93-6

Bruera E (2012) Palliative sedation: when and how? *Journal of Clinical Oncology*, 30(12): 1258-9

Bruinsma S M, Rietjens J A C, Seymour J E, Anquinet L & van der Heide A (2012) The experiences of relatives with the practice of palliative sedation: a systematic review. *Journal of Pain and Symptom Management*, 44(3): 431-45

Buchanan A (1978) Medical paternalism. *Philosophy and Public Affairs*, 7(4): 371-90

Buchanan A (1984) The right to a decent minimum of health care. *Philosophy and Public Affairs*, 13(1), Winter: 55-78

Buchanan A E & Brock D W (1989) *Deciding for others: the ethics of surrogate decision-making*. Cambridge University Press, Cambridge

Budde E, Heichel S, Hurka S & Knill C (2018a) Partisan effects in morality policy making. *European Journal of Political Research*, 57(2): 427-49

Budde E T, Knill C, Fernández-i-Marín X & Preidel C (2018b) A matter of timing: the religious factor and morality policies. *Governance*, 31: 45-63

Budić M (2018). Suicide, euthanasia and the duty to die: a Kantian approach to euthanasia. *Philosophy and Society*, 29(1): 88-114

Bulletti C, Palagiano A, Pace C, Cerni A, Borini A & de Ziegler D (2011) The artificial womb. *Reproductive Science*, 1221: 124-8

Bullivant B M (1981) *Race, ethnicity and curriculum*. Macmillan, Melbourne

Bullivant B M (1984) *Pluralism, cultural maintenance and evolution*. Bank House, Clevedon, Avon

Bullock A & Trombley S (eds) (1999) *The new Fontana dictionary of modern thought*. Harper Collins, London

Bullock K (2011) The influence of culture on end-of-life decision making. *Journal of Social Work in End-Of-Life and Palliative Care*, 7(1): 83-98

Buppert C & Klein T (2008) Dilemmas in mandatory reporting for nurses: how to report. *Medscape Nurses*. Article 585562 (posted 22 December 2008)

Burdekin B, Guilfoyle M & Hall D (1993) *Human rights and mental illness: report of the National Inquiry into the Human Rights of People with Mental Illness*. Australian Government Publishing Service, Canberra

Burnett J, Jackson S L, Sinha A K, Aschenbrenner A R, Murphy K P, Xia R & Diamond P M (2016) Five-year all-cause mortality rates across five categories of substantiated elder abuse occurring in the community. *Journal of Elder Abuse and Neglect*, 28(2): 59-75

Burston G R (1975) Granny battering. *British Medical Journal*, 3: 592

Busch-Geertsema V, Culhane D & Fitzpatrick S (2016) Developing a global framework for conceptualising and measuring homelessness. *Habitat International*, 55: 124-32

Bute J J, Petronio S & Torke A M (2015) Surrogate decision makers and proxy ownership: challenges of privacy management in health care decision making. *Health Communication*, 30(8): 799-809. doi: 10.1080/10410236.2014.900528

Butler R (1989) Dispelling ageism: the cross-cutting intervention. *Annals of the American Academy of Political & Social Science*, 503: 138-47

Caccialanza R, Constans T, Cotogni P, Zaloga G P & Pontes-Arruda A (2018) Subcutaneous infusion of fluids for hydration or nutrition: a review. *Journal of Parenteral and Enteral Nutrition*, 42(2): 297-307

Callaghan S & Ryan C J (2016) An evolving revolution: evaluating Australia's compliance with the Convention on the Rights of Persons with Disabilities in mental health law. *UNSW Law Journal*, 39(2): 596-624

Callahan D (1995) Bioethics. In: W T Reich (ed) *Encyclopedia of bioethics, revised edn*. Simon & Schuster, New York, pp 247-56

Callahan D (2009) *Taming the beloved beast: how medical technology costs are destroying our health care system*. Princeton University Press, Princeton and Oxford

Callahan E J, Hazarian S, Yarborough M & Sánchez J P (2014) Eliminating LGBTIQQ health disparities: the associated roles of electronic health records and institutional culture. *Hastings Center Report*, 44 (5): S48-S52

Callahan S (1988) The role of emotion in ethical decision-making. *Hastings Center Report*, 18(3): 9-14

Çam O & Yalçıner N (2018) Mental illness and recovery. *Journal of Psychiatric Nursing*, 9(1): 55-60

Came H & Griffith D (2018) Tackling racism as a "wicked" public health problem: enabling allies in anti-racism praxis. *Social Science and Medicine*, 199: 181-8

Came H, Doole C, McKenna B & McCreanor T (2018) Institional racism in public health contracting: findings of a nationwide survey from New Zealand. *Social Science and Medicine*, 199: 132-9

Cameron D (2005) Logging out of life. *The Age*, 4 June: 6

Cameron D (2006) Japan fears deaths are suicide plague: website pacts indicate creeping despair among young. *The Age*, 17 March: 11

Campbell A & Huxtable R (2003) The position statement and its commentators: consensus, compromise or confusion? *Palliative Medicine*, 17: 180-3

Campbell C S (1992) Religious ethics and active euthanasia in a pluralistic society. *Kennedy Institute of Ethics Journal* 2(3): 253-77

Campbell D (2012) Doctors back denial of treatment for smokers and the obese. *The Observer*, 29 April. Online. Available: http://www.theguardian.com/society/2012/apr/28/doctors-treatment-denial-smokers-obese

Campbell K M, Gulledge J, McNeill J R, Podesta J, Ogden P, Fuerth L, Wolsey R J, et al (2007) *The age of consequences: the foreign policy and national security implications of global climate change*. Center for Strategic and International Studies, Washington DC. Online. Available: http://csis.org/files/media/csis/pubs/071105_ageofconsequences.pdf

Campbell L (2016) The limits of autonomy: an exploration of the role of autonomy in the debate about assisted suicide. In: M Donnelly & C Murray (eds) *Ethical and legal debates in Irish healthcare: confronting complexities*. Manchester University Press, Manchester, Chapter 4, pp 55-70

Campbell L & Kisely S (2009) Advance treatment directives for people with severe mental illness. *Cochrane Database of Systematic Reviews*, 1: CD005963. doi: 10.1002/14651858.CD005963.pub2

Campbell T (2006) *Rights: a critical introduction*. Routledge, London and New York

Canadian Centre for Elder Law (2011) *A practical guide to elder abuse and neglect law in Canada*. British Columbia Law Institute, Vancouver

Canadian Nurses Association (CAN) (2017) *Code of ethics for registered nurses*. Canadian Nurses Association, Ottawa, ON.

Candib L (2002) Truth telling and advance planning at the end of life: problems with autonomy in a multicultural world. *Family Systems and Health*, 20(3): 213-28

Canetti D (2016) Threatened or threatening? How ideology shapes asylum seekers' immigration policy attitudes in Israel and Australia. *Journal of Refugee Studies*, 29(4): 583-606

Cantor N L (2004) Life, quality of: III. Quality of life in legal perspective. In: S G Post (ed) *Encyclopedia of Bioethics*, 3rd edn. Macmillan Reference USA, New York, pp 1397-402

Caplan A L, Perry C, Plante L, Saloma J & Balzer F (2007) Moving the womb. *Hastings Center Report*, 37(3): 18-20

Capron A (1974) Informed consent in catastrophic disease and treatment. *University of Pennsylvania Law Review* 123, December: 364-76

Capron A (1997) Foreword. In: M Zucker & H Zucker (eds) *Medical futility and the evaluation of life-sustaining interventions*. Cambridge University Press, Cambs, pp ix-xiii.

Card C (ed) (1991) *Feminist ethics*. University of Kansas Press, Lawrence, KS

Carlton W (1978) *'In our professional opinion ...': the primacy of clinical judgment over moral choice*. University of Notre Dame Press, Paris

Carlyle K E, Guidry J P D, Williams K, Tabaac A & Perrin P B (2018) Suicide conversations on Instagram™: contagion or caring? *Journal of Communication in Healthcare*, 11(1): 12-18

Carnevale F (1998) The utility of futility: the construction of biomedical problems. *Nursing Ethics*, 5(6): 509-17

Carney M A & Kenworthy N J (eds) (2017) Special issue section: austerity, health and wellbeing: transnational perspectives. *Social Science and Medicine*, 187(August): 203-311

Carper B A (1979) The ethics of caring. *Advances in Nursing Science* 1(3): 11-19

Carr J M & Clarke P (1997) Development of the concept of family vigilance. *Western Journal of Nursing Research*, 19(6): 726-40

Carr J M & Fogarty J (1999) Families at the bedside: an ethnographic study of vigilance. *Journal of Family Practice*, 48(6): 433-8

Carr W (1995) *For education: towards critical educational inquiry*. Open University Press, Milton Keynes, Bucks

Carrick P (1985) *Medical ethics in antiquity*. D Reidel, Dordrecht

Carrigan C (2014) Flying under the radar: The health of refugees and asylum seekers in Australia. *Australian Nursing and Midwifery Journal*, 21(9): 22-7

Carter R Z, Detering K M, Silvester W & Sutton E (2016) Advance care planning in Australia: what does the law say? *Australian Health Review*, 40(4): 405-14

Casali G & Day G (2010) Treating an unhealthy organisational culture: the implications of the Bundaberg Hospital Inquiry for managerial ethical decision making. *Australian Health Review*, 34: 73-9

Cassell E (1991) *The nature of suffering and the goals of medicine*. Oxford University Press, New York

Centers for Disease Control and Prevention (CDC) (2017) *Bioterrorism*. Online. Available: https://www.cdc.gov/healthcommunication/toolstemplates/entertainmented/tips/Bioterrorism.html

Chabris C & Simons D (2010) *The invisible gorilla: and other ways our intuitions deceive us*. Crown Archetype, New York. Online. Available: http://www.theinvisiblegorilla.com/gorilla_experiment.html

Chadwick R, Levitt M & Shickle D (eds) (2014) *The right to know and the right not to know: genetic privacy and responsibility (Cambridge Bioethics and Law)*, 2 edn. Cambridge University Press, Cambridge

Chamberlain C & MacKenzie D (1992) Understanding contemporary homelessness: issues of definition and meaning. *Australian Journal of Social Issues*, 27(4): 274-97

Chamberlain C & MacKenzie D (2009). *Counting the homeless 2006*. Cat. no. HOU 207. AIHW, Canberra

Chan M (2010) Foreword. *Equity, social determinants and public health programmes* (eds E Blak & A Sivasankara Kurup). WHO, Geneva, pp 1-2

Chan M (2017) *Ten years in public health, 2007–2017*: report by Dr Margaret Chan, Director-General, World Health Organization. WHO, Geneva. Online. Available: https://www.who.int/publications/10-year-review/dg-letter/en/

Chan S (2014) Hidden anthropocentrism and the "benefit of the doubt": problems with the "origins" approach to moral status. *American Journal of Bioethics*, 14(2): 18-20

Chandler J (2001) Transplant row widens. *The Age*, 9 February: 9

Chang E & Daly J (eds) (2015) *Transitions in nursing: preparing for professional practice*, 4th edn. Churchill Livingstone / Elsevier, Sydney

Chang L (2001) Family at the bedside: strength of the Chinese family or weakness of hospital care? *Current Sociology*, 49(3): 155-73

Chappell T (2009) *Ethics and experience: life beyond moral theory*, Acumen, Durham, Co Durham

Chase P G (2006) *The emergence of culture: the evolution of a uniquely human way of life*, Springer, New York

Chater K & Tsai C T (2008) Palliative care in a multicultural society: a challenge for western ethics. *Australian Journal of Advanced Nursing*, 26(2): 95-100

Chavkin W, Leitman L & Polin K (2013) Conscientious objection and refusal to provide reproductive healthcare: a White Paper examining prevalence, health consequences, and policy responses. *International Journal of Gynecology and Obstetrics*, 123: S41-S56

Chen J, Hillman K, Bellomo R, Flabouris A, Finfer S, Cretikos M; MERIT Study Investigators for the Simpson Centre; ANZICS Clinical Trials Group (2009) The impact of introducing medical emergency team system on the documentations of vital signs. *Resuscitation*, 80(1): 35-43

Chen L P, Murad M H, Paras M L, Colbenson K M, Sattler A L, Goranson E N, Elamin M B, et al (2010) Sexual abuse and lifetime diagnosis of psychiatric disorders: systematic review and meta-analysis. *Mayo Clinic Proceedings*, 85(7): 618-29

Cherny N I & Portenoy R K (1994) Sedation in the management of refractory symptoms: guidelines for evaluation and treatment. *Journal of Palliative Care*, 10(2): 31-8

Cherny N, Radbruch L & Board of the European Association for Palliative Care (2009) European Association for Palliative Care (EAPC) recommended framework for the use of sedation in palliative care. *Palliative Medicine*, 23(7): 581-93

Chiappetta-Swanson C (2005) Dignity and dirty work: nurses' experiences in managing genetic termination for fetal anomaly. *Qualitative Sociology*, 28(1): 93-116

Childress J F (1979) Appeals to conscience. *Ethics*, 89: 315-35

Childress J F (1982) *Who should decide? Paternalism in health care*. Oxford University Press, New York

Ching M (1993) The use of touch in nursing practice. *Australian Journal of Advanced Nursing*, 10(4): 4-9

Cholbi M (2015) Kant on euthanasia and the duty to die: clearing the air. *Journal of Medical Ethics*, 41(8): 607-10

Chopra D (1989) *Quantum healing: exploring the frontiers of mind / body medicine*. Bantam, New York

Chorus C G (2015) Models of moral decision making: Literature review and research agenda for discrete choice analysis. *Journal of Choice Modelling*, 16: 69-85

Christensen D & Lackey J (eds) (2013) *The epistemology of disagreement: new essays*. Oxford University Press, Oxford

Chugh D & Kern M C (2016) A dynamic and cyclical model of bounded ethicality. *Research in Organizational Behavior*, 36: 85-100

Chunn D & Gavigan S (2004) Welfare law, welfare fraud, and the moral regulation of the 'never deserving' poor. *Social and Legal Studies*, 13(2): 219-43

Churcher S (1999) Mum tests professor of death. *Herald-Sun*, 15 September: 19

Churchill L (1989) Reviving a distinctive medical ethic. *Hastings Center Report*, May–June, 19(3): 28–34

Claessens P, Menten J, Schotsmans P & Broeckaert B (2008) Palliative sedation: a review of the research literature. *Journal of Pain and Symptom Management*, 36(3): 310-33

Clarke M (2005) Preface to D Wepa (ed) *Cultural safety in Aotearoa New Zealand*. Pearson Education New Zealand, Auckland, pp v-vii

Clayton J M, Hancock K, Parker S, Butow P, Walder S, Carrick S, Currow D, et al (2008) Sustaining hope when communicating with terminally ill patients and their families: a systematic review. *Psycho-Oncology*, 17: 641-59

Cleary S (2014) *Nurse whistleblowers in Australian hospitals: a critical case study*. Unpublished study completed as fulfilment of the requirements for the degree of Doctor of Philosophy (PhD), Deakin University, Melbourne

Clemons J (ed) (1990) *Perspectives on suicide*. Westminster/John Knox Press, Louisville, KY

Close E, Willmott L & White B P (2018) Charlie Gard: in defence of the law. *Journal of Medical Ethics*, 44(7): 476-80. doi: 10.1136/medethics-2017-104721

Clouser K D (1978) Bioethics. In: W T Reich (ed) *Encyclopedia of bioethics*, vol 1. Free Press, New York, pp 115-27

Clouser K D (1995) Common morality as an alternative to principlism. *Kennedy Institute of Ethics Journal*, 5(3): 219-36

Coady C (1996) On regulating ethics. In: M Coady & S Bloch (eds) *Codes of ethics and the professions*. Melbourne University Press, Melbourne, pp 269-87

Cockrill K & Hessini L (2014) Introduction: bringing abortion stigma into focus. *Women and Health*, 54(7): 593-8

Code L, Mullett S & Overall C (eds) (1998) *Feminist perspectives: philosophical essays on methods and morals*. University of Toronto Press, Toronto

Coghlan A (2013) Austerity's toxic genetic legacy, *New Scientist*, 2912 (13 April): 6-7

Cogliano J (1999) The medical futility controversy: bioethical implications for the critical care nurse. *Critical Care Nursing Quarterly*, 22(3): 81-8

Cohen I G (2017) Artificial wombs and abortion rights. *Hastings Center Report*, 47(4): inside back cover

Cohen Y A (1968) *Man in adaptation: the cultural present*. Aldine, Chicago, IL

Cohon R (2003) Disability: I. Ethical and societal perspectives. In. S G Post (ed) *Encyclopedia of bioethics*, vol 5, 3rd edn. Macmillan Reference USA, New York, pp 655-68

Cole C A (2012) Implied consent and nursing practice: ethical or convenient? *Nursing Ethics*, 19(4): 550-7

Cole E B & Coultrap-McQuin S (eds) (1992) *Explorations in feminist ethics: theory and practice*. Indiana University Press, Bloomington and Indianapolis, IN

Coleman S (2004) *The ethics of artificial uteruses: implications for reproduction and abortion*. Ashgate, Aldershot, Hants

Coleman S (2005) *The ethics of artificial uteruses: implications for reproduction and abortion*. Ashgate, Burlington VT

Coles C (2002) Developing professional judgement. *Journal of Continuing Education in the Health Professions*, 22: 3-10

Collier K (1999) Nurse fired over patient's death. *Herald Sun*, 18 May: 2

Collins H & Khaitan T (2018) Indirect discrimination law: controversies and critical questions. In: H Collins & T Khaitan (eds) *Foundations of indirect discrimination*. Hart/Bloomsbury, London. Chapter 1, pp 1-30

Collins Australian Dictionary, 11th edn (2011) Harper Collins Australia, Sydney

Collins English Dictionary (2018) Harper Collins, London. Online. Available: http://www.collinsdictionary.com/dictionary/english/judgement

Colt G H (1991) *The enigma of suicide*. Simon & Schuster, New York

Commonwealth of Australia, Department of Health (2017) *The fifth national mental health and suicide prevention plan*. Commonwealth of Australia, Department of Health, Canberra

Commission on Social Determinants of Health (CSDH) (2008) *Closing the gap in a generation: health equity through action on the social determinants of health*. Final report of the Commission on Social Determinants of Health. World Health Organization, Geneva.

Condon B B (2013) Honoring quality of life. *Nursing Science Quarterly*, 26(2): 124

Connetica (2016) *Suicide in Australia – key facts*. Online. Available: https://www.connetica.com.au/s/media_backgrounder_-_suicide-suicide_prevention_australia_may_24_final.pdf

Conyers L M, Richardson L A, Datti P A, Koch L C & Misrok M (2017) A critical review of health, social, and prevention outcomes associated with employment for people living with HIV. *AIDS Education and Prevention*, 29(5): 475-90

Cook J W (1999) *Morality and cultural differences*, Oxford University Press, New York

Cook L M (2013) Can nurses trust nurses in recovery reentering the workplace? *Nursing*, 43(3): 21-4

Cooley D (2007) A Kantian moral duty for the soon-to-be demented to commit suicide. *American Journal of Bioethics*, 7(6): 37-44

Coonan E (2016) Medical futility: a contemporary review. *Journal of Clinical Ethics*, 27(4): 359-61

Cooper M (1991) Principle-orientated ethics and the ethic of care: a creative tension. *Advances in Nursing Science*, 14(2): 22-31

Corby B, Shemmings D & Wilkins D (2012) *Child abuse: an evidence base for confident practice*, 4th edn. Open University Press / McGraw-Hill Education, Maidenhead, Berks

Corley M (2002) Nurse moral distress: a proposed theory and research agenda. *Nursing Ethics*, 9(6): 636-50

Corring D, O'Reilly R & Sommerdyk C (2017) A systematic review of the views and experiences of subjects of community treatment orders. *International Journal of Law and Psychiatry*, 52: 74-80

Cortese A (1990) *Ethnic ethics: the restructuring of moral theory*. State University of New York Press, Albany, NY

Cortina A & Conill J (2016) Ethics of vulnerability. In: A Masferrer & E García-Sánchez (eds) *Human dignity of the vulnerable in the age of rights*. Ius Gentium: Comparative Perspectives on Law and Justice series, vol. 55. Springer International, Basel, pp 45-61

Costello K & Hodson G (2009) Exploring the roots of dehumanization: the role of animal-human similarity in promoting immigrant humanization. *Group Processes and Intergroup Relations*, 13(1): 3-22

Council of Australian Governments (COAG) (2009) *Protecting children is everyone's business: National framework for protecting Australia's children 2009–2020*. Commonwealth of Australia, Canberra.

Council of Australian Governments (COAG) (2012) *The roadmap for national mental health reform 2012–2022*. Council of Australian Governments, Department of Health, Canberra

Council on Ethical and Judicial Affairs, American Medical Association (1999) Medical futility in end-of-life care: report of the Council on Ethical and Judicial Affairs. *Journal of the American Medical Association*, 281(10): 937-41

Courier-Mail (1995) 13 May, Queenslander supports killing doctors who perform abortion. Reprinted in *Monash Bioethics Review*, 14(3): 11

Coventry C, Flabouris A, Sundararajan K & Cramey T (2013) Rapid response team calls to patients with a pre-existing not for resuscitation order. *Resuscitation*, 84: 1035-9

Coventry L & Branley D (2018) Cybersecurity in healthcare: a narrative review of trends, threats and ways forward. *Maturitas*, 113: 48-52

Coward H & Ratanakul P (eds.) (1999) *A cross-cultural dialogue on health care ethics*. Wilfrid Laurier University Press, Ontario

Coyle A (2007) Standards in prison health: the prisoner as a patient. In: L Moller, H Stover, R Jurgens, A Gatherer & H Nikogosian (eds) *Health in prisons: a WHO guide to the essentials in prison health*, WHO Regional Office for Europe, Copenhagen, pp 7-13

Coyne C (2003) Whistleblowing and problem solving: a 5-step approach. *Physiotherapy*, 11(2): 42-8

Craig G (1994) On withholding nutrition and hydration in the terminally ill: has palliative medicine gone too far? *Journal of Medical Ethics*, 20(3): 139-43

Craig G (1996) On withholding artificial hydration and nutrition from terminally ill: sedated patients. The debate continues. *Journal of Medical Ethics*, 22(3): 147-53

Craig O (1989) How doctors decide which patient gets a 'black dot'. *The Sun-Herald*, 12 March

Crimston D, Hornsey M J, Bain P G & Bastian B (2016) Moral expansiveness: examining variability in the extension of the moral world. *Journal of Personality and Social Psychology*, 111(4): 636-53

Crimston D, Hornsey M J, Bain P G & Bastian B (2018) Toward a psychology of moral expansiveness. *Current Directions in Psychological Science*, 27(1): 14-19

Cross T, Barzon J, Dennis K, & Isaacs R (1989) *Towards a culturally competent system of care: A monograph on effective services for minority children who are severely emotionally disturbed*. CASSP Technical Assistance Center, Georgetown University Child Development Center, Washington, DC

Cuca R (1993) Ulysses in Minnesota: first steps toward a self-binding psychiatric advance directive statute. *Cornell Law Review*, 78(6): 1152-86

Cuman G & Gastmans C (2017) Minors and euthanasia: a systematic review of argument based ethics literature. *European Journal of Pediatrics*, 176(7): 837-43

Curiel TJ (2006) Murder or mercy? Hurricane Katrina and the need for disaster training. *New England Journl of Medicine*, 355: 2067-9

Curzer H (1993) Is care a virtue for health care professionals? *Journal of Medicine and Philosophy*, 18(1): 51-69

Cusack P, Cusack F P, McAndrew S, McKeown M & Duxbury J (2018) An integrative review exploring the physical and psychological harm inherent in using restraint in mental health inpatient settings. *International Journal of Mental Health Nursing*, 27(3): 1162-76

Cutcliffe J R & Links P S (2008a) Whose life is it anyway? An exploration of five contemporary ethical issues that pertain to the psychiatric nursing care of the person who is suicidal: part one. *International Journal of Mental Health Nursing*, 17(4): 236-45. doi: 10.1111/j.1447-0349.2008.00539.x

Cutcliffe J R & Links P S (2008b) Whose life is it anyway? An exploration of five contemporary ethical issues that pertain to the psychiatric nursing care of the person who is suicidal: part two. *International Journal of Mental Health Nursing*, 17(4): 246-54. doi: 10.1111/j.1447-0349.2008.00540.x

D'Oronzio J C (2001) A human right to healthcare access: returning to the origins of the patients' rights movement. *Cambridge Quarterly of Healthcare Ethics*, 10(3): 285-98

Daigle M & Myrttinen H (2018) Bringing diverse sexual orientation and gender identity (SOGI) into peacebuilding policy and practice. *Gender and Development*, 2(1): 103-20

Daley D W (1983) Tarasoff and the psychotherapist's duty to warn. In: S Gorovitz, R Macklin, A L Jameton, J M O'Connor & A Sherwin (eds) *Moral problems in medicine*, 2nd edn. Prentice Hall, Englewood Cliffs, NJ, pp 234-46

Dalla-Vorgia P, Katsouyanni K, Garanis T N, Touloumi G, Drogari P & Koutselinis A (1992) Attitudes of a Mediterranean population to the truth-telling issue. *Journal of Medical Ethics*, 18(2): 67-74

Damasio A (1994) *Descartes' error: emotion, reason, and the human brain*. Avon Books, New York

Damasio A (1999) *The feeling of what happens: body and emotion in the making of consciousness*. Harcourt Brace, New York

Damasio A (2007) Neuroscience and ethics: intersections. *American Journal of Bioethics*, 7(1): 3-7

Dancy J (1993) *Moral reasons*. Blackwell, Oxford and Cambridge, MA

Daniels N (2006) Equity and population health: toward a broader bioethics agenda. *Hastings Center Report*, 36(4): 22-35

Danis M & Patrick D L (2002) Health policy, vulnerability, and vulnerable populations. In: M Danis, C Clancy & L R Churchill (eds) *Ethical dimensions of health policy*, pp 310-34. Oxford University Press, New York

Danjoux M N, Lawless B & Hawryluck L (2009) Conflicts in the ICU: perspectives of administrators and clinicians. *Intensive Care Medicine*, 35(12): 2068-77

Darbyshire P & McKenna L (2013) Nursing's crisis of care: what part does nursing education own? *Nurse Education Today*, 33: 305-7

Das S (1996) Lawyer calls for euthanasia acquittal. *The Age*, 19 December: 7

Davies A N, Waghorn M, Webber K, Johnsen S, Mendis J & Boyle J (2018) A cluster randomised feasibility trial of clinically assisted hydration in cancer patients in the last days of life. *Palliative Medicine*, 32(4): 733-43

Davies J (2002) Unafraid to die, scared to live; Nancy states her case. *The Age*, 27 March: 1, 8. Online. Available: http://www.theage.com.au/articles/2002/03/26/1017089535087.html

Davis A (1992) Suicidal behaviour among adolescents: its nature and prevention. In: R Kosky, H Eshkevari & G Kneebone (eds) *Breaking out: challenges in adolescent mental health in Australia*. Australian Government Publishing Service, Canberra

Davis L (2004) Which morals matter? Freeing moral reasoning from ideology. *University of California Law Review*, 37: 81-94

Davis-Floyd R & Arvidson P S (eds) (1997) *Intuition: the inside story. Interdisciplinary perspectives*. Routledge, New York

de Beauvoir S (1987 edn) *A very easy death (originally printed in 1964)*. Penguin, Harmondsworth, Middlesex

de Bono E (1985) *Conflicts: a better way to resolve them*. Penguin, London

de Bruijne C A N, van Rosse F, Uiters E, Droomers M, Suurmond J, Stronks K & Essink-Bot M-L (2013) Ethnic variations in unplanned readmissions and excess length of hospital stay: a nationwide record-linked cohort study. *European Journal of Public Health* 23(6): 964-71

de Chesnay M & Anderson B A (2012) *Caring for the vulnerable: perspectives in nursing theory, practice, and research*, 3rd edn. Jones & Bartlett, Boston MA

De Gendt C, Bilsen J, Vander Stichele R, Van Den Noortgate N, Lambert M & Deliens L (2007) Nurses' involvement in 'do not resuscitate' decisions on acute elder care wards. *Journal of Advanced Nursing*, 57(4): 404-9

de Graeff A & Dean M (2007) Palliative sedation therapy in the last weeks of life: a literature review and recommendations for standards. *Journal of Palliative Medicine*, 10(1): 67-85

De Vries K & Plaskota M (2017) Ethical dilemmas faced by hospice nurses when administering palliative sedation to patients with terminal cancer. *Palliative and Supportive Care*, 15(2): 148-57

Dean MM, Cellarius V, Henry B, Oneschuk D; Librach Canadian Society of Palliative Care Physicians Task Force SL (2012) Framework for continuous palliative sedation therapy in Canada. *Palliative Medicine*, 15(8): 870-9

Dean R & Allanson S (2003) Abortion in Australia: access versus protest. *Journal of Law and Medicine*, 11(4): 510-15

Death with Dignity Act (1997) *Oregon State*

Declaration of Alma Mata (1978). Online. Available: http://www.who.int/publications/almaata_declaration_en.pdf

Deech R (2017) Reproductive autonomy and regulation – coexistence. in action. Just reproduction: reimagining autonomy in reproductive medicine, special report. *Hastings Center Report*, 47(6): S57-S63

DeGrazia D (2014) Persons, dolphins, and human-nonhuman chimeras. *American Journal of Bioethics*, 14(2): 17-18

Degrie L, Gastman C, Mahieu L, Dierckx de Casterlé B & Denier Y (2017) How do ethnic minority patients experience the intercultural care encounter in hospitals? A systematic review of qualitative research. *BMC Medical Ethics*, 18(1): 2. doi: 10.1186/s12910-016-0163-8

Dekker S (2012) *Just culture: balancing safety and accountability*. CRC, Boca Raton

del Río M, Shand B, Bonati P, Palma A, Maldonado A, Taboada P & Nervi F (2012) Hydration and nutrition at the end of life: a systematic review of emotional impact, perceptions, and decision-making among patients, family, and health care staff. *Psychooncology*, 21(9): 913-21

Denniss D L (2016) Legal and ethical issues associated with Advance Care Directives in an Australian context. *Internal Medicine Journal*, 46(12): 1375-80

Denniston L (1993) US abortion clinics lose civil rights protection, *Baltimore Sun* 14 January: 1. Online. Available: http://articles.baltimoresun.com/1993-01-14/news/1993014095_1_history-of-abortion-abortion-rights-abortion-clinics

Department of Corrections, New Zealand (2018) *Prison facts and statistics* – September 2017. Online. Available: http://www.corrections.govt.nz/resources/research_and_statistics/quarterly_prison_statistics/prison_stats_september_2017.html#total

Department of Health (DoH) Victoria (2012) *Elder abuse prevention and response guidelines for action 2012–2014*. State of Victoria, Department of Health, Melbourne. Online. Available: http://www.health.vic.gov.au/agedcare/downloads/pdf/eap_guidelines.pdf

Department of Health (DoH), Victoria (2014) *Advance care planning: have the conversation. A strategy for Victorian health services 2014–2018*. State of Victoria, Department of Health, Melbourne

Department of Health (DoH), Victoria (2016) *Delivering for diversity – cultural diversity plan 2016–2019*. State of Victoria, Department of Health, Melbourne. Online. Available: https://www2.health.vic.gov.au/about/publications/policiesandguidelines/dhhs-delivering-for-diversity-cultural-diversity-plan-2016-19

Dershowitz A (2004) *Rights from wrongs: a secular theory of the origins of rights*. Basic Books, New York

DeValve M J & Adkinson C D (2008) Mindfulness, compassion, and the police in America: an essay of hope. *Human Architecture: Journal of the Sociology of Self Knowledge*, 6(3): 99-104

Dhaliwal K & Hirst S (2016) Caring in correctional nursing: a systematic search and narrative synthesis. *Journal of Forensic Nursing*, 12(1): 5-12

Dierckx de Casterlé B, Izumi S, Godfrey N S & Denhaerynck K (2008) Nurses' responses to ethical dilemmas in nursing practice: meta-analysis. *Journal of Advanced Nursing*, 63(6): 540-9

Disney G, Teng A, Atkinson J, Wilson N & Blakely T (2017) Changing ethnic inequalities in mortality in New Zealand over 30 years: linked cohort studies with 68.9 million person-years of follow-up. *Population Health Metrics*, 15(1): 15. doi: 10.1186/s12963-017-0132-6

Divi C, Koss R, Schmaltz S & Loeb J (2007) Language proficiency and adverse events in US hospitals: a pilot study. *International Journal for Quality in Health Care*, 19(2): 60-7

Dixon N (1998) On the difference between physician-assisted suicide and active euthanasia. *Hastings Center Report*, 28(5): 25-9

Dock L L (1900) Ethics – or a code of ethics? In: L L Dock (ed) *Short papers on nursing subjects*. M Louise Longeway, New York, pp 37-57

Dodds J A (2017) North Carolina law expands pool of eligible healthcare professionals to oversee executions by lethal injection. *Journal of Medical Ethics*, 4: 2-3

Doder D (1993) Balkans rape babies face life of shame, rejection. *The Age*, 5 July: 8

Dolan M B (1988) Coding abuses hurt nurses, too. *Nursing 88*, 18(12): 47

Donald D (2003) Neutral is not impartial: the confusing legacy of traditional operations thinking. *Armed Forces Society*, 29: 415-48

Donaldson L (2002) Championing patient safety: going global. *Quality and Safety in Health Care*, 11(2): 112

Dong X, Simon M A (2013) Elder abuse as a risk factor for hospitalization in older persons. *Journal of the American Medical Association Internal Medicine*, 173(10): 911-17

Dong X, Simon M A, Beck T T, Farran C, McCann J J, Mendes de Leon C F & Evans D A (2011). Elder abuse and mortality: the role of psychological and social wellbeing. *Gerontology*, 57: 549-58

Donnelly J (ed) (1990) *Suicide: right or wrong?* Prometheus, Buffalo, NY

Donovan P (1990) Neutrality in religious studies. *Religious Studies*, 26: 103-16

Donovan P (1996) Murder-charge nurse bailed. *The Age*, 10 May: 2

Doran C M & Kinchin I (2017) A review of the economic impact of mental illness. *Australian Health Review*, 43(1): 43-8. doi: 10.1071/AH16115

Doran M & Henderson A (2018) Bankers call for urgent financial protections to prevent abuse of elderly Australians. *ABC News*, 8 June. Online: http://www.abc.net.au/news/2018-06-08/bankers-call-for-added-protections-for-elderly-australians/9848056

Dossey L (1982) *Space, time and medicine*. New Science Library, Boston, MA

Dossey L (1991) *Meaning and medicine: a doctor's tales of breakthrough and healing*. Bantam, New York

Dossey L (1993) *Healing words: the power of prayer and the practice of medicine*. HarperSanFrancisco, New York

Dougherty C J & Weber L J (2004) Whistleblowing in healthcare. In: S G Post (ed) *Encyclopedia of Bioethics*, 3rd edn. Macmillan Reference USA, New York, pp 2575-7

Downie J (2017) Medical assistance in dying: lessons for Australia from Canada. *QUT Law Review*, 17(1): 127-46

Downie R S & Calman K C (1987) *Healthy respect: ethics in health care*. Faber & Faber, London

Dresser R (1982) Ulysses and the psychiatrists: a legal and policy analysis of the voluntary commitment contract. *Harvard Civil Rights – Civil Liberties Law Review*, 16(3): 777-854

Dresser R & Robertson J (1989) Quality of life and non-treatment decisions: a critique of the orthodox approach. *Law, Medicine and Health Care*, 17(3): 234-44

Driver T, Katz P, Trupin L & Wachter R (2014) Responding to clinicians who fail to follow patient safety practices: perceptions of physicians, nurses, trainees, and patients, *Journal of Hospital Medicine*, 9(2): 99-105

Dubecki L (2007a) Lost in cyberspace: fears that new networks are breeding grounds for real-life tragedies. *The Age*, 24 April: 1-2

Dubecki L (2007b) Teenagers' secret world. *The Age*, 28 April: 3

Duckett S (2018) Knowing, anticipating, even facilitating but still not intending: another challenge to double effect reasoning. *Journal of Bioethical Inquiry*, 15(1): 33-7

Dudley S & Carr J M (2004) Vigilance: the experience of parents staying at the bedside of hospitalized children. *Journal of Pediatric Nursing*, 19(4): 267-75

Dudzinski D & Shannon E (2006a) Competent patients' refusal of nursing care. *Nursing Ethics*, 13(6): 608-21

Dudzinski D & Shannon E (2006b) Competent refusal of nursing care. *Hastings Center Report* 36(2): 14-15

Dunbar J A, Reddy P, Beresford B, Ramsey W P & Lord R S A (2007) In the wake of hospital enquires: impact on staff and safety. *Medical Journal of Australia*, 186(2): 80-3

Dupré B (2011) *50 political ideas you really need to know*. Quercus, London

Durante C (2018) Bioethics and multiculturalism: nuancing the discussion. *Journal of Medical Ethics*, 44: 77-83

Durkheim E (1952) *Suicide*. Routledge & Kegan Paul, London

Düwell M (2011) Human dignity and human rights. In: P Kaufmann, H Kuch, C Neuhauser & E Webster (eds) *Humiliation, degradation, dehumanization: human dignity violated*. Springer, Dordrecht and NY, pp 215-30

Dworkin G (1972) Paternalism. *Monist*, 56(1): 64-84

Dworkin G (1988) *The theory and practice of autonomy*. Cambridge University Press, New York

Dworkin R (1977) *Taking rights seriously*. Duckworth, London

Dyck A (1984) Ethical aspects of care for the dying incompetent. *Journal of American Geriatric Society*, 32: 661-4

Dyck A J (2005) *Rethinking rights and responsibilities: the moral bonds of community*, revised edn. Georgetown University Press, Washington, DC

Dyer G (2008) *Climate wars*. Scribe, Melbourne

Ebrahim S (2002) Ageing, health and society. *International Journal of Epidemiology*, 31(4): 715-18

Edel M & Edel A (2000) *Anthropology ethics: the quest for moral understanding*, Transaction Pubs, New Brunswick, NJ

Edelstein L M, DeRenzo E G, Waetzig E, Zelizer C & Mokwunye N O (2009) Communication and conflict management training for clinical bioethics committees. *HEC Forum*, 21(4): 341-9

Edwards S D & Hewitt J (2011) Can supervising self-harm be part of ethical nursing practice? *Nursing Ethics*, 18(1): 79-97

Ehlenbach W J & Curtis J R (2011) The meaning of do-not-resuscitation orders: A need for clarity. *Critical Care Medicine*, 39(1): 193-4

Eisenstadt L F & Pacella J (2018) Whistleblowers need not apply. *American Business Law Journal*; Fox School of Business Research Paper No. 18-013; Baruch College Zicklin School of Business Research Paper No. 2018-05-02. Online. Available: https://ssrn.com/abstract=3129731

Elbogen E, Swartz M, Van Dorn R, Swanson J, Kim M & Scheyett A (2006) Clinical decision making and views about psychiatric advance directives. *Psychiatric Services*, 57(3): 350-5

Elder Abuse Victims Act (2009) (US)

Elliott C (1992) Where ethics comes from and what to do about it. *Hastings Center Report*, 22(4): 28-35

Ellison-Loschmann L (2001) Giving a voice to health consumers. *Kai Tiaki Nursing New Zealand*, 7(1): 12-13

Ellison S, Schetzer L, Mullins J, Perry J & Wong K (2004) *Access to justice and legal needs: The legal needs of older people in NSW*. Law and Justice Foundation of New South Wales, Sydney

Elliston F, Keenan J, Lockhart P & van Schaick J (1985) *Whistleblowing research: methodological and moral issues*. Praeger, New York

Emanuel E (2000) Justice and managed care: four principles for the just allocation of health care resources. *Hastings Center Report*, 30(3): 8-16

Enemark C (2017) Drones, risk, and moral injury. *Critical Military Studies*: 1-18. doi: 10.1080/23337486.2017.1384979

Engelhardt H T Jr (1986) *The foundations of bioethics*. Oxford University Press, New York

Engelhardt H T (1989) Harvesting cells, tissues, and organs from fetuses and anencephalic newborns. *Journal of Medicine and Philosophy (special edn)*, 14(1): 1-102

Engelhardt H T (1996) *The foundations of bioethics*, 2nd edn. Oxford University Press, New York

English V & Sheather J C (2017) Withdrawing clinically assisted nutrition and hydration (CANH) in patients with prolonged disorders of consciousness: is there still a role for the courts? *Journal of Medical Ethics*, 43(7): 476-80

Engster D (2014) The social determinants of health, care ethics and just health care. *Contemporary Political Theory*, 13(2): 149-67

Engström J, Bruno E, Holm B & Hellzén O (2007) Palliative sedation at end of life: a systematic literature review. *European Journal of Oncology Nursing*, 11(1): 26-35

Ennis B J (1982) The psychiatric will: Odysseus at the mast. *American Psychologist*, 37(7): 854

Epstein E & Hamric A (2009) Moral distress, moral residue, and the crescendo effect. *Journal of Clinical Ethics*, 20(4): 330-42.

Eren N (2013) Nurses' attitudes toward ethical issues in psychiatric inpatient settings. *Nursing Ethics*, 21(3): 359-73

Eriksson S, Helgesson G, Höglund A T (2007) Being, doing, and knowing: developing ethical competence in health care. *Journal of Academic Ethics* 5: 207-16

Erlen J (1999) What does it mean to blow the whistle? *Orthopaedic Nursing*, 18(6): 67-70

Esses V M, Veenvliet S, Hodson G & Mihic L (2008) Justice, morality, and the dehumanization of refugees. *Social Justice Research*, 21: 4-25

European Federation of National Organisations working with the Homeless (nd) *What is homelessness?* Online. Available: http://www.feantsa.org/

Evans J (2002) The gifts reserved for age. *International Journal of Epidemiology*, 31(4): 792-5

Every D & Augoustinos M (2007) Constructions of racism in the Australian parliamentary debates on asylum seekers. *Discourse and Society*, 18(4): 411-36

Ewin RE (1992) Loyalty and virtues. *Philosophical Quarterly*, 42 (169): 403-19

Faber-Langendoen K & Lanken P (2000) Dying patients in the intensive care unit: forgoing treatment, maintaining care. *Annals of Internal Medicine*, 133(11): 886-93

Faden R R & Beauchamp T L (1986) *A history and theory of informed consent*. Oxford University Press, New York

Fagerlin A & Schneider C E (2004) Enough: the failure of the living will. *Hastings Center Report*, 34(2): 30-42

Falk N, Baigis J & Kopac C (2012) Elder mistreatment and the Elder Justice Act. *Online Journal of Issues in Nursing*, 17(3): 1-12

Fang X, Brown D S, Florence C S & Mercy J A (2012) The economic burden of child maltreatment in the United States and implications for prevention. *Child Abuse and Neglect*, 36(2): 156-65

Farberow N (ed) (1975a) *Suicide in different cultures*. University Park Press, Baltimore MD

Farberow N (1975b) Cultural history of suicide. In: N Farberow (ed) *Suicide in different cultures*. University Park Press, Baltimore, pp 1-15

Farrow T L & O'Brien A J (2003) 'No-suicide contracts' and informed consent: an analysis of ethical issues. *Nursing Ethics*, 10(2): 199-207

Fasching D (1993) *The ethical challenge of Auschwitz and Hiroshima: apocalypse or utopia?* State University of New York Press, Albany NY

Fazel S, Geddes J R & Kushel M (2014) The health of homeless people in high-income countries: descriptive epidemiology, health consequences, and clinical and policy recommendations. *The Lancet*, 384(Oct 25): 1529-40

Feagin J & Bennefield Z (2014) Systemic racism and U.S. health care. *Social Science and Medicine*, 193: 7-14

Feinberg J (1969) *Moral concepts*, Oxford University Press, Oxford, pp 60-73

Feinberg J (1971) Legal paternalism. *Canadian Journal of Philosophy*, 1: 105-24

Feinberg J (1978) Rights. In: W T Reich (ed) *Encyclopedia of bioethics*. The Free Press, New York, pp 1507-11

Feinberg J (1979) The rights of animals and unborn generations. In: R A Wasserstrom (ed) *Today's moral problems*. Macmillan, New York, pp 581-601

Feinberg J (1984) *Harm to others: the moral limits of the criminal law*. Oxford University Press, New York

Felblinger M (2008) Incivility and bullying in the workplace and nurses' shame responses. *Journal of Obstetric, Gynecologic, and Neonatal Nursing*, 37(2): 234-42

Fergusson D M, Boden J M & Horwood J (2006) Examining the intergenerational transmission of violence in a New Zealand birth cohort. *Child Abuse and Neglect*, 30(2): 89-108

Ferrans C E (1990) Quality of life: conceptual issues. *Seminars in Oncology Nursing*, 6(4): 248-54

Fiala C & Arthur J H (2014) "Dishonourable disobedience" – why refusal to treat in reproductive healthcare is not conscientious objection. *Woman – Psychosomatic Gynaecology and Obstetrics*, 1: 12-23

Fida R, Tramontano C, Paciello M, Kangasniemi M, Sili A, Bobbio A & Barbaranelli C (2016) Nurse moral disengagement. *Nursing Ethics*, 23(5): 547-64

Field M (1997) NZ health uproar after life fight fails. *The Age*, 13 October: 10

Fieldhouse P (1986) *Food and nutrition: customs and culture*. Croom Helm, London

Fine M (1990) "The public" in public schools: The social construction/constriction of moral communities. *Journal of Social Issues*, 46(1): 107-19

Fine M (2014) Ageing and the G20- Invited commentary: intergenerational perspectives on ageing, economics and globalisation. *Australasian Journal on Ageing*, 33(4): 220-5

Fine R L (2017) Futility, the multiorganization policy statement, and the Schneiderman response. *Perspectives in Biology and Medicine*, 60(3): 358-66

Firestone R (1997) *Suicide and the inner voice: risk assessment, treatment, and case management*. Sage Publications, Thousand Oaks, CA

Firth-Cozens J, Firth RA & Booth S (2003) Attitudes to and experiences of reporting poor care. *Clinical Governance*, 8(4): 331-6

Fiscella K & Sanders M R (2016) Racial and ethnic disparities in the quality of health care. *Annual Review of Public Health*, 17: 375-94

Fischer G S, Tulsky J A & Arnold R M (2004) Advance directives and advance care planning. In: S G Post (ed) *Encyclopedia of bioethics*, 3rd edn. Macmillan Reference USA, New York, pp 74-9

Fish D & Coles C (1998) *Developing professional judgment in health care: learning through the critical appreciation of practice*. Butterworth-Heinemann, Oxford UK

Fisher M & Raper R (1990a) Withdrawing and withholding treatment in intensive care, Part 1. Social and ethical dimensions. *Medical Journal of Australia*, 153 (20 August): 217-20

Fisher M & Raper R (1990b) Withdrawing and withholding treatment in intensive care, Part 2. Patient assessment. *Medical Journal of Australia*, 153(20 August): 220-2

Fisher M & Raper R (1990c) Withdrawing and withholding treatment in intensive care, Part 3. Practical aspects. *Medical Journal of Australia*, 153(20 August): 222-5

Fitzgerald E M, Myers J G & Clark P (2016) Nurses need not be guilty bystanders: caring for vulnerable immigrant populations. *Online Journal of Issues in Nursing*, 22(1): 8. doi: 10.3912/OJIN.Vol22No01PPT43

Fitzpatrick M J & Hamill S B (2010) Elder abuse: factors related to perceptions of severity and likelihood of reporting. *Journal of Elder Abuse and Neglect*, 23(1): 1-16

Fitzpatrick S, Pawson H, Bramley G, Wilcox S, Watts B & Wood J (2018) *Homeless monitor: England 2018*. Institute for Social Policy, Environment and Real Estate (I-SPHERE), Heriot-Watt University; City Futures Research Centre, University of New South Wales. Online. Available: https://www.crisis.org.uk/media/238700/homelessness_monitor_england_2018.pdf

Fleming V, Ramsayer B & Zakšek T S (2018) Freedom of conscience in Europe? An analysis of three cases of midwives with conscientious objection to abortion. *Journal of Medical Ethics*, 44: 104-8

Fletcher J (1966) *Situation ethics*. SCM Press, Bloomsbury Street, London

Flew A & Priest S (eds) (2002) *A dictionary of philosophy*. Pan, London and Basingstoke

Flood C, Gable L & Gostin L (2005) Introduction: legislating and litigating health care rights around the world. *Journal of Law, Medicine and Ethics*, 33(4): 636-40

Florijn B W (2018) Extending euthanasia to those 'tired of living' in the Netherlands could jeopardize a well-functioning practice of physicians' assessment of a patient's request for death. *Health Policy*, 122(3): 315-19

Fogarty J (1993) *Protective services for children in Victoria: a report*. Justice Fogarty for the Victorian Government, Melbourne

Fogarty J & Sargeant D (1989) *Protective services for children in Victoria – an interim report* (February). Government Printer, Melbourne

Foglia M B & Fredriksen-Goldsen K I (2014) Health disparities among LGBT older adults and the role of nonconscious bias. *Hastings Center Report*, 44 (5): S40-S44

Forbat L, Kunicki N, Chapman M & Lovell C (2017) How and why are subcutaneous fluids administered in an advanced illness population: a systematic review. *Journal of Clinical Nursing*, 26(9-10): 1204-16

Foronda C, Baptiste D L, Reinholdt M M & Ousman K (2016) Cultural humility: a concept analysis. *Journal of Transcultural Nursing*, 27(3): 210-17

Forrester K & Griffiths D (2015) *Essentials of law for health professionals*, 4th edn. Elsevier, Sydney

Forrow L, Arnold R, & Parker L (1993) Preventive ethics: expanding the horizons of clinical ethics, *Journal of Clinical Ethics*, 4(4): 287-94

Fost N (2004) Reconsidering the dead donor: is it imperative that organ donors be dead? *Kennedy Institute of Ethics Journal* 14(3): 249–60

Fourie C & Rid A (2016) *What is enough?: sufficiency, justice, and health*. Oxford University Press, New York

Fox D (2017) Reproductive negligence. *Colorado Law Review*, 117: 149-241

Fox J & Muir R (2016) NFR orders must be understood by all concerned. *Pulse*, March: 8

Fox M (2005) Reconfiguring the animal/human boundary: the impact of xeno technologies. *Liverpool Law Review*, 26(2): 149-67

Frances B (2013) Philosophical renegades. In: D Christensen & J Lackey (eds) *The Epistemology of disagreement*. Oxford University Press, Oxford, pp 121-66

Frankena W (1973) *Ethics*, 2nd edn. Prentice-Hall, Englewood Cliffs, NJ

Franklin M, Stolz G & Griffith C (2002) She died cancer free. *Herald Sun*, 25 May: 1-2

Fraser J A, Mathews B, Walsh K, Chen L & Dunne M (2010) Factors influencing child abuse and neglect recognition and reporting by nurses: a multivariate analysis. *International Journal of Nursing Studies*, 47(2): 146-53

Frati P, Fineschi V, Di Sanzo M, La Russa R, Scopetti M, Severi F M & Turillazzi E (2017) Preimplantation and prenatal diagnosis, wrongful birth and wrongful life: a global view of bioethical and legal controversies. *Human Reproduction Update*, 23(3): 338-57

Freckelton I (1996) Enforcement of ethics. In: M Coady & S Bloch (eds) *Codes of ethics and the professions*. Melbourne University Press, Melbourne, pp 130-65

Freckelton I (2006) Human rights and health law. *Journal of Law and Medicine* 14(1): 7-14

Freckelton I & Flynn J (2004) Paths toward reclamation: therapeutic jurisprudence and the regulation of medical practitioners. *Journal of Law and Medicine*, 12(2): 91-102

Free v Holy Cross Hospital 505 NE2d 1188 (Ill App 1 Dist 1987)

Freedman B (1978) A meta-ethics for professional morality. *Ethics*, 89: 1-19

Freire P (1970) *Cultural action for freedom*. Penguin, Harmondsworth, Middlesex

Freire P (1972) *Pedagogy of the oppressed*. Penguin, London

French M (1998) *A season in hell: a memoir*. Ballantine, New York

Freudenberg N (2001) Jails, prisons, and the health of urban populations: a review of the impact of the correctional system on community health. *Journal of Urban Health*, 78(2): 214-35

Fried C (1982) Equality and rights in medical care. In: T L Beauchamp & L Walters (eds) *Contemporary issues in Bioethics*, 2nd edn. Wadsworth, Belmont, CA, pp 395-401

Fritz Z, Slowther A-M & Perkins G D (2017) Resuscitation policy should focus on the patient, not the decision. *British Medical Journal*, 356: j813.

Fry S T (1989a) The role of caring in a theory of nursing ethics. *Hypatia*, 4(2): 87-103

Fry S T (1989b) Whistleblowing by nurses: a matter of ethics. *Nursing Outlook*, 37(1): 56

Fry S T & Johnstone M-J (2008) *Ethics in nursing practice: a guide to ethical decision making*, 3rd edn. Blackwell Science, London

Fukuda K (2014) Foreword. *Antimicrobial resistance: global report on surveillance*. WHO, Geneva, p ix

Fukuda-Parr S (ed) (2004) *Human development report 2004: cultural liberty in today's diverse world*. United Nations Development Programme (UNDP), New York

Fullinwider R (1996) Professional codes and moral understanding. In: M Coady & S Bloch (eds) *Codes of ethics and the professions*. Melbourne University Press, Melbourne, pp 72-87

Gabbay E, Calvo-Broce J, Meyer K B, Trikalinos T A, Cohen J & Kent D (2010) The empirical basis for determinations of medical futility. *Journal of General Internal Medicine* 25(10): 1083-90

Gaetz S, Dej E, Richter T & Redman M (2016) *The state of homelessness in Canada 2016*. Canadian Observatory on Homelessness Press, Toronto

Gallagher A & Wainwright P (2007) Terminal sedation: promoting ethical nursing practice. *Nursing Standard*, 21(34): 42-6

Ganz FD, Kaufman N, Israel S & Einav S (2012) Resuscitation in general medical wards: who decides? *Journal of Clinical Nursing*, 22(5-6): 848-55

Ganzini L (2006) Artificial nutrition and hydration at the end of life: ethics and evidence. *Palliative and Support Care*, 4: 135-43

Gardiner S M (2010) A perfect moral storm: climate change, intergenerational ethics, and the problem of corruption. In: S M Gardiner, S Caney, D Jamieson & H Shue (eds) *Climate ethics: essential readings*. Oxford University Press, New York, pp 87-98

Gardiner S M (2011) *The perfect moral storm: the ethical tragedy of climate change*. Oxford University Press, New York

Garma C T (2017) Influence of health personnel's attitudes and knowledge in the detection and reporting of elder abuse: an exploratory systematic review. *Psychosocial Intervention*, 26(2): 73-91

Garnett A C (1965) Conscience and conscientiousness. First published in *Rice University Studies*, vol 51. Reprinted in: K Kolenda (ed) (1966), *Insight and vision*. Trinity University Press, San Antonio, TX, pp 71-83. Subsequently reprinted in: J Feinberg (1969), *Moral concepts*. Oxford University Press, Oxford, pp 80-92

Garrett J R (2014) Two agendas for bioethics: critique and integration. *Bioethics*. Online. doi: 10.1111/bioe.12116. [Epub ahead of print] [accessed 24 September 2014]

Garvey J (2008) *The ethics of climate change: right and wrong in a warming world*. Continuum, London

Gastmans C, Dierckx de Casterlé B & Schotsmans P (1998) Nursing considered as moral practice: a philosophical–ethical interpretation of nursing. *Kennedy Institute of Ethics Journal*, 8(1): 43-69

Gatens M (1986) Feminism, philosophy and riddles without answers. In: C O Pateman & E Gross (eds) *Feminist challenges*. Allen & Unwin, Sydney, pp 13-29

Gates G J (2011) *How many people are lesbian, gay, bisexual, and transgender?* Williams Institute, UCLA School of Law, Los Angeles. Online. Available: https://williamsinstitute.law.ucla.edu/wp-content/uploads/Gates-How-Many-People-LGBT-Apr-2011.pdf

Gatherer A (2013) Managing the health of prisoners. *British Medical Journal*, 346: f3463

Gaudine H, LeFort S, Lamb M & Thorne L (2011) Ethical conflicts with hospitals: the perspective of nurses and physicians, *Nursing Ethics*, 18(6): 756-66

Gaut D A (ed) (1992) *The presence of caring in nursing*. National League for Nursing Press, New York

Gaut D A & Leininger M M (eds) (1991) *Caring: the compassionate healer*. National League for Nursing Press, New York

Gauthier D P (1986) *Morals by agreement*. Clarendon Press, Oxford

Gazzaniga M (2005) *The ethical brain: the science of our moral dilemmas*, Harper-Perennial, New York

Gazzaniga M (2011) *Who's in charge? Free will and the science of the brain*. Anniversary 40, imprint of Harper Collins, New York

Gearing R E & Lizardi D (2009) Religion and suicide. *Journal of Religious Health*, 48: 332-41

Geary P & Hawkins J (1991) To cure, to care, or to heal. *Nursing Forum*, 26(3): 5-13

Gelfand S & Shook J R (eds) (2006) *Ectogenesis: artificial womb technology and the future of human reproduction*. Rodopi, Amsterdam

Gellene D (2007) Brain damage can alter moral compass. *The Age*, 23 March: 9

Georgaki S, Kalaidopoulou O, Liarmakopoulos I & Mystakidou K (2002) Nurses' attitudes towards truthful communication with patients with cancer: a Greek study. *Cancer Nursing*, 25(6): 436-41

Geppert C M, Andrews M R, Druyan M E (2010) Ethical issues in artificial nutrition and hydration: a review. *Journal of Parenteral and Enteral Nutrition*, 34(1): 79-88

Gerber L (2013) Bringing home effective nursing care for less. *Nursing* 43(3): 32-8

Gergen K (1994) *Realities and relationships: soundings in social construction*. Harvard University Press, Cambridge, MA

Gerhart K, Koziol-McLain J, Lowenstein S & Whiteneck G (1994) Quality of life following spinal cord injury: knowledge and attitude of emergency care providers. *Annals of Emergency Medicine*, 23(4): 807-12

Gerlach A J (2012) A critical reflection on the concept of cultural safety. *Canadian Journal of Occupational Therapy*, 79(3): 151-8

Gert B & Culver C (1976) Paternalistic behaviour. *Philosophy and Public Affairs*, 6(1): 45-57

Gert B, Culver C & Clouser K D (1997) *Bioethics: a return to fundamentals*. Oxford University Press, New York

Gibbs N (1993) Death giving. *Time Magazine*, 31 May: 49-53

Gibson M (1976) Rationality. *Philosophy and Public Affairs*, 6(3): 193-225

Gilbert P (2013) ANMF support for whistleblower. *On the Record*, November: 9

Giles H & Moule P (2004) 'Do not attempt resuscitation' decision-making: a study exploring the attitudes and experiences of nurses. *Nursing in Critical Care*, 9(3): 115-22

Gilligan C (1982) *In a different voice: psychological theory and women's development*. Harvard University Press, Cambridge, MA

Gillon R (2001) Is there a 'new ethics of abortion'? *Journal of Medical Ethics*, 27 (suppl 2): ii5-ii9

Ginn S & Robinson R (2012a) Prison environment and health. *British Medical Journal*, 345: e5921

Ginn S & Robinson R (2012b) Dealing with mental disorder in prisoners. *British Medical Journal*, 345: e7280

Ginn S & Robinson R (2013) Promoting health in prison. *British Medical Journal*, 346: f2216

Giovannoni J (1982) Mistreated children. In: S Yelaja (ed) *Ethical issues in social work*. Charles C Thomas, Springfield, IL, pp 105-20

Glasson, J, Plows C W, Clarke O W, Cosgriff J H Jr, Kliger C H, Ruff V N, Tenery R M Jr, et al (1995) The use of anencephalic neonates as organ donors. *Journal of the American Medical Association* 273(20): 1614-18

Glendon M A (1991) *Rights talk: the impoverishment of political discourse*. Free Press, New York

Glick H (1992) *The right to die: public policy innovation and its consequences*. Columbia University Press, New York

Glick H & Hutchinson A (1999) The rising agenda of physician assisted suicide: explaining the growth and content of morality policy. *Policy Studies Journal*, 27(4): 750-65

Global Alliance for the Rights of Older People (GAROP) (2015) *In our own words*. GAROP. Online. Available: http://www.rightsofolderpeople.org/new-garop-report-in-our-own-words/

Global Alliance for the Rights of Older People (GAROP) (nd) *Home page*. Online. Available: http://www.rightsofolderpeople.org/

Glover J (1977) *Causing deaths and saving lives*. Penguin, Harmondsworth, Middlesex

Goddard C (1996) *Child abuse and child protection: a guide for health, education and welfare workers*. Churchill Livingstone, Melbourne

Goddard T & Pooley J A (2018) The impact of childhood abuse on adult male prisoners: a systematic review. *Journal of Police and Criminal Psychology*. doi.org/10.1007/s11896-018-9260-6 [Epub ahead of print]

Goethals S, Gastmans C & Dierckx de Casterlé B (2010) Nurses' ethical reasoning and behaviour: a literature review. *International Journal of Nursing Studies*, 47(5): 635-50

Goffman E (1963) *Stigma: notes on the management of spoiled identity*. Penguin, London

Goldberg P (1983) *The intuitive edge*. Jeremy Tarcher, Los Angeles

Goldman A H (1980) *The moral foundations of professional ethics*. Rowman & Littlefield, Totowa, NJ

Goldman D (2006) System failure versus personal accountability – the case for clean hands. *New England Journal of Medicine*, 355(13 July): 121-3

Gonsalves M A (1985) *Right and reason: ethics in theory and practice*, 8th edn. Times Mirror/Mosby College, St Louis, MO

Good P, Richard R, Syrmis W, Jenkins-Marsh S, Stephens J (2014) Medically assisted hydration for adult palliative care patients. *Cochrane Database of Systematic Reviews*, 4: CD006273. doi: 10.1002/14651858.CD006273.pub3

Goodin R E (1985) *Protecting the vulnerable: a reanalysis of our social responsibilities*, University of Chicago Press, Chicago

Goodwin M (2017) *Georgetown Journal of Gender and Law* Volume XVIII Symposium: Dismantling reproductive injustices: the Hyde Amendment and criminalization of self-induced abortion. *Georgetown Journal of Gender and Law*, 18: 279-82

Gostin L (2005) Ethics, the Constitution, and the dying process: the case of Theresa Marie Schiavo. *Journal of the American Medical Association*, 293(19): 2403-7

Gostin L O & Ayala A S (2017) Global health security in an era of explosive pandemic potential. *Journal of National Security Law and Policy*, 9(1): 1-24

Goulet M-H, Larue C & Dumais A (2017) Evaluation of seclusion and restraint reduction programs in mental health: a systematic review. *Aggression and Violent Behavior*, 34: 139-46

Grassi G, Giraldi T, Messina E, Magnani K, Valle E & Cartei G (2000) Physicians' attitudes to and problems with truth-telling to cancer patients. *Support Care Cancer*, 8(1): 40-5

Gray K, Schein C & Ward A F (2014) The myth of harmless wrongs in moral cognition: Automatic dyadic completion from sin to suffering. *Journal of Experimental Psychology General*, 143(4): 1600-15

Greasley K (2017) *Arguments about abortion: personhood, morality and law*. Oxford University Press, Oxford

Greenberg J, Pyszczynski T & Solomon S (1986) The causes and consequences of a need for self-esteem. A terror management theory. In: R F Baumeister (ed) *Public self and private self*. Springer-Verlag, New York, pp 189-212

Greene J (2013) *Moral tribes: emotion, reason, and the gap between us and them*. Atlantic, London

Greenspan P S (1995) *Practical guilt: moral dilemmas, emotions, and social norms*. Oxford University Press, New York

Greenwood J (2001) The new ethics of abortion. *Journal of Medical Ethics*, 27 (suppl 2): ii2-ii4

Gregg J & Saha S (2006). Losing culture on the way to competence: the use and misuse of culture in medical education. *Academic Medicine* 81(6): 542-7

Grennan E (1930) The Somera case. *International Nursing Review* 5 (December/January): 325-33

Griffith C (2002) Killing me softly. *Herald Sun*, 24 May: 4

Grimes D A, Benson J, Singh S, Romero M, Ganatra B, Okonofua F E & Shah I H (2006) Unsafe abortion: the preventable pandemic. *The Lancet*, 368(9550): 1908-19

Grisso T & Appelbaum P S (1995) The MacArthur Treatment Competence Study. III: Abilities of patients to consent to psychiatric and medical treatments. *Law and Human Behavior*, 19(2): 149-74

Grisso T & Appelbaum P (1998) *Assessing competence to consent to treatment: a guide for physicians and other health professionals*. Oxford University Press, New York

Grisso T, Appelbaum P S, Mulvey E P & Fletcher K (1995) The MacArthur Treatment Competence Study. II: Measures of abilities related to competence to consent to treatment. *Law and Human Behavior*, 19(2): 127-48

Grisso T, Appelbaum P & Hill-Fotouhi, C (1997). The MacCAT-T: A clinical tool to assess patients' capacities to make treatment decisions. *Psychiatric Services (Washington, D.C.)*, 48(11): 1415-19. doi: 10.1176/ps.48.11.1415.

Groh A & Linden R (2011) Addressing elder abuse: the Waterloo Restorative Justice Approach to Elder Abuse Project. *Journal of Elder Abuse and Neglect*, 23(2): 127-46

Gross E (1986) Conclusions: what is feminist theory? In: C Pateman & E Gross (eds) *Feminist challenges: social and political theory*. Allen & Unwin, Sydney, pp 190-204

Gruskin S, Grodin M, Annas G & Marks S (eds) (2005) *Perspectives on health and human rights*. Routledge, New York and London

Gundersen Lutheran Medical Foundation (2007) *Respecting Choices® – an advanced care planning system that works! History/overview*. Gundersen Lutheran Medical Foundation, La Crosse, WI. Online. Available: http://www.respectingchoices.org/

Gurschick L, Mayer D K & Hanson L C (2015) Palliative sedation: an analysis of international guidelines and position statements. *American Journal of Hospice and Palliative Medicine*, 32(6): 660-71

Gustafsson L K, Wigerblad A & Lindwall L (2014) Undignified care: Violation of patient dignity in involuntary psychiatric hospital care from a nurse's perspective. *Nursing Ethics*, 21(2): 176-86

Gysels M, Evans N, Meñaca A, Andrew E, Toscani F, Finetti S, Pasman HR, et al (2012) Culture and end of life care: a scoping exercise in seven European countries, *PLoS ONE*, 7(4): e34188 (16 pp)

Haas A P, Eliason M, Mays V M, Mathy R M, Cochran S D, D'Augelli A R, Silverman M M, et al (2011) Suicide and suicide risk in lesbian, gay, bisexual, and transgender populations: review and recommendations. *Journal of Homosexuality*, 58(1): 10-51

Hadley J (1996) *Abortion: between freedom and necessity*. Virago Press, London

Hagens M, Onwuteaka-Philipsen B D & Pasman H R W (2017) Trajectories to seeking demedicalised assistance in suicide: a qualitative in-depth interview study. *Journal of Medical Ethics*, 43: 543-8

Haidt J (2001) The emotional dog and its rational tail: a social intuitionist approach to moral judgment. *Psychological Review*, 108(4): 814-34

Haidt J (2012) *The righteous mind: why good people are divided by politics and religion*. Penguin Books, London

Haidt J (2013) The new science of morality: an edge Conference. In: J Brockman (ed) *Thinking: the new science of decision-making, problem-solving, and prediction*. Harper-Perennial/HarperCollins, New York, pp 295-311

Haidt J & Björklund F (2008) Social intuitionists answer six questions about moral psychology. In: W Sinnott-Armstrong (ed.) *Moral psychology. Volume 2: The cognitive science of morality: intuition and diversity*. MIT, London: pp 181-217

Haidt J, Björklund F & Murphy S (2000) *Moral dumbfounding: when intuition finds no reason*. Unpublished manuscript, University of Virginia.

Halstead J M (2007) Islamic values: a distinctive framework for moral education? *Journal of Moral Education*, 36(3): 283-96

Ham K (2004) Principled thinking: a comparison of nursing students and experienced nurses. *Journal of Continuing Education in Nursing*, 35(2): 66-73

Hamilton C & Maddison S (eds) (2007) *Silencing dissent: how the Australian government is controlling public opinion and stifling debate*. Allen & Unwin, Sydney

Hamilton H (1995) *Euthanasia: an issue for nurses*. Royal College of Nursing, Australia, Canberra.

Hamlyn-Harris J H (2017) Three reasons why pacemakers are vulnerable to hacking. *The Conversation* (4 September). Online. Available: https://theconversation.com/three-reasons-why-pacemakers-are-vulnerable-to-hacking-83362

Hammell K W (2007) Quality of life after spinal cord injury: a meta-synthesis of qualitative findings. *Spinal Cord* 45: 124-39

Hammes B (2003) Update on Respecting choices four years on. *Innovations in End-of-Life Care*, 5(2): 1-12.

Hammes B & Rooney B (1998) Death and end-of-life planning in one Midwestern community. *Archives of Internal Medicine*, 158(4): 383-90

Hamric A B, Borchers C T & Epstein E G (2012) Development and testing of an instrument to measure moral distress in healthcare professionals. *AJOB Primary Research* 3(2): 1-9

Handwerker W P (2009) *The origin of cultures: how individual choices make cultures change*. Left Coast Press, Walnut Creek, CA

Hanssen I (2004) From human ability to ethical principle: an intercultural perspective on autonomy. *Medicine, Health Care and Philosophy*, 7(3): 269-79

Harding S & Hintikka M B (eds) (1983) *Discovering reality*. D Reidel, Dordrecht

Hardwig J (ed) (2000) *Is there a duty to die? And other essays in bioethics*. Routledge, New York

Hardwig J (2014) Dying at the right time: reflections on (un)assisted suicide. In: H LaFollette (ed) *Ethics in practice: an anthology*, 4th edn. John Wiley & Sons, Chichester, pp 101-11

Hardy J R, Haberecht J, Maresco-Pennisi D & Yates P (2007) Audit of the care of the dying in a network of hospitals and institutions in Queensland. *Internal Medicine Journal*, 37(5): 315-19

Hare R M (1963) *Freedom and reason*. Oxford University Press, London (see in particular Chapter 9 'Toleration and fanaticism')

Hare R M (1964) *The language of morals*. Oxford University Press, Oxford

Hare R M (1981) *Moral thinking: its levels, methods and point*. Clarendon Press, Oxford

Harmon G (1977) *The nature of morality*. Oxford University Press, New York

Harris C, Green S, Ramsey W, Allen K & King R (2017) Sustainability in health care by allocating resources effectively (SHARE) 1: introducing a series of papers reporting an investigation of disinvestment in a local healthcare setting. *BMC Health Services Research*, 17(1): 323 doi.org/10.1186/s12913-017-2210-7

Harris L F, Halpern J, Prata N, Chavkin W & Gerdts C (2018) Conscientious objection to abortion provision: why context matters. *Global Public Health*, 13(5): 556-66

Harris L T & Fiske S T (2006) Dehumanizing the lowest of the low. *Psychological Science*, 17(10): 847-53

Harrison J (1954) When is a principle a moral principle? *Aristotelian Society*, 28 (suppl): 111-34

Harrison R (2005) Democracy. In: E Craig (ed) *The shorter Routledge encyclopedia of philosophy*. Routledge, London and New York, pp 165-70

Hart H L A (1958) Positivism and the separation of law and morals. *Harvard Law Review*, 71(1–4): 593-629

Hart H L A (1961) *The concept of law*. Oxford University Press (Clarendon Law Series), Oxford

Hart H L A (1963) *Law, liberty, and morality*. Stanford University Press, Stanford, CA

Hartvigsson T, Munthe C & Forsander G (2018) Error trawling and fringe decision competence: Ethical hazards in monitoring and address patient decision capacity in clinical practice. *Clinical Ethics*, 13(3): 126-36. doi: 10.1177/1477750917749955

Harvey A & Salter B (2012) Anticipatory governance: bioethical expertise for human / animal chimeras. *Science as Culture*, 21(3): 291-313

Haslam N (2006) Dehumanization: an integrative review. *Personality and Social Psychology Review*, 10(3): 252-64

Haslam N (2013) What is dehumanization? In: P G Bain, J Vaes & J P Leyens (eds) *Advances in understanding humanness and dehumanization*. Taylor & Francis, Hoboken, NJ, pp 34-48

Haslam N & Loughnan S (2014) Dehumanization and infrahumanization. *Annual Review of Psychology*, 65(1): 399-423

Haslam N, Loughnan S, Kashima Y & Bain P (2008) Attributing and denying humanness to others. *European Review of Social Psychology*, 19(1): 55-85

Hastings Center Report (1982a) Case studies: can a subject consent to a 'Ulysses contract'? *Hastings Center Report*, 12(4): 26

Hastings Center Report (1982b) Does 'doing everything' include CPR? *Hastings Center Report* 12(5): 27–8

Hauerwas S (1986) *Suffering presence*. University of Notre Dame Press, South Bend, IN

Hawking S (2011) Foreword. *World report on disability: summary*. WHO and World Bank, Geneva, p ix.

Hawse S & Wood L N (2018) Fostering wise judgement: professional decisions in development programmes for early career engineers. *Journal of Vocational Education and Training*, 70(2): 297-312

Hayes B (2010) Trust and distrust in CPR decisions. *Bioethical Inquiry*, 7: 111-22

Hayes B (2012) Clinical model for ethical cardiopulmonary resuscitation decision-making. *Internal Medicine Journal*, 43(1): 77-83

Häyry M & Takala T (2001) Genetic information, rights and autonomy. *Theoretical Medicine*, 22: 403-14

Health and Disability Commissioner (HDC) (2012) *Code of Health and Disability Services Consumers' Rights*. Online. Available: https://www.hdc.org.nz/your-rights/the-code-and-your-rights/

Health Care Complaints Commission (HCCC) (2003) *Investigation report: Campbelltown and Camden Hospitals MacArthur Health Service*. HCCC, Sydney

Health Practitioner Regulation National Law Act 2009 (Qld). Online. Available: https://www.ahpra.gov.au/documents/default.aspx?record=WD10%2F1563&dbid=AP&chksum=b1YsKvtKyhHdnDKio5ERFA%3D%3D

Health Practitioner Regulation National Law Act (2018). Online. Available: https://www.legislation.act.gov.au/a/db_39269/current/pdf/db_39269.pdf.

Health Practitioners Competence Assurance Act. New Zealand (2003) Online. Available: http://www.legislation.govt.nz/act/public/2003/0048/latest/DLM203312.html

Health4LGBTI: State-of-the-art synthesis report (SSR) (2017) *European Union*. Online. Available: http://eprints.brighton.ac.uk/17562/1/stateofart_report_en.pdf

Heckler R (1994) *Waking up alive: the descent to suicide and return to life*. Piatkus, London

Heffernan M (2011) *Willful blindness: why we ignore the obvious at our peril*. Doubleday Canada, Toronto

Hehir B (2013) Report 'A crisis of compassion: who cares?' Battle of Ideas, 20–1 October 2012, London. *Nursing Ethics*, 20(1): 109-11

Heikkinen A, Lemonidou C, Petsios K, Sala R, Barazzetti G, Radaelli S & Leino-Kilpi H (2006) Ethical codes in nursing practice: the viewpoint of Finnish, Greek and Italian nurses. *Journal of Advanced Nursing*, 55(3): 310-19

Heisenberg W (1990) *Physics and philosophy*. Penguin, London

Hekman S (1995) *Moral voices, moral selves: Carol Gilligan and feminist moral theory*. Polity Press, Cambridge, Cambs

Helft P, Siegler M & Lantos J (2000) The rise and fall of the futility movement. *The New England Journal of Medicine*, 343(4): 293-6

Helman C (1990) *Culture, health and illness*. Wright, London

HelpAge International (2001) *Equal treatment, equal rights: ten actions to end age discrimination*. HelpAge International, London

HelpAge International (HAI) (2015) *A new convention on the rights of older people: a concrete proposal*. HAI, London. Online. Available: https://social.un.org/ageing-working-group/documents/sixth/HelpAgeInternational.pdf

HelpAge International (nd) *Towards a convention on the rights of older people*. Online. Available: http://www.helpage.org/what-we-do/rights/towards-a-convention-on-the-rights-of-older-people/

Hem M H, Gjerberg E, Husum T L & Pedersen R (2018) Ethical challenges when using coercion in mental healthcare: a systematic literature review. *Nursing Ethics*, 25(1): 92-110

Hendin H (1998) *Seduced by death: doctors, patients, and assisted suicide*. W W Norton & Co, New York

Herman J (1992) *Trauma and recovery: the aftermath of violence – from domestic abuse to political terror*. Basic Books, a Division of HarperCollins, New York

Herndon M (1992) The fairness factor: business lessons from the LA riots. *Management Review*, 81(10): 45-7

Hertogh C (2009) The role of advance euthanasia directives as an aid to communication and shared decision-making in dementia. *Journal of Medical Ethics*, 35(2): 100-3

Heuberger R A (2010) Artificial nutrition and hydration at the end of life. *Journal of Nutrition for the Elderly*, 29(4): 347-85

Hewitt T, Chreim S & Forster A (2017) Sociocultural factors influencing incident reporting among physicians and nurses: understanding frames underlying self- and peer-reporting practices. *Journal of Patient Safety*, 13(3): 129-37

Heyd D & Bloch S (1981) The ethics of suicide. In: S Bloch & P Chodoff (eds) *Psychiatric ethics*. Oxford University Press, Oxford, pp 185-202

Heyland D K, Frank C, Groll D, Pichora D, Dodek P, Rocker G & Gafni A (2006) Understanding cardiopulmonary resuscitation decision making: perspectives of seriously ill hospitalized patients and family members. *Chest*, 130(2): 419-28

Hicken M T, Jackson J S, Kravitz-Wirtz N & Durkee M (2018) Racial inequalities in health: framing future research. *Social Science and Medicine*, 199: 11-18

Hickson G B, Pichert J W, Webb L E & Gabbe S G (2007) A complementary approach to promoting professionalism: identifying, measuring, and addressing unprofessional behaviors. *Academic Medicine*, 82(11): 1040-8

Hilario C T, Browne A J & McFadden A (2018) The influence of democratic racism in nursing inquiry. *Nursing Inquiry*, 25(1): E12213. doi: 10.1111/nin.12213 [Epub ahead of print]

Hillman K (2009) *Vital signs: stories from intensive care*, University of New South Wales, Sydney

Hindle D, Braithwaite J, Travaglia J & Iedema R (2006) *Patient safety: a comparative analysis of eight enquiries in six countries*. Centre for Clinical Governance Research in Health, University of New South Wales, Sydney

Hindriks F (2015) How does reasoning (fail to) contribute to moral judgment? Dumbfounding and disengagement. *Ethical Theory and Moral Practice*, 18(2): 237-50

Hinman L (1994) *Ethics: a pluralistic approach to moral theory*. Harcourt Brace Jovanovich, Fort Worth, TX

Hobbes T (1968) *Leviathan* (reprinted from 1651 edition with notes by C B Macpherson). Pelican, Harmondsworth, Middlesex

Hobbs P (2007) The limitations of advance directives and statements in mental health. *Australasian Psychiatry*, 15(1): 22

Hodson G & Costello K (2007) Interpersonal disgust, ideological orientations, and dehumanization as predictors of intergroup attitudes. *Psychological Science*, 18(8): 691-8

Hodson G, MacInnis C C & Costello K (2013) (Over)Valuing "humanness" as an aggravator of intergroup prejudices an discrimination. In: Bain P G, Vaes J & Leyens J P (eds) *Advances in understanding humanness and dehumanization*. Taylor & Francis, Hoboken, NJ, pp 86-110

Hoffmaster B (2006) What does vulnerability mean? *Hastings Center Report*, 36(2): 38-45

Hofmann B (2017) The overdiagnosis of what? On the relationship between the concepts of overdiagnosis, disease, and diagnosis. *Medicine, Health Care and Philosophy*, 20: 453-64

Holden W (1994) *Unlawful carnal knowledge: the true story of the Irish 'X' case*. HarperCollins, London

Homeless World Cup Foundation (nd) *Global homelessness statistics*. Online. Available: https://homelessworldcup.org/homelessness-statistics/

Homelessness Australia (2016) *Homelessness in Australia. Fact Sheet*. Online. Available: https://www.homelessnessaustralia.org.au/sites/homelessnessaus/files/2017-07/Homelessness%20in%20Australiav2.pdf

Homelessness Australia (nd) *Home page*. Online. Available: https://www.homelessnessaustralia.org.au/

Honan S, Helseth C, Bakke J, Karpiuk K, Krsnak G & Torkelson R (1991) Perception of 'No Code' and the role of the nurse. *Journal of Continuing Education in Nursing*, 22(2): 54-61

Hook J N, Davis D E, Owen J, Worthington E L & Utsey S O (2013) Cultural humility: measuring openness to culturally diverse clients. *Journal of Counselling Psychology*, 60(3): 353-66

Hooker C, Leask J & King C (2012) Media ethics and infectious disease. In: C Enemark & M J Selgelid (eds) *Ethics and security aspects of infectious disease control*. Ashgate, Farnham, Surrey, pp 161-77

Horsfall L (2016) The nocebo effect. *SAAD Digest*, 32 (January): 55-7. Online. Available: https://www.saad.org.uk/Digest/LinkedSAADDigest2016FINAL.pdf

Hough A (2013) Grandfather dies after doctors 'misdiagnosed pea on lung for cancer'. *The Telegraph* 22 April. Online. Available: https://www.telegraph.co.uk/news/health/news/10009756/Grandfather-dies-after-doctors-misdiagnosed-pea-on-lung-for-cancer.html

Houkamau C A, Stronge S & Sibley C G (2017) The prevalence and impact of racism towards Indigenous Māori in New Zealand. *International Perspectives in Psychology: Research, Practice, Consultation*, 6(2): 61-80

Howe A & Healy J (2005) Generational justice in aged care policy in Australia and the United Kingdom. *Australasian Journal on Ageing*, 24(1 – June suppl): S12-S18

Hudson F (2002) 21 Clap as Nancy dies. *Herald Sun*, 24 May: 1, 4

Hughes J (1995) Ultimate justification: Wittgenstein and medical ethics. *Journal of Medical Ethics*, 21: 25-30

Hughes M (2018) Health and well being of lesbian, gay, bisexual, transgender and intersex people aged 50 years and over. *Australian Health Review*, 42: 146-51

Hui D, Dev R & Bruerra E (2015) The last days of life: symptom burden and impact on nutrition and hydration in cancer patients. *Current Opinion in Supportive and Palliative Care*, 9(4): 346-54

Hui K (2014) Moral anthropocentrism is unavoidable. *American Journal of Bioethics*, 14(2): 25

Hume D (1888 edn) *Treatise of human nature* (ed L A Selby-Bigge). Oxford University Press, London

Huntington A (2002) Working with women experiencing mid-trimester termination of pregnancy: the integration of nursing and feminist knowledge in the gynaecological setting. *Journal of Clinical Nursing*, 11(2): 273-9

Hurka S, Knill C & Rivière L (2018) Four worlds of morality politics: the impact of institutional venues and party cleavages. *West European Politics*, 41(2): 428-47

Hursthouse R (1999) *On virtue ethics*. Oxford University Press, Oxford

Hursthouse R (2007) Virtue theory. In: H LaFollette (ed) *Ethics in practice: an anthology*, 3rd edn. Blackwell, Oxford, pp 45-55

Hursthouse R (2014a). Virtue theory. In: H LaFollette, (ed) *Ethics in practice: an anthology* (4th edn). John Wiley & Sons, Chichester, Sussex, pp 60-9

Hursthouse R (2014b) Virtue theory and abortion (revised) In: H LaFollette (ed) *Ethics in practice: an anthology*, 4th edn. John Wiley & Sons, Chichester, Sussex, pp 160-8

Huxtable R & Möller M (2007) 'Setting a principled boundary'? Euthanasia as a response to 'life fatigue'. *Bioethics* 21(3): 117-26

Hyatt J (2017) Recognizing moral disengagement and its impact on patient safety. *Journal of Nursing Regulation*, 7(4): 15-21

Idrees N, Ullah Z & Zeb Khan M (2018) Impact of ethical conflict on job performance: the mediating role of proactive behavior. *Asian Journal of Business Ethics*, 7(1): 103-16

Iliffe J (2002) Whistleblowing: a difficult decision. *Australian Nursing Journal*, 9(7): 1

Imai K, Morita T, Yokomich N, Mori M, Naito A S, Tsukuura H, Yamauchi T, et al (2018) Efficacy of two types of palliative sedation therapy defined using intervention protocols: proportional vs. deep sedation. *Supportive Care in Cancer*, 26(6): 1763-71

In re alleged unfair dismissal of Ms K Howden by the City of Whittlesea 6/9/90 (Case no 90/3672, decision D90/1933) IRCV (unreported)

Independent (1992) Jubilation in Ireland as abortion ban lifted. *The Age*, 28 February: 6

Independent Commission Against Corruption (ICAC) (2005a) *Report on investigation into the alleged mistreatment of nurses.* ICAC, Sydney

Independent Commission Against Corruption (ICAC) (2005b) *Report on investigation into various allegations relating to the former South Western Sydney Area Health Service.* ICAC, Sydney

Infoplease-Ethnicity and race by countries. Online. Available: https://www.infoplease.com/ethnicity-and-race-countries

Inghelbrecht E, Bilsen J, Mortier F & Deliens L (2011) Continuous deep sedation until death in Belgium: a survey among nurses. *Journal of Pain and Symptom Management*, 41(5): 870-9

Institute for Criminal Policy Research (2016) *World Prison Population List*, 11th edn. Online. Available: https://prisonstudies.org/sites/.../world_prison_population_list_11th_edition_0.pdf

Inter-Agency Standing Committee (IASC) (2007) *Inter-agency contingency planning guidelines for humanitarian assistance.* IASC, Geneva

International Association of Forensic Nurses (2017) *Correctional nursing.* Online. Available: http://www.forensicnurses.org/?page=correctionalnursing

International Committee of Medical Journal Editors (ICMJE) Guideline: *Recommendations for the conduct, reporting, editing, and publication of scholarly work in medical journals*. Online. Available: www.icmje.org.

International Council of Nurses (ICN) (1973) *Code for nurses*. ICN, Geneva

International Council of Nurses (ICN) (2007) *Vision for the future of nursing*. ICN, Geneva

International Council of Nurses (ICN) (2009) *Nursing matters fact sheet: The health of indigenous people: A concern for nursing*. ICN, Geneva

International Council of Nurses (ICN) (2011a) *Position statement: Nurses and human rights*. ICN, Geneva

International Council of Nurses (ICN) (2011b) *Position statement: Nurses' role in the care of detainees and prisoners*. ICN, Geneva

International Council of Nurses (ICN) (2012a) *The ICN code of ethics for nurses*. ICN, Geneva

International Council of Nurses (ICN) (2012b) *Position statement: patient safety*. ICN, Geneva

International Council of Nurses (ICN) (2018) *Position statement: Health of migrants, refugees and displaced persons*. ICN, Geneva

International Council of Prison Medical Services (1979) *The Oath of Athens*. Online. Available: http://www.medekspert.az/ru/chapter1/resources/The_Oath_of_Athens.pdf

International Work Group for Indigenous Affairs (IWGIA) (2013) *The indigenous world 2013* (compiled and edited by Cæcilie Mikkelsen). IWGIA, Copenhagen. Online. Available: http://www.iwgia.org/iwgia

International Work Group for Indigenous Affairs (IWGIA) (2017) *The indigenous world 2017* (compiled and co-edited by: K B Hansen, K Jepsen & P L Jacquelin). IWGIA, Copenhagen. Online. Available: https://www.iwgia.org/images/documents/indigenous-world/indigenous-world-2017.pdf

Irwin J (2007) Culture attack on the cancer taboo. *Northcote Leader*, 17 July: 9

Irwin v Ciena Health Care Management Inc. (2013). Unpublished opinion, Nos. 305878; 306013. Oakland Circuit Court (LC No. 2008-093145-CD). Online. Available: http://www.michiganemploymentlawadvisor.com/wp-content/uploads/sites/341/2013/10/Irwin-v-Ciena-Health-Care.2013_100313_55492.pdf

Jackson D, Peters K, Andrews S, Edenborough M, Halcomb E, Luck L, Salamonson Y, et al (2010a) Understanding whistleblowing: qualitative insights from nurse whistleblowers. *Journal of Advanced Nursing*, 66(10): 2194-201

Jackson D, Peters K, Andrews S, Edenborough M, Halcomb E, Luck L, Salamonson Y, et al (2010b) Trial and retribution: A qualitative study of whistleblowing and workplace relationships in nursing. *Contemporary Nurse*, 36(1-2): 34-44

Jackson D, Hickman L D, Hutchinson M, Andrew S, Smith J, Potgieter I, Cleary M, et al (2014) Whistleblowing: an integrative literature review of data-based studies involving nurses. *Contemporary Nurse*, 48(2): 240-52

Jackson S L (2016a) The shifting conceptualization of elder abuse in the United States: from social services, to criminal justice, and beyond. *International Psychogeriatrics*, 28(1): 1-8

Jackson S L (2016b) All elder abuse perpetrators are not alike: the heterogeneity of elder abuse perpetrators and implications for intervention. *International Journal of Offender Therapy and Comparative Criminology*, 60(3): 265-85

Jackson S L & Hafemeister T L (2013) How do abused elderly persons and their adult protective caseworkers view law enforcement involvement and criminal prosecution, and what impact do these views have on case processing? *Journal of Elder Abuse and Neglect*, 25(3): 254-80

Jackson T (2013) The inside story on prison health. *British Medical Journal*, 346: f3471

Jafarey A M & Farooqui A (2005) Informed consent in the Pakistani milieu: the physician's perspective. *Journal of Medical Ethics*, 31(2): 93-6

Jaggar A M & Tobin T W (2013) Situating moral justification: rethinking the mission of moral epistemology. *Metaphilosophy*, 44(4): 383-408

James S (1994) Reconciling international human rights and cultural relativism: the case of female circumcision. *Bioethics*, 8(1): 1-26

Jameton A (1984) *Nursing practice: the ethical issues*. Prentice-Hall, Englewood Cliffs, NJ

Jameton A (1993) Dilemmas of moral distress: moral responsibility and nursing practice. *AWHONN's Clinical Issues*, 4: 542-51

Jamieson D (2010) Climate change, responsibility, and justice. *Science and Engineering Ethics*, 16: 431-45

Jansen L & Friedman Ross L (2000) Patient confidentiality and the surrogate's right to know. *Journal of Law, Medicine and Ethics*, 28(2): 137-43

Jastrow J (1899) The mind's eye. *Popular Science Monthly*, 54: 299–312

Jecker N & Schneiderman L (1995) When families request that 'everything possible' be done. *Journal of Medicine and Philosophy*, 20(2): 146-63

Jecker N, Jonsen A & Pearlman R (2007) *Bioethics: an introduction to the history, methods, and practice*, 2nd edn. Jones and Bartlett, Boston MA

Jego M, Abcaya J, Stefan D E, Calvet-Montredon C & Gentile S (2018) Improving health care management in primary care for homeless people: a literature review. *International Journal of Environmental Research and Public Health*,15(2).pii: E309

Jenkins R (2011) Moral imperialism. Entry in: *Encyclopedia of global justice* (ed Deen K Chatterjee). Springer Science and Business Media, Dordrecht/New York, pp 721-3

Jennings B (1991) Possibilities of consensus: toward democratic moral discourse. *Journal of Medicine and Philosophy*, 16(4): 447-63

Jennings B (ed) (2014) *Encyclopedia of bioethics*, 4th edn. Gale-Macmillan Reference USA, New York

Jennings B (2016) Reconceptualizing autonomy: a relational turn in bioethics. *Hastings Center Report*, 46(3): 11-16

Jenniskens K, de Groot JAH, Reitsma JB, Moons KGM, Hooft L & Naaktgeboren C A (2017) Overdiagnosis across medical disciplines: a scoping review. *BMJ Open*, 7: e018448. doi: 10.1136/bmjopen-2017-018448

Jin P & Hakkarinen M (2017) Highlights in bioethics through 40 years: a quantitative analysis of top-cited journal articles. *Journal of Medical Ethics*, 43: 339-45. doi: 10.1136/medethics-2016-103658

John M & Bailey L L (2018) Neonatal heart transplantation. *Annals of Cardiothoracic Surgery*, 7(1): 118-25

Johns J (1996) Advance directives and opportunities for nurses. *Image: Journal of Nursing Scholarship*, 28(2): 149-53

Johnson B R, Mishra V, Lavelanet A F, Khosla R & Ganatra B (2017) A global database of abortion laws, policies, health standards and guidelines. *Bulletin of the World Health Organization*, 95: 542-4

Johnson S, Kerridge I, Butow P N & Tattersall M H (2017) Advance Care Planning: is quality end of life care really that simple? *Internal Medicine Journal*, 47(4): 390-4

Johnson N P A S & Mueller J (2002) Updating the accounts: global mortality of the 1918–1920 "Spanish" influenza pandemic. *Bulletin of the History of Medicine*, 76(1): 105-15

Johnston P (1989) *Wittgenstein and moral philosophy*. Routledge, London

Johnstone G (2002) *Restorative justice: ideas, values, debates*. Willan, Oregon

Johnstone G & Van Ness D W (eds) (2007) *Handbook of restorative justice*. Willan, Cullompton, Devon and Portland, OR

Johnstone M-J (1988) The nature and moral implications of 'Not For Resuscitation' orders. In: *Proceedings of the Conference Nursing Law and Ethics, First Victorian State Conference, theme: matters of life and death*. School of Nursing, Phillip Institute of Technology, Melbourne, 30th September, pp 26-48

Johnstone M-J (1989a) 'Dying with dignity', *New Zealand Nursing Journal* 81(12): 34, 37 (ch 7)

Johnstone M-J (1989b) *Bioethics: a nursing perspective*. W B Saunders/Baillière Tindall, Sydney (ch 9)

Johnstone M-J (1989c) The nature and moral implications of 'Not For Resuscitation' orders. *Bioethics News*, 8(2): 26-44

Johnstone M-J (1989d) 'Not For Resuscitation [NFR]' orders – the nurse's dilemma, the nurse's demise. In: Australian Nursing Federation (ANF) (eds) *Ethics: nursing perspectives*, vol. 2. ANF, Melbourne, pp 23-8

Johnstone M-J (1994a) *Nursing and the injustices of the law*. W B Saunders/Baillière Tindall, Sydney

Johnstone M-J (1994b) The legal invalidation of professional nursing ethics. In: M-J Johnstone, *Nursing and the injustices of the law* (pp 251-67). W B Saunders/Baillière Tindall, Sydney

Johnstone M (1995) Invited guest editorial: the scandalous neglect of mental health care ethics. *Contemporary Nurse*, 4(4): 142-4

Johnstone M-J (ed) (1996a) *The politics of euthanasia: a nursing response*. Royal College of Nursing, Australia, Canberra

Johnstone M-J (1996b) The politics of euthanasia: an introduction. In: M-J Johnstone (ed) *The politics of euthanasia: a nursing response*. Royal College of Nursing, Australia, Canberra, pp 13-19

Johnstone M-J (1999a) *Bioethics: a nursing perspective*, 3rd edn. Harcourt/Saunders, Sydney

Johnstone M-J (1999b) *Reporting child abuse: ethical issues for the nursing profession and nurse regulating authorities: a report to the Nurses Board of Victoria*. Department of Nursing and Public Health, RMIT University, Melbourne

Johnstone M-J (2001) Stigma, social justice and the rights of the mentally ill: challenging the status quo. *Australian and New Zealand Journal of Mental Health Nursing*, 10: 200-9

Johnstone M-J (2002) Poor working conditions and the capacity of nurses to provide moral care. *Contemporary Nurse*, 12(1): 7-15

Johnstone M-J (2004a) *Effective writing for health professionals*. Allen & Unwin, Sydney, pp 3-4

Johnstone M-J (2004b) Patient safety, ethics and whistleblowing: a nursing response to the events at the Campbelltown and Camden Hospitals. *Australian Health Review*, 28(1): 13-19

Johnstone M-J (2007a) Research ethics, reconciliation, and strengthening the research relationship in Indigenous health domains: an Australian perspective. *International Journal of Intercultural Relations*, 31(3): 391-406

Johnstone M-J (2007b) Patient safety ethics and human error management in ED contexts. Part II: accountability and the challenge to change. *Australasian Emergency Nurses Journal*, 10(2): 80-5

Johnstone M-J (2008) Questioning nursing ethics. *Australian Nursing Journal*, 15(7): 19

Johnstone M-J (2009a) Ethics and human vulnerability. *Australian Nursing Journal* 16(10): 23

Johnstone M-J (2009b) Health care disaster ethics: a call to action. *Australian Nursing Journal*, 17(1): 27

Johnstone M-J (2010) Equitable health care form and end-of-life care. *Australian Nursing Journal* 18(2): 22

Johnstone M-J (2011) Nursing and justice as a basic human need. *Nursing Philosophy*, 12: 34-44

Johnstone M-J (2012a) Unethical professional conduct. *Australian Nursing Journal*, 19(11): 34

Johnstone M-J (2012b) Bioethics, cultural differences and the problem of moral disagreements in end-of-life care: a terror management theory. *Journal of Medicine and Philosophy*, 37(4): 181-200

Johnstone M-J (2012c) Organization position statements and the stance of 'Studied Neutrality' on euthanasia in palliative care. *Journal of Pain and Symptom Management*, 44(6): 896-907

Johnstone M-J (2012d) Nurses and ethical conflicts with employer organisations. *Australian Nursing Journal*, 19(9): 29

Johnstone M-J (2013a) *Alzheimer's disease, media representations and the politics of euthanasia: constructing risk and selling death in an aging society*. Ashgate, Farnham, Surrey

Johnstone M-J (2013b) Moral distress. *Australian Nursing Journal* 20(12): 25

Johnstone M-J (2013c) Ageism and the moral exclusion of older people. *Australian Nursing and Midwifery Journal* 21(3): 27

Johnstone M-J (2013d) Climate change. *Australian Nursing Journal*, 20(8): 24

Johnstone M-J (2014a) Media manipulation and the euthanasia debate. *Australian Nursing and Midwifery Journal*, 21(7): 32

Johnstone M-J (2014b) 'Moral luck' and the question of autonomy, choice, and control in end-of-life decision making. *Progress in Palliative Care*, 23(3): 126-32

Johnstone M-J (ed) (2015a) *Nursing ethics. Volume 1: developing theoretical foundations for nursing ethics*. Sage Publications, Oxford

Johnstone M-J (ed) (2015b) *Nursing ethics. Volume 2: nursing ethics pedagogy and praxis*. Sage Publications, Oxford

Johnstone M-J (ed) (2015c) *Nursing ethics. Volume 3: politics and future directions of nursing ethics*. Sage Publications, Oxford

Johnstone M-J (2016a) Key milestones in the operationalisation of professional nursing ethics in Australia: a brief historical overview. *Australian Journal of Advanced Nursing*, 33(4): 35-45

Johnstone M-J (2016b) Academic dishonesty and unethical behaviour in the workplace. *Australian Nursing and Midwifery Journal*, 23(1): 33

Johnstone M-J (2016c) Professional ethics, bullying and workplace cliques. *Australian Nursing and Midwifery Journal*, 23(9): 14

Johnstone M-J (2017) Honesty and integrity in authorship attribution. *Australian Nursing and Midwifery Journal*, 24(10): 30

Johnstone M-J & Crock E (2015) Dealing with ethical issues in nursing practice. In: E Chang & J Daly (eds) *Transitions in nursing: preparing for professional practice*, 4th edn. Churchill Livingstone/Elsevier Australia, Sydney

Johnstone M-J & Hutchinson A (2015) Moral distress in nursing – time to abandon a flawed nursing construct? *Nursing Ethics*, 22(1): 5-14. doi: 10.1177/0969733013505312

Johnstone M-J & Kanitsaki O (1991) Some moral implications of cultural and linguistic diversity in health care. *Bioethics News*, 10(2): 22-32

Johnstone M-J & Kanitsaki O (2006a) Culture, language and patient safety: making the link. *International Journal for Quality in Health Care*, 18(5): 383-8

Johnstone M-J & Kanitsaki O (2006b) The ethics and practical importance of defining, distinguishing and disclosing nursing errors: a discussion paper. *Journal of Nursing Studies*, 43(3): 367-76

Johnstone M-J & Kanitsaki O (2007a) Health care provider and consumer understandings of cultural safety and cultural competency in health care: an Australian study. *Journal of Cultural Diversity*, 14(2): 96-104

Johnstone M-J & Kanitsaki O (2007b) An exploration of the notion and nature of 'cultural safety' and its applicability to the Australian health care context. *Journal of Transcultural Nursing*, 18(3): 247-56

Johnstone M & Kanitsaki O (2007c) Clinical risk management and patient safety education for nurses: a critique. *Nurse Education Today*, 27(3): 185-91

Johnstone M-J & Kanitsaki O (2008a) Cultural racism, language prejudice and discrimination in hospital contexts: an Australian study. *Diversity in Health and Social Care*, 5(1): 19-30

Johnstone M-J & Kanitsaki O (2008b) The problem of failing to provide culturally and linguistically appropriate healthcare. In: S Barrowclough and H Gardner (eds) *Analysing Australian health policy: a problem orientated approach*. Elsevier Australia, Sydney, pp 176-87

Johnstone M-J & Kanitsaki O (2008c) Ethnic aged discrimination and disparities in health and social care: a question of social justice. *Australasian Journal on Ageing*, 27(3): 110-15

Johnstone M-J & Kanitsaki O (2009a) Ethics and advance care planning in a culturally diverse society. *Journal of Transcultural Nursing*, 20(4): 405-16

Johnstone M-J & Kanitsaki O (2009b) Engaging patients as safety partners: some considerations for ensuring a culturally and linguistically appropriate approach, *Health Policy*, 90(1): 1-7

Johnstone M-J & Kanitsaki O (2010) The neglect of racism as an ethical issue in health care. *Journal of Immigrant and Minority Health*, 12(6): 489-95

Johnstone M-J & Turale S (2014) Nurses' experiences of ethical preparedness for public health emergencies and healthcare disasters: a systematic review of qualitative evidence. *Nursing and Health Sciences*, 16(1): 67-77

Johnstone M-J, Hutchinson A, Rawson H & Redley B (2016) Nursing strategies for engaging families of older immigrants hospitalised for end-of-life care: an Australian study. *Journal of Patient Experience*, 3(3): 57-63

Joint Centre for Bioethics Pandemic Influenza Working Group (2005) *Stand on guard for thee: ethical considerations in preparedness for pandemic influenza*. University of Toronto Joint Centre for Bioethics, Toronto

Jones A & Johnstone M-J (2017) Inattentional blindness and failures to rescue the deteriorating patient in critical care, emergency and perioperative settings: four case scenarios. *Australian Critical Care*, 30: 219-23

Jones A & Kelly D (2014) Whistle-blowing and workplace culture in older peoples' care: qualitative insights from the healthcare and social care workforce. *Sociology of Health and Illness*, 36(7): 986-1002

Jones A, Johnstone M-J & Duke M (2016) Recognizing and responding to "cutting corners" when providing nursing care: a qualitative study. *Journal of Clinical Nursing*, 25(15-16): 2126-33

Jones E, Farina A, Hastorf A, Marcus H, Miller D & Scott R (1984) *Social stigma: the psychology of marked relationships*. Freeman & Co, New York

Jones J & Hoffman T (2005) 'I had to act': in conversation with a whistleblower. *Australian Journal of Advanced Nursing*, 23(1): 4-6

Jones T (1991) Ethical decision making by individuals in organizations: an issue-contingent model. *Academy of Management*, 16(2): 366-95

Jones T M, Nurius P, Song C & Fleming C M (2018) Modeling life course pathways from adverse childhood experiences to adult mental health. *Child Abuse and Neglect*, 80: 32-40

Jonsen A (1993) The birth of bioethics. *Hastings Center Report, Special Supplement*, 23(6): S1–S4

Jonson-Reid M, Kohl P L & Drake B (2012) Child and adult outcomes of chronic child maltreatment. *Pediatrics*, 129(5): 839-45

Jordens C, Little M, Kerridge I & McPhee J (2005) Ethics in medicine, from advance directives to advance care planning: current legal status, ethical rationales and a new research agenda. *Internal Medicine Journal*, 35(9): 563-6

Jørgensen M B (2012) *Dependent, deprived or deviant? The construction of deserving and undeserving groups: the case of single mothers in Denmark*. CoMID Working Paper Series, No. 2. Online. Available: http://vbn.aau.dk/files/66950697/CoMID_wp_2.pdf

Joseph R (2011) Hospital policy on medical futility- Does it help in conflict resolution and ensuring good end-of-life care? *Annals Academy of Medicine Singapore*, 40(1): 19-25

Jubb M & Shanley E (2002) Family involvement: the key to opening locked wards and closed minds. *International Journal of Mental Health Nursing*, 11(1): 47-53

Kahn D & Steeves R (1986) The experience of suffering: conceptual clarification and theoretical definition. *Journal of Advanced Nursing*, 11(6): 623-31

Kairys D (ed) (1997) *The politics of law: a progressive critique*, 2nd edn. Pantheon, New York

Kälvemark S, Höglund A T, Hansson M G, Westerholm P & Arnetz B (2004) Living with conflicts-ethical dilemmas and moral distress in the health care system. *Social Science and Medicine*, 58: 1075-84

Kanitsaki O (1989a) *Health–illness–suffering experiences of a sample of Greek-born members of 12 Greek–Australian families living in Melbourne*. Minor thesis completed in partial fulfilment of the requirements for the Degree of Master of Educational Studies, Faculty of Education, Monash University, Melbourne

Kanitsaki O (1989b) Cross-cultural sensitivity in palliative care. In: P Hodder & A Turley (eds) *The creative option of palliative care: a manual for health professionals*. Melbourne City Mission, Melbourne, pp 68–71

Kanitsaki O (1994) Cultural and linguistic diversity. In: J Romanini & J Daly, *Critical care nursing: Australian perspectives.* W B Saunders/Baillière Tindall, Sydney, pp 94–125

Kanitsaki O (2000) Diverse cultural care: a critical approach to care and caring (book chapter). In: C Taylor & J Crisp (eds) *Fundamentals of nursing.* Harcourt Australia, Sydney, pp 114-37

Kanitsaki O (2002) Mental health, culture and spirituality: implications for the effective psychotherapeutic care of Australia's ageing migrant population. *Journal of Religious Gerontology*, 13(3/4): 17-37

Kanitsaki O (2003) Transcultural nursing and challenging the status quo. *Contemporary Nurse*, 15(3): v-x

Kant I (1930 edn) *Lectures on ethics* (transl L Infield & J MacMurray). Methuen, London (see in particular 'Conscience', pp 129-35)

Kant I (1959 edn) *Fundamental principles of the metaphysics of ethics* (transl T Kingmill Abbott). Longmans, London

Kant I (1972 edn) *The moral law* (transl H J Paton). Hutchinson University Press, London

Kaplan K & Schwartz M (1993) *A psychology of hope: an antidote to the suicidal pathology of Western civilization.* Praeger, Westport, Connecticut

Kappel K (2018) How moral disagreement may ground principled moral compromise. *Politics, Philosophy and Economics*, 17(1): 75-96

Karim K (2002) *A grounded theory study of truth-telling in cancer: perceptions of white British and British South Asian Community Workers.* Universal, Boca Raton, FL

Kaspiew R, Carson R & Rhoades H (2016) *Elder abuse: understanding issues, frameworks and responses.* Australian Institute of Family Studies, Melbourne

Kass L (1993) Is there a right to die? *Hastings Center Report*, 23(1): 34-43

Kaufman S R (2015) *Ordinary medicine: extraordinary treatments, longer lives and where to draw the line.* Duke University Press, Durham (NC)

Kaufmann P, Kuch H, Neuhauser C & Webster E (eds) (2011a) *Humiliation, degradation, dehumanization: human dignity violated,* Springer, Dordrecht

Kaufmann P, Kuch H, Neuhauser C & Webster E (2011b) Human dignity violated: a negative approach – introduction. In: P Kaufmann, H Kuch, C Neuhauser & E Webster (eds) *Humiliation, degradation, dehumanization: human dignity violated,* Springer, Dordrecht and NY, pp 1-5

Kaustubh J (2003) Psychiatric advance directives. *Journal of Psychiatric Practice*, 9(4): 303-6

Kavanagh A, Wielding S, Cochrane R, Sim J, Johnstone A & Cameron S (2018) 'Abortion' or 'termination of pregnancy'? Views from abortion care providers in Scotland, UK. *BMJ Sexual and Reproductive Health*, 44(2): 122-7

Kavussanu M & Stanger N (2017) Moral behavior in sport. *Current Opinion in Psychology*, 16: 185-92

Kazdaglis G A, Arnaoutoglou C, Karypidis D, Memekidou G, Spanos G & Papadopoulos O (2010) Disclosing the truth to terminal cancer patients: a discussion of ethical and cultural values. *Eastern Mediterranean Health Journal*, 16(4): 442-7

Kelly D & Jones A (2013) When care is needed: the role of whistleblowing in promoting best standards from an individual and organizational perspective. *Quality in Ageing and Older Adults*, 14(3): 180-91

Kempe C H, Silverman F, Steele B, Droegemuller W & Silver H (1962) The battered-child syndrome. *Journal of the American Medical Association*, 181(1): 17-24

Kenny K, Fotaki M & Scriver S (2018) Mental health as a weapon: whistleblower retaliation and normative violence. *Journal of Business Ethics*. Online. Available: https://doi.org/10.1007/s10551-018-3868-4

Kentikelenis K, Karanikolos M, Reeves A, McKee M, Stuckler D (2014) Greece's health crisis: from austerity to denialism. *The Lancet*, 383 (22 Feb): 748-53

Kerridge I, Mitchell K & Myser C (1994) The decision to withhold resuscitation in Australia: problems, hospital policy and legal uncertainty. *Journal of Law and Medicine*, 2 (November): 125-30

Kerridge I, Lowe M & McPhee J (2013) *Ethics and law for the health profession*, 4th edn. Federation Press, Sydney

Khaitan T (2018) Indirect discrimination. In: K Lippert-Rasmussen (ed) *Routledge handbook of the ethics of discrimination.* Routledge, Milton Park, Abingdon, pp 30-41

Khan F & Lea B (2009) *Paging King Solomon: towards allowing parents to donate organs of anencephalic infants.* Online. Available: http://digitalcommons.law.uga.edu/fac_artchop/560

Kieny M-P, Evans D B, Schmets G & Kadandale S (2014) Health-system resilience: reflection on the Ebola crisis in western Africa. *Bulletin of the World Health Organization*, 92(12): 850

Kim M, Van Dorn R, Scheyett A, Elbogen E, Swanson J, Swartz M & McDaniel L (2007) Understanding the personal and clinical utility of advance directives: a qualitative perspective. *Psychiatry: Interpersonal and Biological Processes*, 70(1): 19-29

King G (1997) The effects of interpersonal closeness and issue seriousness on blowing the whistle. *International Journal of Business Communication*, 34(4): 419-36

King G (2001) Perceptions of intentional wrongdoing and peer reporting behaviour among registered nurses. *Journal of Business Ethics*, 34(1): 1-13

King G & Hermodson A (2000) Peer reporting of coworker wrongdoing: a qualitative analysis of observer attitudes in the decision to report versus not report unethical behaviour. *Journal of Applied Communication Research*, 28(4): 309-29

King G & Scudder J N (2013) Reasons registered nurses report serious wrongdoings in a public teaching hospital. *Psychological Reports*, 112(2): 626-36

King M, Semlyen J, Tai S S, Killaspy H, Osborn D, Popelyuk D & Nazareth I (2008) A systematic review of mental disorder, suicide, and deliberate self harm in lesbian, gay and bisexual people. *BMC Psychiatry*, 8: 70

Kingsley M J (2017) Digital lives in psychotherapy: 'the other in the room'. *Psychoanalytic Psychotherapy*, 31(2): 160-75

Kittay E F & Meyers D T (eds) (1987) *Women and moral theory*. Rowman & Littlefield, Totowa, NJ

Kleinman A, Eisenberg L & Good B (1978) Culture, illness, and care: clinical lessons from anthropologic and cross-cultural research. *Annals of Internal Medicine*, 88(2): 251-8

Klemke E D (ed) (1981) *The meaning of life*. Oxford University Press, New York

Klonoff D C (2015) Cybersecurity for connected diabetes devices. *Journal of Diabetes Science and Technology*, 9(5): 1143-7

Klotzko A (1995) CQ interview: Arlene Judith Klotzko and Dr Boudewijn Chabot discuss assisted suicide in the absence of somatic illness. *Cambridge Quarterly of Health Care Ethics Journal*, 4(2): 239-49

Kluckhohn C (1962) *Culture and behavior*. Free Press, New York

Knight J (1992) The suffering of suicide: the victim and family considered. In: P Starck & J McGovern (eds) *The hidden dimension of illness: human suffering*. National League for Nursing Press, New York, pp 245-68

Koenigs M, Young L, Adolphs R, Tranel D, Cushman F, Hauser M & Damasio A (2007) Damage to the prefrontal cortex increases utilitarian moral judgments. *Nature*, 446(7138): 908-11

Kohn L, Corrigan J & Donaldson M (eds) (2000) *To err is human: building a safer health system*. National Academy Press, Washington, DC

Kopelman L (1995) Conceptual and moral disputes about futile and useful treatments. *Journal of Medicine and Philosophy*, 20(2): 109-21

Kordig C R (1976) Pseudo-appeals to conscience. *Journal of Value Inquiry*, 10: 7-17

Korean Nurses Association (KNA) (2013) *Korean Nurses' declaration of ethics*. Online. Available: http://en.koreanurse.or.kr/about_KNA/ethical.php

Kottow M (2003) The vulnerable and the susceptible. *Bioethics*, 17(5-6): 460-71

Kottow M (2004) Vulnerability: what kind of principle is it? *Medicine, Health Care and Philosophy*, 7(3): 281-7

Koubaridis A (2018) *Irish abortion vote leaves UK Prime Minister Theresa May with a big problem. news.com.au* (29 May). Online. Available: http://www.news.com.au/world/europe/irish-abortion-vote-leaves-uk-prime-minister-theresa-may-with-big-problem/news-story/e999e6a2e292e1f3b6d19fd460409eec

Koutantji M, Davis R, Vincent C & Coulter A (2005) The patient's role in patient safety: engaging patients, their representatives, and health professionals. *Clinical Risk*, 11(3): 99-104

Kozeniecki M, Ewy M & Patel J J (2017) Nutrition at the end of life: it's not what you say, it's how you say it. *Current Nutrition Reports*, 6(3): 261-5

Krein SL, Mayer J, Harrod M, Gregory L, Petersen L, Samore M H & Drews F A (2018) Identification and characterization of failures in infectious agent transmission precaution practices in hospitals: a qualitative study. *JAMA Internal Medicine*, 178(8): 1051-7. doi: 10.1001/jamainternmed.2018.1898

Kreitman N (1977) *Parasuicide*. John Wiley, Chichester

Kreslake J, Sarfaty M, Roser-Renouf C, Leiserowitz A & Maibach E (2018) The critical roles of health professionals in climate change prevention and preparedness. *American Journal of Public Health*, 108(S2): S68-S69

Krieger E, Moritz S, Weil R & Nagel M (2018) Patients' attitudes towards and acceptance of coercion in psychiatry. *Psychiatry Research*, 260: 478-85

Krisberg K (2017) Public health increasingly facing cybersecurity threats: Health field a top target for attacks. *The Nation's Health*, 47(4): 1-12

Kroeber A L, Kluckhohn C & Untereiner W (1952) *Culture: a critical review of concepts and definitions*. Vintage Books, New York

Kruschwitz R & Roberts R (1987) *The virtues: contemporary essays on moral character*. Wadsworth, Belmont, CA

Kruse C S, Frederick B, Jacobson T, Monticone D (2017) Cybersecurity in healthcare: a systematic review of modern threats and trends. *Technology and Health Care*, 25(1): 1-10

Kuczewski M (1996) Reconceiving the family: the process of consent in medical decision making. *Hastings Center Report*, 26(2): 30-7

Kuhse H (1987a) A modern myth. That letting die is not the intentional causation of death: some reflections on the trial and acquittal of Dr Leonard Arthur. *Journal of Applied Philosophy*, 1(1): 21-38

Kuhse H (1987b) *The sanctity-of-life doctrine in medicine: a critique*. Clarendon Press, Oxford

Kuhse H & Singer P (1985) *Should the baby live?* Oxford University Press, Oxford

Kultgen J (1982) The ideological use of professional codes. *Business and Professional Ethics Journal*, 1(3): 53-69

Kumar A, Hessini L & Mitchell E M H (2009) Conceptualising abortion stigma. *Culture, Health and Sexuality*, 11(6): 625-63

Kwak J & Haley W E (2005) Current research findings on end-of-life decision making among racially or ethnically diverse groups. *The Gerontologist*, 45(5): 634-41

La Cerra C, Sorrentino M, Franconi I, Notarnicola I, Petrucci C & Lancia L (2017) Primary care program in prison: a review of the literature. *Journal of Correctional Health Care*, 23(2): 147-56

Ladd J (1967) Loyalty. Entry in D M Borchert (ed) (2006) *The encyclopedia of philosophy*, 2nd edn. Macmillan Reference USA, New York, pp 595-6

LaFollette H (ed) (2014) *Ethics in practice: an anthology*, 4th edn. John Wiley & Sons, Chichester

Lakoff G & Rockridge Institute (2006) *Thinking points: communicating our American values and vision*. Farrar, Straus and Giroux, New York

Lamont L (2003) $727,000 payout for infected wife. *The Age*, 11 June: 1

Lamperd R (2013) Court told how a nursing home went to extraordinary lengths to hide the truth about death of someone's mum. *Herald Sun*. Online. Available: http://www.heraldsun.com.au/news/victoria/court-told-how-a-nursing-home-went-to-extraordinary-lengths-to-hide-the-truth-about-the-death-of-someone8217s-mum/story-fni0fit3-1226733529877

Lane H, Sarkies M, Martin J & Haimes T (2017) Equity in healthcare resource allocation decision making: a systematic review. *Social Science and Medicine*, 175: 11-27

Langford S (2008) An end of abortion? A feminist critique of the 'ectogenetic solution' to abortion. *Women's Studies International Forum*, 31(4): 263-9

Lantos J (2004) Child abuse. In: S G Post (ed) *The encyclopedia of bioethics*, 3rd edn. Macmillan Reference, New York, pp 43-7

Lantos J (2017) Intractable disagreements about futility. *Perspectives in Biology and Medicine*, 60(3): 390-9

Larsen C (2008) The institutional logic of welfare attitudes, *Comparative Political Studies*, 41(2): 145-68

Larsen C A & Dejgaard T E (2013) The institutional logic of images of the poor and welfare recipients: a comparative study of British, Swedish and Danish newspapers. *Journal of European Social Policy*, 23(3): 287-99

Latimer T, Roscamp J & Papanikitas A (2017) Patient-centredness and consumerism in healthcare: an ideological mess. *Journal of the Royal Society of Medicine*, 110(11): 425-7

Laycock D (1990) Formal, substantive, and disaggregated neutrality toward religion. *Depaul Law Review*, 39: 993-1018

Leach M (2003) "Disturbing practices": dehumanizing asylum seekers in the refugee "crisis" in Australia, 2001-2002. *Refuge*, 21(3): 25-33

Leape, L L, Shore M F, Dienstag J L, Mayer R J, Edgman-Levitan S, Meyer G S & Healey G B (2012) Perspective: a culture of respect. Part 2: creating a culture of respect. *Academic Medicine*, 87: 1-6

'Lectric Law Library, version 2011. Online. Available: http://www.lectlaw.com/

Lee A & Wu H (2002) Diagnosis disclosure in cancer patients – when the family says 'no!' *Singapore Medical Journal*, 43(10): 533-8

Lee D (2002) Whistle blowing. *British Journal of Perioperative Nursing*, 12(9): 314-15

Lee J S, Pérez-Stable E J, Gregorich S E, Crawford M H, Green A, Livaudais-Toman J & Karliner L S (2017) Increased access to professional interpreters in the hospital improves informed consent for patients with limited English proficiency. *Journal of General Internal Medicine*, 32: 863-70

Lee J-W (2003) *Foreword to The World Health Report 2003: shaping the future*. WHO, Geneva, pp vii-viii

Lee M-J, Heland M, Romios P, Naksook C, & Silvester W (2003) Respecting patient choices: advance care planning to improve patient care at Austin Health. *Health Issues*, 77: 23-6

Lee S Y & Kwon Y (2018) Twitter as a place where people meet to make suicide pacts. *Public Health*, 159: 21-6

Lee V K & Harris L T (2013) Dehumanized perception: psychological and neural mechanisms underlying everyday dehumanization. In: P G Bain, J Vaes & J P Leyens (eds) (2013) *Advances in understanding humanness and dehumanization*. Taylor & Francis, Hoboken, NJ, pp 68-85

Leffers J & Butterfield P (2018) Nurses play essential roles in reducing health problems due to climate change. *Nursing Outlook*, 66(2): 210-13

Leftwich R (1993) Care and cure as healing processes in nursing. *Nursing Forum*, 28(3): 13-17

Legal Dictionary 2016 *Moral turpitude*. Online. Available: http://legal-dictionary.thefreedictionary.com/Moral+Turpitude

Lehrer J (2009) *The decisive moment: how the brain makes up its mind*. The Text Publishing Company, Melbourne

Leininger M M (1990a) *Ethical and moral dimensions of care*. Wayne State University Press, Detroit, MI

Leininger M M (1990b) Culture: the conspicuous missing link to understanding ethical and moral dimensions of human care. In: M Leininger (ed) *Ethical and moral dimensions of care*. Wayne State University Press, Detroit, MI, pp 49-66

Leininger M M (ed) (1991) *Culture care diversity and universality: a theory of nursing*. National League for Nursing Press, New York

Leininger M M (1994) Quality of life from a transcultural nursing perspective. *Nursing Science Quarterly*, 7(1): 22-8

Lemmens T, Heesoo K & Kurz E (2018) Canada's venture into medical assistance in dying: why its federal law should be c(h)arter compliant and what it may help to avoid. *McGill Journal of Law and Health*, 11(1): 61-148

Lemmon E J (1987) Moral dilemmas. In: C W Gowans (ed) *Moral dilemmas*. Oxford University Press, New York, pp 101-14

Leo J (1983) Sharing the pain of abortion. *Time Magazine*, 26 September: 59

Leplège A & Hunt S (1997) The problem of quality of life in medicine. *Journal of the American Medical Association*, 278(1): 47-50

Leslie C (2010) The "psychiatric masquerade": the mental health law exception in New Zealand abortion law. *Feminist Legal Studies*, 18(1): 1-23

Leuter C, La Cerra C, Calisse S, Dosa D, Petrucci C & Lancia L (2017) Ethical difficulties in healthcare: a comparison between physicians and nurses. *Nursing Ethics*, 20(3): 348-58. doi: 10.1177/0969733016687158

Levin P D & Sprung C L (1999) End of life decisions in intensive care. *Intensive Care Medicine*, 25(9): 893-95

Levine C & Zuckerman C (2000) Hands on/hands off: why health care professionals depend on families but keep them at arm's length. *Journal of Law, Medicine and Ethics*, 28: 5–18

Levinson M, Mills A, Barrett J, Srithara G & Gellie A (2018) 'Why didn't you write a not-for-cardiopulmonary resuscitation order?' Unexpected death or failure of process? *Australian Health Review*, 42: 53-8

Levitt P (2014) Challenging the systems approach: why adverse event rates are not improving. *BMJ Quality and Safety*, 23: 1051-2.

Lewin L (1994) Child abuse: ethical and legal concerns. *Journal of Psychosocial Nursing and Mental Health Services* 32(12): 15-18

Lewin Group (2002) *Indicators of cultural competence in health care delivery organizations: an organizational cultural competency assessment profile*. US Department of Health and Human Services Health Resources and Services Administration, Washington, DC

Lewis P (2001) Rights discourse and assisted suicide. *American Journal of Law, Medicine and Ethics*, 27(1): 45-99

Lewis P (2007) The empirical slippery slope from voluntary to non-voluntary euthanasia. *Journal of Law, Medicine and Ethics*, 35(1): 197-210

Leyens J P, Paladino P M, Rodriguez-Torres R, Vaes J, Demoulin S, Rodriguez-Perez A & Gaunt R (2000) The emotional side of prejudice: the attribution of secondary emotions to ingroups and outgroups. *Personality and Social Psychology Review*, 4(2): 186-97

Leyens J P, Demoulin S, Vaes J, Gaunt R & Paladino P M (2007) Infrahumanization: the wall of group differences. *Social Issues and Policy Review*, 1: 139-72

Liamputtong P (2007) *Researching the vulnerable*. Sage Publications, London

Liberman A (2017) Wrongness, responsibility, and conscientious refusals in health care. *Bioethics*, 31(7): 495-504

Liccardi G, Senna G, Russo M, Bonadonna P, Crivellaro M, Dama A, D'Amato M, et al (2004) Evaluation of the nocebo effect during oral challenge in patients with adverse drug reactions. *Journal of Investigational Allergology and Clinical Immunology*, 14(2): 104-7

Lichtenberg J (1996) What are codes of ethics for? In: M Coady & S Bloch (eds) *Codes of ethics and the professions*. Melbourne University Press, Melbourne, pp 13-27

Liddell G (1994) Pugmire and the dilemma of disclosure. *Otago Bioethics Report*, 3(2): 14-16

Lifton B (1979) *The broken connection*. Simon & Schuster, New York

Light E M, Robertson M D, Kerridge I H, Boyce P, Carney T, Rosen A, Cleary M, et al (2016) Reconceptualizing involuntary outpatient psychiatric treatment: from "capacity" to "capability". *Philosophy, Psychiatry and Psychology*, 23(1): 33-45

Lim C R, Zhang M W B, Hussain S F & Ho R C M (2017) The consequences of whistle-blowing: an integrative review. *Journal of Patient Safety*, Jun 30. doi: 10.1097/PTS.0000000000000396 [Epub ahead of print]

Lines L E, Hutton A E & Grant J (2017) Integrative review: nurses' roles and experiences in keeping children safe. *Journal of Advanced Nursing*, 73(2): 302-22

Link B & Phelan J (2006) Conceptualizing stigma. *Annual Review of Sociology*, 27: 363-85

Link B, Yang L, Phelan J & Collins P (2004) Measuring mental illness stigma. *Schizophrenia Bulletin*, 30(3): 511-41

Lipscomb M (2016) Editorial: Dishonesty and deception in nursing. *Nursing Philosophy*, 17(3): 157-62

Lithwick M, Beaulieu M, Gravel S & Straka SM (2000) The mistreatment of older adults: perpetrator–victim relationships and interventions. *Journal of Elder Abuse and Neglect*, 11(4): 95-112

Little M (1996) Why a feminist approach to bioethics? *Kennedy Institute of Ethics Journal*, 6(1): 1-18

Little M (2001) On knowing the 'why': particularism and moral theory. *Hastings Center Report*, 31(4): 32-40

Little M O (2014) The moral permissibility of abortion. In: H LaFollette (ed) *Ethics in practice: an anthology*, 4th edn. John Wiley & Sons, Chichester, pp 151-9

Lo B (2000) *Resolving ethical dilemmas: a guide for clinicians,* 2nd edn. Lippincott Williams & Wilkins, Philadelphia, Chapter 9: Futile interventions.

Locatelli C, Piselli P, Cicerchia M & Repetto L (2013) Physicians' age and sex influence breaking bad news to elderly cancer patients. Beliefs and practices of 50 Italian oncologists: the G.I.O Ger study, *Psycho-Oncology*, 22: 1112-19

Loewy E H (1991) Involving patients in Do Not Resuscitate (DNR) decisions: an old issue raising its ugly head. *Journal of Medical Ethics*, 17(1): 156-60

Loewy E H & Carlson R (1993) Futility and its wider implications: a concept in need for further examination. *Archives of Internal Medicine*, 153(4): 429-31

Long A, Long A & Smyth A (1998) Suicide: a statement of suffering. *Nursing Ethics*, 5(1): 3-15

Louw E (2010) *The media and political process*, Sage Publications, London

Lowe P & Hayes G (2018) Anti-abortion clinic activism, civil inattention and the problem of gendered harassment. *Sociology* (first published 23 March 2018). https://doi.org/10.1177/003803851876207 [Epub ahead of print]

Lowther W (1988) Father seeks right to stop wife's abortion. *The Age*, 26 August: 8

Lynn J & Teno J (1995) Advance directives. In: W T Reich (ed) *Encyclopedia of bioethics*, revised edn. Simon & Schuster Macmillan, New York/Simon & Schuster and Prentice Hall International, pp 572-7

McCarthy M M, Taylor P, Norman R E, Pezzullo L, Tucci J & Goddard C (2016) The lifetime economic and social costs of child maltreatment in Australia. *Children and Youth Services Review*, 71: 217-26

McCarthy J, O'Donnell K, Campbell L & Dooley D (2018) Ethical arguments for access to abortion services in the Republic of Ireland: recent developments in the public discourse. *Journal of Medical Ethics*, 44(8): 513-17. doi: 10.1136/medethics-2017-104728

McCloskey H J (1980) Privacy and the right to privacy. *Philosophy*, 55: 17-38

MacCormick FM, Emmett C, Paes P & Hughes J C (2018) Resuscitation decisions at the end of life: medical views and the juridification of practice. *Journal of Medical Ethics*, 44(6): 376-83. doi: 10.1136/medethics-2017-104608

McCulley M G (1988) The male abortion: the putative father's right to terminate his interests in and obligations to the unborn child. *Journal of Law and Policy*, 7(1): 1-55

McCullough L (1995) Preventive ethics, professional integrity, and boundary setting: the clinical management of moral uncertainty. *Journal of Medicine and Philosophy*, 20(1): 1-11

McDonald S (2002) Physical and emotional effects of whistle blowing. *Journal of Psychosocial Nursing and Mental Health Services*, 40(1): 14-27

McDonald-Gibson C (2014) World first as Belgium allows euthanasia for children with terminal illness. *The Independent*, 14 February. Online. Available: https://www.independent.co.uk/life-style/health-and-families/health-news/world-first-as-belgium-allows-euthanasia-for-children-with-terminal-illness-9127078.html

McGee P (2011) Foreword. In: M R Matiti & L Baillie (eds) *Dignity in healthcare: a practical approach for nurses and midwives*. Radcliffe, London/New York, pp ix-xi

McGill J (2014) So what: sexual orientation, gender identity and human rights discourse at the United Nations. *Canadian Journal of Human Rights*, 3: 1

McGuire C (1987) Euthanasia without consent. *The Age*, Letter to the Editor, 19 October: 12

Machan T (1983) Individualism and the problem of political authority. *The Monist*, 66(4), October: 500-16

McHugh C, McGann M, Igou E R & Kinsella E L (2017) Searching for moral dumbfounding: identifying measurable indicators of moral dumbfounding. *Collabora Psychology* 3(1): 23. doi: 10.1525/collabra.79

MacIntyre A (1985) *After virtue: a study in moral theory*, 2nd edn. Duckworth, London

MacIntyre A (1988) *Whose justice? Which rationality?* Duckworth, London

MacIntyre A (2016) *After virtue: a study in moral theory*, 3rd edn. Duckworth, London

McKenna B, McEvedy S, Maguire T, Ryan J & Furness T (2017) Prolonged use of seclusion and mechanical restraint in mental health services: a statewide retrospective cohort study. *International Journal of Mental Health Nursing*, 26(5): 491-9

MacKenzie D (2009) Preparing for the storm ahead. *New Scientist* 2707 (9 May): 4-5

MacKenzie M A, Smith-Howell E, Bomba P A & Meghani S H (2018) Respecting choices and related models of advance care planning: a systematic review of published evidence. *American Journal of Hospice and Palliative Medicine*, 35(6): 897-907

McKibbin W & Sidorenko A (2006) *Global macroeconomic consequences of pandemic influenza*. Lowy Institute for International Policy, Sydney

Mackie J L (1977) *Ethics: inventing right and wrong*. Penguin, Harmondsworth, Middlesex

McKie A & Swinton J (2000) Community, culture and character: the place of the virtues on psychiatric nursing practice. *Journal of Psychiatric and Mental Health Nursing*, 7(1): 35-42

McKillop A, Sheridan N & Rowe D (2013) New light through old windows: nurses, colonists and indigenous survival. *Nursing Inquiry*, 20(3): 265-76

MacKinnon C A (1987) *Feminism unmodified: discourses on life and law*. Harvard University Press, Cambridge, MA

Macklin R (1998) Ethical relativism in a multicultural society. *Kennedy Institute of Ethics Journal*, 8(1): 1-22

Macklin R (2003) Bioethics, vulnerability, and protection. *Bioethics*, 17(5-6): 472-86

Macklin R (2016) Not all cultural traditions deserve respect. *Journal of Medical Ethics*, 42(3): 155

MacLennan N (2002) The Pacific 'non solution'. *Pacific Journalism Review*, 8: 145-54

MacLeod A M (2008) The search for moral neutrality in same sex-marriage decisions. *BYU Journal of Public Law*, 23: 1-58

McMahon M (2006) Re-thinking confidentiality. In: I Freckelton & K Petersen (eds) *Disputes and dilemmas in health law*. Federation Press, Sydney, pp 563-603

McMurray A (2007) *Community health and wellness: a socio-ecological approach*, 3rd edn. Mosby Elsevier, Sydney

MacNair R (1992) Ethical dilemmas of child abuse reporting: implications for mental health counsellors. *Journal of Mental Health Counselling*, 14(2): 127-36

McNaughton D (1988) *Moral vision: an introduction to ethics*. Basil Blackwell, Oxford/New York

MacRae A, Thomson N, Anomie, Burns J, Catto M, Gray C, Levitan L, et al (2013) *Overview of Australian Indigenous health status, 2012*. Australian Indigenous HealthInfoNet, Mount Lawley, WA. Online. Available: http://www.healthinfonet.ecu.edu.au/uploads/docs/overview_of_indigenous_health_2012.pdf

McSherry B (2012) Time to rethink mental health laws for treatment without consent. *The Conversation*, 5 October. Online. Available: http://theconversation.com/time-to-rethink-mental-health-laws-for-treatment-without-consent-9302

McStay R (2003) Terminal sedation: palliative care for intractable pain, post Gluckberg and Quill. *American Journal of Law and Medicine*, 29(1): 45-76

McTavish J R, Kimber M, Devries K, Colombini M, MacGregor J C D, Wathen C N, Agarwal A, et al (2017) Mandated reporters' experiences with reporting child maltreatment: a meta-synthesis of qualitative studies. *BMJ Open*, 7: e013942. doi: 10.1136/bmjopen-2016-013942

McTier L, Botti M & Duke M (2013) Patient participation in medication safety during an acute care admission. *Health Expectations*, Dec 17. doi: 10.1111/hex.12167 [Epub ahead of print]

Madden E E, Ryan S, Aguiniga D M, Killian M & Romanchik B (2018) The relationship between time and birth mother satisfaction with relinquishment. *Families in Society*, 99(2): 170-83

Mademoiselle and the doctor (dir. Janine Hoskings, 2009) Icarus Films, Brooklyn, NY [film]

Magazanik M (1998) Fatal choice: his wife or his faith. *Weekend Australian*, 28-9 November: 1-2

Magelssen M (2017) Professional and conscience-based refusals: the case of the psychiatrist's harmful prescription. *Journal of Medical Ethics*, 43: 841-4

Magnusson R (2002) *Angels of death: exploring the euthanasia underground*. Melbourne University Press, Melbourne

Makkai T & Braithwaite J (1994) Reintegrative shaming and compliance with regulatory standards. *Criminology*, 32(2): 361-85

Makri A (2018) Ireland to vote on a referendum to repeal the Eighth. *The Lancet*, 391(10129): 1466-7

Malia C & Bennett M I (2011) What influences patients' decisions on artificial hydration at the end of life? A Q-methodology study. *Journal of Pain and Symptom Management*, 42(2): 192-201

Malmedal W, Hammervold R & Saveman B-I (2009) To report or not report? Attitudes held by Norwegian nursing home staff on reporting inadequate care carried out by colleagues. *Scandinavian Journal of Public Health*, 37(7): 744-50

Maltoni M, Scarpi E, Rosati M, Derni S, Fabbri L, Martini F, Amadori D, et al (2012) Palliative sedation in end of life care and survival: a systematic review. *Journal of Clinical Oncology*, 30(12): 1378-83

Maltoni M, Scarpi E & Nanni O (2013) Palliative sedation in end of life care. *Current Opinion in Oncology*, 25(4): 360-7

Maltoni M, Scarpi E & Nanni O (2014) Palliative sedation for intolerable suffering. *Current Opinion in Oncology*, 26(4): 389-94

Mann J (1996) Health and human rights: broadening the agenda for health professionals. *Health and Human Rights*, 2(1): 1-5

Mann J (1997) Medicine and public health, ethics and human rights. *Hastings Center Report*, 27(3): 6-13

Mansbach A (2009) Keeping democracy vibrant: whistleblowing as truth-telling in the workplace. *Constellations*, 16(3): 363-76

Mann J, Gostin L, Gruskin S, Brennan T, Lazzarine Z & Fineberg H (1994) Health and human rights. *Health & Human Rights*, 1(1): 7-24

Mann J, Gruskin S, Grodin M & Annas G (1999) *Health and human rights: a reader*. Routledge, New York / London

Manne R (ed) (2005) *Do not disturb: is the media failing Australia?* Black Inc. Agenda, Melbourne

Manning J & Paterson R (2005) 'Prioritization': rationing health care in New Zealand. *Journal of Law, Medicine and Ethics*, 33(4): 681-97

Marcus E L, Clarfield A M & Moses A E (2001) Ethical issues relating to the use of antimicrobial therapy in older adults. *Clinical Infectious Diseases* 33(15 November): 1697-705

Margolis J (1975) Suicide. Reprinted in T L Beauchamp & S Perlin (1978), *Ethical issues in death and dying*. Prentice Hall, Englewood Cliffs, NJ, pp 92–7 (with permission from Charles & Merrill Publishing Company)

Markel H, Lipman H B, Navarro J A, Sloan A, Michalsen J R, Stern A M & Cetron M S (2007) Nonpharmaceutical interventions implemented by US cities during the 1918–1919 influenza pandemic, *Journal of the American Medical Association*, 298(6): 644-55

Marks S (2002) The evolving field of health and human rights: issues and methods. *Journal of Law, Medicine and Ethics*, 30(4): 739-54

Marquis D (2014) An argument that abortion is wrong. In: H LaFollette (ed) *Ethics in practice: an anthology*, 4th edn. John Wiley & Sons, Chichester, pp 141-50

Marshall P A (1992) Anthropology and bioethics. *Medical Anthropology Quarterly*, 6(1): 49–73

Martin B (2007) Energising dissent. *Dissent*, 24(Spring): 62-4

Martin D, Emanuel L & Singer P (2000) Planning for the end of life. *The Lancet*, 356(9242): 1672-6

Martin G, Martin P, Hankin C, Darzi A & Kinross J (2017). Cybersecurity and healthcare: how safe are we? *British Medical Journal*, 358: j3179

Martin L A, Hassinger J A, Debbink M & Harris L H (2017) Dangertalk: voices of abortion providers. *Social Science and Medicine*, 184: 75-83

Martin L A, Hassinger J A, Seewald M & Harris L H (2018) Evaluation of abortion stigma in the workforce: development of the revised abortion providers stigma scale. *Women's Health Issues*, 28(1): 59-67

Martin R (2017) Conceptions of rights in recent Anglo-American philosophy. In: M Sellers & S Kirste (eds) *Encyclopedia of the philosophy of law and social philosophy*. Springer, Dordrecht

Martin R & Nickel J W (1980) Recent work on the concepts of rights. *American Philosophical Quarterly*, 17(3): 165-80

Martin R D, Cohen M A, Weiss Roberts L, Batista S M, Hicks D & Bourgeois J (2007) DNR Versus DNT: clinical implications of a conceptual ambiguity: a case analysis. *Psychosomatics*, 48(1): 10-15

Martin T (2001) *Interests in abortion: a new perspective on foetal potential and the abortion debate*. Routledge, Taylor & Francis, London

Martinez-Martin P (2017) What is quality of life and how do we measure it? Relevance to Parkinson's disease and movement disorders. *Movement Disorders*, 32(3): 382-92

Maruca A T & Shelton D (2016) Correctional nursing interventions for incarcerated persons with mental disorders: an integrative review. *Issues in Mental Health Nursing*, 37(5): 285-92

Marx D (2001) *Patient safety and the "just culture": a primer for health care executives*. David Marx Consulting/Trustees of Columbia University in the City of New York. Online. Available: https://psnet.ahrq.gov/resources/resource/1582/patient-safety-and-the-just-culture-a-primer-for-health-care-executives

Masferrer A & García-Sánchez E (eds) (2016) *Human dignity of the vulnerable in the age of rights: interdisciplinary perspectives*. Ius Gentium: Comparative Perspectives on Law and Justice series, vol. 55. Springer International, Basel

Mastroianni A C (2009) Slipping through the net: social vulnerability in pandemic planning. *Hasting Center Report*, 39(5): 11-12

Mathews B & Kenny M C (2008) Mandatory reporting legislation in the United States, Canada, and Australia: a cross-jurisdictional review of key features, differences, and issues. *Child Maltreatment*, 13(1): 50-63

Maxwell G & Morris A (2006) Meeting human needs: the potential of restorative justice. In: A Taylor (ed) *Justice as a basic human need*. Nova Science, New York, pp 71-84

May T & Spellecy R (2006) Autonomy, full information, and genetic ignorance in reproductive medicine. *The Monist*, 89(4): 466-81

May W F (1975) Code, covenant, contract or philanthropy. *Hastings Center Report*, 5(6): 29-37

Mayer K H, Bradford J B, Makadon H J, Stall R, Goldhammer H & Landers S (2008) Sexual and gender minority health: what we know and what needs to be done. *American Journal of Public Health*, 98(6): 989-95

Maylea C & Ryan C J (2017) Decision-making capacity and the Victorian Mental Health Tribunal. *International Journal of Mental Health and Capacity Law*, 24: 87-108

Mead M (1955) *Cultural patterns and technical change*. Mentor, New York

Medical Assistance in Dying Act (MAiD) Act, SC 2016, c 3, s 241.1. Online. Available: http://laws-lois.justice.gc.ca/PDF/2016_3.pdf

Medina R A (2018) 1918 influenza virus: 100 years on, are we prepared against the next influenza pandemic? *Nature Reviews. Microbiology*, 16(2): 61-2

Meeberg G A (1993) Quality of life: a concept analysis. *Journal of Advanced Nursing*, 18: 32-8

Meinke S A (1989) *Anencephalic infants as potential organ sources: ethical and legal issues: Scope Notes 12*. Kennedy Institute of Ethics, Georgetown University, Washington, DC

Mendelson D (1997) Quill, Glucksberg and palliative care: does alleviation of pain necessarily hasten death? *Journal of Law and Medicine*, 5 (November): 110-13

Mendelson D & Wolf G (2017) Health privacy and confidentiality. In: I Petersen & K Freckelton (eds) *Tensions and traumas in health law*. Federation Press, Annandale NSW, Chapter 14, pp 266-82

Mental Health (Compulsory Assessment and Treatment) Act 1992 (New Zealand) Online. Available: http://www.legislation.govt.nz/act/public/1992/0046/latest/whole.html

Mental Health Consumers Outcomes Task Force (1991) *Mental health statement of rights and responsibilities*. Australian Government Publishing Service, Canberra

Meredith S (2005) *Policing pregnancy: the law and ethics of obstetric conflict*. Ashgate, Aldershot, Hants

Meter D J & Bauman S (2018) Moral disengagement about cyberbullying and parental monitoring: effects on traditional bullying and victimization via cyberbullying involvement. *Journal of Early Adolescence*, 38(3): 303-26

Meulenbergs T, Verpeet E, Schotsmans P & Gastmans C (2004) Professional codes in a changing nursing context: literature review. *Journal of Advanced Nursing*, 46(3): 331-6

Meyer I H (2003) Prejudice, social stress, and mental health in lesbian, gay and bisexual populations: conceptual issues and research evidence. *Psychological Bulletin*, 129(5): 674-97

Meyers T, Eichhorn D, Guzzetta C, Clark A & Taliaferro E (2004) Family presence during invasive procedures and resuscitation: the experience of family members, nurses, and physicians. *Topics in Emergency Medicine*, 26(1): 61-73

Midgley M (1991a) *Can't we make moral judgements?* Bristol Press, Bristol, Avon

Midgley M (1991b) The origins of ethics. In: P Singer (ed) *A companion to ethics*. Basil Blackwell, Cambridge, MA, pp 3-13

Mill J S (1962) Utilitarianism (reprinted from 1861 edn). In: M Warnock (ed) *Utilitarianism*. Fontana Library/Collins, London, pp 251-342

Miller C (1988) Nurses told, let sick die. *The Herald*, 30 September: 3

Miller C (1989) *NFR system is 'dangerous'*. The Australian Dr Weekly, 20 January

Miller F G (2016) Should a legal option of physician-assisted death include those who are "tired of life"? *Perspectives in Biology and Medicine*, 59(3): 351-63

Miller J (ed) (1992) *On suicide: great writers on the ultimate question*. Chronicle, San Francisco

Miller L A (2013) What you should know before you "blow". *Journal of Perinatal and Neonatal Nursing*, 27(3): 201-2

Miller R & Weinstock R (1987) Conflict of interest between therapist–patient confidentiality and the duty to report sexual abuse of children. *Behavioral Sciences and the Law*, 5(2): 161-74

Miller T, Kanai T, Kebritchi M, Grendell R & Howard T (2015) Hiring nurses re-entering the workforce after chemical dependence. *Journal of Nursing Education and Practice*, 5(11): 65-72

Mills A, Walker A, Levinson M, Hutchinson A M, Stephenson G, Gellie A, Heriot G, et al (2017) Resuscitation orders in acute hospitals: a point prevalence study. *Australasian Journal on Ageing*, 36(1): 32-7

Milo R (1986) Moral deadlock. *Philosophy*, 61: 453-71

Milton C L (2013) The ethics of defining quality of life. *Nursing Science Quarterly*, 26(2): 121-3

Mindframe (2017) *Facts and stats about suicide in Australia (updated 27 September)*. Online. Available: http://www.mindframe-media.info/for-media/reporting-suicide/facts-and-stats

Ministry of Health (2011) *Advance care planning: a guide for the New Zealand health care workforce*. Ministry of Health, Wellington

Ministry of Health (2012) *Rising to the challenge: the mental health and addiction service development plan 2012–2017*. Ministry of Health, Wellington

Ministry of Health (2015) *Ngā mana hauora tūtohu: health status indicators*. Online. Available: https://www.health.govt.nz/our-work/populations/maori-health/tatau-kahukura-maori-health-statistics/nga-mana-hauora-tutohu-health-status-indicators

Ministry of Health (2017) *Suicide facts: 2015 data*. NZ Ministry of Health, Wellington. Online. Available: https://www.health.govt.nz/publication/suicide-facts-2015-data

Ministry of Health (2018) *Life expectancy*. Online. Available: https://www.health.govt.nz/our-work/populations/maori-health/tatau-kahukura-maori-health-statistics/nga-mana-hauora-tutohu-health-status-indicators/life-expectancy

Minow M (1990) *Making all the difference: inclusion, exclusion, and American law*. Cornell University Press, Ithaca/London

Mo H N, Shin D W, Woo J H, Choi J Y, Kang J, Baik Y J, Huh Y R, et al (2012) Is patient autonomy a critical determinant of quality of life in Korea? End-of-life decision making from the perspective of the patient. *Palliative Medicine*, 26(3): 222-31

Mockford G, Fritz Z, George R, Court R, Grove A, Clarke B, Field R, et al (2015) Do not attempt cardiopulmonary resuscitation (DNACPR) orders: a systematic review of the barriers and facilitators of decision-making and implementation. *Resuscitation*, 88: 99-113

Moe C, Kvig E I, Brinchmann B & Brinchmann B S (2012) 'Working behind the scenes': an ethical view of mental health nursing and first-episode psychosis. *Nursing Ethics*, 20(5): 517-27

Mold A (2012) Patients' rights and the national health service in Britain 1960–1980. *American Journal of Public Health*, 102(11): 2030-8

Mollarahimi-Maleki F, Nojomi M & Rostami M-R (2016) Attitude about cancer disclosure and quality of life of patients with cancer. *International Journal of Medical Research and Health Sciences*, 5(7S): 457-66

Molodynski A, Turnpenny L, Rugkåsa J, Burns T, Moussaoui D & The World Association of Social Psychiatry International Working Group on Coercion (2014) Coercion and compulsion in mental healthcare – an international perspective. *Asian Journal of Psychiatry*, 8: 2-6

Moloney B, Cameron I, Bake B, Feeney J, Korner A, Kornhaber R, Cleary M, et al (2018) Implementing a trauma-informed model of care in a community acute mental health team. *Issues in Mental Health Nursing*, 39(7): 547-53. doi: 10.1080/01612840.2018.1437855

Monroe T & Kenaga H (2010) Don't ask don't tell: substance abuse and addiction among nurses. *Journal of Clinical Nursing*, 20(3-4): 504-9

Montello M (2017) Introduction to the special issue. *Perspectives in Biology and Medicine*, 60(3): 293-4

Moody H (1992) *Ethics in an aging society*. John Hopkins University Press, Baltimore, MD

Mooney C (1999) The politics of morality policy: symposium editor's introduction. *Policy Studies Journal*, 27(4): 675-800

Mooney C & Schuldt R (2008) Does morality policy exist? Testing a basic assumption. *Policy Studies Journal*, 36(2): 199-217

Moons P, Budts W & De Geest S (2006) Critique on the conceptualisation of quality of life: A review and evaluation of different conceptual approaches. *International Journal of Nursing Studies*, 43: 891-901

Moons P, Jaarsma T & Norekval T M (2010) Requirements for quality of life reports. *European Journal of Cardiovascular Nursing*, 9(3): 141-3

Moore C (2008) Moral disengagement in processes of organizational corruption. *Journal of Business Ethics*, 80: 129-39

Moore C (2015) Moral disengagement. *Current Opinion in Psychology*, 6: 199-204

Moore C & Gino F (2013) Ethically adrift: how others pull our moral compass from true North, and how we can fix it. *Research in Organizational Behavior*, 33: 53-77

Moore C, Detert J R, Trevino L K, Baker V L & Mayer D M (2012) Why employees do bad things: moral disengagement and unethical organizational behavior. *Personnel Psychology* 65: 1-48

Moore G, Gerdtz M F & Manias E (2007) Homelessness, health status and emergency department use: an integrated review of the literature. *Australasian Emergency Nursing Journal*, 10(4): 178-85

Moore G, Manias E & Gerdtz M F (2011) Complex health service needs for people who are homeless. *Australian Health Review*, 35(4): 480-5

Moore N & Komras H (1993) *Patient-focused healing: integrating caring and curing in health care*. Jossey-Bass, San Francisco, CA

Moratti S (2009) The development of "medical futility": towards a procedural approach based on the role of the medical profession. *Law, Ethics and Medicine*, 35(6): 369-72

Moreno J (1995) *Deciding together: bioethics and moral consensus*. Oxford University Press, New York

Morgan D & Allen R (1998) Indigenous health: a special moral imperative. *Australian and New Zealand Journal of Public Health*, 22(6): 731-2

Morgan D J, Dhruva, S S, Coon E R, Wright S M & Korenstein D (2018) 2017 Update on medical overuse: a systematic review. *JAMA Internal Medicine*, 178(1): 110-15

Morreim E H (2004) Life, quality of: II. Quality of life in healthcare allocation. In: S G Post (ed) *Encyclopedia of bioethics*, vol. 3, 3rd edn. Macmillan Reference USA, New York, pp 1394-7

Morrow L (1991) When one body can save another. *Time Magazine*, 17 June: 46-50

Mortensen R (2002) Lawyers' character, moral insight and ethical blindness. *Queensland Lawyer*, 22: 166-78

Mortier T (2013) Paying the price for their autonomy. *Mercator Net*, 4 October, Online. Available: http://www.mercatornet.com/articles/view/paying_the_price_for_autonomy

Moser P K & Carson T L (2001) *Moral relativism: a reader*. Oxford University Press, New York

Motto J (1983) The right to suicide: a psychiatrist's view. In: S Gorovitz, R Macklin, A L Jameton, J M O'Connor & A Sherwin (eds) *Moral problems in medicine*. Prentice Hall, Englewood Cliffs, NJ, pp 443-6

Moumtzoglou A (2010) Factors impeding nurses from reporting adverse events. *Journal of Nursing Management*, 18(5): 542-7

Mucciaroni G (2011) Are debates about "morality policy" really about morality? Framing opposition to gay and lesbian rights. *Policy Studies Journal*, 39(2): 187-215

Mueller P S, Strand J J, Tilburt J C (2018) Voluntarily stopping and eating and drinking among patients with serious advanced illness – a label in search of a problem? *JAMA Internal Medicine*, 178(5): 726-7

Murphy S & Genuis S J (2013) Freedom of conscience in health care: distinctions and limits. *Bioethical Inquiry*, 10: 347-54

Muskett C (2014) Trauma-informed care in inpatient mental health settings: a review of the literature. *International Journal of Mental Health Nursing*, 23(1): 51-9

Musto L & Rodney P (2018) What we know about moral distress. In: C M Ulrich & C Grady (eds.) *Moral distress in the health professions*. Springer International, Basel, pp 9-20

Mystakidou K, Liossi C, Vlachos L & Padadimitriou J (1996) Disclosure of diagnostic information to cancer patients in Greece. *Journal of Palliative Medicine*, 10(3): 195-200

Nader C (2007) Abortion clinic protesters face $1000 fines. *The Age*, 26 January. Online. Available: http://www.theage.com.au/news/national/abortion-clinic-protesters-face-1000-fines/2007/01/25/1169594432339.html

Nagakawa T, Zollinger C, Chao J, Hill R, Angle S & Pilot M (2017) Anencephalic infants as organ donors after circulatory death. *Transplantation*, 101: S60. doi: 10.1097/01.tp.0000525071.97665.cb

Nagel T (1991) *Mortal questions*, Canto edn. Cambridge University Press, Cambridge, Cambs

Nagra M K, Pillinger T, Prata-Ribeiro H, Khazaal Y & Molodynski A (2016) Community treatment orders – a pause for thought. *Asian Journal of Psychiatry*, 24: 1-4

Narayan A J, Kalstabakken A W, Labella M H, Nerenberg L S, Monn A R & Masten A S (2017). Intergenerational continuity of adverse childhood experiences in homeless families: unpacking exposure to maltreatment versus family dysfunction. *American Journal of Orthopsychiatry*, 87(1): 3-14

National Abortion Federation (NAF) (2017) *2017 Violence and disruption statistics*. Online. Available: https://prochoice.org/wp-content/uploads/2017-NAF-Violence-and-Disruption-Statistics.pdf

National Abortion Federation (NAF) (nd) *Anti-abortion extremists*. Online. Available: https://prochoice.org/education-and-advocacy/violence/anti-abortion-extremists/

National Law Center on Homelessness and Poverty (NLCHP) (2014) *No safe place: the criminalization of homelessness in US cities*. National Law Center on Homelessness and Poverty, Washington, DC. Online. Available: http://www.nlchp.org/reports

Nayda R (2005) Australian nurses and child protection: practices and pitfalls. *Collegian*, 12(1): 25-8

Neal T M S & Crammer R J (2017) Moral disengagement in legal judgments. *Journal of Empirical Legal Studies*, 14(4): 745-61

Near J P & Miceli M P (1985) Organizational dissidence: the case of whistle-blowing. *Journal of Business Ethics*, 4(1): 1-16

Neimeyer R (ed) (2001) *Meaning reconstruction and the experience of loss*. American Psychological Association, Washington, DC

Neisser U (1979) The control of information pickup in selective looking. In: A Pick (ed.) *Perception and its development: a tribute to Eleanor J Gibson*. Erlbaum, Hillsdale, NJ: pp 201-19

Nelkin D K & Rickless S C (2016) The relevance of intention to criminal wrongdoing. *Criminal Law and Philosophy*, 10(4): 745-62

Nelson S (2003) 'Do everything!': encountering 'futility' in medical practice. *Ethics and Medicine*, 19(2): 103-13

Nelson S, Simons L E & Logan D (2018) The incidence of adverse childhood experiences (ACEs) and their association with pain-related and psychosocial impairment in youth with chronic pain. *Clinical Journal of Pain*, 34(5): 402-8

Nelson W, Neily J, Mills P & Weeks W B (2008) Collaboration of ethics and patient safety programs: opportunities to promote quality care. *HEC Forum*, 20(1): 15-27

Nelson W, Gardent P, Shulman E & Splaine M (2010) Preventing ethics conflicts and improving healthcare quality through system redesign. *Quality and Safety in Health Care*, 19: 526-30

Neves M P (2004) Cultural context and consent: an anthropological view. *Medicine, Health Care and Philosophy*, 7(1): 93-8

New Oxford dictionary of English (2001) (ed J Pearsall) Oxford University Press, Oxford.

New Zealand Health and Disability Commissioner (HDC) (2012) *Code of health and disability services consumers' rights*. HDC, Auckland. Online. Available: https://www.hdc.org.nz/your-rights/the-code-and-your-rights/

New Zealand Human Rights Commission (nd). *Enquires and complaints*. Online. Available: https://www.hrc.co.nz/files/3214/2371/4082/22-Mar-2010_12-45-34_Enq_and_Comps_English.html

New Zealand Medical Association (NZMA) (nd) *Advance directives*. NZMA, Wellington. Online https://www.nzma.org.nz/patients-guide/advance-directive

New Zealand Nurses Organisation (NZNO) (2013) *Code of ethics*. NZNO, Wellington. Available: http://www.nzno.org.nz/resources/nzno_publications

New Zealand Nurses Organisation (NZNO) (2016) *Position statement: climate change, 2016*. NZNO, Wellington

Nicaise P, Lorant V & Dubois V (2013) Psychiatric advance directives as a complex and multistage intervention: a realist systematic review. *Health and Social Care in the Community*, 21(1): 1-14

Nicholas P K & Breakey S (2017) Climate change, climate justice, and environmental health: implications for the nursing profession. *Journal of Nursing Scholarship*, 49: 606-16

Nielsen K (1989) *Why be moral?* Prometheus, Buffalo, New York

Nightingale F (1980) *Notes on nursing: what it is, and what it is not*. Gerald Duckworth & Co, London (first published in 1859 by Harrison and Sons)

Noddings N (1984) *Caring: a feminine approach to ethics and moral education*. University of California Press, Berkeley, CA

Noonan J T (1983) From 'an almost absolute value in history'. In: S Gorovitz, R Macklin, A L Jameton, J M O'Connor & A Sherwin (eds) *Moral problems in medicine*, 2nd edn. Prentice Hall, Englewood Cliffs, NJ, pp 303-8

Norrander B & Wilcox C (1999) Public opinion and policymaking in the States: the case of post-Roe abortion policy. *Policy Studies Journal*, 27(4): 702-22

Northoff G (2006) Neuroscience of decision making and informed consent: an investigation in neuroethics. *Journal of Medical Ethics*, 32(2): 70-3

Northridge v Central Sydney Area Health Service [2000] NSWSC 1241 revised – 17/01/2001, 50 NSWLR 549

Nortvedt P (2003) Subjectivity and vulnerability: reflections on the foundation of ethical sensibility, *Nursing Philosophy*, 4(2): 222-30

Norvoll R & Pedersen R (2018) Patients' moral views on coercion in mental healthcare. *Nursing Ethics*, 25(6): 796-807. doi: 10.1177/0969733016674768

Nowell-Smith P H (1954) *Ethics*. Penguin, Harmondsworth, Middlesex

Nozick R (2007) The entitlement theory of justice. In: H LaFollette (ed) *Ethics in practice: an anthology*, 3rd edn. Blackwell, Oxford, pp 578-90

Nuccetelli S (2017) Abortion for fetal defects: two current arguments. *Medicine, Health Care and Philosophy*, 20(3): 447-50

Numminen O, van der Arend A & Leino-Kilpi H (2009) Nurses' codes of ethics in practice and education: a review of the literature. *Scandinavian Journal of Caring Sciences*, 23(2): 380-94

Nunes R, Nunes S B & Rego G (2017) Health care as a universal right. *Journal of Public Health*, 25: 1-9

Nurses and Midwives Board of New South Wales (2010) *Professional conduct: a case book of disciplinary decisions relating to professional conduct matters*, 2nd edn. Nurses and Midwives Board of New South Wales, Sydney

Nursing and Midwifery Board of Australia (NMBA) (2008a) *Code of ethics for nurses in Australia*. NMBA, Canberra

Nursing and Midwifery Board of Australia (NMBA) (2008b) *Code of professional conduct for nurses in Australia*. NMBA, Canberra

Nursing and Midwifery Board of Australia (NMBA) (2010) *A nurse's guide to professional boundaries*. NMBA, Canberra. Online. Available: http://www.nursingmidwiferyboard.gov.au/Codes-Guidelines-Statements/Codes-Guidelines.aspx#codesofethics

Nursing and Midwifery Board of Australia (NMBA) (2014) *Nurse practitioner standards for practice*. NMBA, Canberra. Online. Available: https://www.nursingmidwiferyboard.gov.au/Codes-Guidelines-Statements/Professional-standards.aspx

Nursing and Midwifery Board of Australia (NMBA) (2016) *Registered nurse standards for practice*. NMBA, Canberra. Online. Available: http://www.nursingmidwiferyboard.gov.au/Codes-Guidelines-Statements/Professional-standards/registered-nurse-standards-for-practice.aspx

Nursing and Midwifery Board of Australia (NMBA) (2017) *Code of conduct for nurses*. NMBA, Canberra. Online. Available: http://www.nursingmidwiferyboard.gov.au/Codes-Guidelines-Statements/Professional-standards.aspx

Nursing and Midwifery Board of Australia (NMBA) (2018a) *Code of conduct for nurses*. NMBA, Canberra. Online. Available: https://www.nursingmidwiferyboard.gov.au/Codes-Guidelines-Statements/Professional-standards.aspx

Nursing and Midwifery Board of Australia (NMBA) (2018b) *Code of conduct for midwives*. NMBA, Canberra. Online. Available: https://www.nursingmidwiferyboard.gov.au/Codes-Guidelines-Statements/Professional-standards.aspx

Nursing and Midwifery Board of Australia v Seijbel-Chocmingkwan [2015] QCAT 283. Online. Available: http://www8.austlii.edu.au/cgi-bin/viewdoc/au/cases/qld/QCAT/2015/283.html

Nursing and Midwifery Council (NMC) (2015) *The code: professional standards of practice and behaviour for nurses and midwives*. NMC, London

Nursing Council of Hong Kong (NCHK) (2015) *Code of ethics and professional conduct for nurses in Hong Kong*. NCHK, Hong Kong (China)

Nursing Council of New Zealand (NCNZ) (2011) *Guidelines for cultural safety, the Treaty of Waitangi and Māori health in nursing education and practice*. NCNZ, Wellington. Online. Available: http://www.nursingcouncil.org.nz/Publications/Standards-and-guidelines-for-nurses

Nursing Council of New Zealand (NCNZ) (2012a) *Code of conduct for nurses*. NCNZ, Wellington. Online. Available: http://www.nursingcouncil.org.nz/Nurses/Code-of-Conduct

Nursing Council of New Zealand (NCNZ 2012b) *Competencies for nurse practitioners*. NCNZ, Wellington. Online. Available: http://www.nursingcouncil.org.nz/Publications/Standards-and-guidelines-for-nurses

Nursing Council of New Zealand (NCNZ) (2012c) *Guidelines: professional boundaries*. NCNZ, Wellington. Online. Available: http://www.nursingcouncil.org.nz/Publications/Standards-and-guidelines-for-nurses

Nursing Council of New Zealand (NCNZ) (2012d) *Guidelines: social media and electronic communication*. NCNZ, Wellington. Online. Available: http://www.nursingcouncil.org.nz/Publications/Standards-and-guidelines-for-nurses

Nursing Council of New Zealand (NCNZ) (2016) *Competencies for registered nurses*. NCNZ, Wellington. Online. Available: http://www.nursingcouncil.org.nz/Publications/Standards-and-guidelines-for-nurses

Nursing Council of New Zealand (NCNZ) (2016) *Code of conduct*. Online. Available: http://www.nursingcouncil.org.nz/Nurses/Code-of-Conduct.

Nursing Philosophy (2016) *Special issue: Dishonesty and deception in nursing*, 17(3): 155-224. https://onlinelibrary.wiley.com/toc/1466769x/17/3

Nussbaum M (2006) *Frontiers of justice: disability, nationality, species membership*. Belknap Press of Harvard University Press, Boston, MA

O'Brien J G (2010) A physician's perspective: elder abuse and neglect over 25 years. *Journal of Elder Abuse and Neglect*, 22(1-2): 94-104

O'Connor N, Kotze B & Wright M (2011) Blame and accountability 1: understanding blame and blame pathologies. *Australasian Psychiatry*, 19(2): 113-18

O'Connor R C & Armitage C J (2003) Theory of planned behaviour and parasuicide: an exploratory study. *Current Psychology*, 22: 247-56

Office of the Public Advocate (OPA) & Queensland Law Society (QLS) (2010) *Elder abuse: how well does the law in Queensland cope?* Office of the Public Advocate & Queensland Law Society, Brisbane

Officer A & de la Fuente-Núñez V (2018) A global campaign to combat ageism. *Bulletin of the World Health Organization*, 96: 299-300

Ogilvie A & Potts S (1994) Assisted suicide for depression: the slippery slope in action? *British Medical Journal*, 309(20-7 August): 492-3

Ohnishi K, Hayama Y, Asai A & Kosugi S (2008) The process of whistleblowing in a Japanese psychiatric hospital. *Nursing Ethics*, 15(5): 631-42

Okoroh J S, Uribe E F & Weingart S (2017) Racial and ethnic disparities in patient safety. *Journal of Patient Safety*, 13(3): 153-61

Oliver J (1993) Intergenerational transmission of child abuse: rates, research and clinical implications. *American Journal of Psychiatry*, 150(9): 1315-24

Olshansky B (2007) Placebo and nocebo in cardiovascular health. *Journal of the American College of Cardiology* 49(4): 415-21

Open Congress 2009. Online. Available: https://www.congress.gov/bill/111th-congress/house-bill/448

Opotow S (1990a) Moral exclusion and injustice: an introduction. *Journal of Social Issues*, 46(1): 1-20

Opotow S (1990b) Deterring moral exclusion. *Journal of Social Issues*, 46(1): 173-82

Opotow S (1993) Animals and the scope of justice. *Journal of Social Issues*, 49(1): 71-85

Osterholm M T (2017) Global health security – an unfinished journey. *Emerging Infectious Diseases*, 23(13): S225-S227

Ouliaris C & Kealy-Bateman W (2017) Psychiatric advance directives in Australian mental-health legislation. *Australasian Psychiatry*, 25(6): 574-7

Outka G (1972) *Agape: an ethical analysis*. Yale University Press, New Haven, CT and London

Oxford English dictionary (2014 edn). Oxford University Press, Oxford. Online. Available: http://www.oed.com/

Oxford English dictionary (2018 edn). Oxford University Press, Oxford. Online. Available: http://www.oed.com

PA (1987) Law Lords reject father's plea to stop abortion. *The Age*, 26 February: 8

Page K (2012) The four principles: can they be measured and do they predict ethical decision making? *BMC Medical Ethics*, 13: (10 pp). Online. Available: https://doi.org/10.1186/1472-6939-13-10

Palliative Care Australia (2010) *Health system reform and care at the end of life: a guidance document*. Palliative Care Australia, Canberra

Palmer A (2012) Moral judgments about treating smokers or obese patients have no place in the health service. *The Telegraph*, 10 March. Online. Available http://www.telegraph.co.uk/health/9135184/Moral-judgments-about-treating-smokers-or-obese-patients-have-no-place-in-the-health-service.html

Papps E (2005) Cultural safety: daring to be different. In: D Wepa (ed) *Cultural safety in Aotearoa New Zealand*. Pearson Education New Zealand, Auckland, pp 20-8

Papps E & Ramsden I (1996) Cultural safety in Nursing: the New Zealand experience. *International Journal for Quality in Health Care*, 8(5): 491-7

Paras M L, Murad M H, Chen L P, Goranson E N, Sattler A L, Colbenson K M, Elamin M B, et al (2009) Sexual abuse and lifetime diagnosis of somatic disorders: a systematic review and meta-analysis. *Journal of the American Medical Association*, 302(5): 550-61

Paris J J, Ahluwalia J, Cummings B M, Moreland M P & Wilkinson D J (2017) The Charlie Gard case: British and American approaches to court resolution of disputes over medical decisions. *Journal of Perinatology*, 37: 1268-71

Pariser L (2011) *The filter bubble: what the internet is hiding from you*. Penguin, London

Park H & Lewis D (2018) The negative health effects of external whistleblowing: A study of some key factors. *Social Science Journal*, 55(4): 387-95. doi: 10.1016/j.soscij.2018.04.002

Parker R (1974) A definition of privacy. *Rutgers Law Review*, 27(2): 275-96

Parker R (1990) Nurses stories: the search for a relational ethic of care. *Advances in Nursing Science*, 13(1): 31-40

Parliamentary Library & Information Services, Department of Parliamentary Services (2017). *Voluntary Assisted Dying Bill 2017*. Parliament of Victoria, Melbourne. Online. Available: https://www.parliament.vic.gov.au/publications/research-papers/download/36-research-papers/13834-voluntary-assisted-dying-bill-2017

Parse R R (1994) Quality of life: sciencing and living the art of human becoming. *Nursing Science Quarterly*, 7(1): 16-21

Parse R R (2007) A human becoming perspective on quality of life. *Nursing Science Quarterly*, 20(1): 217

Patten S B, Wilkes T C R, Williams J V A, Lavorato D H, el-Guebaly N, Schopflocher D, Wild C, et al (2015) Retrospective and prospectively assessed childhood adversity in association with major depression, alcohol consumption and painful conditions. *Epidemiology and Psychiatric Sciences*, 24: 158-65

Pattison S (2001) Are nursing codes or practice ethical? *Nursing Ethics* 8(1): 5-18

Pavlish C, Brown-Saltzman K, Fine A & Jakel P (2013) Making the call: a proactive ethics framework. *HEC Forum*, 25(3): 269-83

Pavlish C, Brown-Saltzman K, Jakel P & Fine A (2014) The nature of ethical conflicts and the meaning of moral community in oncology practice. *Oncology Nursing Forum*, 41(2): 130-40

Paxman A (2017) 'Pretty tense': What it's like to run the gauntlet of anti-abortion protesters. *Sydney Morning Herald*, 6 June. Online. Available; https://www.smh.com.au/lifestyle/pretty-tense-what-its-like-to-run-the-gauntlet-of-antiabortion-protesters-20170605-gwkqbr.html

Pedersen A & Hartley L K (2015) Can we make a difference? Prejudice towards asylum seekers in Australia and the effectiveness of anti-prejudice interventions. *Journal of Pacific Rim Psychology*, 9(1): 1-14

Pellegrino E (1992) Is truth telling to the patient a cultural artefact? *Journal of the American Medical Association*, 268(13): 1734-5

Pellegrino E (1995) Toward a virtue-based normative ethics for the health professions. *Kennedy Institute of Ethics Journal*, 5(3): 253-77

Pena A (2015) Preventing the predictable. *American Journal of Bioethics*, 15(1): 72-4

Pence G (1984) Recent work on virtues. *American Philosophical Quarterly*, 21(4): 281-97

Pence G (1991) Virtue theory. In: P Singer (ed) *A companion to ethics*. Basil Blackwell, Oxford, pp 249–58

People's Health Movement (2000) *People's charter for health*. Online. Available: http://archive.phmovement.org/en/resources/charters/peopleshealth

Pereira-Salgado A, Mader P & Boyd L M (2018) Advance care planning, culture and religion: an environmental scan of Australian-based online resources. *Australian Health Review*, 42: 152-63

Perkins G D, Griffiths F, Slowther A-M, George R, Fritz Z, Satherley P, Williams B, et al (2016) Do-not-attempt-cardiopulmonary-resuscitation decisions: an evidence synthesis. *Health Services and Delivery Research*, 4(11). Online. Available: https://www.ncbi.nlm.nih.gov/books/NBK355498/

Perkins H S (2007) Controlling death: the false promise of advance directives. *Annals of Internal Medicine*, 147(1): 51-7

Perry J, Churchill L & Kirshner H (2005) The Terri Schiavo case: legal, ethical, and medical perspectives. *Annals of Internal Medicine*, 143(10): 744-8

Perry R & Adar Y (2005) Wrongful abortion: a wrong in search of a remedy. *Yale Journal of Health Policy, Law, and Ethics*, 5(2): 507-86

Persily N (2017) The 2016 U.S. election: can democracy survive the internet? *Journal of Democracy*, 28(2): 63-76

Peters K, Luck L, Hutchinson M, Wilkes L, Andrew S & Jackson D (2011) The emotional sequelae of whistleblowing: findings from a qualitative study. *Journal of Clinical Nursing*, 20: 2907-14

Peto T, Srebnik D, Zick E & Russo J (2004) Support needed to create psychiatric advance directives. *Administration and Policy in Mental Health*, 31(5): 409-19

Pham J C, Girard T & Pronovost P J (2013) What to do with healthcare incident reporting systems. *Journal of Public Health Research*, 2(3): e27. doi: 10.4081/jphr.2013.e27

Phillips B, Taylor R, Morrell S, Daniels J, Woodward A & Blakely T (2017) Mortality trends in Australian Aboriginal peoples and New Zealand Māori. *Population Health Metrics*, 15(1): 25. doi: 10.1186/s12963-017-0140-6

Piel J L & Opara R (2018) Does Volk v DeMeerleer conflict with the AMA code of medical ethics on breaching patient confidentiality to protect third parties? *AMA Journal of Ethics*, 20(1): 10-18

Pilcher H (2009) Beware witchdoctors: are you a victim of placebo's evil twin? *New Scientist* 2708: 30-3

Pincoffs E (1971) Quandary ethics. *Mind*, 80(320): 552-71

Pinheiro P S (2006) *World report on violence against children. United Nations Secretary General's study on violence against children*. United Nations, Geneva

Pinto A & Upshur R (2013) *An introduction to global health ethics*, Routledge, Abingdon, Oxon

Piotrowska M (2014) Transferring morality to human-nonhuman chimeras. *American Journal of Bioethics*, 14(2): 4-12

Pitman A L, Osborn D P J, Rantell K & King M B (2016) Bereavement by suicide as a risk factor for suicide attempt: a cross-sectional national UK-wide study of 3432 young bereaved adults. *BMJ Open*, 6(1): e009948. doi: 10.1136/bmjopen-2015-009948

Planned Parenthood of Central Missouri v. Danforth (No. 74-1151), 428 U.S. 52 (1976). Online. Available: https://www.law.cornell.edu/supremecourt/text/428/52

Planès S, Villier C & Mallaret M (2016) The nocebo effect of drugs. *Pharmacology Research and Perspectives*, 4(2): e00208. doi: 10.1002/prp2.208

Plato (1886 edn). *The trial and death of Socrates, being the Euthyphro, Apology, Crito, and Phaedo of Plato* (transl F J Church). Macmillan, London

Plato (1955 edn). *The republic* (transl H D P Lee). Penguin, Harmondsworth, Middlesex

Ploeg J, Fear J, Hutchison B, MacMillan H & Bolan G (2009) A systematic review of interventions for elder abuse. *Journal of Elder Abuse and Neglect*, 21(3): 187-210

Plummer M & Molzahn A E (2009) Quality of life in contemporary nursing theory: a concept analysis. *Nursing Science Quarterly*, 22(2): 134-40

Podnieks E & Thomas C (2017) The consequences of elder abuse. In: X Dong (ed) *Elder abuse*. Springer, Champaign, pp 109-23

Pojman L & Beckwith F (eds) (1994) *The abortion controversy: a reader*. Jones and Bartlett, Boston, MA

Pope T M (2009) Legal briefing: medical futility and assisted suicide. *Journal of Clinical Ethics*, 20(3): 274-86

Pope T M (2012) Review of Wrong medicine: doctors, patients, and futile treatment, 2nd edn by Lawrence J Schneiderman and Nancy S Jecker. *American Journal of Bioethics*, 12(1): 49-51

Porter E (1991) *Women and moral identity*. Allen & Unwin, Sydney, pp 19-44

Porter M E (2010) What is value in health care? *New England Journal of Medicine*, 363(26): 2477-81

Post S (ed) (2004) *Encyclopedia of bioethics*, 3rd edn. Macmillan Reference USA, New York

Potter V (1971) *Bioethics: bridge to the future*. Prentice-Hall, Englewood Cliffs, NJ

Powell T & Foglia M B (2014) The time is now: bioethics and LGBT issues. *Hastings Center Report*, 44 (5): S2-S3

Powers A, Fani N, Pallos A, Stevens J, Ressler K J & Bradley B (2014) Childhood abuse and the experience of pain in adulthood: the mediating effects of PTSD and emotion dysregulation on pain levels and pain-related functional impairment. *Psychosomatics*, 55(5): 491-9

Powers M & Faden R (2006) *Social justice: the moral foundations of public health and health policy*. Oxford University Press, New York

Prado B L, Bugano D, Gomes D, Serrano P L, Junior U, Taranto P, Franca M S, et al (2018) Continuous palliative sedation for patients with advanced cancer at a tertiary care cancer center. *BMC Palliative Care*, 17(1): 13. doi: 10.1186/s12904-017-0264-2

Price M R & Williams T C (2018) When doing wrong feels so right: normalization of deviance. *Journal of Patient Safety*, 14(1): 1-2

Price-Robertson R, Rush P, Wall L & Higgins D (2013) *Rarely an isolated incident: acknowledging the interrelatedness of child maltreatment, victimisation and trauma*. CFCA Paper No. 15 2013. Australian Government & Australian Institute of Family Studies, Child Family Community Australia (CFCA), Canberra

Priebe S, Giacco D & El-Nagib R (2016) *Public health aspects of mental health among migrants and refugees: a review of the evidence on mental health care for refugees, asylum seekers and irregular migrants in the WHO European Region* (Health Evidence Network (HEN) Synthesis Report 47). WHO Regional Office for Europe, Copenhagen. Online. Available: http://www.euro.who.int/__data/assets/pdf_file/0003/317622/HEN-synthesis-report-47.pdf

Prinz J (2012) *Beyond human nature: how culture and experience shape our lives*, Allen Lane, London

Promotion of National Unity and Reconciliation Act, 1995 (available for viewing at: www.doj.gov.za/trc/)

Prowse C (2008) A mockery of human rights. *Herald Sun*, 09 September. Online. Available: http://www.heraldsun.com.au/news/opinion/a-mockery-of-human-rights/story-e6frfifo-1111117428257

Puka B (1989) The liberation of caring: a different voice for Gilligan's 'different voice'. In: M Brabeck (ed) *Who cares? Theory, research, and educational implications of the ethic of care.* Praeger, New York, pp 19-44

Puran N (2005) Ulysses contracts: bound to treatment or free to choose? *The York Scholar*, 2, Spring: 42-51

Purdy I (2004) Vulnerable: a concept analysis. *Nursing Forum*, 39(4): 25-33

Pyszczynski T, Wicklund R, Floresku S, Koch H, Gauch G, Solomon S & Greenberg G J (1996) Whistling in the dark: exaggerated consensus estimates in response to incidental reminders of mortality. *Psychological Science*, 7(6): 332-6

Quammen D (2014) *Ebola: the natural and human history.* Bodley Head/Random House, London

Queensland State Archives Agency (2005) *ID10821, Queensland Public Hospitals Commission of Inquiry.* Queensland Government, State Archives Agency, Runcorn, QLD. Online. Available: http://www.qphci.qld.gov.au/

Quick J D & Fryer B (2018) *The end of epidemics: the looming threat to humanity and how to stop it.* Scribe, Melbourne

Quill T (2005) Terri Schiavo – a tragedy compounded. *New England Journal of Medicine*, 352(16): 1630-3

Quill T E, Arnold R & Back A L (2009) Discussing treatment preferences with patients who want "everything". *Annals of Internal Medicine*, 151(5): 345-49

Quill T E, Ganzini L, Truog R D & Pope T M (2018a) Voluntarily stopping eating and drinking among patients with serious advanced illness – clinical, ethical, and legal aspects. *JAMA Internal Medicine*, 178(1): 123-7

Quill T E, Ganzini L, Truog R D & Pope T M (2018b) Voluntary stopping and eating and drinking among patients with serious advanced illness – a label in search of a problem? – reply. *JAMA Internal Medicine*, 178(5): 727

Quinlan C (2017) Policing women's bodies in an illiberal society: the case of Ireland. *Women and Criminal Justice*, 27(1): 51-72. doi: 10.1080/08974454.2016.1259600

Rachels J (1988) Can ethics provide answers? In: D Rosenthal & F Shehadi (eds) *Applied ethics and ethical theory.* University of Utah Press, Salt Lake City, UT, pp 3-24

Rady M Y & Verheijde J L (2014) Nonconsensual withdrawal of nutrition and hydration in prolonged disorders of consciousness: authoritarianism and trustworthiness in medicine. *Philosophy, Ethics, and Humanities in Medicine* (Open access), 9(1): 16

Raes K (1995) Neutrality of what? Public morality and the ethics of equal respect. *Philosophica*, 2: 133-68

Raijmakers N J H, Fradsham S, van Zuylen L, Mayland C, Ellershaw J E & van der Heide A (2011a) Variation in attitudes towards artificial hydration at the end of life: a systematic literature review. *Current Opinion in Supportive and Palliative Care*, 5(3): 265-72

Raijmakers N J H, van Zuylen L, Constantini M, Caraceni A, Clark J, Lunquist G, Voltz R, et al (2011b) Artificial nutrition and hydration in the last week of life in cancer patients. A systematic literature review of practices and effects. *Annals of Oncology*, 22(7): 1478-86

Räikkä J (1998) Freedom and a right (not) to know. *Bioethics*, 12(1): 49-63

Rajagopal S (2004) Suicide pacts and the internet. *British Medical Journal*, 329(7478): 1298-9

Ramsden I (2002) *Cultural safety and nursing education in Aotearoa and Te Waipounamu.* Unpublished Doctor of Philosophy in Nursing thesis. Victoria University of Wellington, Wellington

Rathod S, Pinninti N, Irfan M, Gorczynski P, Rathod P, Gega L & Naeem F (2017) Mental health service provision in low-and middle-income countries. *Health Service Insights*, 10: 1-7

Raus K (2016) The extension of Belgium's euthanasia law to include competent minors. *Journal of Bioethical Inquiry*, 13(2): 305-15

Raus K, Brown K, Seale C, Rietjens J A C, Janssens R, Bruinsma S, Mortier F, et al (2014) Continuous sedation until death: the everyday moral reasoning of physicians, nurses and family caregivers in the UK, The Netherlands and Belgium. *BMC Medical Ethics*, 15(1): 14

Rawls J (1971) *A theory of justice.* Oxford University Press, Oxford

Rawls J (1993) *Political liberalism.* Columbia University Press, New York

Raz A, Schües C, Wilhelm N & Rehmann-Sutter C (2017) Saving or subordinating life? Popular views in Israel and Germany of donor sibling created through PGD. *Journal of Medical Humanities*, 38(2): 191-207

Raz M (2017) Unintended consequences of expanded mandatory reporting laws. *Pediatrics*, 139(4): e20163511. doi 10.1542/peds.2016-3511

Reason J (2000) Human error: models and management. *British Medical Journal*, 320(7237): 768-70

Rees M & Head M (2001) Killing at Australian abortion clinic raises disturbing questions. *World Socialist Web Site*. Online. Available: http://www.wsws.org/en/articles/2001/08/abor-a20.html

Regan L & Glasier A (2017) The British 1967 Abortion Act – still fit for purpose? *The Lancet*, 390(10106): 1936-7

Reiber D T (2010) The morality of artificial womb technology. *National Catholic Bioethics Quarterly*, 10(3): 515-28

Reich W T (ed) (1978a) *Encyclopedia of bioethics*. Free Press, New York

Reich W T (1978b) Quality of life. In: W T Reich (ed) *Encyclopedia of bioethics*. Free Press, New York, pp 829-39

Reich W T (1994) The word 'bioethics': its birth and the legacies of those who shaped it. *Kennedy Institute of Ethics Journal*, 4(4): 319-35

Reich W T (1995a) *Introduction to the encyclopedia of bioethics*, 2nd edn. Simon & Schuster Macmillan, New York / Simon & Schuster and Prentice Hall International

Reich W T (1995b) The word 'bioethics': the struggle over its earliest meanings. *Kennedy Institute of Ethics Journal*, 5(1): 19-34

Reid B (2002) The nocebo effect: placebo's evil twin. *Washington Post*, April 30: HE01

Reid L (2005) Diminishing returns? Risk and the duty to care on the SARS epidemic. *Bioethics*, 19(4): 348-61

Renner L & Slack K S (2006) Intimate partner violence and child maltreatment: understanding intra- and intergenerational connections. *Child Abuse and Neglect*, 30(6): 599-617

Renvoize J (1993) *Innocence destroyed: a study of child sexual abuse*. Routledge, London / New York

Report of the Royal Commission into Deep Sleep Therapy (1990) Government Printer, Sydney

Reuter's Health (2005) Australian nurse feared for job in 'Dr Death' case. 27 June [no longer available online]

Reuters (1990a) Belgian king steps down over legalising abortion. *The Age*, 5 April: 7

Reuters (1990b) Abortion issue threatens German treaty. *The Age*, 31 August: 7

Reyners M (2004) Health consequences of female genital mutilation. *Reviews in Gynaecological Practice*, 4(4): 242-51

Rhoades H, Rusow J A, Bond D, Lanteigne A, Fulginiti A & Goldbach J T (2018) Homelessness, mental health and suicidality among LGBTQ youth accessing crisis services. *Child Psychiatry and Human Development*, 49(4): 643-51. doi: 10.1007/s10578-018-0780-1

Rhodes R (1998) Genetics links, family ties, and social bonds: rights and responsibilities in the face of genetic knowledge. *Journal of Medicine and Philosophy*, 23(1): 10-30

Ribeiro J D, Huang X, Fox K R & Franklin J C (2018) Depression and hopelessness as risk factors for suicide ideation, attempts and death: meta-analysis of longitudinal studies. *British Journal of Psychiatry*, 212: 279-86

Rice S (1988) *Some doctors make you sick: the scandal of medical incompetence*. Angus & Robertson, Sydney

Richards B & Coggon J (2018) Assisted dying in Australia and limiting court involvement in withdrawal of nutrition and hydration. *Bioethical Inquiry*, 15(1): 15-18

Richardson S (2003) Aotearoa / New Zealand nursing: from eugenics to cultural safety. *Nursing Inquiry*, 11(1): 35-42

Rietjens J A C, Sudore R L, Connolly M, van Delden J J, Drickamer M A, Droger M, van der Helde A, et al (2017) Definition and recommendations for advance care planning: an international consensus supported by the European Association for Palliative Care. *Lancet Oncology*, 18(9): e543-e551

Right to Life New Zealand Inc v Abortion Supervisory Committee [2008] 2 NZLR 825 (HC)

Rights of the Terminally Ill Act 1995 (NT)

Rivers F (1996) *The way of the owl: succeeding with integrity in a conflicted world*. HarperSanFrancisco, New York

Roach M S (1987) *The human act of caring: a blueprint for the health professions*. Canadian Hospital Association, Ottawa, Ontario Roach

Robbins D (1983) Breaking the conspiracy of silence. *Journal of Emergency Nursing*, 9(2): 109

Roberts M (2017) A critical analysis of the failure of nurses to raise concerns about poor patient care. *Nursing Philosophy*, 18(3): e12149. doi:10.1111/nup.12149

Roberts M & Ion R (2014) A critical consideration of systemic moral catastrophe in modern health care systems: a big idea from an Arendtian perspective, *Nurse Education Today*, 34: 673-75

Robertson G (1981) Informed consent to medical treatment. *Law Quarterly Review*, 97(January): 102-26

Robinson B A (2004) Abortion access: violence and harassment at US abortion clinics. *Ontario Consultants on Religious Tolerance*. Online. Available: http://www.religioustolerance.org/abo_viol.htm

Roche M A, Duffield C, Smith J, Kelly D, Cook R, Bichel-Findlay J, Saunders C & Carter D J (2017) Nurse-led primary health care for homeless men: a multimethods descriptive study. *International Nursing Review*, 65(3): 392-9.

Rodrigues P, Crokaert J & Gastmans C (2018) Palliative sedation for existential suffering: a systematic review of argument-based ethics literature. *Journal of Pain and Symptom Management*, 55(6): 1577-90

Rodriguez A (2017) A new rhetoric for a decolonial world. *Postcolonial Studies* 20(2): 176-86

Rodriguez F, Hong C, Chang Y, Oertel L B, Singer D E, Green A R & Lopez L (2013) Limited English proficient patients and time spent in therapeutic range in a warfarin anticoagulation clinic. *Journal of the American Heart Association*, 2: e000170. doi: 10.1161/JAHA.113.000170

Rodriguez-Prat A, Monforte-Royo C & Balaguer A (2018) Ethical challenges for an understanding of suffering: voluntary stopping of eating and drinking and the wish to hasten death in advanced patients. *Frontiers in Pharmacology*, 9: 294. doi: 10.3389/fphar.2018.00294

Rohter L (1993) Anti-abortion protester kills doctor. *The Age*, 12 March: 7

Rosen L (1999) Whistle blowing. *Today's Surgical Nurse*, 21(1): 41-2

Rosenstein A (2017) Disruptive and unprofessional behaviors. In: K Brower & M Riba (eds) *Physician mental health and well-being: integrating psychiatry and primary care*. Springer, Champaign IL, pp 61-86

Ross S D (1972) *Moral decision: an introduction to ethics*. Freeman, Cooper & Co, San Francisco, CA

Ross W D (1930) *The right and the good*. Oxford University Press, London

Roth L H, Meisel A & Lidz C W (1977) Tests of competency to consent to treatment. *American Journal of Psychiatry*, 134(4): 279-84

Rowland R (1992) *Living laboratories: women and reproductive technologies*. Pan Macmillan, Sydney

Royal College of Nursing, Australia (RCNA) (1996) *Position statement on voluntary euthanasia / assisted suicide*. RCNA, Canberra

Royal College of Nursing, Australia (RCNA) (1999) *Position statement: voluntary euthanasia / assisted suicide*. RCNA, Canberra.

Royal College of Physicians (2013) *Prolonged disorders of consciousness*. National clinical guidelines. RCP, London

Royal Dutch Medical Association (KNMG) (2009) *KNMG – guidelines for palliative sedation*. Online. Available: https://palliativedrugs.com/download/091110_KNMG_Guideline_for_Palliative_sedation_2009__2_%5B1%5D.pdf

Royzman E B, Kim K & Leeman R F (2015) The curious tale of Julie and Mark: unraveling the moral dumbfounding effect. *Judgment and Decision Making*, 10(4): 296-313

Ruckert A & Labonté R (2017) Health inequities in the age of austerity: the need for social protection policies. *Social Science and Medicine*, 187: 306-11

Rumbold B E (2015) Review article: the moral right to health: a survey of available conceptions. *Critical Review of International Social and Political Philosophy*, 20(4): 508-28

Runciman W, Hibbert P, Thomson R, Van Der Schaaf T, Sherman H & Lewalle P (2009) Towards an international classification for patient safety: key concepts and terms. *International Journal for Quality in Health Care*, 21(1): 18-26

Ruof M C (2004) Vulnerability, vulnerable populations, and policy. *Kennedy Institute of Ethics Journal*, 14(4): 411-25

Rurup M L, Onwuteaka-Philipsen B D, Pasman H R W, Ribbe M W & van der Wal G (2006) Attitudes of physicians, nurses and relatives towards end-of-life decisions concerning nursing home patients with dementia. *Patient Education and Counseling*, 61(3): 372-80

Rüsch N, Angermeyer M & Corrigan P (2005) Mental illness stigma: concepts, consequences, and initiatives to reduce stigma. *European Psychiatry*, 20(8): 529-39

Sachs-Ericsson N, Cromer K, Hernandez A & Kendall-Tackett K (2009) A review of childhood abuse, health, and pain-related problems: the role of psychiatric disorders and current life stress. *Journal of Trauma & Dissociation*, 10(2): 170-88

Sachs-Ericsson N J, Sheffler J L, Stanley I H, Piazza J R & Preacher K J (2017) When emotional pain becomes physical: adverse childhood experiences, pain, and the role of mood and anxiety disorders. *Journal of Clinical Psychology*, 73: 1403-28

Sade R M (1983) Medical care as a right: a refutation. In: S Gorovitz, R Macklin, A L Jameton, J M O'Connor & A Sherwin (eds) *Moral problems in medicine*, 2nd edn. Prentice Hall, Englewood Cliffs, NJ, pp 532-5

Sadler K (2012) Palliative sedation to alleviate existential suffering at end-of-life: Insight into a controversial practice. *Canadian Oncology Nursing Journal*, 22(3): 195-9

Safranek J (1998) Autonomy and assisted suicide: the execution of freedom. *Hastings Center Report*, 28(4): 32-6

Salloch S, Vollmann J & Schildmann J (2014) Ethics by opinion poll? The functions of attitudes research for normative deliberations in medical ethics. *J Med Ethics*, 40(9): 597-602. doi: 10.1136/medethics-2012-101253.

Samanta J (2015) Children and euthanasia: Belgium's controversial new law. *Diversity and Equality in Health and Care*, 12(1): 4-5

Sandel MJ (2004) Embryo ethics – the moral logic of stem-cell research. *New England Journal of Medicine*, 351(3): 207-9

Sanders A, Schepp M & Baird M (2011) Partial do-not-resuscitate orders: A hazard to patient safety and clinical outcomes? *Critical Care Medicine,* 39(1): 14-18

Sapienza J (2009) 'Baby Killers' graffiti, bomb found at medical clinic. *WA Today*. Online. Available: https://www.watoday.com.au/national/western-australia/baby-killers-graffiti-bomb-found-at-medical-centre-20090107-7bji.html

Sarafis P, Tsounis A, Malliarou M & Lahana E (2014) Disclosing truth: a dilemma between instilling hope and respecting patient autonomy in everyday clinical practice. *Global Journal of Health Science*, 6(2): 128-37

Sartorius N (2014) A hidden human rights emergency, *Lundbeck Magazine: Progress in the Mind* 2014–2015: 6-9

Sass H (1998) Advance directives. In: R Chadwick (ed) *Encyclopedia of applied ethics*, vol. 3. Academic Press, a division of Harcourt Brace & Co, San Diego, CA, pp 41-9

Sasso L, Stievano A, Jurado G & Rocco G (2008) Code of ethics and conduct for European nursing, *Nursing Ethics*, 15(6): 821-36

Sato R, Beppu H, Iba N & Sawada A (2012) The meaning of life prognosis disclosure for Japanese cancer patients: a qualitative study of patients' narratives, *Chronic Illness*, 8(3): 225-36

Saunders M (2003a) Heads roll over horror hospitals. *The Australian*, 12 December: 1

Saunders M (2003b) No escaping that foul hospital smell. *The Australian*, 12 December: 4

Savage C L, Lindsell C J, Gillespie G L, Dempsey A, Lee R J & Corbin A (2006) Health care needs of homeless adults at a nurse-managed clinic. *Journal of Community Health Nursing*, 23(4): 225-34

Schildmann E & Schildmann J (2014) Palliative sedation therapy: a systematic literature review and critical appraisal of available guidance on indication and decision making. *Journal of Palliative Medicine*, 17(5): 601-11

Schildmann E, Schildmann J & Kiesewetter I (2015) Medication and monitoring in palliative sedation therapy: a systematic review and quality assessment of published guidelines. *Journal of Pain and Symptom Management*, 49(4): 734-46

Schildmann E, Pörnbacher S, Kalies H & Bausewein C (2018) 'Palliative sedation'? A retrospective cohort study on the use and labelling of continuously administered sedatives on a palliative care unit. *Palliative Medicine*, 32(7): 1189-97. doi: 10.1177/0269216318764095

Schmeidel A N, Daly J M, Rosenbaum M E, Schmuch G A & Jogerst J G (2012) Health care professionals' perspectives on barriers to elder abuse detection and reporting in primary care settings. *Journal of Elder Abuse and Neglect*, 24(1): 17-36

Schneiderman L J (2011) Rationing just medical care. *American Journal of Bioethics*, 11(7): 7-14

Schneiderman L J & Jecker N S (2011) *Wrong medicine: doctors, patients and futile treatment*, 2nd edn. Johns Hopkins University Press, Baltimore and London

Schneiderman L J, Jecker N S & Jonsen A R (2017) The abuse of futility. *Perspectives in Biology and Medicine*, 60(3): 295-313

Schoenly L (nd) *What's in a name – correctional or forensic nursing?* Online. Available: https://correctionalnurse.net/whats-in-a-name-correctional-or-forensic-nursing

Schoenly L & Knox C M (eds) (2013) *Essentials of correctional nursing*, Springer, New York

Schofield M J, Powers J R & Loxton D (2013) Mortality and disability outcomes of self-reported elder abuse: a 12 year prospective Investigation. *Journal of the American Geriatriatrics Society*, 61: 679-85

Schrecker T (2018) Priority setting: right answer to a far too narrow question? Comment on "Global developments in priority setting in health". *International Journal of Health Policy Management*, 7(1): 86-8

Schumpeter P (1988) No-resuscitation rules are unclear: lecturer. *The Age*, 1 October: 21

Schwappach D L B, Massetti C M & Gehring K (2012) Communication barriers in counselling foreign-language patients in public pharmacies: threats to patient safety? *International Journal of Clinical Pharmacy*, 34(5): 765-72

Scoccia D (2010) Physician-assisted suicide, disability, and paternalism. *Social Theory and Practice*, 36(3): 479-98

Scofield G R (1991) Is consent useful when resuscitation isn't? *Hastings Center Report*, 21(6): 28-36

Scott D & O'Neil D (1996) *Beyond child rescue: developing family-centred practice at St Luke's*. Allen & Unwin / Institute of Public Affairs, Sydney

Scott I (2014) Ten clinical-driven strategies for maximising value of Australian health care. *Australian Health Review*, 38(2): 125-33

Scott P A (2014) Lack of care in nursing: is character the missing ingredient? *International Journal of Nursing Studies*, 51: 177-80

Seachris J W (ed) (2013) *Exploring the meaning of life: an anthology and guide*. Wiley-Blackwell, Oxford

Seal M (2007) Patient advocacy and advance care planning in the acute hospital setting. *Australian Journal of Advanced Nursing*, 24(4): 29-36

Seary v State Bar of Texas (1980), 604 SW2d 256 at 258

Seedhouse D (1988) *Ethics: the heart of health care*. John Wiley & Sons, Chichester, Sussex

Seeskin K R (1978) Genuine appeals to conscience. *Journal of Value Inquiry*, 12: 296-300

Seixas B V, Mitton C, Danis M, Williams I, Gold M & Baltussen R (2017) Should priority setting also be concerned about profound socio-economic transformations? A response to recent commentary. *International Journal of Health Policy Management*, 6(12): 733-4

Selgelid M J (2008) Ethics, tuberculosis and globalizations, *Public Health Ethics* 1(1): 10-20

Selgelid M J, Battin M P & Smith C B (eds) (2006) *Ethics and infectious diseases*. Blackwell, Oxford

Sellars M, Fullam R, O'Leary C, Mountjoy R, Mawren D, Weller P, Newton R, et al (2017) Australian psychiatrists' support for psychiatric advance directives: responses to a hypothetical vignette. *Psychiatry, Psychology and Law*, 24(1): 61-73

Sen A (2009) *The idea of justice*, Allen Lane/Penguin, London

Senate Select Committee on a Certain Maritime Incident (2002) *Report on a certain maritime incident*. Commonwealth of Australia, Canberra, p xxi. Online. Available: http://www.aph.gov.au/binaries/senate/committee/maritime_incident_ctte/report/report.pdf

Sepper E (2012) Taking conscience seriously. *Virginia Law Review*, 98(7): 1501-75

Seyedrasooly A, Rahmani A, Zamanzadeh V, Aliashrafi Z, Nikanfar A-R & Jasemi M (2014) Association between perception of prognosis and spiritual well-being among cancer patients. *Journal of Caring Sciences*, 3(1): 47-55

Shadmi E (2013) Quality of hospital to community care transitions: the experience of minority patients. *International Journal of Quality in Health Care*, 25(3): 255-60

Shanley C & Wall S (2004) Promoting patient autonomy and communication through advance care planning: a challenge for nurses in Australia. *Australian Journal of Advanced Nursing*, 21(3): 32-8

Shariff M J (2012) Assisted death and the slippery slope-finding clarity amid advocacy, convergence, and complexity. *Current Oncology*, 19(3): 143-54

Shariff M J & Gingerich M (2018) Endgame: philosophical, clinical and legal distinctions between palliative care and termination of life. *Supreme Court Law Review (2d)*, 85: 225-93

Sharkey A (1994) Killing for life. *The Age* (extra): 3-4

Sharpe E (ed) (2004) *Accountability: patient safety and policy reform*. Georgetown University Press, Washington, DC

Sheehan M & Wells D (1985) The allocation of medical resources. In: C L Buchanan & E W Prior (eds) *Medical care and markets: conflicts between efficiency and justice*. George Allen & Unwin, Sydney, pp 55-69

Shewmon D A, Capron A C, Peacock W J & Schulman B L (1989) The use of anencephalic infants as organ sources: a critique. *Journal of the American Medical Association*, 261(12): 1773-81

Shneidman E (1985) *Definition of suicide*. Wiley, New York

Shneidman E (1993) *Suicide as psychache: a clinical approach to self-destructive behaviour*. Jason Aronson, Northvale, NJ

Shojania K G & Dixon-Woods M (2013) 'Bad apples': time to redefine as a type of systems problem? *BMJ Quality & Safety*, 22: 528-31

Sibbald B (2003) Right to refuse work becomes another SARS issue. *Canadian Medical Association Journal*, 169(2): 141

Sidhu N S, Dunkley M E & Egan M J (2007) 'Not-for-resuscitation' orders in Australian public hospitals: policies, standardised order forms and patient information leaflets. *Medical Journal of Australia*, 186(2): 72-5

Sifris R & Belton S (2017) Australia: abortion and human rights. *Health and Human Rights Journal*, 19(1): 8209-20

Sikka S (2011) *Herder on humanity and cultural difference: enlightened relativism*, Cambridge University Press, Cambridge, Cambs

Silber TJ (1989) Justified paternalism in adolescent health care: cases of anorexia nervosa and substance abuse. *Journal of Adolescent Health Care*, 10(6): 449-53

Silberbauer G (1991) Ethics in small-scale societies. In: P Singer (ed) *A companion to ethics*. Basil Blackwell, Cambridge, MA, pp 14-28

Sim S (2004) *Fundamentalist world: the new dark age of dogma*. Icon, Cambridge, Cambs

Siminoff L (2004) Death and organ procurement: public beliefs and attitudes. *Kennedy Institute of Ethics Journal* 14(3): 217-34

Simon-Davies J (2011) *Background note: suicide in Australia* (29 July) Parliamentary Library. Australian Parliament House, Department of Parliamentary Services, Canberra

Singapore Nurses Board (SNB) (2018a) *Code for nurses and midwives*. SNB, Singapore

Singapore Nurses Board (SNB) (2018b) *Core competencies and generic skills for Registered Nurses*. SNB, Singapore

Singapore Nurses Board (SNB) (2018c) *Core competencies of advanced practice nurses*. SNB, Singapore

Singer P (ed) (1991) *A companion to ethics*. Basil Blackwell, Cambridge, MA

Singer P (1993) *Practical ethics*, 2nd edn. Cambridge University Press, Cambridge, Cambs

Singer P (1994) *Rethinking life & death: the collapse of our traditional ethics*. Text Publishing Company, Melbourne

Singer P, Martin D, Lavery J, Thiel E, Kelner M & Mendelssohn D (1998) Reconceptualizing advance care planning from the patient's perspective. *Archives of Internal Medicine*, 158(8): 879-84

Singer P A, Benatar S R, Bernstein M, Daar A S, Dickens B, Scholl W, MacRae S K, et al (2003) Ethics and SARS: lessons from Toronto. *British Medical Journal*, 327(7427): 1342-4

Skene L (1996) A legal perspective on codes of ethics. In: M Coady & S Bloch (eds) *Codes of ethics and the professions*. Melbourne University Press, Melbourne, pp 111-29

Skinner B F (1973) *Beyond freedom and dignity*. Penguin, Harmondsworth, Middlesex

Slavich G M & Cole S W (2013) The emerging field of human social genomics. *Clinical Psychological Science*, 1(3): 331-48

Slavich G M, Way B M, Eisenberger N I & Taylor S E (2010) Neural sensitivity to social rejection is associated with inflammatory responses to social stress. *Proceedings of the National Academy of Sciences, USA*, 107(33): 14817-22

Smart J J C & Williams B (1973) *Utilitarianism: for and against*. Cambridge University Press, Cambridge, MA

Smedley B, Stith A & Nelson A (eds) (2003) *Unequal treatment: confronting racial and ethnic disparities in health care*. National Academies Press, Washington, DC

Smith C B, Battin M P, Jacobson J A, Francis L P, Botkin J R, Asplund E P, Domek G J, et al (2006) Are there characteristics of infectious diseases that raise special ethical issues. In: M J Selgelid, M-P Battin & C B Smith (eds) *Ethics and infectious diseases*. Blackwell, Oxford, pp 20-34

Smith P (2017) State of Victoria will allow voluntary euthanasia from mid 2019. *British Medical Journal*, 359: j5571

Smith P T (2015) Distinguishing terminal sedation from euthanasia: a philosophical critique of Torbjörn Tannsjö's model. *National Catholic Bioethics Quarterly*, 15(2): 287-301

Snelling PC (2016) The metaethics of nursing codes of ethics and conflict. *Nursing Philosophy*, 17(4): 239-49

Soares M, Barbosa M, Matos R & Mendes S M (2018). Public protest and police violence: Moral disengagement and its role in police repression of public demonstrations in Portugal. *Peace and Conflict: Journal of Peace Psychology*, 24(1): 27-35

Social Development Committee, Parliament of Victoria (1986) *First report on inquiry into options for dying with dignity*, March. Government Printer, Melbourne

Social Development Committee, Parliament of Victoria (1987) *Inquiry into options for dying with dignity: second and final report*, April. Government Printer, Melbourne

Solomon M Z & Jennings B (2017) Bioethics and populism: how should our field respond? *Hastings Center Report*, 47(2): 11-16. doi: 10.1002/hast.684

Solomon R C & Murphy M C (eds) (1990) *What is justice? Classic and contemporary readings*. Oxford University Press, New York

Solomon W D (1978) Rules and principles. In: W T Reich (ed) *Encyclopedia of bioethics*. Free Press, New York, pp 407-12

Sonenshein S (2007) The role of construction, intuition, and justification in responding to ethical issues at work: the sensemaking-intuitive model. *Academy of Management Review*, 32(4): 1022-40

Sorokin P (1957) *Social and cultural dynamics*. Extending Horizons Books–Porter Sargent, Boston, MA

Spellecy R (2003) Reviving Ulysses contracts. *Kennedy Institute of Ethics Journal*, 13(4): 373-92

Spelman E (1997) *Fruits of sorrow: framing our attention to suffering*. Beacon Press, Boston, MA

Spies-Butcher B & Stebbing A (2018) Mobilising alternative futures: generational accounting and the fiscal politics of ageing in Australia. *Ageing and Society*, 1-27. doi: 10.1017/S0144686X18000028

Spillane A, Larkin C, Corcoran P, Matvienko-Sikar K, Riordan F & Arensman E (2017) Physical and psychosomatic health outcomes in people bereaved by suicide compared to people bereaved by other modes of death: a systematic review. *BMC Public Health*, 17(1): 939. doi: 10.1186/s12889-017-4930-3

Spittal M J, Studdert D M, Paterson R & Bismark M M (2016) Outcomes of notifications to health practitioner boards: a retrospective cohort study. *BMC Medicine*, 14: 198. doi: 10.1186/s12916-018-1030-x

Spooner K (2015) The legal and ethical principles of medical confidentiality are far from absolute. *New England Law Review*, 3: 60-7

Springer K, Sheridan J, Kuo D & Carnes M (2007) Long-term physical and mental health consequences of childhood physical abuse: results from a large population-based sample of men and women. *Child Abuse and Neglect*, 31(5): 517-30

Srebnik D (2005) Issues in applying advance directives to psychiatric care in the United States. *Australasian Journal of Ageing*, 24 (suppl 1): S42-5

Srebnik D & Brodoff L (2003) Implementing psychiatric advance directives: service provider issues and answers. *Journal of Behavioural Health Services and Research*, 30(3): 253-8

Sreenivasan G (2007) Health care and equality of opportunity. *Hastings Center Report*, 37(2): 21-31

Sritharan G, Mills A C, Levinson M R & Gellie A L (2016) Doctors' attitudes regarding not for resuscitation orders. *Australian Health Review* 41(6): 680-7. doi.org/10.1071/AH16161

Stafford A & Wood L (2017) Tackling health disparities for people who are homeless? Start with social determinants. *International Journal of Environmental Research and Public Health*, 14(12): e1535. doi: 10.3390/ijerph14121535

Stahl D & Tomlinson T (2017) Is there a right not to know? *Nature Reviews Clinical Oncology*, 14(5): 259-60

Starck P & McGovern J (eds) (1992) *The hidden dimension of illness: human suffering*. National League for Nursing Press, New York

Statistics New Zealand (2015) *New Zealand definition of homelessness: 2015 update*. Statistics New Zealand, Wellington. Online. Available: http://archive.stats.govt.nz/browse_for_stats/people_and_communities/housing/homelessness-defn-update-2015.aspx.

Staub E (1990) Moral exclusion, personal goal theory, and extreme destructiveness. *Journal of Social Issues*, 46(1): 47-64

Staunton P & Chiarella M (2017) *Law for nurses and midwives, 8th edn*. Elsevier, Sydney, NSW.

Steine I M, Winje D, Skogen J C, Krystal J H, Milde A M, Bjorvatn B, Nordhus I H, et al (2017) Posttraumatic symptom profiles among adult survivors of childhood sexual abuse: a longitudinal study. *Child Abuse and Neglect*, 67: 280-93

Steiner N (1998) Methods of hydration in palliative care patients. *Journal of Palliative Care*, 14(2): 6-13

Stengel E (1970) *Suicide and attempted suicide*. Penguin, Harmondsworth, Middx

Stewart C (2006) Advance directives; disputes and dilemmas. In: I Freckelton & K Petersen (eds) *Disputes and dilemmas in health law*. Federation Press, Sydney, pp 38–53

Stier M (2013) Normative preconditions for the assessment of mental disorder. *Frontiers in Psychology*, 4: 611. doi: 10.3389/fpsyg.2013.00611

Stokes F (2017) The emerging role of nurse practitioners in physician-assisted death. *Journal for Nurse Practitioners*, 13(2): 150-5

Stout J (1988) *Ethics after Babel: the languages of morals and their discontents*. Beacon Press, Boston, MA

Stratton-Lake P (ed) (2002) *Ethical intuitionism: re-evaluations*. Oxford University Press, Oxford

Strong R (nd) *Discussion paper: living wills – a response*. Independent Consumer Consultant. Mental Health and Disability Issues. Brunswick, Victoria

Stroud C, Altevogt B M, Nadig L & Hougan M (2010) *Crisis standards of care: summary of a workshop series*. National Academies Press, Washington, DC

Strueber D, Lueck M & Roth G (2007) The violent brain. *Scientific American Mind*, 17(3): 20-7

Stubbs D (1994) Foreword. In: R Heckler, *Waking up alive: the descent to suicide and return to life*. Piatkus, London, pp xi–xiv

Stuckler D, Reeves A, Loopstra R, Karanikolos M & McKee M (2017); Austerity and health: the impact in the UK and Europe; *European Journal of Public Health*, 27(suppl 4): 18-21

Studlar D T & Cagossi A (2018) Institutions and morality policy in western democracies. *Review of Policy Research*, 35(1): 61-88

Su Z, Khoshnood K & Forster S H (2015) Assessing impact of community health nurses on improving primary care use by homeless/ marginally housed persons. *Journal of Community Health Nursing*, 32(3): 161-9

Sudore R L, Lum H D, You J L, Hanson L C, Meier D E, Pantilat S Z, Matlock D D, et al (2017) Defining advance care planning for adults: a consensus definition from a multidisciplinary Delphi panel. *Journal of Pain and Symptom Management*, 53(5): 821-32

Sue D (2001a) Multidimensional facets of cultural competence. *Counseling Psychologist* 29(6): 790-821

Sue D (2001b) The superordinate nature of cultural competence. *Counseling Psychologist* 29(6): 850-7

Sugirtharjah S. (1994) The notion of respect in Asian traditions. *British Journal of Nursing*, 3(14): 739-41

Sullivan D & Tifft L (2005) *Restorative justice: healing foundations of our everyday lives.* Willow Free Press, New York

Sullivan D & Tifft L (2006) *Handbook of restorative justice: a global perspective.* Routledge, London / New York

Sullivan-Marx E & McCauley L (2017) Climate change, global health, and nursing scholarship. *Journal of Nursing Scholarship*, 49: 593-5

Summerfield D (2000) Conflict and health: war and mental health: a brief overview. *British Medical Journal*, 321(7255): 232-5

Sunstein C R (1992) Neutrality in constitutional law (with special reference to pornography, abortion, and surrogacy). *Colum. L. Rev*, 92: 1-52

SUPPORT Principal Investigators (1995) A controlled trial to improve care for seriously ill hospital patients. The Study to Understand Prognosis and Preferences for Outcomes and Risks of Treatment (SUPPORT). *Journal of the American Medical Association*, 274(20): 1591-636

Supported Accommodation Assistance Act 1994 (Commonwealth)

Surbone A (1992) Truth telling to the patient. *Journal of American Medical Association*, 268(13): 1661-2

Suurmond J, Uiters E, de Bruijne M, Stronks K & Essink-Bot M-L (2010) Explaining ethnic disparities in patient safety: a qualitative analysis. *American Journal of Public Health*, 100 (S1): S113-S117

Suurmond J, Uiters E, de Bruijne M C, Stronks K & Essink-Bot M L (2011) Negative health care experiences of immigrant patients: a qualitative study. *BMC Health Services Research*, 11: 10. doi: 10.1186/1472-6963-11-10

Swanson J W, Swartz M S, Elbogen E B, Van Dorn R A, Ferron J, Wagner H R, McCauley B J, et al (2006a) Facilitated psychiatric advance directives: A randomized trial of an intervention to foster advance treatment planning among persons with severe mental illness. *American Journal of Psychiatry*, 163(11): 1943-51

Swanson J, Swartz M, Ferron J, Elbogen E & Van Dorn R (2006b) Psychiatric advanced directives among public mental health consumers in five US cities: prevalence, demand, and correlates. *Journal of the American Academy of Psychiatry and Law*, 34(1): 43-57

Swanson J, Van McCrary S, Swartz M, Elbogen E & Van Dorn R (2006c) Superseding psychiatric advanced directives: ethical and legal considerations. *Journal of the American Academy of Psychiatry and Law*, 34(3): 385-94

Swanson J, Van McCrary S, Swartz M, Van Dorn R & Elbogen E (2007) Overriding psychiatric advance directives: factors associated with psychiatrists' decisions to preempt patients' advance refusal of hospitalization and medication. *Law and Human Behaviour*, 31(1): 77-90

Swanson K (1993) Nursing as informed caring for the wellbeing of others. *IMAGE: Journal of Nursing Scholarship*, 25(4): 352-7

Swanton C (1987) The rationality of ethical intuitionism. *Australasian Journal of Philosophy*, 65(2 – June): 172-81

Swartz L & Drennan G (2000) The cultural construction of healing in the Truth and Reconciliation Commission: implications for mental health practice. *Ethnicity and Health*, 5(3/4): 205-13

Swartz M, Swanson J, Van Dorn R, Elbogen E & Shumway M (2006) Patient preferences for psychiatric advance directives. *International Journal of Forensic Mental Health*, 5(1): 67-81

Swenson D F (1981) The dignity of human life. In: E D Klemke (ed) *The meaning of life.* Oxford University Press, New York, pp 20-30

Sykes N (1990) The last 48 hours of life: caring for patient, family and doctor. *Geriatric Medicine*, 20(9): 22-4

Synnes O & Malterud K (2018) Queer narratives and minority stress: stories from lesbian, gay and bisexual individuals in Norway. *Scandinavian Journal of Public Health*, Mar 1: 1403494818759841. doi: 10.1177/1403494818759841 [Epub ahead of print]

Szasz T (1971) The ethics of suicide. *Antioch Review*, 31(1): 7-17

Szasz T (1982) The psychiatric will. *American Psychologist*, 37: 762-70

Szasz T (1988) The ethics of suicide. In: T Szasz *The theology of medicine.* Syracuse University Press, New York, pp 68-85

Tabuenca A A, Trallero J A, Orna T A G & Bretón M G O (2018) Mortality risk factors after percutaneous gastrostomy: who is a good candidate? *Clinical Nutrition*, pii: S0261-5614(18)30081-5. doi: 10.1016/j.clnu.2018.02.018 [Epub ahead of print]

Tadd G (1998) *Ethics and values for care workers.* Blackwell Science, Oxford

Tadd W, Clarke A, Lloyd L, Leino-Kilpi H, Strandell C, Lemonidou C, Petsios K, et al (2006) The value of nurses' codes: European nurses' views. *Nursing Ethics*, 13(4): 376-93

Tai C-T & Lin C S (2001) Developing a cultural relevant bioethics for Asian people. *Journal of Medical Ethics*, 27(1): 51-4

Tajfel H & Turner J C (1979) An integrative theory of intergroup conflict. In: W G Austin & S Worchel (eds) *The social psychology of intergroup relations*. Brooks/Cole, Monterey, CA, pp 33-47

Taira BR (2018) Improving communication with patients with limited English proficiency. *JAMA Internal Medicine*, 178(5): 605-6. doi: 10.1001/jamainternmed.2018.0373

Takala T (1999) The right to genetic ignorance confirmed. *Bioethics*, 13(3/4): 288-93

Takala T (2001) Genetic ignorance and reasonable paternalism. *Theoretical Medicine*, 22(5): 485-91

Tännsjö T (ed) (2004a) *Terminal sedation: euthanasia in disguise?* Kluwer Academic, Dordrecht

Tännsjö T (2004b) Introduction. In: T Tännsjö (ed) *Terminal sedation: euthanasia in disguise?* Kluwer Academic, Dordrecht, pp xiii-xxiii

Tarasoff v Regents of the University of California 13 Cal. 3d 177, 529 P.2d 553, 118 Cal. Rptr. 129 (1974)

Tarrant C, Leslie M, Bion J & Dixon-Woods M (2017) A qualitative study of speaking out about patient safety concerns in intensive care units. *Social Science and Medicine*, 193: 8-15

Taubenberger J K & Morens D M (2006) 1918 influenza: the mother of all pandemics. *Emerging Infectious Diseases*, 12(1): 15-22

Taylor A (2003) Justice as a basic human need. *New Ideas in Psychology*, 21: 209-19

Taylor A (ed) (2006) *Justice as a basic human need*. Nova Science, New York

Taylor C (1998) Reflections on 'nursing considered as moral practice'. *Kennedy Institute of Ethics Journal*, 8(1): 71-82

Taylor R & Lantos J (1995) The politics of medical futility. *Issues in Law and Medicine*, 11(1): 4-12

Taylor T (2001) Surgery ban on smokers. *Herald Sun*, 8 February: 1, 4

Telegraph Reporter (2014) Superbugs pose graver threat than climate change: scientists. *The Telegraph*, 22 May 7 pm. Online. Available: https://www.telegraph.co.uk/news/health/news/10849686/Superbugs-pose-graver-threat-than-climate-change-scientists.html

ten Have H (2005) End-of-life decision making in the Netherlands. In: R Blank & J Merrick (eds) *End-of-life decision making: a cross-national study*. MIT Press, Cambridge, MA, pp 147-68

Tenbrunsel A E & Messick D M (2004) Ethical fading: The role of self-deception in unethical behavior. *Social Justice Research*, 17: 223-36

Tenbrunsel A E, Diekmann KA, Wade-Benzoni K A & Bazerman M H (2010). The ethical mirage: a temporal explanation as to why we are not as ethical as we think we are. *Research in Organizational Behavior*, 30: 153-73

Ter Meulen R (2011) How 'decent' is a decent minimum of health care? *Journal of Medicine and Philosophy*, 36(6): 612-23

Tervalon M & Murray-Garcia J (1998) Cultural humility versus cultural competence: a critical distinction in defining physician training outcomes in multicultural education. *Journal of Health Care for the Poor and Underserved*, 9(2): 117-25

Tetlock P E (2003) Thinking the unthinkable: sacred values and taboo cognitions. *Trends in Cognitive Sciences*, 7: 320-4

Thailand Nursing and Midwifery Council (TNMC) (nd) *Competencies of registered nurses*. TNMC, Amphur Muang, Nonthaburi. Available: http://www.tnc.or.th/en

The Age (2003) *Editorial: Confidentiality and responsible medicine*. 12 June: 14

The Standard (Warrnambool) (1989) Patient wishes 'need care', 24 February: 5

Thom K, O'Brien A J & Tellez J J (2015) Service user and clinical perspectives of psychiatric advance directives in New Zealand. *International Journal of Mental Health Nursing*, 24(6): 554-60

Thomas D (2004). *Reading doctors' writing: race, politics and power in Indigenous health research 1870–1969*. Aboriginal Studies Press, Canberra

Thomas H (2007) *Sick to death: a manipulative surgeon and a health system in crisis – a disaster waiting to happen*. Allen & Unwin, Sydney

Thomas R L, Zubair M Y, Hayes B & Ashby M A (2014) Goals of care: a clinical framework for limitation of medical treatment. *Medical Journal of Australia*, 201(8): 452-5

Thomasma D (1990) Establishing the moral basis of medicine: Edmund D Pellegrino's philosophy of medicine. *Journal of Medicine and Philosophy*, 15(3): 245-67

Thompson I, Melia K & Boyd K (2006) *Nursing ethics*, 5th edn (first published in 1983). Churchill Livingstone, Edinburgh

Thomson J J (1971) A defense of abortion. *Philosophy and Public Affairs*, 1(1): 47-66

Thomson J J (1975) The right to privacy. *Philosophy and Public Affairs*, 4(4): 295-314

Thornberg R, Wänström L, Pozzoli T & Gini G (2016) Victim prevalence in bullying and its association with teacher–student and student–student relationships and class moral disengagement: a class-level path analysis. *Educational Psychology*, 37(5): 524-36

Thorne L (2010) The association between ethical conflict and adverse outcomes. *Journal of Business Ethics*, 92(2): 269-76

Thorne S (2017) Isn't it time we talked openly about racism? *Nursing Inquiry*, 24(4): 1-2

Thornicroft G, Deb T & Henderson C (2016) Community mental health care worldwide: current status and further developments. *World Psychiatry*, 15(3): 276-86

Timms N (1983) *Social work values: an enquiry*. Routledge & Kegan Paul, London (see in particular Chapter 3, 'Conscience in social work: towards the practice of moral judgment', pp 33-44)

Tingleff E B, Bradley S K, Gildberg F A, Munksgaard G & Hounsgaard L (2017) "Treat me with respect". A systematic review and thematic analysis of psychiatric patients' reported perceptions of the situations associated with the process of coercion. *Journal of Psychiatric and Mental Health Nursing*, 24(9–10): 681-98

Tobias M, Blakely T, Matheson D, Rasanathan K, & Atkinson J (2009) Changing trends in indigenous inequalities in mortality: lessons from New Zealand. *International Journal of Epidemiology*, 38(6): 1711-22

Tobin T W (2011) The relevance of trust for moral justification. *Social Theory and Practice*, 37(4): 599-628

Tobin T W & Jaggar A M (2013) Naturalizing moral justification: rethinking the method of moral epistemology. *Metaphilosophy*, 44(4): 409-37

Tomes N (2006) The patient as a policy factor: a historical case study of the consumer/survivor movement in mental health. *Health Affairs*, 25(3): 720-9

Tomlinson R & Brody H (1990) Futility and the ethics of resuscitation. *Journal of the American Medical Association*, 264(10): 1276-80

Tonelli M R (2005) Waking the dying: must we always attempt to involve critically ill patients in end-of-life decisions? *Chest*, 127(2): 637-42

Toner R (1993) President in move to reverse policy on abortion. *The Age*, 25 January: 6

Tong R (1995) Towards a just, courageous, and honest resolution of the futility debate. *Journal of Medicine and Philosophy*, 20(2): 165-89

Tong R (2006) Competent refusal of nursing care: commentary. *Hastings Center Report* 36(2): 15

Tooley M (1972) Abortion and infanticide. *Philosophy and Public Affairs*, 2(1): 37-65

Tricarico P, Castriotta L, Battistella C, Bellomo F, Cattani G, Grillone L, Degan S, et al (2017) Professional attitudes toward incident reporting: can we measure and compare improvements in patient safety culture? *International Journal for Quality in Health Care*, 29(2): 243-9

Trigg R (2017) Conscientious objection and "effective referral". *Cambridge Quarterly of Healthcare Ethics*, 26(1): 32-43

Tronto J C (1993) *Moral boundaries: a political argument for an ethic of care*. Routledge, New York/London

Tropman E (2009) Renewing moral intuitionism. *Journal of Moral Philosophy*, 6(4): 440-63

Tropman E (2011) Non-inferential moral knowledge. *Acta Analytica* 26: 355-66

Tuffrey-Wijne I, Curfs L, Finlay I & Hollins S (2018) Euthanasia and assisted suicide for people with an intellectual disability and/or autism spectrum disorder: an examination of nine relevant euthanasia cases in the Netherlands (2012–2016). *BMC Medical Ethics*, 19(1): 17. doi: 10.1186/s12910-018-0257-6

Tung J, Barreiroa L B, Johnson Z P, Hansen K D, Michopoulos V, Toufexis D, Michelinia K, et al (2012) Social environment is associated with gene regulatory variation in the rhesus macaque immune system. *Proceedings of the National Academy of Sciences, USA*, 109(7): 6490-5

Turner C (2009) The burden of knowledge. *Georgia Law Review*, 43(2): 297-365

Tutu D (1999) *No future without forgiveness*. Rider/Ebury Press/Random House, London

Tweeddale M (2002) Grasping the nettle – what to do when patients withdraw their consent for treatment: (a clinical perspective on the case of Ms B). *Journal of Medical Ethics*, 28(4): 236-7

Tyler E (1871) *Primitive culture*. John Murray, London

Uberoi D & Galli B (2017) In pursuit of a balance: the regulation of conscience and access to sexual reproductive health care. *Human Rights Review*, 18(3): 283-304

United Nations (UN) (1949) *United Nations Universal Declaration of Human Rights 1948*. UN, New York

United Nations (UN) (1955) *Standard Minimum Rules for the Treatment of Prisoners: Adopted by the First United Nations Congress on the Prevention of Crime and the Treatment of Offenders, held at Geneva in 1955, and approved by the Economic and Social Council by its resolutions 663 C (XXIV) of 31 July 1957 and 2076 (LXII) of 13 May 1977*. UN, New York.

Online. Available: https://www.unodc.org/pdf/criminal_justice/UN_Standard_Minimum_Rules_for_the_Treatment_of_Prisoners.pdf

United Nations (UN) (1966) *International Covenant on Economic, Social and Cultural Rights*. UN, New York. Online. Available: http://www.ohchr.org/EN/ProfessionalInterest/Pages/CESCR.aspx

United Nations (UN) (1978) *The International Bill of Human Rights*. UN, New York

United Nations (UN) (1982) *Principles of medical ethics relevant to the role of health personnel, particularly physicians, in the protection of prisoners and detainees against torture and other cruel, inhuman or degrading treatment or punishment*. UN, New York. Online. Available: https://www.ohchr.org/EN/ProfessionalInterest/Pages/MedicalEthics.aspx

United Nations (UN) (1990) *General Assembly basic principles for the treatment of prisoners*. UN, New York. Online. Available: http://www.un.org/documents/ga/res/45/a45r111.htm

United Nations (UN) (1991) *Principles for the protection of persons with mental illness and for the improvement of mental health care*. Adopted by General Assembly HYPERLINK "http://www.un-documents.net/a46r119.htm" resolution 46/119. UN, New York. Online. Available: http://www.un-documents.net/pppmi.htm

United Nations (UN) (2006a) *Convention of the Rights of Persons with Disabilities*. UN, New York. Online. Available: https://www.un.org/development/desa/disabilities/convention-on-the-rights-of-persons-with-disabilities.html

United Nations (UN) (2006b) Part 1: Treatment of prisoners. In: *Compendium of United Nations standards and norms in crime prevention and criminal justice*. UN, New York, pp 3-50. Online. Available: https://www.unodc.org/pdf/criminal_justice/Compendium_UN_Standards_and_Norms_CP_and_CJ_English.pdf

United Nations (UN) (nd) *United Nations Declaration on the Rights of Indigenous Peoples*. UN, New York. Online. Available: https://www.un.org/development/desa/indigenouspeoples/declaration-on-the-rights-of-indigenous-peoples.html

United Nations Committee on Economic, Social and Cultural Rights (CESCR) (2000) *General comment no. 14: the right to the highest attainable standard of health (article 12 of the International Covenant on Economic, Social and Cultural Rights)*. 11 August 2000, E/C.12/2000/4. UN, New York. Online. Available: http://www.refworld.org/docid/4538838d0.html

United Nations, Department of Economic and Social Affairs (UN DESA), Population Division (2015). *World Population Ageing 2015 (ST/ESA/SER.A/390)*. UN, New York.

United Nations Department of Economic and Social Affairs (UN DESA), Population Division (2017a). *World population prospects: the 2017 revision, key findings and advance tables*. Working Paper No. ESA/P/WP/248, UN, New York. Online. Available: https://esa.un.org/unpd/wpp/Publications/Files/WPP2017_KeyFindings.pdf

United Nations, Department of Economic and Social Affairs (UN DESA), Population Division (2017b). *World population ageing 2017 – highlights (ST/ESA/SER.A/397)*. UN, New York. Online: http://www.un.org/en/development/desa/population/publications/pdf/ageing/WPA2017_Highlights.pdf

United Nations Office of the High Commissioner for Human Rights (UNOHCHR) (2004) *Istanbul protocol: manual on the effective investigation and documentation of torture and other cruel, inhuman or degrading treatment or punishment*. Professional training series no. 8/rev.1. UNHCR, Geneva. Online. Available: https://www.ohchr.org/Documents/Publications/training8Rev1en.pdf

United Nations High Commissioner for Refugees (UNHCR) (2011a) *The 1951 Convention Relating to the Status of Refugees and its 1967 Protocol*. UNHCR, Geneva.

United Nations High Commissioner for Refugees (UNHCR) (2011b) *UNHCR resettlement handbook*, revised edn. UNHCR, Geneva

United Nations High Commissioner for Refugees (UNHCR) (2014a) *Protecting refugees and the role of UNHCR*. UNHCR, Geneva. Online. Available: http://www.unhcr.org/en-au/about-us/background/509a836e9/protecting-refugees-role-unhcr.html

United Nations High Commissioner for Refugees (UNHCR) (2014b) *Global forced displacement tops 50 million for first time since World War II – UHNCR Report*. Press release, 20 June 2014.

United Nations High Commissioner for Refugees (UNHCR) (2014c) *Preventing and reducing statelessness: the 1961 Convention on the Reduction of Statelessness*. UNHCR, Geneva

United Nations High Commissioner for Refugees (UNHCR) (2016) *The global report*. Online. Available: http://www.unhcr.org/en-au/the-global-report.html

United Nations High Commissioner for Refugees (UNHCR) (2017) *Global trends: forced displacement in 2016*. Online. Available: http://www.refworld.org/docid/594aa38e0.html

United Nations Office on Drugs and Crime (UNODC) *The United Nations standard minimum rules for the treatment of prisoners (the Nelson Mandela rules)*. UN, Vienna. Online. Available: http://www.unodc.org/documents/justice-and-prison-reform/GA-RESOLUTION/E_ebook.pdf

United Nations Population Fund (UNFPA) and HelpAge International (2012) *Ageing in the 21st century: a celebration and a challenge*. United Nations Population Fund (UNFPA) and HelpAge International, New York and London. Online. Available: https://www.unfpa.org/publications/ageing-twenty-first-century

United Nations Statistics Division (2018) *Ethnocultural characteristics*. United Nations Statistics Division. Online: https://unstats.un.org/unsd/demographic/sconcerns/popchar/popcharmethods.htm

United States (US) Department of Housing and Urban Development (2017) *The 2017 annual homeless assessment report (AHAR) to Congress: Part 1. Point-in-time estimates of homelessness*. US Department of Housing and Urban Development, Washington, DC. On line. Available: https://www.hudexchange.info/resources/documents/2017-AHAR-Part-1.pdf

United States (US) Health and Human Services Office of Minority Health (2013) *The national standards for culturally and linguistically appropriate services in health and health care (the National CLAS Standards: Fact Sheet)*. US Health and Human Services Office of Minority Health, Washington, DC

Unwin N (1985) Relativism and moral complacency. *Philosophy*, 60: 205-14

Urmson J O (1958) Saints and heroes. In: A I Melden (ed) *Essays in moral philosophy*. University of Washington Press, pp 198-216

Valent P (1993) *Child survivors: adults living with childhood trauma*. William Heinemann Australia, Melbourne

van Delden J J M (2004) The unfeasibility of requests for euthanasia in advance directives. *Journal of Medical Ethics*, 30(5): 447-52

Van Der Weyden M B (2005) The Bundaberg Hospital scandal: the need for reform in Queensland and beyond. *Medical Journal of Australia*, 183(6): 284-5

van Hooft S (2006) *Understanding virtue ethics*. Acumen, Chesham, Bucks

van Hooft S, Athanassoulis N, Kawall J, Oaksley J, Saunders N & van Zyl L (2013) *The handbook of virtue ethics*. Acumen, Durham

Van Keer R-L, Deschepper R, Francke A L, Huyghens L & Bilsen J (2015) Conflicts between healthcare professionals and families of a multi-ethnic patient population during critical care: an ethnographic study. *Critical Care*, 19: 441. doi: 10.1186/s13054-015-1158-4

van Oorschot W & Roosma F (2015) *The social legitimacy of differently targeted benefits*. ImPRovE Working Papers 15/11. Herman Deleeck Centre for Social Policy, University of Antwerp, Antwerp. Online. Available: http://www.centrumvoorsociaalbeleid.be/ImPRovE/Working%20Papers/ImPRovE%20WP%201511_1.pdf

van Oorschot W, Roosma F, Meuleman B, & Reeskens T (eds) (2017) *The social legitimacy of targeted welfare: attitude to welfare deservingness*. Edward Elgar, Northampton, MA

van Rosse F, de Bruijne M, Suurmond J, Essink-Bot M-L & Wagner C (2016) Language barriers and patient safety risks in hospital care. A mixed methods study. *International Journal of Nursing Studies*, 54: 45-53

van Wijngaarden E, Leget C & Goossensen A (2015) Ready to give up on life: the lived experience of elderly people who feel life is completed and no longer worth living. *Social Science and Medicine*, 138: 257-64

Vandekerckhove W & Phillips A (2017) Whistleblowing as a protracted process: a study of UK whistleblowers. *Journeys Journal of Business Ethics*, 1-19. doi: 10.1007/s10551-017-3727-8

Vardey L (1995) *Mother Teresa: a simple path*. Rider, London

Varekamp I (2004) Ulysses directives in The Netherlands: opinions of psychiatrist and clients. *Health Policy*, 70(3): 291-301

Vatican (1980) *Declaration on Euthanasia*. Vatican Polyglot Press, Vatican City

Veatch R M (2017) Why some "futile" care is "appropriate": the implications for conscientious objection to contraceptive services perspectives. *Biology and Medicine*, 60(3): 438-48

Veatch R M & Fry S T (1987) *Case studies in nursing ethics*. J B Lippincott, Philadelphia

Velissaris H (2014) Grieve in peace: suicide stigma still prevails in the community. *Neos Kosmos*, 10 May: 1, 4-5

Vermeulen H (2015) Language barriers and patient safety risks in hospital care: a mixed method study. *Nederlands Tijdschrift voor Evidence Based Practice*, 13(2): 14-15

Victorian Hospital Association Report (1988) 'Stickers recommended', 42, August– September: 3

Vincent C (2001) Introduction. In: C Vincent (ed) *Clinical risk management*, 2nd edn. BMJ Books, London, pp 1–6

Vinten G (1994) Whistle while you work in the health-related professions? *Journal of the Royal Society of Health*, 114(5): 256-62

Voluntary Assisted Dying Bill (2017) State of Victoria. Online. Available: https://www.parliament.vic.gov.au/publications/research-papers/download/36-research-papers/13834-voluntary-assisted-dying-bill-2017

Voss M J (2018) Contesting sexual orientation and gender identity at the UN Human Rights Council. *Human Rights Review*, 19: 1-22

Wachter R & Pronovost P J (2009) Balancing "no blame" with accountability for patient safety, *New England Journal of Medicine*, 361(14): 1401-6

Waitemata District Health Board (2013) *Best practice principles: CALD competency standards and framework*. Waitemata District Health Board, Auckland NZ. Online. Available: http://www.comprehensivecare.co.nz/wp-content/uploads/2013/03/Best-Practice-CALD-Cultural-Competency-Standards-Framework-Jun13.pdf

Waithe M E (ed) (1987) *A history of women philosophers. Volume I: Ancient women philosophers, 600 BC–500AD*. Martinus Nijhoff, Dordrecht

Walker M (1998) *Moral understandings: a feminist study in ethics*. Routledge, New York

Walker R, Cromarty H, Kelly L & St Pierre-Hansen N (2009) Achieving cultural safety in Aboriginal health services: implementation of a cross-cultural safety model in a hospital setting. *Diversity in Health and Care*, 6(1): 11-22

Walsh B & Pirrie M (1996) Nurse faces murder charge. *Herald Sun*, 8 May: 1-2

Walter J J (2004) Life, quality of: quality of life in clinical decisions. In: S G Post (ed) *Encyclopedia of bioethics*, vol. 3, 3rd edn. Macmillan Reference USA, New York, pp 1380-94

Walton M (2004) Creating 'no blame' culture: have we got the balance right? *Quality and Safety in Health Care*, 13(3): 162-7

Wang C, Ryoo J H, Sweare S M, Turner R & Goldberg T S (2017) Longitudinal relationships between bullying and moral disengagement among adolescents. *Journal of Youth and Adolescence*, 46(6): 1304-7

Wang S-B, Wang Y-Y, Ungvari G S, Ng C H, Wu R-R, Wang J & Xiang Y-T (2017) The MacArthur Competence Assessment Tools for assessing decision-making capacity in schizophrenia: a meta-analysis. *Schizophrenia Research*, 183: 56-63

Warnock G J (1967) *Contemporary moral philosophy*. Macmillan Education, Basingstoke, Hants

Warren M A (1973) On the moral and legal status of abortion. *The Monist*, 57(1): 43-61

Warren M A (1977) Do potential people have moral rights? *Canadian Journal of Philosophy*, 7(2): 275-89

Warren M A (1997) On the moral and legal status of abortion. In: H LaFollette (ed) *Ethics in practice: an anthology*. Blackwell, Boston, MA, pp 79-90

Warren M A (2007) On the legal and moral status of abortion. In H LaFollette (ed) *Ethics in practice: an anthology*, 3rd edn. Blackwell Publishing, Melbourne, pp 126-36

Warren M A (2014) On the moral and legal status of abortion (revised). In: H LaFollette (ed) *Ethics in practice: an anthology*, 4th edn. John Wiley & Sons, Chichester, Sussex, pp 132-40

Warrender D (2017) Borderline personality disorder and the ethics of risk management: The action/consequence model. *Nursing Ethics*, 25(7): 918-27. doi: 10.1177/0969733016679467

Warthen v Toms River Community Memorial Hospital 488 A 2d 299 (NJ Super AD 1985)

Warthen v Toms River Community Memorial Hospital, Superior Court of New Jersey, AD, 8/1/85–14/2/85. (1985) In: *Atlantic Reporter*, 2nd Series, NJ, pp 205, 229-34

Waterfield B (2013) Euthanasia twins 'had nothing to live for'. *The Telegraph*, 14 January. Online. Available: http://www.telegraph.co.uk/news/worldnews/europe/belgium/9801251/Euthanasia-twins-had-nothing-to-live-for.html

Waters R A & Buchanan A (2017) An exploration of person-centred concepts in human services: a thematic analysis of the literature. *Health Policy*, 121:1031–9

Watson C L & O'Connor T (2017) Legislating for advocacy: the case of whistleblowing. *Nursing Ethics*, 24(3): 305-12

Watson J (1985) *Nursing: human science and human care*. Appleton-Century-Crofts, Norwalk, CT

Watt H (2017) Double effect reasoning: why we need it. *Ethics and Medicine: An International Journal of Bioethics*, 33(1): 13-19

Watts B, Fitzpatrick S & Johnsen S (2018) Controlling homeless people? Power, interventionism and legitimacy. *Journal of Social Policy*, 47(2): 235-52. doi: 10.1017/S0047279417000289

Watts L L & Buckley R M J (2017) A dual-processing model of moral whistleblowing in organizations. *Journal of Business Ethics*, 146(3): 669-83

Wax A L (2007) Traditionalism, pluralism, and same-sex marriage. *Rutgers Law Review*, 59: 377-412

Wax J W, An A W, Kosier N & Quill T E (2018), Voluntary stopping eating and drinking. *Journal of the American Geriatratrics Society*, 66(3): 441-5

Webb E & Somes T (2017) How can we prevent financial abuse of the elderly? *The Conversation* (3 October). Online: https://theconversation.com/how-can-we-prevent-financial-abuse-of-the-elderly-84991

Webb M, Heisler D, Call S, Chickering S A & Colburn T A (2007) Shame, guilt, symptoms of depression, and reported history of psychological maltreatment. *Child Abuse and Neglect*, 31(11-12): 1143-53

Weenink J W, Westert G P, Schoonhoven L, Wollersheim H & Kool R B (2014) Am I my brother's keeper? A survey of 10 healthcare professions in the Netherlands about experiences with impaired and incompetent colleagues. *British Medical Journal Quality and Safety*, 24(1): 56-64. doi: 10.1136/bmjqs-2014-003068

Wegman, H L & Stetler C (2009). A meta-analytic review of the effects of childhood abuse on medical outcomes in adulthood. *Psychosomatic Medicine*, 71(8): 805-12

Weingart S, Pagovich O, Sands D, Li J, Aronson M, Davis R, Bates D, et al (2005) What can hospitalized patients tell us about adverse events? Learning from patient-reported incidents. *Journal of General Internal Medicine*, 20(9): 830-6

Wekerle C (2013) Resilience in the context of child maltreatment: Connections to the practice of mandatory reporting. *Child Abuse and Neglect*, 37(2-3): 93-101

Welch H G, Schwartz L M & Woloshin S (2011) *Over diagnosis: making people sick in the pursuit of health*, Beacon Press, Boston, MA

Welch-McCaffrey D (1985) Cancer, anxiety, and quality of life. *Cancer Nursing*, 8(3): 151-8

Wells R E & Kaptchuk T J (2012) To tell the truth, the whole truth, may do patients harm: the problem of the nocebo effect for informed consent. *American Journal of Bioethics*, 12(3): 22-9

Wennberg R (1989) *Terminal choices: euthanasia, suicide, and the right to die*. William B Eerdmans, Grand Rapids, MI / Paternoster Press, Exeter, Devon

Wepa D (ed) (2005) *Cultural safety in Aotearoa New Zealand*. Pearson Education, Auckland

Werner R (1979) Abortion: the ontological and moral status of the unborn. In: R A Wasserstrom (ed) *Today's moral problems*, 2nd edn. Macmillan, New York, pp 51-74

Westerlund M (2011) The production of pro-suicide content on the internet: a counter-discourse activity. *New Media & Society*, 14(5): 764-80

Westeson J (2013) Reproductive health information and abortion services: standards developed by the European Court of Human Rights. *International Journal of Gynecology and Obstetrics*, 122(2): 173-6

White D B & Pope T M (2012) The courts, futility, and the ends of medicine. *Journal of the American Medical Association*, 307(2): 151-2

Whitton L (1997) Ageism: paternalism and prejudice. *DePaul Law Review*, 46: 453-82

Whyte L (2018) *Has Trump's White House 'resurrected' Army of God anti-abortion extremists?* Online. Available: https://www.opendemocracy.net/5050/lara-whyte/army-of-god-anti-abortion-terrorists-emboldened-under-trump

Wicclair M R (2000) Conscientious objection in medicine. *Bioethics*, 14: 205-27

Wicclair M R (2011) *Conscientious objection in health care: an ethical analysis*. Cambridge University Press, New York

Wicks W (2015) The consequences of euthanasia legislation for disabled people. *Policy Quarterly*, 11(3): 38-40

Widdershoven G & Berghmans R (2001) Advance directives in psychiatric care: a narrative approach. *Journal of Medical Ethics*, 27(2): 92-7

Wikipedia: The Free Encyclopedia (2018a) *Moral turpitude*. Online. Available: http://en.wikiped.ia.org/wiki/Moral_turpitude (ch 1)

Wikipedia: The Free Encyclopedia (2018b) *Demographics of sexual orientation*. Online. Available: https://en.wikipedia.org/w/index.php?title=Demographics_of_sexual_orientation&oldid=838435707 (ch 6)

Wikipedia: The Free Encyclopedia (2018c) *Sexual minorities*. Online. Available: http://en.wikipedia.org/wiki/ (ch 6)

Wikipedia: The Free Encyclopedia (2018d) *Suicide methods*. Online. Available: https://en.wikipedia.org/wiki/Suicide_methods (ch 8)

Wikipedia: The Free Encyclopedia (2018e) *Anti-abortion violence*. Online. Available: http://www.wikipedia.org/wiki/Anti-abortion_violence

Wikipedia: The Free Encyclopedia (2018f). *Peter Singer*. Online. Available: https://en.wikipedia.org/w/index.php?title=Peter_Singer&oldid=842174644

Wikipedia: The Free Encyclopedia (2018g) *Deep sleep therapy (DST)*. Online. Available: http://en.wikipedia.org/wiki/Deep_sleep_therapy

Wikipedia: The Free Encyclopedia (2018h) *Wisdom*. Online. Available: http://en.wikipedia.org/wiki/Wisdom (ch 11)

Wikipedia: The Free Encyclopedia (2018i) *Cardinal virtues*. Online. Available: http://en.wikipedia.org/wiki/Cardinal_virtues (ch 11)

Wiley M O (2017) Adoption research, practice, and societal trends: ten years of progress. *American Psychologist*, 72(9): 985-95

Wilkes L M, Peters K, Weaver R & Jackson D (2011) Nurses involved in whistleblowing incidents: sequelae for their families. *Collegian*, 18: 101-6

Wilkinson R & Marmot M (eds) (2003) *Social determinants of health: the solid facts*, 2nd edn. World Health Organization Regional Office for Europe, Denmark

Williams A (2002) Issues of consent and data collection in vulnerable populations. *Journal of Neuroscience Nursing*, 34(4): 211-17

Williams A R (2016) Opportunities in reform: bioethics and mental health ethics. *Bioethics*, 30(4): 221-6

Williams B (1973) Ethical consistency. In: C W Gowans (ed) (1987) *Moral dilemmas*. Oxford University Press, New York, pp 115-37

Williams B (1985) *Ethics and the limits of philosophy*. Fontana / Collins, London

Williams C (1993) Children of rape in Bosnia trapped by new policy. *The Age*, 26 July: 8

Williams M (1997) *Cry of pain: understanding suicide and self-harm*. Penguin, London

Williams P (2009) Age discrimination in the delivery of health care services to our elders. *Marquette Law Scholarly Commons, Faculty Publications*, paper 70. Online. Available: http://scholarship.law.marquette.edu/facpub/79/

Williams R (1999) Cultural safety – what does it mean for our work practice? *Australian and New Zealand Journal of Public Health*, 23(2): 213-14

Willmott L & White B (2017) Persistent vegetative state and minimally conscious state: ethical, legal and practical dilemmas. *Journal of Medical Ethics*, 43(7): 425-6

Willmott L, White B, Smith M & Wilkinson D (2014) Withholding and withdrawing life sustaining treatment in a patient's best interests: Australian judicial deliberations. *Medical Journal of Australia*, 201: 545-7

Willmott L, White B, Parker M, Cartwright C & Williams G (2016) Is there a role for law in medical practice when withholding and withdrawing life-sustaining medical treatment? Empirical findings on attitudes of doctors. *Journal of Law and Medicine*, 24: 342-55

Wilson J (2005) To know or not to know? Genetic ignorance, autonomy and paternalism. *Bioethics*, 19(5–6): 492-504

Wilson A, Hutchinson M & Hurley J (2017) Literature review of trauma-informed care: Implications for mental health nurses working in acute inpatient settings in Australia. *International Journal of Mental Health Nursing*, 26: 326-43

Wilson-Stronks A, Lee K K, Cordero C L, Kopp A L & Galvez E (2008) *One size does not fit all: meeting the health care needs of diverse populations*. Joint Commission, Oakbrook Terrace, IL. Online. Available: https://www.jointcommission.org/assets/1/6/HLCOneSizeFinal.pdf

Windt P (1980) The concept of suicide. In: M Pabst Battin & D Mayo (eds) *Suicide: the philosophical issues*. Peter Owen, London, pp 39-47

Winslade W (2004) Confidentiality. In: W T Reich (ed) *Encyclopedia of bioethics*, 3rd edn, vol 1. Macmillan Reference, New York / Simon & Schuster and Prentice Hall International, pp 494-503. Gale Virtual Reference Library. Available: http://link.galegroup.com/apps/doc/CX3402500115

Winslow G R (1984) From loyalty to advocacy: a new metaphor for nursing. *Hastings Center Report*, 14(3), June: 32-40

Winter G F (2017) The future of artificial wombs. *British Journal of Midwifery*, 25(7): 416

Wlodarczyk D & Lazarewicz M (2011) Frequency and burden with ethical conflicts and burnout in nurses. *Nursing Ethics*, 18(6): 847-61

Wolenberg K M, Yoon J D, Rasinski K A & Curlin F A (2013) Religion and United States physicians' opinions and self-predicted practices concerning artificial nutrition and hydration. *Journal of Religious Health*, 52(4): 1051-65

Wolf S (ed) (1996) *Feminism and bioethics: beyond reproduction*. Oxford University Press, New York

Wolf S (2010) *The meaning in life and why it matters*. Princeton University Press, Princeton, NJ

Wolf S M, Wright Clayton E & Lawrenz F (2018) The past, present, and future of informed consent in research and translational medicine. *Journal of Law, Medicine and Ethics*, 46(1): 7-11

Wolff R P, Moore B & Marcuse H (1969) *A critique of pure tolerance*. Beacon Press, Boston, MA

Wong B M & Ginsburg S (2017) Speaking up against unsafe unprofessional behaviours: the difficulty in knowing when and how. *BMJ Quality and Safety*, 26: 859-62

Wong D (1992) Coping with moral conflict and ambiguity. *Ethics*, 102(4): 763-84

Wong J S & Waite L J (2017) Elder mistreatment predicts later physical and psychological health: results from a national longitudinal study. *Journal of Elder Abuse and Neglect*, 29(1): 15-42

Woodall J (2016) A critical examination of the health promoting prison two decades on. *Critical Public Health*, 26(5): 615-21

Woodall J & Dixey R (2015) Advancing the health-promoting prison: a call for global action. *Global Health Promotion*, 24(1): 58-61

Woods S (2004) Terminal sedation: a nursing perspective. In: T Tännsjö (ed) *Terminal sedation: euthanasia in disguise?* Kluwer Academic, Dordrecht, pp 43-56

World Health Assembly (WHA) (2001) Fifty-fourth World Health Assembly Resolutions and decisions: *WHA54.16 International decade of the world's Indigenous people*. Online. Available: http://www.who.int/hhr/WHA54.16.pdf; also available at: http://www.who.int/hhr/activities/indigenous/en/

World Health Organization (WHO) (1978) *Declaration of Alma-Ata*. International Conference on Primary Health Care, Alma-Ata, USSR, 6–12 September 1978. WHO, Geneva. Online. Available: http://www.who.int/publications/almaata_declaration_en.pdf.

World Health Organization (WHO) (1981) *Global strategy for health for all by the year 2000*. "Health for all" series, no 3. WHO, Geneva

World Health Organization (WHO) (1995) *Violence. A public health priority*. WHO, Geneva

World Health Organization (WHO) (1998) *Health 21: health for all in the 21st century*. WHO, Geneva

World Health Organization (WHO) (1999) *Report of the consultation on child abuse prevention*, 29–31 March 1999. WHO, Geneva.

World Health Organization (WHO) (2000) *Social development and ageing: crisis or opportunity?* WHO, Geneva

World Health Organization (WHO) (2001a) *The world health report 2001: mental health: new understanding, new hope*. WHO, Geneva

World Health Organization (WHO) (2001b) *WHA 54.16 International decade of the world's indigenous people*, WHO 54th World Health Assembly, WHA54.16, WHO, Geneva

World Health Organization (WHO) (2002a) *World report on violence and health* (eds E G Krug, L L Dahlberg, J A Mercy, A B Zwi & R Lozano). WHO, Geneva, Chapter 3: Child abuse and neglect by parents and other caregivers, pp 59–86

World Health Organization (WHO) (2002b) *Active ageing, a policy framework*. WHO, Geneva

World Health Organization (WHO) (2002c) *The Toronto Declaration on the Global Prevention of Elder Abuse* (2002). World Health Organization, Geneva. Online. Available: http://www.who.int/ageing/publications/toronto_declaration/en/

World Health Organization (WHO) (2003) *The world health report 2003: shaping the future*. WHO, Geneva.

World Health Organization (WHO) (2005a) *Project to develop the international patient safety event taxonomy. Final report of the WHO World Alliance for Patient Safety Drafting Group*. WHO, Geneva

World Health Organization (WHO) (2005b) *WHO draft guidelines for adverse event reporting and learning systems*. WHO, Geneva

World Health Organization (WHO) (2006a) *Project to develop the international patient safety event classification: final report of the second meeting of the WHO World Alliance for Patient Safety Drafting Group*. WHO, Geneva

World Health Organization (WHO) (2006b) *Preventing child maltreatment: a guide to taking action and generating evidence*. WHO, Geneva.

World Health Organization (WHO) (2007a) *Health of indigenous peoples*. WHO Fact Sheet no 326, October. WHO, Geneva

World Health Organization (WHO) (2007b) *Health in prisons: a WHO guide to the essentials in prison health* (eds L Moller, H Stover, R Jurgens, A Gatherer & H Nikogosian). WHO Regional Office for Europe, Copenhagen

World Health Organization (WHO) (2007c) *Suicide prevention (SUPRE)*. WHO, Geneva

World Health Organization (WHO) (2007d) *Ethical considerations in developing a public health response to pandemic influenza*. WHO, Geneva

World Health Organization (WHO) (2007e) *Pandemic influenza preparedness and response: a WHO guidance document*. WHO, Geneva

World Health Organization (WHO) (2008) *A global response to elder abuse and neglect: building primary health care capacity to deal with the problem worldwide: main report*. WHO, Geneva

World Health Organization (WHO) (2010) *Equity, social determinants and public health programmes* (eds E Blas & A Sivasankara Kurup). WHO, Geneva

World Health Organization (WHO) (2011a) *Mental health atlas 2011*. WHO, Geneva

World Health Organization (WHO) (2011b) *World report on disability: summary*, WHO, Geneva

World Health Organization (WHO) (2012a) *Risks to mental health: an overview of vulnerabilities and risk factors. Background paper by WHO Secretariat for the development of a comprehensive mental health action plan (27 August)*, WHO, Geneva. Online. Available: http://www.who.int/mental_health/mhgap/risks_to_mental_health_EN_27_08_12.pdf

World Health Organization (WHO) (2012b) *WHO quality rights tool kit*. WHO, Geneva. Online. Available: http://www.who.int/mental_health/publications/QualityRights_toolkit/en/

World Health Organization (WHO) (2012c) *Quality rights project–flier*. WHO, Geneva

World Health Organization (WHO) (2012d) *Safe abortion: technical and policy guidance for health systems*, 2nd edn. WHO, Geneva. Online. Available: http://www.who.int/reproductivehealth/publications/unsafe_abortion/9789241548434/en/

World Health Organization (WHO) (2013a) *Mental health action plan 2013–2020*, WHO, Geneva. Online. Available: http://www.who.int/mental_health/publications/action_plan/en/

World Health Organization (WHO) (2013b) *Comprehensive mental health action plan 2013–2020*, WHO 66th World Health Assembly, WHA66/8, WHO, Geneva. Online. Available: http://www.who.int/mental_health/action_plan_2013/en/

World Health Organization (WHO) (2014a) *Prisons and health*. WHO, Geneva. Online. Available: http://www.euro.who.int/en/health-topics/health-determinants/prisons-and-health/publications/2014/prisons-and-health

World Health Organisation (WHO) (2014b) *Preventing suicide: a global imperative*.

World Health Organization (WHO) (2014c) *Minimal information model for patient safety. Working paper WHO/HIS/SDS/2014.7*. WHO Online. Available: http://www.who.int/patientsafety/implementation/information_model/en/

World Health Organisation (WHO) (2014d) *Global status report on violence prevention 2014*. WHO, Geneva.

World Health Organisation (WHO) (2014e) *Antimicrobial resistance: global report on surveillance*, WHO, Geneva

World Health Organisation (WHO) (2014f) *Antimicrobial resistance: fact sheet*. Online. Available: http://www.who.int/mediacentre/factsheets/fs194/en/

World Health Organization (WHO) (2015) *2014 mental health atlas*. WHO, Geneva

World Health Organization (WHO) (2016) *Questions and answers about extensively drug-resistant tuberculosis (XDR-TB)*. Online. Available: http://www.who.int/features/qa/extensively-resistant-tuberculosis/en/

World Health Organization (WHO) (2017a) *Global strategy and action plan on ageing and health*. WHO, Geneva. Licence: CC BY-NC-SA 3.0 IGO. Online. Available: https://www.who.int/ageing/global-strategy/en/

World Health Organization (WHO) (2017b) *Depression and other common mental disorders: global health estimates*. WHO, Geneva. Licence: CC BY-NC-SA 3.0 IGO. Online. Available: http://apps.who.int/iris/bitstream/handle/10665/254610/WHO-MSD-MER-2017.2-eng.pdf?sequence=1

World Health Organization (WHO) (2017c) *Fact sheet: Human rights and health* (29 December 2017). WHO, Geneva. Online. Available: https://www.who.int/news-room/fact-sheets/detail/human-rights-and-health

World Health Organization (WHO) (2018a) *Female genital mutilation: fact sheet no. 241* (updated January 2018). WHO, Geneva. Online. Available: http://www.who.int/mediacentre/factsheets/fs241/en/

World Health Organization (WHO) (2018b) *Ageism*. WHO, Geneva. Online. Available: http://www.who.int/ageing/ageism/en/).

World Health Organization (WHO) (2018c) *Ageing and health, key facts* (5 February). WHO, Geneva. Online. Available: http://www.who.int/en/news-room/fact-sheets/detail/ageing-and-health

World Health Organization (WHO) (2018d) *Tuberculosis (TB)*. WHO, Geneva. Online. Available: http://www.who.int/tb/areas-of-work/drug-resistant-tb/en/

World Health Organization (WHO) (nd) *Definitions*. WHO, Geneva. Online. Available: http://www.who.int/hac/about/definitions/en/

World Health Organization (WHO) and International Society for the Prevention of Child Abuse and Neglect (ISPCAN) (2006) *Preventing child maltreatment: a guide to taking action and generating evidence* (by A Butchart & A Harvey). WHO, Geneva

World Medical Association (WMA) (1983 edn) *WMA international code of medical ethics*. WMA, Ferney-Voltaire

World Medical Association (WMA) (2006 edn) *WMA international code of medical ethics*. WMA, Ferney-Voltaire. Online. Available: https://www.wma.net/policies-post/wma-international-code-of-medical-ethics/

Wuthnow R, Hunter J D, Bergesen A & Kurzweil E (1984) *Cultural analysis*. Routledge & Kegan Paul, London

Wyatt J (2001) Medical paternalism and the fetus. *Journal of Medical Ethics*, 27(suppl 2): ii15-ii20

Wynia M (2007) Ethics and public health emergencies: encouraging responsibility. *American Journal of Bioethics*, 7(4): 1-4

Yakren S (2017) 'Wrongful birth' claims and the paradox of parenting a child with a disability. *Fordham Law Review*, 87. Online. Available: https://ssrn.com/abstract=3146669

Yamin A E & Lander F (2015) Implementing a Circle of Accountability: a proposed framework for judiciaries and other actors in enforcing health-related rights. *Journal of Human Rights*, 14(3): 312-31

Yarling R & McElmurry B (1986) Rethinking the nurse's role in 'Do Not Resuscitate' orders: a clinical policy proposal in nursing ethics. In: P Chinn (ed) *Ethical issues in nursing*. Aspen Systems, Rockville, MD, pp 123-34

Yeager K A & Bauer-Wu S (2013) Cultural humility: essential foundation for clinical researchers. *Applied Nursing Research*, 26(4): 251-6. doi: 10.1016/j.apnr.2013.06.008

Yetzer A M, Pyszczynski T & Greenberg J (2018) A stairway to heaven: a Terror Management Theory perspective on morality. In: K Gray & J Graham (eds.) *Atlas of moral psychology*. Guilford Press, New York, pp 241-51

Yon Y, Mikton C R, Gassoumis D & Wilber K H (2017) Elder abuse prevalence in community settings: a systematic review and meta-analysis. *Lancet Global Health*, 5: e147-e156

Young I M (1990) *Justice and the politics of difference*. Princeton University Press, Princeton, NJ

Young I M (2007) Displacing the distributive paradigm. In: H LaFollette (ed) *Ethics in practice: an anthology*, 3rd edn. Blackwell, Oxford, pp 591-601

Youngner S J (1987) Do-not-resuscitate orders: no longer secret, but still a problem. *Hastings Center Report*, 17(1): 24-33

Youngner S J (2004) Medical futility. In S G Post (ed) *Encyclopedia of bioethics*, vol. 3, 3rd edn. Macmillan Reference USA, New York

Yuko E I (2012) *Is the development of artificial wombs ethically desirable?* PhD thesis, Dublin City University. Online. Available: http://doras.dcu.ie/17451/

Zaal-Schuller I H, Willems D L, de Vos M A, Ewals F V P M & van Goudoever J B (2018) Considering quality of life in end-of-life decisions for severely disabled children. *Research in Developmental Disabilities*, 73: 67-75

Zamanzadeh V, Rahmani A, Valizadeh L, Ferguson C, Hassankhani H, Nikanfar A R & Howard F (2013) The taboo of cancer: the experiences of cancer disclosure by Iranian patients, their family members and physicians, *Psycho-Oncology*, 22: 396-402

Zapolski T C B, Banks D E, Lau K S L & Aalsma M C (2018) Perceived police injustice, moral disengagement, and aggression among juvenile offenders: utilizing the General Strain Theory Model. *Child Psychiatry and Human Development*, 49(2): 290-7

Zelle H, Kemp K & Bonnie R J (2015a) Advance directives in mental health care: evidence, challenges and promise. *World Psychiatry*, 14(3): 278-80

Zelle H, Kemp K & Bonnie R J (2015b) Advance directives for mental health care: innovation in law, policy, and practice. *Psychiatric Services*, 66(1): 7-9

Zhang W & Webster R G (2017) Can we beat influenza? *Science*, 357(6347): 111

Zhu Z, Rooney D & Phillips N (2016) Practice-based wisdom theory for integrating institutional logics: a new model for social entrepreneurship learning and education. *Academy of Management Learning and Education*, 15(3): 607-25

Zohar D (1991) *The quantum self*. Flamingo, London

Zohar D & Marshall I (1993) *The quantum society*. Flamingo, London

Zohar D & Marshall I (2000) *SQ Spiritual intelligence: the ultimate intelligence*. Bloomsbury, London

Zucker M & Zucker H (eds) (1997) *Medical futility and the evaluation of life-sustaining interventions*. Cambridge University Press, Cambridge, Cambs

Zuniga J M, Marks S P & Gostin L O (eds) (2013) *Advancing the human right to health*. Oxford University Press, Oxford

Zwartz B (2008) Archbishop's abortion threat. *The Age*, 23 September: 1-2

Index

Page numbers followed by 'f' indicate figures, and 'b' indicate boxes.

A

abortion, 270–303
  adoption and, 275
  in Australia, 282
  case scenario on, 308b
  conservative position on, 273–274, 277f
  definition of, 273
  EC and, 281
  in Ireland, 270–271, 281
  liberal position on, 276–277, 277f
  moderate position on, 274–276, 277f
  moral politics of, 269–270
  moral rights of women, fetuses, and fathers in, 277–281
  morality policy for, 268–269
  in New Zealand, 271
  personhood and, 277
  politics and the broader community, 281–282
  reproductive rights and, 271
  right to life and, 279
  in United States, 280
  WHO on, 270
  wrongful abortion suits, 272
  wrongful birth, 272
absolute confidentiality, 190–191
absolute rights, 53
abuse. see also child abuse; elder abuse
  euthanasia and, 292–293
  prevention, 368
ACN. see Australian College of Nurses
adequacy, measured by, 39
adoption, 275
advance care planning, 260–262
  RPC and, 261–262
advance directives
  culture relating to, 258–259
  definition and description of, 256–257
  in end-of-life care, 256–260
  psychiatric, 215–221
  risks and benefits of, 258–260
aesthetics, 142
ageing population. see also elder abuse; end-of-life care
  protecting, 359–361
  as vulnerable population, 352
ageism, 145
aggregate vulnerability, 132–133
Alma Ata Declaration, 378
altruism, euthanasia and, 288, 290–291

amoralism, 104
AMR. see antimicrobial resistance
Anglo-American moral philosophy, 76
animalistic dehumanisation, 135
animals, dehumanisation and, 138
ANMF. see Australian Nursing and Midwifery Federation
anti-abortion violence, 282
antimicrobial resistance (AMR), 377–378
anti-paternalism, 188
apartheid, morality of laws during, 19
appropriate action, 311–340
appropriate care, 179
appropriate disagreement, 337–338
Aristotle, 14–15
Aroskar, Mila, 102
artificial heart, 226
assisted suicide. see also euthanasia
  definition of, 284–286
  views for and against, 286–297
asylum seekers, 28
  definition of, 152
  dehumanisation of, 137, 153
  rights of, 153
  vulnerability of, 152–154
Australia
  abortion in, 282
  Bundaberg Base Hospital case in, 332
  Chelmsford Private Hospital, 97
  euthanasia in, 13–14, 283
  homeless people in, 162–164
  Indigenous peoples of, 157
  MacArthur Health Service case in, 330–331
  mental health problems in, 149
  Moylan case in, 329
  Palliative Care Australia, 263
Australian College of Nurses (ACN), 2–4
Australian Nursing and Midwifery Federation (ANMF), 2–4
  in conscientious objection, 326–327
authoritarianism, 138
autonomy
  cross-cultural ethics and, 78
  ethical principlism relating to, 41–42
  euthanasia and, 287–289
  informed consent and, 182
  mental health disorders, harm, and, 215–216
  reproductive, 277
  suicide and, 229–232

451

B

Baby Boom Generation, of LGBTIQ people, 166
Bailey, Dr Harry, 97
Bardenilla case, 330
Baudouin, King, 281
Beauchamp, Tom, 33
Beecher, Henry, 15
beneficence
　cross-cultural ethics and, 77
　ethical principlism and, 43–44
　non-maleficence compared with, 42
　obligatory, 43–44
benefit paternalism, 187
benefits, 45–47
Bentham, Jeremy, 64
bio-error, 376–377
bioethical thinking, two more ambitious agendas of, 105–106
bioethics
　defining, 15–17
　development of, 15–16
　task of, 31–33
bioterrorism, 376
blood transfusion, 201b
Buddha, 58
Bundaberg Base Hospital case, 332
burdens, 45–47
bystanders, 141

C

cadavers, 108
Cambridge Analytica, 28, 141–142
Canadian Nurses Association, *Code of ethics for registered nurses*, 317
CANH. *see* clinically assisted nutrition or hydration
cardiopulmonary resuscitation (CPR), 241
caring, virtuous, 60
Chabot, Boudewijn, 294–295
character virtues, 61–62
Chelmsford Private Hospital, 97
child abuse
　case scenario on, 369b–370b
　confidentiality relating to, 365–366
　considerations against reporting, 362–365
　criticisms relating to, 365–368
　defining, 353
　family relating to, 363–364, 367–368
　incidence of, 353–354
　maltreatment, as moral issue, 360
　moral duty to report and prevent, 361
　neglect and, 352–355
　politics and, 367
　professional-client relationship relating to, 363, 367
　protecting against, 359–361
　redressing, 354–355
　reporting of, 351–352, 363–364
child vulnerability, 352
children overboard incident, 28, 137
Childress, James, 33

choice
　based on rational reasons, 210
　evidencing, 209
　imprudent, 293–294
　reasonable outcome of, 209–210
　in treatment, 254
Christian ethics, 45
city-based university teaching hospitals, 77
claims rights
　making, 54
　problems with, 55–56
clarity, 27–28
Clark, Barney, 226
climate change, 373–375
climate justice, 374
'climate wars', 374
clinical decision-making, 19, 21f
clinical governance, 336
clinical risk management, whistleblowing and, 335–336
clinical settings, types of decisions, 21f
clinical situations, in moral distress, 114
clinically assisted nutrition or hydration (CANH), 300
　withholding or withdrawing, 301–303
Code of conduct for nurses, 315–316
codes of conduct, 24–25
codes of ethics, 22–24
　in Australia, 3b, 86, 181, 191, 198, 345
　Canadian Nurses Association, 317
　ICN, 314
　for ICN, 2, 23–24, 86, 162, 181, 191, 198, 345
　jurisdictions outside Australia, 3b
　in New Zealand, 2, 86, 198
　nursing, 3b
coherence, 27–28
coherent cluster of attitudes, 140
committed suicide, 227
common humanity, 50–51
common morality, 13
community, abortion and, 281–282
comparative justice, 47
competency, 209
　ability to understand, 210
　actual understanding, 210
　choice based on rational reasons, 210
　cultural, 86–90
　to decide, 207–215, 213f
　rationally incompetent, 212–213, 213f
　reasonable outcome of choice, 209–210
　surrogate decision-making, 211–212
　test, 209
competing interests, in moral dilemma, 112
competing moral duties, 110
completed suicide, 227
comprehensiveness, 27–28
compromise view, 326
concealability, 142

conceptual diversity, 109
confidentiality
    as absolute principle, 191–193
    child and elder abuse relating to, 365–366
    patient rights to, 190–195
    as prima-facie principle, 193–195
    right to privacy, 190–195
conflicting interests, in moral dilemma, 112
conflicts
    ethics, preventing, 336–338
    of interest, in moral conflict, 314
    moral, 109–110
    problem of, in personal values, 323–324
Confucianism, 58
conscience
    definition of, 319
    function of, 320–321
    as moral feelings, 320
    as moral reasoning, 319–320
    nature of, 319–320
    voice of, 319–320
conscience absolutism, 326
conscientious judgments, 319–320
conscientious objection
    bogus and genuine claims of, 321–324
    case scenario on, 323b–324b
    to controversial directives of an employer/manager, 322–323
    personal values and, 323–324
    policy considerations and, 324–327
    professional judgment and, 316–327
conservative view, in conscientious objection, 325
contextual issues, 89
CPR. see cardiopulmonary resuscitation
cross-cultural ethics, 71–92
    case scenario on, 91b–92b
    cultural competency, 86–90
    cultural humility, 86–90
    cultural safety and, 86–90
    culture, relating to ethics, 74–75
    implications of, 75–82
    moral diversity and moral pluralism, 82–83
    nursing and, 73–74
    problems associated with, 83–86
cultural competency, 86–90
cultural humility, 86–90
cultural issues, 89
cultural liberty, 200
cultural perception, in moral decision-making, 116
cultural safety, 86–90
cultural-language incongruence, 72
culturally and linguistically diverse communities, 150–151
culture
    advance directives relating to, 258–259
    defining, 73–74, 76
    ethics relating to, 74–75
    no blame, 347–348
    socio-cultural environment and abuse prevention, 368

cybercrime, 386
cybersecurity, 386
cybersuicide, 221–222

D
Damasio, Antonio, on emotion and moral decision-making, 120
death, right to choose, 288–289
decision-making. see also moral decision-making
    clinical, 19, 21f
    competency, to decide, 207–215, 213f
    for DNR directives, 240–241
    ethical, 20–21
    informed decisions, 181–190
    legal, 20
    moral justification relating to, 39
    surrogate, 211–212
deep sleep therapy (DST), 97
dehumanisation, 131–171
    addressing root causes of, 139–140
    animalistic, 135
    of asylum seekers, 137, 153
    authoritarianism relating to, 138
    bystanders relating to, 141
    consequences of, 138–139
    defining, 135–142
    deterring, 139–142
    energising dissent, 141–142
    expressions of, 136–137
    forms of, 135–136
    of homeless people, 163
    humanness, vulnerability, and, 134–144
    instances of, 141
    "inter-species" empathy and concern, 138
    mechanistic, 136
    moral exclusion and, 141
    moral inclusion and, 140–141
    occurrence of, 137–138
    superhumanisation, 136
delegitimisation, 136
demand to be treated fairly, euthanasia and, 290
democracy, 28–29
deontology, 63
dependence, 13–14
depression, 230
descriptive ethics, 15
detainees. see prisoners and detainees
dignity
    definition of, 195–197
    euthanasia and, 287, 289–290
    Hobbes on, 196
    Kant on, 196
    Oregon State's Death with Dignity Act, 286
    patient rights to, 195–198
    rights to, 197
    violations of, 197–198
disabilities, vulnerable populations and, 154–156
disadvantage, 144
disclosure, 190

discrimination
    against ethnic minorities, 151
    euthanasia and, 293
    against immigrants, 151
    of older people, 145
    prejudice and, 143–144
    vulnerability and, 144–145
displaced people, 152–154. *see also* asylum seekers
disputes, dealing with, 124
disrespect, 199
disruptiveness, 142
dissent, energising, 141–142
distress, moral, 114–115
distributive justice, 45–46
divine command, 50
Do Not Resuscitate (DNR) directives, 100
    case scenario on, 264b–265b
    CPR relating to, 241–248
    decision-making
        criteria and guidelines, 244–245
        and patient exclusion, 245
    documentation and communication problems in, 246
    implementation concerns and problems, 246–247
    improving practices of, 247–248
    issues with, 243–244
    medical futility and, 248–251
    misinterpretation of, 245
Dock, Lavinia, 22
doctrine of double effect, 297–298
DST. *see* deep sleep therapy
duty. *see also* moral duty
    conflict in, 111
    Kant on, 63
duty to die, euthanasia and, 288, 290–291

E

EC. *see* European Community
economic impact, of mental health problems, 148
economy, 378–379
elder abuse
    case scenario on, 369b–370b
    confidentiality relating to, 365–366
    considerations against reporting, 362–365
    criticisms relating to, 365–368
    defining, 356–357
    family relating to, 363–364, 367–368
    incidence of, 357
    maltreatment, as moral issue, 360
    moral duty to report and prevent, 361
    neglect and, 355–359
    politics and, 367
    professional-client relationship relating to, 363, 367
    protecting against, 359–361
    redressing, 357–359
    reporting of, 351–352, 355, 363–364
emergency preparedness, 372–378, 382–384
emotions
    basic, 135
    complex, 135
    moral decision-making and, 118–121, 124

empathy, 138
employer, controversial directives of, conscientious objection to, 322–323
end-of-life care, 237–266. *see also* Do Not Resuscitate directives
    advance care planning, 260–262
    advance directives in, 256–260
    case scenarios on, 264b–265b
    improving and rethinking, 262–263
    medical futility, 248–251
    NFT directives, 239–241
    quality of life in, 251–256
energising dissent, 141–142
Engelhardt Jr., Tristram, 33
equity, justice as, 45–46
ethical blindness, 98
ethical decision-making process, 86–87
ethical decisions, 20, 21f. *see also* decision-making
ethical dilemma, 95, 110
ethical fading, 103–104
ethical loading, 78
ethical practice
    of nursing, moral theory and, 37–69
    theoretical perspectives informing, 40–66
ethical principlism
    autonomy relating to, 41–42
    beneficence and, 43–44
    defining ethical principles, 41
    informed consent and, 184
    justice relating to, 45–48
    moral rules and, 48, 49f
    moral theory and, 41–49
    non-maleficence and, 42–43
    problems with, 49
ethical professional conduct, 5
    following orders, 31
    professional etiquette, 25–26
ethical professional practice, critical inquiry into, 13
ethical rationalism, 63
ethical standards, in internal moral disagreement, 108
ethical terms, 12
ethics, 11–35, 86–90, 131–171. *see also* nursing ethics
    bioethics, 15–17, 31–33
    of care, in nursing, 61–62
    case scenario on, 34b
    child and elder protection relating to, 359–361
    codes of, 22–24
    conflicts of, preventing, 336–338
    critical inquiry into, 13
    cross-cultural, 71–92
    culture relating to, 74–75
    defining, 14–15
    descriptive, 15
    etiquette relating to, 25
    hospital or institutional policy and, 26
    ideology relating to, 30
    importance of, 12
    law and, 20
    mental health, 222
    metaethics, 15

normative, 15
nursing codes of, 3b
by opinion, 29
public opinion and, 27–29
questioning, 6–7
spaceship, 67
sub-fields of, 15
subway, 67
of suicide prevention, 232–234
task of, 31–33
virtue, 40
    decline of, 57
    ethic of care, in nursing, 61–62
    moral theory on, 56–62
    problems with, 62
ethics-quality linkage, 337
ethnic minorities
    discrimination against, 151
    IOM on, 150
    vulnerability of, 150–152
etiquette, 25
    hospital, 25–26
    professional, 25–26
European Community (EC), 281
euthanasia, 282–283
    abuse and, 292–293
    altruism and, 288, 290–291
    arguments against, 291–297
    assisted suicide, 286
    in Australia, 13–14, 27
    autonomy and, 287–289
    case scenario on, 308b
    categories of, 285f
    definition of, 284–286
    dignity and, 287, 289–290
    discrimination and, 293
    doctrine of double effect in, 297–298
    duty to die and, 288, 290–291
    Exit International and, 296
    involuntary, 285
    irrational, mistaken, or imprudent choice in, 293–294
    law on, 18–19
    mercy killing, 286, 385b
    misdiagnosis and, 291–292
    moral justification relating to, 39
    moral politics of, 267–309
    non-partisan (neutral) stance in, 304–306
    non-voluntary, 284–286
    nurse practitioners and, 297
    Oregon State's Death with Dignity Act, 286
    palliative sedation and, 298–301
    partisan stance, 304
    passive, 285
    position statements in, 303–307
    prognostic uncertainty and, 291–292
    sanctity-of-life doctrine and, 291
    significance of, for nurses, 283–284
    slippery slope argument and, 294–297
    suffering and, 287–288, 290
    suicide compared with, 228
    systematic response to, 306–307
    views for and against, 286–297
    voluntary, 284–285
Euthyphro (Plato), 351
evidencing choice, 209
existential suffering, 300–301
Exit International, 296
explanatory power, 27–28
extended-family members, 84
external constraints, in moral distress, 114

F
failure to disclose, 192
fairness, 45–46
fake news, 28
family
    child and elder abuse relating to, 363–364, 367–368
    extended-family member visitation, 84
    informed consent relating to, 186
    patient desires *vs.*, 83
fathers, moral rights of, abortion and, 277–281
feelings. *see* emotions
Feinberg, Joel, 51, 52f
feminist moral perspective, in dilemma, 112
fetuses. *see also* abortion
    moral rights of, abortion and, 277–281
    potentiality of, 278
'filter bubbles', 28
five-step decision-making process, 117
following orders, 31
'fossilised' culture, 80
Free, Frances, 318
French, Marilyn, 291
Fried, Charles, 177
'frozen' culture, 80
fundamental conflict, in internal moral disagreement, 107
fundamental requisite, 43

G
Gauthier, David, 33
gender identities, 166
genetic ignorance, 184
genomics, 381–382
Glover, Jonathan, 229
God, 63. *see also* religion
good nursing, 59–60
goodness, self-evident property of, 121
Greatest Generation, of LGBTIQ people, 166
Greece, 79
    austerity measures, impact on health, 381
grief, 113–114
grievous wrongs, 52–53
Gunn, Dr David, 126

H
Halappanavar, Savita, 281
Hare, Richard
    on intuition and moral decision-making, 122
    on moral fanaticism, 106–107
    on morality, 33

harm, 42
    from failure to disclose, 192
    mental health disorders, autonomy, and, 215–216
    notion of, 361–362
    paternalism, 187
    preventing, 215
harmony, justice as, 45
Hawking, Steven, 156
health care
    appropriate care, 179
    challenges posed by rights to, 180–181
    contexts, moral fanaticism in, 107
    decent minimum of, 177
    equal access to, 178–179
    inequality, 378–382
    paternalistic principle in, 189–190
    patient rights to, 176–181
    quality care, 179–180
    safe care, 180
    whistleblowing in, 327–336
heart, artificial, 226
Hobbes, Thomas
    on dignity, 196
    on morality, 32
Hoffman, Toni, 332
homeless people
    in Australia, 162–164
    dehumanisation of, 163
    four categories of, 163
    homelessness
        causes of, 164–165
        defining, 163–164
    in New Zealand, 164
    rights of, 165
    as vulnerable populations, 162–165
homelessness
    causes of, 164–165
    defining, 163–164
hospital etiquette, 25–26
hospital policy, 26
houselessness, 163
human experience, 52–53
human inventions, 73
human nature, 135
human rights
    grievous wrongs relating to, 52
    mental health ethics, vulnerability, and, 205–207
    United Nations Declaration of Human Rights, 53, 178
human uniqueness, 135
humanity, 50–51
humanness
    defining, 134–135
    dehumanisation and vulnerability and, 134–144
Hume, David
    on emotion and moral decision-making, 118–119
    on morality, 32
humility, cultural, 86–90
Hurricane Katrina, 385b

hurt
    attachment and, 112
    avoiding, 113
    grief and, 113–114

I
ICN. see International Council of Nurses
ideology
    about poverty, 30
    distinguishing feature of, 30
    ethics relating to, 30
    politics and, 30
Iliffe, Jill, 102
immigrants
    definition of, 153
    discrimination against, 151
    ICN on, 151
    IOM on, 150
    vulnerability of, 150–152
immoral conduct, 105
immoralism, 104–105
impairment
    moral, 6
    practitioner/student, reporting of, 342–351, 343b
impartiality, 45–46
inadequate housing, living in, 163
inalienable rights, 53
inattentional blindness, 98
incompatibility thesis, 325
incompetence, moral, 6
incongruence, cultural-language, 72
Indigenous peoples
    of Australia, 157
    health disparities in, 156
    IWGIA and, 156
    of New Zealand, 157–158, 169b
    as vulnerable populations, 156–159
individual vulnerability, 132–133
industrialised large-scale society, 76
inequality, 378–382
influenza, 375–377
informed consent
    analytic components and elements of, 183
    autonomy and, 182
    competency, to decide, 207–215, 213f
    defining, 182–183
    ethical principlism and, 184
    family relating to, 186
    mental health disorders relating to, 207–208
    nursing care and, 190
    paternalism and, 186–188, 189f
    sovereignty and, 186
informed decisions, 181–190
infrahumanisation, 136–137
initial moral distress, 114
insecure housing, living in, 163
Institute of Medicine (IOM), 150
institutional policy, 26
instructional directive, 217

interests
  competing, 112
  moral rights relating to, 51–52
  person's, 43
internal constraints, in moral distress, 114
internal moral disagreement, 107–108
International Council of Nurses (ICN), 2
  codes of ethics for, 23–24
  on conscientious objection, 323
  on immigrants, 151
  on prisoners, 162
  on professional judgment, 314–316
  on safety, 180
  on whistleblowing, 327–328
International Work Group for Indigenous Affairs (IWGIA), 156
interpersonal professional relationships, 349
inter-species empathy, 138
intuition, moral decision-making and, 121–124
IOM. *see* Institute of Medicine
Ireland, abortion in, 270–271, 281
irrevocability, during crisis, 217
Islam, 58
isolation, 169
  cross-cultural ethics and, 78
IWGIA. *see* International Work Group for Indigenous Affairs

J

Jameton, Andrew, 114
Jehovah's Witness, 63, 201*b*
justice
  as basic human need, 45
  comparative, 47
  cross-cultural ethics and, 77
  different conceptions of, 45
  distributive, 46
  as equal distribution of benefits and burdens, 45–47
  as equity, 45–46
  ethical principlism relating to, 45–48
  euthanasia and, 290
  as fairness, 45–46
  as harmony, 45
  as impartiality, 45–46
  as love, 45
  as mercy, 45
  non-comparative, 47
  as reconciliation and reparation, 45, 47–48
  restorative, 47
  as revenge, 45
  as therapeutic jurisprudence, 47–48
  as what is deserved, 45
justificatory power, 27–28

K

Kant, Immanuel
  on dignity, 196
  on duty, 63
  on ethical rationalism, 63
  on morality, 32
  on rationality, 51
  on reason and moral decision-making, 118
  on respect, 199
Kawa Whakaruruhau, 88
Knight, Peter, 126
knowledge
  of moral theories, 116
  right, to not know, 184–185
  self-, 116

L

language
  barriers, 75–76
  moral, 13–14
  rights relating to, 56
large-scale society, 76
law
  ethics and, 18–19
  on euthanasia, 27
  legal regulation, of PADs, 220–221
  moral, 32
  natural, 50
  on reporting wrongdoing, 342–345
  traditional view of, 19
legal decisions, 19–20, 21*f*
legal-moral conflict, problem of, 323
LGBTIQ people. *see* sexual minorities
liberal view, in conscientious objection, 326
liberty, cultural, 200
life experience, moral decision-making and, 123–124
linguistic issues, 89
literacy, medical, 89
logical incompatibility, moral dilemmas and, 110
love, justice as, 45
loyalty, 350
lying, 48

M

MacArthur Health Service case, 330–331
MacIntyre, Alasdair, on emotion and moral decision-making, 119
Mackie, John, 32–33
Mademoiselle and the Doctor, 296
managers and supervisors
  conscientious objection to, 322–323
  following orders of, 31
Mann, Jonathan, 17, 197
Māori, 88, 157–158, 169*b*
McEwan, John, 209
mechanistic dehumanisation, 136, 138
media constructions, 27
medical futility, 248–251
medical literacy, 89
medical/biomedical senses, of bioethics, 17
medically hopeless cases, 239–240
mental health care
  autonomy, harm, and, 215–216
  case scenario on, 234*b*

mental health care *(Continued)*
  ethical issues in, 203–235
    human rights, vulnerability, and, 205–207
    informed consent relating to, 207–208
    psychiatric advance directives, 215–221
    vulnerabilities, of mentally ill, 205–207
mental health ethics, 222
mental health problems
  in Australia, 149
  economic impact of, 148
  of prisoners, 160–161
  stigmatisation of, 142–143
  vulnerabilities, and mental illness, 148–150
  WHO on, 148
mentally ill, 205–207
mercy, justice as, 45
mercy killing, 284–286. *see also* euthanasia
  after Hurricane Katrina, 385*b*
metaethics, 15
migrant, 153. *see also* asylum seekers
Mill, John Stuart, 55, 64
misdiagnosis, 291–292
moderate view, in conscientious objection, 326
modern moral philosophy, 33
moral
  blindness, 98–101, 99*f*–100*f*
  character, 24
    reflection, 24
  child and elder protection relating to, 360
  complacency, 105–106
  delinquency, 6, 105
  differences, 125
  dilemmas, 95, 110–114
  disengagement, 102–103
    cause of, 114
  distress, 114–115
  diversity, 82–83
    pluralism, 82–83
  dumbfounding, 106
  fading, 103–104
  fanaticism, 106–107
  heroes, 58
  impairment, 6
  incompetence, 6, 96–98
  indifference, 101–102
  insensitivity, 101–102
  intuitionism, 121–122
  language, 13–14
  life, 57
  obligations, 65–66
  professional standards and, 6–7
  responsibility, 31
  rules, 48, 49*f*
  saints, 58
  stupefaction, 106
  superiority, 82
  thinking, 32
  turpitude, 6, 105
  unaccountability, 31
  unpreparedness, 96–98
moral challenge, of suicide, 222–224
moral conflict, 109–110
  common situations involving, 314
moral deadlock, 107
moral decision-making, 93–129
  case scenario on, 128*b*–129*b*
  definition of, 116
  emotion and, 118–121, 124
  intuition and, 121–124
  life experience and, 123–124
  points of view in, 124–126
  processes for, 116–124, 117*f*
  reason and, 118, 124
moral disagreements, 82, 107–109
  appropriate, 337–338
  critical moral thinking and, 109
  dealing with, 124
  internal, 107–108
  moral conflict and professional judgment, 312–313
  radical, 108–109
moral duty, 64–65
  competing, 110
  to report and prevent child and elder abuse, 361
moral exclusion, 141
moral fascism, 82
moral feelings, conscience as, 320
moral imperialism, 75–76
moral inaction, 104
moral inclusion, 140–141
moral issue, 28–29
moral judgments, correct, 313–314
moral justification, 38–40, 104
  appeal and, 49*f*
  decision-making relating to, 39
  euthanasia relating to, 39
  moral theory and, 67–68
  problems with, 40
  relevance and, 39
moral law, 32
moral neglect, 104
moral philosophy, 14–15
moral policy, 29
moral politics, abortion and, 269–270
moral principles, 77
moral problems, 93–129
  amoralism in, 104
  case scenario on, 128*b*–129*b*
  definition of, 94
  distinguishing, 94–95
  ethical fading in, 103–104
  everyday, 126–127
  immoralism in, 105
  kinds of, 95–115
  moral blindness in, 98–101, 99*f*–100*f*
  moral complacency in, 105–106
  moral disagreements in, 107–109
  moral disengagement in, 102–103

moral dumbfounding/stupefaction in, 106
moral fading in, 103–104
moral fanaticism in, 106–107
moral incompetence in, 96–98
moral indifference and insensitivity in, 101–102
moral unpreparedness in, 96–98
moral project, nursing as, 7
moral quandaries, 311–340
moral reasoning, conscience as, 319–320
moral residue, 114
moral rights
    abortion and, 277–281
    claims
        making, 54
        problems with, 55–56
    defining, 50
    divine command relating to, 50
    grievous wrongs relating to, 52–53
    human experience relating to, 52–53
    humanity relating to, 50–51
    interests relating to, 51–52, 52f
    natural law based, 50
    rationality based, 51
    rights and responsibilities, 54–55
    theory on, 49–56
    types of, 53–54
moral robots, 57
moral standards, in internal moral disagreement, 107
moral theory
    case scenarios on, 68b–69b
    criteria for, 27–28
    deontology, 63
    ethical practice of nursing and, 37–69
    ethical principlism and, 41–49
    knowledge of, 116
    limitations and weaknesses of, 66–67
    on moral duties and obligations, 64–66
    moral justification and, 67–68
    on moral rights, 49–56
    teleology, 63–64
    theoretical perspectives informing, 40–66
    on virtue ethics, 56–62
morality
    common, 13
    defining, 14
    ethics compared with, 14
    Hare on, 33
    Hobbes on, 32
    Hume on, 32
    Kant on, 32
    in large-scale society, 76
    modern moral philosophy, 33
    quantum, 124–125
    Ross on, 33
    in small-scale society, 76
morality policy, abortion and, 268–269
Mother Teresa, 58
Moylan case, 329

multidrug-resistant bacteria, 382
myocardial infarction, 264b

N

natural law, 50
need, 95
neglect
    child abuse and, 352–355
    elder abuse and, 355–359
neutrality, 304
New Zealand
    abortion in, 271
    cultural safety in, 88
    homeless people in, 164
    Indigenous peoples of, 157–158, 169b
    Pugmire case in, 329–330
NFR directives. *see* Not For Resuscitation directives
NFT directives. *see* Not For Treatment directives
Nightingale, Florence, 328
no blame culture, 347–348
nocebo effect, 79
non-abuse, 39
non-comparative justice, 47
non-maleficence, 110
    beneficence compared with, 42
    cross-cultural ethics and, 77
    ethical principlism and, 42–43
non-Māori, 89
non-traditional large-scale society, 76
non-voluntary euthanasia, 284–286
normalisation of deviance, 98
normative ethics, 15
Not For Resuscitation directives, 100. *see also* Do Not Resuscitate directives
Not For Treatment (NFT) directives, 239–241
    medically hopeless cases, 239–240
notifiable conduct, 342–351, 343b
nudging, choice and, 251
    choice architecture, 251
nurse whistleblower, notion of, 333
nurses
    euthanasia and its significance for, 283–284
    palliative sedation and, 300–301
nurses' preparedness
    for climate change, 374
    for inequality, 382
    for public health emergencies, 372–378
nursing
    codes of ethics, 3b
    cross-cultural ethics and, 73–74
    ethic of care in, 61–62
    good, 59–60
    as moral project, 7
    in remote locations, 77
nursing care, informed consent and, 190
nursing ethics, 371–372, 382
    case scenarios on, 384b–385b
    climate change relating to, 373–375
    defining, 17–18

nursing ethics *(Continued)*
　future of, 371–386
　on inequality, 378–382
　for public health emergencies, 372–378
　task of, 31–33
　virtue theory and, 59–61
　vulnerability and, 133–134
　wellbeing relating to, 61

O
objectivity, 46
obligations, 65–66
obligatory beneficence, 43–44
older people
　discrimination against, 145
　rights of, 147–148
　safety of, 146
　vulnerability of, 145–148
opinions. *see* public opinion
Oregon State's Death with Dignity Act, 286
organisational aggravators, 104
organisational values, disagreement with, in moral conflict, 314
origin, 142
output power, 27–28
over-diagnosis, 176

P
PADs. *see* psychiatric advance directives
Palliative Care Australia, 263
palliative sedation, 298–301
　definition, purpose and intention of, 299–300
　existential suffering, 300
　nurses and, 300–301
pandemic influenza, 375–377
parasuicide, 221–234. *see also* suicide
partial radical moral disagreement, 108
participant-neutrality, 305
Patel, Jayant, 332
paternalism
　anti-, 188
　benefit, 187
　definition of, 186–187
　harm, 187
　informed consent and, 186–188
　justification for, 188–189
　prima-facie, 188–189, 189f
　pro-, 188
　strong, 187
　types of, 187
　weak, 187
paternalistic principle, 189–190
patient safety. *see* safety
patients' rights, 173–202
　to appropriate care, 179
　case scenario on, 201b
　charters and bills of, 175b
　to confidentiality, 190–195
　to cultural liberty, 200
　defining, 175–200

　to dignity, 195–198
　to health care, 176–181
　informed decisions and, 181–190
　not to know, 184–185
　personal lives, 4
　to quality care, 179–180
　to respect, 198–200
　to safe care, 180
People's Health Movement (PHM), 56
peril, 142
personal lives, patient rights, 4
personal values, conscientious objection and the problem of conflict in, 323–324
personhood, 134, 277
PHM. *see* People's Health Movement
placebo effect, 79
Plato, 14–15, 32–33
　Euthyphro, 351
plausibility, 39
pluralism, moral, 75
Poddar, Prosenjit, 192
policies
　considerations, conscientious objection and, 324–327
　disagreement with, in moral conflict, 314
　hospital or institutional, 26
　morality, 268–269
'political priority', 378
politics
　abortion and, 281–282
　child abuse, elder abuse, and, 367
　ideology and, 30
　moral, 269–270
populism, 27–29
poverty, 30
practicability, 27–28
practical feasibility, 39
practical wisdom, 315
practice issues, 89
practitioner wrongdoing, 342–345
preferences, 95
prejudice, 143–144
preparedness. *see* nurses' preparedness
prescription, 217
preventive ethics, 336–337
prima-facie confidentiality, 193–195
prima-facie paternalism, 188–189, 189f
prima-facie rights, 53–54
principle of autonomy, 41
principle of beneficence, 43
principle of justice, 45
principlism. *see* ethical principlism
prisoners and detainees
　ICN on, 162
　mental health problems of, 160–161
　rights of, 161, 161b
　as vulnerable populations, 159–162, 161b
privacy. *see* confidentiality
professional conduct. *see* ethical professional conduct
professional etiquette, 25–26

professional judgment, 311–340
  case scenario on, 338b–339b
  conscientious objection and, 316–327
  'correct' moral judgments and, 313–314
  ICN in, 314
  moral conflict and, 312–316
  nature and moral importance of, 315–316
  preventing ethics conflicts, 336–338
professional misconduct
  definition of, 5
  unethical professional conduct and, 6
  unprofessional conduct and, 4–6
professional performance, unsatisfactory, 5–6
professional relationships
  with clients, 363, 367
  interpersonal, 349
professional standards, 1–9
  case scenarios on, 8b
  codes of ethics as, 22
  ethical professional conduct, 6
  ethical professional practice, 13
  following orders, 31
  morals and, 6–7
  nursing as moral project, 7
  nursing codes of ethics and position statements, 3b
  professional misconduct, 5
  questioning requirement of, 6–7
  requirement to uphold, 4
  unprofessional conduct, 5
  unsatisfactory professional performance, 5–6
Promotion of National Unity and Reconciliation Act, 47
pro-paternalism, 188
proscription, 217
proxy directives, 217
'pseudo-interaction', 27
psychiatric advance directives (PADs), 215–221
  anticipated benefits of, 218–219
  anticipated risks of, 219
  current trends in, 220–221
  forms and function of, 217–218
  legal regulation of, 220–221
  origin, rationale, and purpose of, 216–217
  Ulysses contract, 217
psychiatric wills, 217
psychotropic medication, 207
public health emergencies
  antimicrobial resistance, 377–378
  nurses' preparedness for, 372–378
  nursing ethics for, 372–378
  pandemic influenza, 375–377
public opinion
  democracy relating to, 28–29
    polls, 27
  ethics and, 27–29
publics, 27
public-stigma, 143
Pugmire case, 329–330

Q

quality care, 179–180
quality of life, 13–14
  defining, 251–252
  descriptive sense of, 254
  different conceptions of, 252–254
  in end-of-life care, 251–256
  evaluative sense of, 254–255
  phrase origins, 251
  prescriptive sense of, 255–256
  senses of, 254–256
  treatment choices relating to, 254
quantum morality, 124–125
Quinlan, Karen Ann, 15–16

R

racism/discrimination, 89
radical moral disagreement, 108–109
rampant individualism, 54
rationalism, 63
rationality, 51
  Kant on, 51
Rawls, John, 46
reactive moral distress, 114
reason, moral decision-making and, 118, 124
reasonable outcome of choice, 209–210
reconciliation, 45, 47–48
reflective judgment, 86
refugees, 137, 152–154. *see also* asylum seekers
relevance, measured by, 39
religion
  Buddha and, 58
  Confucianism, 58
  deontology and God, 63
  divine command, 50
  Islam, 58
  Jehovah's Witness, 63, 201b
reparation, 45
reporting harmful behaviours. *see under* child abuse; elder abuse; harm; impairment; student wrongdoing
reproductive autonomy, 277
reproductive rights, 271
rescue principle, 176
resources, in moral conflict, 314
respect
  disrespect, 199
  Kant on, 199
  lack of, in moral conflict, 314
  patient rights to, 198–200
Respecting Patient Choices (RPC), 261–262
responsibilities, 54–55
restorative justice, 47
retributive justice, 45
returnees, definition of, 153. *see also* asylum seekers
revenge, justice as, 45
right to life, 279
rights. *see also* human rights; moral rights; patients' rights
  absolute, 53
  of asylum seekers, 153
  to dignity, 197

rights *(Continued)*
    duty compared with, 66
    of homeless people, 165
    human
        grievous wrongs relating to, 52
        United Nations Declaration of Human Rights, 53
    human, mental health ethics, vulnerability, and, 205–207
    inalienable, 53
    language relating to, 56
    moral
        defining, 50
        divine command relating to, 50
        grievous wrongs relating to, 52–53
        human experience relating to, 52–53
        humanity relating to, 50–51
        interests relating to, 51–52, 52*f*
        making rights claims, 54
        natural law based, 50
        problems with rights claims, 55–56
        rationality based, 51
        rights and responsibilities, 54–55
        theory on, 49–56
        types of, 53–54
    of older people, 147–148
    PHM and, 56
    prima-facie, 53–54
    of prisoners, 161, 161*b*
    to privacy, 193–194
    of stateless people, 153
    to suicide, 229–232
role-neutrality, 305
rooflessness, 163
Ross, Stephen, 33
RPC. *see* Respecting Patient Choices
rules, disagreement with, in moral conflict, 314

S
safe care, 180
safety, 341–370. *see also* child abuse; elder abuse
    attitudes and experiences of reporting concerns in, 348–351
    cultural, 86–90
    International Council of Nurses on, 180
    no blame culture and, 347–348
    of older people, 146
    patient safety literature, 31
    reporting wrongdoing and, 342–345
    supportive socio-cultural environment and abuse prevention, 368
same-sex marriage, 167
sanctity-of-life doctrine, 291
SARS. *see* severe acute respiratory syndrome
SBDs. *see* self-binding directives
scientism, 57
sedation, palliative, 298–301
self-binding directives (SBDs), 217
self-conscious moral reflection, 24
self-knowledge, in moral decision-making, 116

self-stigma, 143
sentience, 274, 277–278
    definition of, 278
    as bedrock of ethics, 51–52. *see also* moral rights
severe acute respiratory syndrome (SARS), 373
sexual minorities (LGBTIQ people)
    biases against, 167
    demographics of, 165
    generations of, 166
    same-sex marriage and, 167
    as vulnerable populations, 165–168
sexual orientation, 166
Silberbauer, 77
Silent Generation, of LGBTIQ people, 166
'sliding scale' framework, 213
slippery slope argument, 294–297
small-scale society, 76
social cooperation, 46
social dominance orientation, 138
society
    large-scale, 76
    small-scale, 76
socio-cultural environment, 368
Socrates, 14–15
Somera, Lorenza, 31
sound justification, 38
sovereignty, 186
spaceship ethics, 67
standards, in internal moral disagreement
    ethical, 108
    moral, 107
stateless people, 152–154. *see also* asylum seekers
stigma
    public-, 143
    self-, 143
    vulnerability and, 133, 142–143
stigmatisation
    of mental health problems, 142–143
    process of, 142–143
    of suicide, 222
'stringentness', 42–43
strong paternalism, 187
student wrongdoing, reporting of, 342–345
suburban isolation, 169
subway ethics, 67
suffering
    euthanasia and, 287–288, 290
    existential, palliative sedation in, 300
suicide
    autonomy and right to, 229–232
    committed, 227
    completed, 227
    cybersuicide, 221–222
    defining, 224–228
    depression and, 230
    ethical dimensions of, 228–234
    ethical issues in, 221–234
    euthanasia compared with, 228
    moral challenge of, 222–224

parasuicide, 221–234
  prevention of, 232–234
  problem, scope of, 221
  rates, 221
  stigmatisation of, 222
superhumanisation, 136
supervisors. *see* managers and supervisors
surrogate decision-making, 211–212
  designation, 217
survival, problems of, 15
systematic step-by-step decision-making process, 117
systemic issues, 89
Szasz, Thomas, 222

T

Tarasoff v Regents of the University of California, 192
taxes, 19
teleology, 63–64
terror management theory (TMT), 73
therapeutic jurisprudence, 47–48
Thomson, Judith Jarvis, 274–276
TMT. *see* terror management theory
Tooley, Michael, 276, 278
total radical moral disagreement, 108
'toxic service', 72
traditions, cultural, 81
treatment choices, 254
triangular thinking, 109
truth telling, 48, 79
tuberculosis, 377–378

U

UK Nursing and Midwifery Council (NMC), 317
Ulysses contract, 217
uncertainty, 291–292, 307
understanding. *see* competency
UNDP. *see* United Nations Development Programme
unethical conduct, 105
unethical professional conduct, 6
United Nations Declaration of Human Rights, 53, 178
United Nations Development Programme (UNDP), 71–72
United States (US)
  abortion in, 280
  Bardenilla case, 330
  Oregon State's Death with Dignity Act, 286
unprofessional conduct, 5
  professional misconduct and, 4–6
unsatisfactory professional performance, 5–6
US. *see* United States
usability, 39
utilitarianism, 52, 64

V

value, 87
violence, anti-abortion, 282
virtue
  of character, 61–62
  notion of, 58
  theory, 59–61

virtue ethics, 40
  decline of, 57
  ethic of care, in nursing, 61–62
  moral theory on, 56–62
  problems with, 62
Virtues Project, 58
virtuous caring, 60
virtuous person, 58–59
voluntary euthanasia, 284–285
voluntary notification, 344*b*
vulnerability, 132–134
  aggregate, 132–133
  of children, 352
  defining, 132
  disadvantage and, 144
  as guide to action, 133
  humanness, dehumanisation and, 134–144
  individual, 132–133
  mental health ethics, human rights, and, 205–207
  nursing ethics and, 133–134
  prejudice and discrimination and, 143–144
  stigma and, 133, 142–143
vulnerable populations, 131–171
  ageing population as, 352
  case scenarios on, 169*b*
  define, 133
  with disabilities, 154–156
  homeless people as, 162–165
  identifying, 132–133, 144–168
  immigrants and ethnic minorities as, 150–152
  Indigenous peoples as, 156–159
  with mental health problems and mental illness, 148–150
  mentally ill people, 205–207
  older people as, 145–148
  prisoners and detainees as, 159–162, 161*b*
  refugees, asylum seekers, displaced people, stateless people and returnees, 152–154
  sexual minorities (LGBTIQ people) as, 165–168

W

want, 95
Warren, Mary Anne, 276–277
Warthen, Corrine, 318
weak paternalism, 187
wellbeing
  nursing ethics relating to, 61
  person's, 43
Western moral thinking, 32
whistleblowers, notion of, 332–333
whistleblowing
  act of, 333
  in Bardenilla case, 330
  in Bundaberg Base Hospital case, 332
  clinical risk management and, 335–336
  deciding to 'go public', 333–334
  in health care, 327–336
  as last resort, 336
  in MacArthur Health Service case, 330–331

whistleblowing *(Continued)*
    in Moylan case, 329
    notion of, 332–333
    in Pugmire case, 329–330
    risks of, 334–335
    WHO on, 335
WHO. *see* World Health Organization
willful blindness, 98–99
Williams, Rau, 169*b*
wills, 217. *see also* advance directives
wisdom, practical, 315
withholding clinically assisted nutrition and hydration, 301–303
women, moral rights of, abortion and, 277–281
World Health Organization (WHO)
    abortion and, 270
    on disabled populations, 154
    on inequality, in health care, 378
    on mental health problems, 148
    on whistleblowing and clinical risk management, 335
wrongdoing. *see also* whistleblowing
    grievous wrongs, 52–53
    impairment, 343*b*
    legal requirements for reporting, 342–345
    notifiable conduct, 342–351, 343*b*
    by practitioner or student, 342–351
    professional requirements to report, 345–346
    safety and reporting, 342–351
    voluntary notification, about students, 344*b*
    voluntary notification grounds, 345*b*
wrongful abortion suits, 272
wrongness, self-evident property of, 121